KU-453-732

Cochrane Handbook for Systematic Reviews of Interventions

Cochrane Handbook for Systematic Reviews of Interventions

Second Edition

Edited by Julian P.T. Higgins, James Thomas, Jacqueline Chandler, Miranda Cumpston, Tianjing Li, Matthew J. Page and Vivian A. Welch

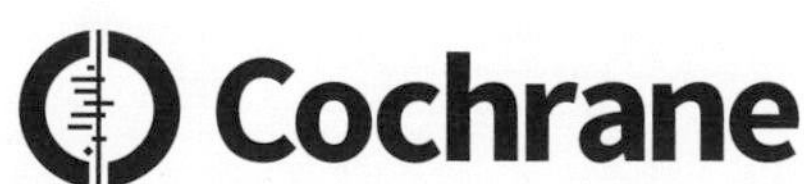

WILEY Blackwell

This work is a co-publication between The Cochrane Collaboration and John Wiley & Sons Ltd.

Edition History
1e The Cochrane Collaboration

Registered Office(s)
John Wiley & Sons, Inc., 111 River Street, Hoboken, NJ 07030, USA
John Wiley & Sons Ltd, The Atrium, Southern Gate, Chichester, West Sussex, PO19 8SQ, UK

Editorial Office
9600 Garsington Road, Oxford, OX4 2DQ, UK

For details of our global editorial offices, customer services, and more information about Wiley products visit us at www.wiley.com.

Wiley also publishes its books in a variety of electronic formats and by print-on-demand. Some content that appears in standard print versions of this book may not be available in other formats.

Library of Congress Cataloging-in-Publication Data

Names: Higgins, Julian P. T., editor. | Cochrane Collaboration, issuing body.
Title: Cochrane handbook for systematic reviews of interventions / edited by Julian P.T. Higgins, James Thomas, Jacqueline Chandler, Miranda Cumpston, Tianjing Li, Matthew J. Page, Vivian A. Welch.
Other titles: Cochrane book series.
Description: Second edition. | Hoboken, NJ : Wiley-Blackwell, 2019. | Series: Cochrane book series | Includes bibliographical references and index. | “This work is a co-publication between The Cochrane Collaboration and John Wiley & Sons Ltd.”–ECIP title page verso.
Identifiers: LCCN 2019024539| ISBN 9781119536628 (hardback) | ISBN 9781119536611 (adobe pdf) | ISBN 9781119536659 (epub)
Subjects: | MESH: Outcome and Process Assessment (Health Care) | Evidence-Based Medicine–methods | Meta-Analysis as Topic | Systematic Reviews as Topic
Classification: LCC RA427.3 | NLM W 84.41 | DDC 362.1–dc23 LC record available at https://lccn.loc.gov/2019024539

Cover image: © ittipon2002/iStock.com, © Eraxion/iStock.com, © Raycat/iStock.com, © atoss/iStock.com, © anmbph/iStock.com, © shapecharge/iStock.com, © adventtr/iStock.com, © PeopleImages/iStock.com, © Abel Mitja Varela/iStock.com, © kiankhoon/iStock.com, © Wavebreakmedia/iStock.com, © 9comeback/iStock.com, © leoniepow/iStock.com
Cover design by Wiley

Set in 10/12pt SourceSansPro by SPi Global, Pondicherry, India

Printed in the UK by Bell & Bain Ltd, Glasgow

HB printing 10 9 8 7 6 5 4 3

Contents

Contributors

Akl, Elie A
Department of Internal Medicine
American University of Beirut Medical Center
Beirut
Lebanon

Altman, Douglas G[*]
Centre for Statistics in Medicine
University of Oxford
Oxford
UK

Aluko, Patricia
Institute of Health and Society
Newcastle University
Newcastle upon Tyne
UK

Askie, Lisa M
NHMRC Clinical Trials Centre
University of Sydney
Sydney
Australia

Beaton, Dorcas E
Institute for Work & Health
Toronto, Ontario
Canada

Berlin, Jesse A
Department of Epidemiology
Johnson & Johnson
Titusville, NJ
USA

Bhaumik, Soumyadeep
The George Institute for Global Health
New Delhi
India

Bingham III, Clifton O
Department of Rheumatology
Johns Hopkins University
Baltimore, MD
USA

Boers, Maarten
Department of Epidemiology and Biostatistics
Amsterdam UMC
Vrije Universiteit Amsterdam
Amsterdam
The Netherlands

Booth, Andrew
School of Health and Related Research
University of Sheffield
Sheffield
UK

Boutron, Isabelle
METHODS team, Centre of Research in Epidemiology and Statistics (CRESS-UMR1153), INSERM/Paris Descartes University;

[*] Deceased 3 June 2018

Centre d' Epidémiologie Clinique
Assistance Publique des hôpitaux de Paris;
Cochrane France
Paris
France

Brennan, Sue E
Cochrane Australia
School of Public Health and Preventive Medicine
Monash University
Melbourne
Australia

Briel, Matthias
Department of Clinical Research
University of Basel
Basel
Switzerland

Briscoe, Simon
College of Medicine and Health
University of Exeter
Exeter
UK

Busse, Jason W
Department of Anesthesia
McMaster University
Hamilton, Ontario
Canada

Caldwell, Deborah M
Population Health Sciences
Bristol Medical School
University of Bristol
Bristol
UK

Cargo, Margaret
Health Research Institute
University of Canberra
Canberra
Australia

Carrasco-Labra, Alonso
Department of Health Research Methods, Evidence and Impact (HEI)
McMaster University
Hamilton, Ontario
Canada
Department of Oral and Craniofacial Health Science
University of North Carolina at Chapel Hill
Chapel Hill, NC
USA

Chaimani, Anna
METHODS team Centre of Research in Epidemiology and Statistics Sorbonne Paris Cité (CRESS-UMR1153), INSERM/Paris Descartes University
Paris
France

Chandler, Jacqueline
Wessex Academic Health Science Network
University Hospital Southampton
Southampton
UK

Christensen, Robin
Musculoskeletal Statistics Unit
The Parker Institute
Bispebjerg and Frederiksberg Hospital
Copenhagen
Denmark

Clarke, Mike
Northern Ireland Methodology Hub
Centre for Public Health
Queen's University Belfast
Belfast
Northern Ireland

Craig, Dawn
Institute of Health and Society
Newcastle University
Newcastle upon Tyne
UK

da Costa, Bruno R
Applied Health Research Centre
St. Michael's Hospital
Toronto, Ontario
Canada

Deeks, Jonathan J
Institute of Applied Health Research
University of Birmingham
Birmingham
UK

Devji, Tahira
Department of Health Research Methods, Evidence and Impact (HEI)
McMaster University
Hamilton, Ontario
Canada

Drummond, Michael
Centre for Health Economics
University of York
York
UK

Elbers, Roy G
Population Health Sciences
Bristol Medical School
University of Bristol
Bristol
UK

El Dib, Regina
Institute of Science and Technology
UNESP - Univ Estadual Paulista
São José dos Campos
Brazil

Eldridge, Sandra
Centre for Primary Care and Public Health
Blizard Institute
Barts and The London
School of Medicine and Dentistry
Queen Mary University of London
London
UK

Elliott, Julian H
Cochrane Australia
Monash University
Melbourne
Australia

Flemming, Kate
Department of Health Sciences
University of York
York
UK

Gagnier, Joel J
Department of Orthopaedic Surgery
Epidemiology
University of Michigan
Ann Arbor, MI
USA

Garside, Ruth
European Centre for Environment and Human Health
University of Exeter Medical School University of Exeter
Truro
UK

Ghersi, Davina
Research Policy and Translation
National Health and Medical Research Council
Canberra
Australia

Glanville, Julie
York Health Economics Consortium
York
UK

Glasziou, Paul
Institute for Evidence-Based Healthcare
Bond University
Queensland
Australia

Golder, Su
Department of Health Sciences
University of York
York
UK

Graybill, Erin
Department of Economics
Newcastle University
Business School
Newcastle upon Tyne
UK

Guyatt, Gordon H
Department of Health Research Methods, Evidence and Impact (HEI)
McMaster University
Hamilton, Ontario
Canada

Hannes, Karin
Social Research Methodology Group
Faculty of Social Sciences
KU Leuven
Leuven
Belgium

Harden, Angela
Institute of Health and Human Development
University of East London
London
UK

Harris, Janet
School of Health and Related Research
University of Sheffield
Sheffield
UK

Hartling, Lisa
Department of Pediatrics, Faculty of Medicine & Dentistry
University of Alberta
Edmonton, Alberta
Canada

Henderson, Catherine
Personal Social Services Unit
London School of Economics and Political Science
London
UK

Hernán, Miguel A
Departments of Epidemiology and Biostatistics
Harvard T.H. Chan School of Public Health
Boston, MA
USA

Higgins, Julian PT
Population Health Sciences
Bristol Medical School
University of Bristol
Bristol
UK

Hróbjartsson, Asbjørn
Centre for Evidence-Based Medicine Odense (CEBMO)
Odense University Hospital
Odense
Denmark

Johnston, Bradley C
Department of Community Health and Epidemiology
Dalhousie University
Halifax, Nova Scotia
Canada

Johnston, Renea V
Monash Department of Clinical Epidemiology, Cabrini Institute
School of Public Health and Preventive Medicine, Monash University
Melbourne
Australia

Jull, Janet
School of Rehabilitation Therapy
Queen's University
Kingston, Ontario
Canada

Junqueira, Daniela R
Faculty of Medicine and Dentistry
University of Alberta
Edmonton, Alberta
Canada

Klassen, Terry
Manitoba Institute of Child Health
Winnipeg, Manitoba
Canada

Kneale, Dylan
EPPI-Centre, Institute of Education
University College London
London
UK

Kristjansson, Elizabeth
School of Psychology
Faculty of Social Sciences
University of Ottawa
Ottawa, Ontario
Canada

Lasserson, Toby J
Editorial & Methods Department
Cochrane Central Executive
London
UK

Lefebvre, Carol
Lefebvre Associates Ltd
Oxford
UK

Li, Tianjing
Department of Epidemiology
Johns Hopkins Bloomberg School of Public Health
Baltimore, MD
USA

Littlewood, Anne
Cochrane Oral Health
University of Manchester
Manchester
UK

Loke, Yoon Kong
Norwich Medical School
University of East Anglia
Norwich
UK

Lundh, Andreas
Centre for Evidence-Based Medicine Odense (CEBMO)
Odense University Hospital
Odense
Denmark

Lyddiatt, Anne
Ingersoll, Ontario
Canada

Marshall, Chris
Institute of Health and Society
Newcastle University
Newcastle upon Tyne
UK

Maxwell, Lara J
University of Ottawa
Ottawa, Ontario
Canada

McAleenan, Alexandra
Population Health Sciences
Bristol Medical School
University of Bristol
Bristol
UK

McKenzie, Joanne E
School of Public Health and Preventive Medicine
Monash University
Melbourne
Australia

Metzendorf, Maria-Inti
Institute of General Practice
Medical Faculty of the Heinrich-Heine-University Düsseldorf
Düsseldorf
Germany

Noel-Storr, Anna
Radcliffe Department of Medicine
University of Oxford
Oxford
UK

Noyes, Jane
School of Health Sciences
Bangor University
Bangor
UK

Ostelo, Raymond W
Department of Epidemiology and Biostatistics
Amsterdam UMC
Vrije Universiteit Amsterdam
Amsterdam
The Netherlands

Page, Matthew J
School of Public Health and Preventive Medicine
Monash University
Melbourne
Australia

Pantoja, Tomás
Department of Family Medicine
Faculty of Medicine
Pontificia Universidad Católica de Chile
Santiago
Chile

Pardo Pardo, Jordi
Cochrane Musculoskeletal Group
University of Ottawa
Ottawa, Ontario
Canada

Patrick, Donald L
Health Services and Epidemiology
University of Washington
Seattle, WA
USA

Peryer, Guy
University of East Anglia
Norwich
UK

Petkovic, Jennifer
Bruyère Research Institute
University of Ottawa
Ottawa, Ontario
Canada

Petticrew, Mark
Faculty of Public Health and Policy
London School of Hygiene and Tropical Medicine
London
UK

Rader, Tamara
Evidence Standards
Canadian Agency for Drugs and Technologies in Health
Ottawa, Ontario
Canada

Reeves, Barnaby C
Translational Health Sciences
Bristol Medical School
University of Bristol
Bristol
UK

Rehfuess, Eva
Pettenkofer School of Public Health
Institute for Medical Information Processing, Biometry and Epidemiology
LMU Munich
Munich
Germany

Robalino, Shannon
Institute of Health and Society
Newcastle University
Newcastle upon Tyne
UK

Ryan, Rebecca E
Cochrane Consumers and Communication Group
Centre for Health Communication and Participation
La Trobe University
Melbourne
Australia

Salanti, Georgia
Institute of Social and Preventive Medicine
University of Bern
Bern
Switzerland

Santesso, Nancy
Department of Health Research Methods Evidence and Impact (HEI)
McMaster University
Hamilton, Ontario
Canada

Savović, Jelena
Population Health Sciences
Bristol Medical School
University of Bristol
Bristol
UK

Schünemann, Holger J
Departments of Health Research Methods, Evidence, and Impact (HEI) and of Medicine
McMaster University
Hamilton, Ontario
Canada

Shea, Beverley
Department of Medicine, Ottawa Hospital Research Institute;
School of Epidemiology and Public Health, University of Ottawa
Ottawa, Ontario
Canada

Shemilt, Ian
EPPI-Centre
University College London
London
UK

Shokraneh, Farhad
Cochrane Schizophrenia Group
Division of Psychiatry and Applied Psychology
Institute of Mental Health
School of Medicine
University of Nottingham
Nottingham
UK

Simmonds, Mark
Centre for Reviews and Dissemination
University of York
York
UK

Singh, Jasvinder
School of Medicine
University of Alabama at Birmingham
Birmingham, AL
USA

Skoetz, Nicole
Department of Internal Medicine
University Hospital of Cologne
Cologne
Germany

Sterne, Jonathan AC
Population Health Sciences Bristol Medical School
University of Bristol
Bristol
UK

Stewart, Lesley A
Centre for Reviews and Dissemination
University of York
York
UK

Stott, David J
Academic Section of Geriatric Medicine
Institute of Cardiovascular and Medical Sciences
University of Glasgow
Glasgow
UK

Takwoingi, Yemisi
Institute of Applied Health Research
University of Birmingham
Birmingham
UK

Terwee, Caroline B
Department of Epidemiology and Biostatistics
Amsterdam Public Health Research Institute
Amsterdam UMC
Vrije Universiteit Amsterdam
Amsterdam
The Netherlands

Thomas, James
EPPI-Centre, Department of Social Science
University College London
London
UK

Thomson, Denise
Department of Pediatrics
Faculty of Medicine and Dentistry
University of Alberta
Edmonton, Alberta
Canada

Thomson, Hilary J
MRC/CSO Social and Public Health Sciences Unit
University of Glasgow
Glasgow
UK

Tierney, Jayne F
MRC Clinical Trials Unit at UCL
Institute of Clinical Trials and Methodology
London
UK

Tugwell, Peter
Department of Medicine & School of Epidemiology and Public Health, Faculty of Medicine, University of Ottawa;
Clinical Epidemiology Program, Ottawa Hospital Research Institute
Ottawa, Ontario
Canada

Ueffing, Erin
Centre for Practice-Changing Research
Ottawa Hospital Research Institute
Ottawa, Ontario
Canada

Vale, Luke
Health Economics Group
Institute of Health and Society
Newcastle University
Newcastle upon Tyne
UK

Vist, Gunn E
Department of Preventive, Health Promotion and Organisation of Care
Norwegian Institute of Public Health
Oslo
Norway

Vohra, Sunita
Department of Pediatrics
Faculty of Medicine & Dentistry
University of Alberta
Edmonton, Alberta
Canada

Welch, Vivian A
Bruyère Research Institute
Ottawa, Ontario
Canada

Wells, George A
School of Epidemiology and Public Health, University of Ottawa;
University of Ottawa Heart Institute
Ottawa, Ontario
Canada

Wieland, L Susan
Center for Integrative Medicine
Department of Family and Community Medicine
University of Maryland School of Medicine
Baltimore, MD
USA

Williams, Katrina
Department of Paediatrics, Monash University;
Developmental Paediatrics, Monash Children's Hospital;
Neurodisability and Rehabilitation, Murdoch Children's Research Institute
Melbourne
Australia

Williamson, Paula R
Department of Biostatistics
University of Liverpool
Liverpool
UK

Wilson, Edward CF
Health Economics Group Norwich Medical School
University of East Anglia
UK

Young, Camilla
Institute of Cardiovascular and Medical Sciences
University of Glasgow
Glasgow
UK

Preface

'First, do no harm' is a principle to which those who would intervene in the lives of other people are often called to ascribe. However, in this era of data deluge, it is not possible for individual decision makers to ensure that their decisions are informed by the latest, reliable, research knowledge; and without reliable information to guide them, they can cause harm, even though their intentions may be good. This is the core problem that the founder of Cochrane, Sir Iain Chalmers, aimed to address through the provision of systematic reviews of reliable research.

By synthesizing the results of individual studies, systematic reviews present a summary of all the available evidence to answer a question, and in doing so can uncover important knowledge about the effects of healthcare interventions. Systematic reviews undertaken by Cochrane (Cochrane Reviews) present reliable syntheses of the results of multiple studies, alongside an assessment of the possibility of bias in the results, contextual factors influencing the interpretation and applicability of results, and other elements that can affect certainty in decision making. They reduce the time wasted by individuals searching for and appraising the same studies, and also aim to reduce research waste by ensuring that future studies can build on the body of studies already completed.

A systematic review attempts to collate all empirical evidence that fits pre-specified eligibility criteria in order to answer a specific research question. It uses explicit, systematic methods that are selected with a view to minimizing bias, thus providing more reliable findings from which conclusions can be drawn and decisions made. The key characteristics of a systematic review are:

- a clearly stated set of objectives with pre-defined eligibility criteria for studies;
- an explicit, reproducible methodology;
- a systematic search that attempts to identify all studies that meet the eligibility criteria;
- an assessment of the validity of the findings of the included studies, for example through the assessment of risk of bias; and
- a systematic presentation, and synthesis, of the characteristics and findings of the included studies.

For twenty-five years, Cochrane Reviews have supported people making healthcare decisions, whether they are health professionals, managers, policy makers, or individuals making choices for themselves and their families. The *Cochrane Handbook for*

Systematic Reviews of Interventions (the *Handbook*) provides guidance to authors for this work.

About Cochrane

Cochrane is a global network of health practitioners, researchers, patient advocates and others, with a mission to promote evidence-informed health decision making by producing high quality, relevant, accessible systematic reviews and other synthesized research evidence (www.cochrane.org). Founded as The Cochrane Collaboration in 1993, it is a not-for-profit organization whose members aim to produce credible, accessible health information that is free from commercial sponsorship and other conflicts of interest.

Cochrane works collaboratively with health professionals, policy makers and international organizations such as the World Health Organization (WHO) to support the development of evidence-informed guidelines and policy. WHO guidelines on critical public health issues such as breastfeeding (2017) and malaria (2015), and the WHO Essential Medicines List (2017) are underpinned by dozens of Cochrane Reviews.

There are many examples of the impact of Cochrane Reviews on health and health care. Influential reviews of corticosteroids for women at risk of giving birth prematurely, treatments for macular degeneration and tranexamic acid for trauma patients with bleeding have demonstrated the effectiveness of these life-changing interventions and influenced clinical practice around the world. Other reviews of anti-arrhythmic drugs for atrial fibrillation and neuraminidase inhibitors for influenza have raised important doubts about the effectiveness of interventions in common use.

Cochrane Reviews are published in full online in the *Cochrane Database of Systematic Reviews*, which is a core component of the Cochrane Library (www.thecochranelibrary.com). The Cochrane Library was first published in 1996, and is now an online collection of multiple databases.

The evidence for Cochrane methodology

While Cochrane was one of the earliest organizations to produce and publish systematic reviews, there are now many organizations and journals doing so. One of the key elements that sets Cochrane apart is its rigorous methods, and Cochrane has played a unique role in fostering the development of methodology for systematic reviews throughout its history. Cochrane Methods Groups are voluntary collaborations of some of the world's leading methodological researchers in statistics, information retrieval, bias, qualitative methods, and many other specialist areas (see https://methods.cochrane.org). These Methods Groups support and disseminate methods research that identifies the most effective and efficient methods for systematic reviews, minimizing bias and increasing the appropriate analysis and interpretation of results.

The use of these rigorous methods is challenging and often time-consuming, but the recommendations are not made for their own sake. As McKenzie and colleagues wrote, "Our confidence in the findings of systematic reviews rests on the evidence base underpinning the methods we use. Just as there are consequences arising from the choices we make about health and social care interventions, so too are there consequences when we choose the methods to use in systematic reviews." (McKenzie et al, Cochrane Database of Systematic Reviews 2015; 7: ED00010)

With this in mind, the guidance in this *Handbook* has been written by authors who are international leaders in their fields, many of whom are supported by the work of Cochrane Methods Groups.

Ongoing challenges for systematic reviews

The landscape in which systematic reviews are conducted continues to evolve. Old and emerging challenges continue to spark debate, research and innovation.

The time required to complete a full systematic review, which is often more than two years, is a barrier both for author teams (representing a considerable commitment of often volunteer time) and for decision makers (who often require evidence within much shorter time frames). Methodology for undertaking reviews more rapidly is developing quickly. However, difficult choices are required in the trade-off between rigour and speed. The rise of technological solutions offers much potential, including collaboration tools, online crowd sourcing and automation of many aspects of the review process. Alongside consideration of appropriate ways to prioritize work, technology is also supporting more efficient approaches to keeping reviews up to date, with some reviews moving towards a 'living' systematic review model of very frequent, even continuous updates.

Cochrane Reviews have always encompassed complex questions of multi-component interventions, health systems and public health, and the challenging issues that arise from many of these reviews have prompted considerable thought and effort. Cochrane Reviews have always incorporated non-randomized studies where appropriate to the question, and a wider range of data sources is increasingly relevant to reviews, from the unpublished clinical study reports produced by pharmaceutical companies, to novel challenges in appraising and interpreting 'big data' repositories. The use of systematic reviews is expanding, and new methods developing, in areas such as environmental exposure and prognosis.

These conversations will continue, and new questions will continue to arise. Cochrane will continue to contribute actively to methodological development and application in each of these areas, continually striving to improve both the validity and usefulness of the reviews to decision makers.

Undertaking a Cochrane Review

Preparing a Cochrane Review is complex and involves many judgements. Authors work closely with Cochrane editorial teams in the production of reviews, supplying a highly structured format for both its protocols and reviews to guide authors on the information they should report. Cochrane groups and other research groups increasingly use priority-setting methods to engage stakeholders such as patients, the public, policy makers and healthcare professionals to understand from them the most important uncertainties or information gap. Since its inception, Cochrane has advocated for routine updating of systematic reviews to take account of new evidence. In some fast-moving topics frequent updating is needed to ensure that review conclusions remain relevant.

While some authors new to Cochrane Reviews have training and experience in conducting other systematic reviews, many do not. Training for review authors is delivered in many countries by regional Cochrane groups or by the Cochrane Methods Groups responsible for researching and developing the methods used on Cochrane Reviews. In addition, Cochrane produces an extensive range of online learning resources. Detailed information is available via https://training.cochrane.org. Training materials and opportunities for training are continually developed and updated to reflect the evolving Cochrane methods and the needs of contributors.

About this *Handbook*

Work on a handbook to support authors of Cochrane Reviews began in 1993, and the first version was published in May 1994. Since then it has evolved and grown, through the stewardship of several editorial teams, with regular updating of its contents being punctuated by major new editions. This book represents Version 6 of the *Handbook*, the first major revision since the first print edition of the *Handbook* was published in 2008.

The book is divided into three parts. Part One provides the core methodology for undertaking systematic reviews on the effects of health interventions, with a particular emphasis on reviewing randomized trials. Part Two provides considerations for tackling these systematic reviews from different perspectives, such as when thinking about specific populations, or complex interventions, or particular types of outcomes. Part Three covers a range of further topics, including reviewing evidence other than straightforward randomized trials. The online version of the *Handbook* has an addition part, describing the particular organizational and procedural considerations when working specifically with Cochrane.

For this edition, each chapter that provides new or substantively updated guidance has been rigorously peer reviewed to ensure the guidance presented reflects the state of the science and is appropriate and efficient for use by Cochrane authors. The *Handbook* is updated regularly to reflect advances in systematic review methodology and in response to feedback from users. Please refer to https://training.cochrane.org/handbook for the most recent online version, for interim updates to the guidance and for details of previous versions of the *Handbook*. Feedback and corrections to the *Handbook* are also welcome via the contact details on the website.

What's new in this edition

In this edition, every chapter of the *Handbook* has been extensively revised, new chapters added, and authors familiar with previous versions will find it valuable to re-read any chapter of interest.

In particular, this edition incorporates the following major new chapters and areas of guidance:

- Expanded advice on assessing the risk of bias in included studies (Chapter 7), including Version 2 of the Cochrane Risk of Bias tool (Chapter 8) and the ROBINS-I tool for assessing risk of bias in non-randomized studies (Chapter 25).
- New guidance on summarizing study characteristics and preparing for synthesis (Chapters 3 and 9).
- New guidance on network meta-analysis (Chapter 11).
- New guidance on synthesizing results using methods other than meta-analysis (Chapter 12).
- Updated guidance on assessing the risk of bias due to missing results (reporting biases, Chapter 13).
- New guidance addressing intervention complexity (Chapter 17).

How to cite this book

Higgins JPT, Thomas J, Chandler J, Cumpston M, Li T, Page MJ, Welch VA (editors). *Cochrane Handbook for Systematic Reviews of Interventions*. 2nd Edition. Chichester (UK): John Wiley & Sons, 2019.

Acknowledgements

We thank all of our contributing authors and chapter editors for their patience and responsiveness in preparing this *Handbook*. We are also indebted to all those who have contributed to previous versions of the *Handbook*, and particularly to past editors Rachel Churchill, Sally Green, Phil Alderson, Mike Clarke, Cynthia Mulrow and Andy Oxman.

Many contributed constructive and timely peer review for this edition. We thank Zhenggang Bai, Hilda Bastian, Jesse Berlin, Lisa Bero, Jane Blazeby, Jacob Burns, Chris Cates, Nathorn Chaiyakunapruk, Kay Dickersin, Christopher Eccleston, Sam Egger, Cindy Farquhar, Nicole Fusco, Hernando Guillermo Gaitán Duarte, Paul Garner, Claire Glenton, Su Golder, Helen Handoll, Jamie Hartmann-Boyce, Joseph Lau, Simon Lewin, Jane Marjoribanks, Evan Mayo-Wilson, Steve McDonald, Emma Mead, Richard Morley, Sylivia Nalubega, Gerry Richardson, Richard Riley, Elham Shakibazadeh, Dayane Silveira, Jonathan Sterne, Alex Sutton, Özge Tunçalp, Peter von Philipsborn, Evelyn Whitlock, Jack Wilkinson. We thank Tamara Lotfi from the Secretariat for the Global Evidence Synthesis Initiative (GESI) and GESI for assisting with identifying peer referees, and Paul Garner and Taryn Young for their liaison with Learning Initiative for eXperienced Authors (LIXA).

Specific administrative support for this version of the *Handbook* was provided by Laura Mellor, and we are deeply indebted to Laura for her many contributions. We would also like to thank staff at Wiley for their patience, support and advice, including Priyanka Gibbons (Commissioning Editor), Jennifer Seward (Senior Project Editor), Deirdre Barry (Senior Editorial Assistant) and Tom Bates (Senior Production Editor).

We thank Ella Flemyng for her assistance and Elizabeth Royle and Jenny Bellorini at Cochrane Copy Edit Support for their assistance in copy editing some chapters of the *Handbook*. Finally, we thank Jan East for copy editing the whole volume, and Nik Prowse for project management.

This *Handbook* would not have been possible without the generous support provided to the editors by colleagues at the University of Bristol, University College London, Johns Hopkins Bloomberg School of Public Health, Cochrane Australia at Monash University, and the Cochrane Editorial and Methods Department at Cochrane Central Executive. We particularly thank David Tovey (former Editor in Chief, The Cochrane Library), and acknowledge Cochrane staff Madeleine Hill for editorial support, and Jo Anthony and Holly Millward for contributing to the cover design.

Finally, the Editors would like to thank the thousands of Cochrane authors who volunteer their time to collate evidence for people making decisions about health care, and the methodologists, editors and trainers who support them.

The *Handbook* editorial team

Julian P.T. Higgins (*Senior Editor*) is Professor of Evidence Synthesis at the University of Bristol, UK.

James Thomas (*Senior Editor*) is Professor of Social Research & Policy, and Associate Director of the EPPI-Centre at UCL, London, UK.

Jacqueline Chandler (*Managing Editor*) is Evaluation Programme Manager (Qualitative Evaluation) at Wessex Academic Health Science Network, University Hospital Southampton, Southampton, UK.

Miranda Cumpston (*Implementation Editor*) is an Editor at Cochrane Public Health in the School of Medicine and Public Health, University of Newcastle, and the School of Public Health and Preventive Medicine, Monash University, Melbourne, Australia.

Tianjing Li (*Associate Scientific Editor*) is an Associate Professor of Epidemiology at Johns Hopkins Bloomberg School of Public Health, Baltimore, USA. She is a Coordinating Editor for Cochrane Eyes and Vision.

Matthew J. Page (*Associate Scientific Editor*) is a Research Fellow in the Research Methodology Division of the School of Public Health and Preventive Medicine, Monash University, Melbourne, Australia.

Vivian A. Welch (*Associate Scientific Editor*) is Editor in Chief of the Campbell Collaboration, Scientist at Bruyère Research Institute, Ottawa, Canada; Associate Professor at the School of Epidemiology and Public Health, University of Ottawa, Canada.

Part One

Core methods

1

Starting a review

Toby J Lasserson, James Thomas, Julian PT Higgins

KEY POINTS
• Systematic reviews address a need for health decision makers to be able to access high quality, relevant, accessible and up-to-date information. • Systematic reviews aim to minimize bias through the use of pre-specified research questions and methods that are documented in protocols, and by basing their findings on reliable research. • Systematic reviews should be conducted by a team that includes domain expertise and methodological expertise, who are free of potential conflicts of interest. • People who might make – or be affected by – decisions around the use of interventions should be involved in important decisions about the review. • Good data management, project management and quality assurance mechanisms are essential for the completion of a successful systematic review.

1.1 Why do a systematic review?

Systematic reviews were developed out of a need to ensure that decisions affecting people's lives can be informed by an up-to-date and complete understanding of the relevant research evidence. With the volume of research literature growing at an ever-increasing rate, it is impossible for individual decision makers to assess this vast quantity of primary research to enable them to make the most appropriate healthcare decisions that do more good than harm. By systematically assessing this primary research, systematic reviews aim to provide an up-to-date summary of the state of research knowledge on an intervention, diagnostic test, prognostic factor or other health or healthcare topic. Systematic reviews address the main problem with ad hoc searching and selection of research, namely that of bias. Just as primary research studies use methods to avoid bias, so should summaries and syntheses of that research.

This chapter should be cited as: Lasserson TJ, Thomas J, Higgins JPT. Chapter 1: Starting a review. In: Higgins JPT, Thomas J, Chandler J, Cumpston M, Li T, Page MJ, Welch VA (editors). *Cochrane Handbook for Systematic Reviews of Interventions*. 2nd Edition. Chichester (UK): John Wiley & Sons, 2019: 3–12.

A systematic review attempts to collate all the empirical evidence that fits pre-specified eligibility criteria in order to answer a specific research question. It uses explicit, systematic methods that are selected with a view to minimizing bias, thus providing more reliable findings from which conclusions can be drawn and decisions made (Antman et al 1992, Oxman and Guyatt 1993). Systematic review methodology, pioneered and developed by Cochrane, sets out a highly structured, transparent and reproducible methodology (Chandler and Hopewell 2013). This involves: the a priori specification of a research question; clarity on the scope of the review and which studies are eligible for inclusion; making every effort to find all relevant research and to ensure that issues of bias in included studies are accounted for; and analysing the included studies in order to draw conclusions based on all the identified research in an impartial and objective way.

This *Handbook* is about systematic reviews on the effects of interventions, and specifically about methods used by Cochrane to undertake them. Cochrane Reviews use primary research to generate new knowledge about the effects of an intervention (or interventions) used in clinical, public health or policy settings. They aim to provide users with a balanced summary of the potential benefits and harms of interventions and give an indication of how certain they can be of the findings. They can also compare the effectiveness of different interventions with one another and so help users to choose the most appropriate intervention in particular situations. The primary purpose of Cochrane Reviews is therefore to inform people making decisions about health or health care.

Systematic reviews are important for other reasons. New research should be designed or commissioned only if it does not unnecessarily duplicate existing research (Chalmers et al 2014). Therefore, a systematic review should typically be undertaken before embarking on new primary research. Such a review will identify current and ongoing studies, as well as indicate where specific gaps in knowledge exist, or evidence is lacking; for example, where existing studies have not used outcomes that are important to users of research (Macleod et al 2014). A systematic review may also reveal limitations in the conduct of previous studies that might be addressed in the new study or studies.

Systematic reviews are important, often rewarding and, at times, exciting research projects. They offer the opportunity for authors to make authoritative statements about the extent of human knowledge in important areas and to identify priorities for further research. They sometimes cover issues high on the political agenda and receive attention from the media. Conducting research with these impacts is not without its challenges, however, and completing a high-quality systematic review is often demanding and time-consuming. In this chapter we introduce some of the key considerations for review authors who are about to start a systematic review.

1.2 What is the review question?

Getting the research question right is critical for the success of a systematic review. Review authors should ensure that the review addresses an important question to those who are expected to use and act upon its conclusions.

We discuss the formulation of questions in detail in Chapter 2. For a question about the effects of an intervention, the PICO approach is usually used, which is an acronym for Population, Intervention, Comparison(s) and Outcome. Reviews may have additional questions, for example about how interventions were implemented, economic issues, equity issues or patient experience.

To ensure that the review addresses a relevant question in a way that benefits users, it is important to ensure wide input. In most cases, question formulation should therefore be informed by people with various relevant – but potentially different – perspectives (see Chapter 2, Section 2.4).

1.3 Who should do a systematic review?

Systematic reviews should be undertaken by a team. Indeed, Cochrane will not publish a review that is proposed to be undertaken by a single person. Working as a team not only spreads the effort, but ensures that tasks such as the selection of studies for eligibility, data extraction and rating the certainty of the evidence will be performed by at least two people independently, minimizing the likelihood of errors. First-time review authors are encouraged to work with others who are experienced in the process of systematic reviews and to attend relevant training.

Review teams must include expertise in the topic area under review. Topic expertise should not be overly narrow, to ensure that all relevant perspectives are considered. Perspectives from different disciplines can help to avoid assumptions or terminology stemming from an over-reliance on a single discipline. Review teams should also include expertise in systematic review methodology, including statistical expertise.

Arguments have been made that methodological expertise is sufficient to perform a review, and that content expertise should be avoided because of the risk of preconceptions about the effects of interventions (Gøtzsche and Ioannidis 2012). However, it is important that both topic and methodological expertise is present to ensure a good mix of skills, knowledge and objectivity, because topic expertise provides important insight into the implementation of the intervention(s), the nature of the condition being treated or prevented, the relationships between outcomes measured, and other factors that may have an impact on decision making.

A Cochrane Review should represent an independent assessment of the evidence and avoiding financial and non-financial conflicts of interest often requires careful management. It will be important to consider if there are any relevant interests that may constitute real or perceived conflicts. There are situations where employment, holding of patents and other financial support should prevent people joining an author team. Funding of Cochrane Reviews by commercial organizations with an interest in the outcome of the review is not permitted. To ensure that any issues are identified early in the process, authors planning Cochrane Reviews should consult the conflicts of interest policy before starting the review. Authors should make complete declarations of interest at the outset of the review, and refresh these throughout the review life cycle (title, protocol, review, update) or at any point when their circumstances change.

1.3.1 Involving consumers and other stakeholders

Because the priorities of decision makers and consumers may be different from those of researchers, it is important that review authors consider carefully what questions are important to these different stakeholders. Systematic reviews are more likely to be relevant to a broad range of end users if they are informed by the involvement of people with a range of experiences, in terms of both the topic and the methodology (Thomas et al 2004, Rees and Oliver 2017). Engaging consumers and other stakeholders, such as policy makers, research funders and healthcare professionals, increases relevance, promotes mutual learning, improved uptake and decreases research waste.

Mapping out all potential stakeholders specific to the review question is a helpful first step to considering who might be invited to be involved in a review. Stakeholders typically include: patients and consumers; consumer advocates; policy makers and other public officials; guideline developers; professional organizations; researchers; funders of health services and research; healthcare practitioners, and, on occasion, journalists and other media professionals. Balancing seniority, credibility within the given field, and diversity should be considered. Review authors should also take account of the needs of resource-poor countries and regions in the review process (see Chapter 16) and invite appropriate input on the scope of the review and the questions it will address.

It is established good practice to ensure that **consumers** are involved and engaged in health research, including systematic reviews. Cochrane uses the term ‘consumers’ to refer to a wide range of people, including patients or people with personal experience of a healthcare condition, carers and family members, representatives of patients and carers, service users and members of the public. In 2017, a Statement of Principles for consumer involvement in Cochrane was agreed. This seeks to change the culture of research practice to one where both consumers and other stakeholders are joint partners in research from planning, conduct, and reporting to dissemination. Systematic reviews that have had consumer involvement should be more directly applicable to decision makers than those that have not (see online Chapter II).

1.3.2 Working with consumers and other stakeholders

Methods for working with consumers and other stakeholders include surveys, workshops, focus groups and involvement in advisory groups. Decisions about what methods to use will typically be based on resource availability, but review teams should be aware of the merits and limitations of such methods. Authors will need to decide who to involve and how to provide adequate support for their involvement. This can include financial reimbursement, the provision of training, and stating clearly expectations of involvement, possibly in the form of terms of reference.

While a small number of consumers or other stakeholders may be part of the review team and become co-authors of the subsequent review, it is sometimes important to bring in a wider range of perspectives and to recognize that not everyone has the capacity or interest in becoming an author. Advisory groups offer a convenient approach to involving consumers and other relevant stakeholders, especially for topics in which opinions differ. Important points to ensure successful involvement include the following.

- The review team should co-ordinate the input of the advisory group to inform key review decisions.
- The advisory group's input should continue throughout the systematic review process to ensure relevance of the review to end users is maintained.
- Advisory group membership should reflect the breadth of the review question, and consideration should be given to involving vulnerable and marginalized people (Steel 2004) to ensure that conclusions on the value of the interventions are well-informed and applicable to all groups in society (see Chapter 16).

Templates such as terms of reference, job descriptions, or person specifications for an advisory group help to ensure clarity about the task(s) required and are available from INVOLVE. The website also gives further information on setting and organizing advisory groups. See also the Cochrane training website for further resources to support consumer involvement.

1.4 The importance of reliability

Systematic reviews aim to be an accurate representation of the current state of knowledge about a given issue. As understanding improves, the review can be updated. Nevertheless, it is important that the review itself is accurate at the time of publication. There are two main reasons for this imperative for accuracy. First, health decisions that affect people's lives are increasingly taken based on systematic review findings. Current knowledge may be imperfect, but decisions will be better informed when taken in the light of the best of current knowledge. Second, systematic reviews form a critical component of legal and regulatory frameworks; for example, drug licensing or insurance coverage. Here, systematic reviews also need to hold up as auditable processes for legal examination. As systematic reviews need to be both correct, and be seen to be correct, detailed evidence-based methods have been developed to guide review authors as to the most appropriate procedures to follow, and what information to include in their reports to aid auditability.

1.4.1 Expectations for the conduct and reporting of Cochrane Reviews

Cochrane has developed methodological expectations for the conduct, reporting and updating of systematic reviews of interventions (MECIR) and their plain language summaries (Plain Language Expectations for Authors of Cochrane Summaries; PLEACS). Developed collaboratively by methodologists and Cochrane editors, they are intended to describe the desirable attributes of a Cochrane Review. The expectations are not all relevant at the same stage of review conduct, so care should be taken to identify those that are relevant at specific points during the review. Different methods should be used at different stages of the review in terms of the planning, conduct, reporting and updating of the review.

Each expectation has a title, a rationale and an elaboration. For the purposes of publication of a review with Cochrane, each has the status of either 'mandatory' or 'highly desirable'. Items described as mandatory are expected to be applied, and if they are not then an appropriate justification should be provided; failure to implement such items may be used as a basis for deciding not to publish a review in the *Cochrane Database of Systematic Reviews* (CDSR). Items described as highly desirable should generally be implemented, but there are reasonable exceptions and justifications are not required.

All MECIR expectations for the conduct of a review are presented in the relevant chapters of this *Handbook*. Expectations for reporting of completed reviews (including PLEACS) are described in online Chapter III. The recommendations provided in the Preferred Reporting Items for Systematic reviews and Meta-Analyses (PRISMA) Statement have been incorporated into the Cochrane reporting expectations, ensuring compliance with the PRISMA recommendations and summarizing attributes of reporting that should allow a full assessment of the methods and findings of the review (Moher et al 2009).

1.5 Protocol development

Preparing a systematic review is complex and involves many judgements. To minimize the potential for bias in the review process, these judgements should be made as far as possible in ways that do not depend on the findings of the studies included in the review. Review authors' prior knowledge of the evidence may, for example, influence the definition of a systematic review question, the choice of criteria for study eligibility, or the pre-specification of intervention comparisons and outcomes to analyse. It is important that the methods to be used should be established and documented in advance (see MECIR Box 1.5.a, MECIR Box 1.5.b and below MECIR Box 1.5.c).

MECIR Box 1.5.a Relevant expectations for conduct of intervention reviews	
C19: Planning the search (**Mandatory**)	
Plan in advance the methods to be used for identifying studies. Design searches to capture as many studies as possible that meet the eligibility criteria, ensuring that relevant time periods and sources are covered and not restricted by language or publication status.	Searches should be motivated directly by the eligibility criteria for the review, and it is important that all types of eligible studies are considered when planning the search. If searches are restricted by publication status or by language of publication, there is a possibility of publication bias, or language bias (whereby the language of publication is selected in a way that depends on the findings of the study), or both. Removing language restrictions in English language databases is not a good substitute for searching non-English language journals and databases.

MECIR Box 1.5.b Relevant expectations for the conduct of intervention reviews

C20: Planning the assessment of risk of bias in included studies (**Mandatory**)

Plan in advance the methods to be used for assessing risk of bias in included studies, including the tool(s) to be used, how the tool(s) will be implemented, and the criteria used to assign studies, for example, to judgements of low risk, high risk and unclear risk of bias.	Predefining the methods and criteria for assessing risk of bias is important since analysis or interpretation of the review findings may be affected by the judgements made during this process. For randomized trials, use of the Cochrane risk-of-bias tool is Mandatory, so it is sufficient (and easiest) simply to refer to the definitions of low risk, unclear risk and high risk of bias provided in the *Handbook*.

MECIR Box 1.5.c Relevant expectations for conduct of intervention reviews

C21: Planning the synthesis of results (**Mandatory**)

Plan in advance the methods to be used to synthesize the results of the included studies, including whether a quantitative synthesis is planned, how heterogeneity will be assessed, choice of effect measure (e.g. odds ratio, risk ratio, risk difference or other for dichotomous outcomes), and methods for meta-analysis (e.g. inverse variance or Mantel Haenszel, fixed-effect or random-effects model).	Predefining the synthesis methods, particularly the statistical methods, is important, since analysis or interpretation of the review findings may be affected by the judgements made during this process.

C22: Planning sub-group analyses (**Mandatory**)

Predefine potential effect modifiers (e.g. for subgroup analyses) at the protocol stage; restrict these in number, and provide rationale for each.	Pre-specification reduces the risk that large numbers of undirected subgroup analyses will lead to spurious explanations of heterogeneity.

C23: Planning the GRADE assessment and 'Summary of findings' table (**Mandatory**)

Plan in advance the methods to be used for assessing the certainty of the body of evidence, and summarizing the findings of the review.	Methods for assessing the certainty of evidence for the most important outcomes in the review need to be pre-specified. In 'Summary of findings' tables the most important feature is to predefine the choice of outcomes in order to guard against selective presentation of results in the review. The table should include the essential outcomes for decision making (typically up to seven), which generally should not include surrogate or interim outcomes. The choice of outcomes should not be based on any anticipated or observed magnitude of effect, or because they are likely to have been addressed in the studies to be reviewed.

Publication of a protocol for a review that is written without knowledge of the available studies reduces the impact of review authors' biases, promotes transparency of methods and processes, reduces the potential for duplication, allows peer review of the planned methods before they have been completed, and offers an opportunity for the review team to plan resources and logistics for undertaking the review itself. All chapters in the *Handbook* should be consulted when drafting the protocol. Since systematic reviews are by their nature retrospective, an element of knowledge of the evidence is often inevitable. This is one reason why non-content experts such as methodologists should be part of the review team (see Section 1.3). Two exceptions to the retrospective nature of a systematic review are a meta-analysis of a prospectively planned series of trials and some living systematic reviews, as described in Chapter 22.

The review question should determine the methods used in the review, and not vice versa. The question may concern a relatively straightforward comparison of one treatment with another; or it may necessitate plans to compare different treatments as part of a network meta-analysis, or assess differential effects of an intervention in different populations or delivered in different ways.

The protocol sets out the context in which the review is being conducted. It presents an opportunity to develop ideas that are foundational for the review. This concerns, most explicitly, definition of the eligibility criteria such as the study participants and the choice of comparators and outcomes. The eligibility criteria may also be defined following the development of a logic model (or an articulation of the aspects of an extent logic model that the review is addressing) to explain how the intervention might work (see Chapter 2, Section 2.5.1).

A key purpose of the protocol is to make plans to minimize bias in the eventual findings of the review. Reliable synthesis of available evidence requires a planned, systematic approach. Threats to the validity of systematic reviews can come from the studies they include or the process by which reviews are conducted. Biases within the studies can arise from the method by which participants are allocated to the intervention groups, awareness of intervention group assignment, and the collection, analysis and reporting of data. Methods for examining these issues should be specified in the protocol. Review processes can generate bias through a failure to identify an unbiased (and preferably complete) set of studies, and poor quality assurance throughout the review. The availability of research may be influenced by the nature of the results (i.e. reporting bias). To reduce the impact of this form of bias, searching may need to include unpublished sources of evidence (Dwan et al 2013) (MECIR Box 1.5.b).

Developing a protocol for a systematic review has benefits beyond reducing bias. Investing effort in designing a systematic review will make the process more manageable and help to inform key priorities for the review. Defining the question, referring to it throughout, and using appropriate methods to address the question focuses the analysis and reporting, ensuring the review is most likely to inform treatment decisions for funders, policy makers, healthcare professionals and consumers. Details of the planned analyses, including investigations of variability across studies, should be specified in the protocol, along with methods for interpreting the results through the systematic consideration of factors that affect confidence in estimates of intervention effect (MECIR Box 1.5.c).

While the intention should be that a review will adhere to the published protocol, changes in a review protocol are sometimes necessary. This is also the case for a protocol for a randomized trial, which must sometimes be changed to adapt to unanticipated circumstances such as problems with participant recruitment, data collection or event rates. While every effort should be made to adhere to a predetermined protocol, this is not always possible or appropriate. It is important, however, that changes in the protocol should not be made based on how they affect the outcome of the research study, whether it is a randomized trial or a systematic review. Post hoc decisions made when the impact on the results of the research is known, such as excluding selected studies from a systematic review, or changing the statistical analysis, are highly susceptible to bias and should therefore be avoided unless there are reasonable grounds for doing this.

Enabling access to a protocol through publication (all Cochrane Protocols are published in the *CDSR*) and registration on the PROSPERO register of systematic reviews reduces duplication of effort, research waste, and promotes accountability. Changes to the methods outlined in the protocol should be transparently declared.

This *Handbook* provides details of the systematic review methods developed or selected by Cochrane. They are intended to address the need for rigour, comprehensiveness and transparency in preparing a Cochrane systematic review. All relevant chapters – including those describing procedures to be followed in the later stages of the review – should be consulted during the preparation of the protocol. A more specific description of the structure of Cochrane Protocols is provide in online Chapter II.

1.6 Data management and quality assurance

Systematic reviews should be replicable, and retaining a record of the inclusion decisions, data collection, transformations or adjustment of data will help to establish a secure and retrievable audit trail. They can be operationally complex projects, often involving large research teams operating in different sites across the world. Good data management processes are essential to ensure that data are not inadvertently lost, facilitating the identification and correction of errors and supporting future efforts to update and maintain the review. Transparent reporting of review decisions enables readers to assess the reliability of the review for themselves.

Review management software, such as Covidence and EPPI-Reviewer, can be used to assist data management and maintain consistent and standardized records of decisions made throughout the review. These tools offer a central repository for review data that can be accessed remotely throughout the world by members of the review team. They record independent assessment of studies for inclusion, risk of bias and extraction of data, enabling checks to be made later in the process if needed. Research has shown that even experienced reviewers make mistakes and disagree with one another on risk-of-bias assessments, so it is particularly important to maintain quality assurance here, despite its cost in terms of author time. As more sophisticated information technology tools begin to be deployed in reviews (see Chapter 4, Section 4.6.6.2 and Chapter 22, Section 22.2.4), it is increasingly apparent that all review data – including the initial decisions about study eligibility – have value beyond the scope of the individual review. For example, review updates can be made more efficient through (semi-) automation when data from the original review are available for machine learning.

1.7 Chapter information

Authors: Toby J Lasserson, James Thomas, Julian PT Higgins

Acknowledgements: This chapter builds on earlier versions of the *Handbook*. We would like to thank Ruth Foxlee, Richard Morley, Soumyadeep Bhaumik, Mona Nasser, Dan Fox and Sally Crowe for their contributions to Section 1.3.

Funding: JT is supported by the National Institute for Health Research (NIHR) Collaboration for Leadership in Applied Health Research and Care North Thames at Barts Health NHS Trust. JPTH is a member of the NIHR Biomedical Research Centre at University Hospitals Bristol NHS Foundation Trust and the University of Bristol. JPTH received funding from National Institute for Health Research Senior Investigator award NF-SI-0617-10145. The views expressed are those of the author(s) and not necessarily those of the NHS, the NIHR or the Department of Health.

1.8 References

Antman E, Lau J, Kupelnick B, Mosteller F, Chalmers T. A comparison of results of meta-analyses of randomized control trials and recommendations of clinical experts: treatment for myocardial infarction. *JAMA* 1992; **268**: 240–248.

Chalmers I, Bracken MB, Djulbegovic B, Garattini S, Grant J, Gulmezoglu AM, Howells DW, Ioannidis JP, Oliver S. How to increase value and reduce waste when research priorities are set. *Lancet* 2014; **383**: 156–165.

Chandler J, Hopewell S. Cochrane methods – twenty years experience in developing systematic review methods. *Systematic Reviews* 2013; **2**: 76.

Dwan K, Gamble C, Williamson PR, Kirkham JJ, Reporting Bias Group. Systematic review of the empirical evidence of study publication bias and outcome reporting bias: an updated review. *PloS One* 2013; **8**: e66844.

Gøtzsche PC, Ioannidis JPA. Content area experts as authors: helpful or harmful for systematic reviews and meta-analyses? *BMJ* 2012; **345**.

Macleod MR, Michie S, Roberts I, Dirnagl U, Chalmers I, Ioannidis JP, Al-Shahi Salman R, Chan AW, Glasziou P. Biomedical research: increasing value, reducing waste. *Lancet* 2014; **383**: 101–104.

Moher D, Liberati A, Tetzlaff J, Altman D, PRISMA Group. Preferred reporting items for systematic reviews and meta-analyses: the PRISMA statement. *PLoS Medicine* 2009; **6**: e1000097.

Oxman A, Guyatt G. The science of reviewing research. *Annals of the New York Academy of Sciences* 1993; **703**: 125–133.

Rees R, Oliver S. Stakeholder perspectives and participation in reviews. In: Gough D, Oliver S, Thomas J, editors. *An Introduction to Systematic Reviews*. 2nd ed. London: Sage; 2017. p. 17–34.

Steel R. Involving marginalised and vulnerable people in research: a consultation document (2nd revision). INVOLVE; 2004.

Thomas J, Harden A, Oakley A, Oliver S, Sutcliffe K, Rees R, Brunton G, Kavanagh J. Integrating qualitative research with trials in systematic reviews. *BMJ* 2004; **328**: 1010–1012.

2

Determining the scope of the review and the questions it will address

James Thomas, Dylan Kneale, Joanne E McKenzie, Sue E Brennan, Soumyadeep Bhaumik

KEY POINTS

- Systematic reviews should address answerable questions and fill important gaps in knowledge.
- Developing good review questions takes time, expertise and engagement with intended users of the review.
- Cochrane Reviews can focus on broad questions, or be more narrowly defined. There are advantages and disadvantages of each.
- Logic models are a way of documenting how interventions, particularly complex interventions, are intended to 'work', and can be used to refine review questions and the broader scope of the review.
- Using priority-setting exercises, involving relevant stakeholders, and ensuring that the review takes account of issues relating to equity can be strategies for ensuring that the scope and focus of reviews address the right questions.

2.1 Rationale for well-formulated questions

As with any research, the first and most important decision in preparing a systematic review is to determine its focus. This is best done by clearly framing the questions the review seeks to answer. The focus of any Cochrane Review should be on questions that are important to people making decisions about health or health care. These decisions will usually need to take into account both the benefits and harms of interventions (see MECIR Box 2.1.a). Good review questions often take time to develop, requiring engagement with not only the subject area, but with a wide group of stakeholders (Section 2.4.2).

Well-formulated questions will guide many aspects of the review process, including determining eligibility criteria, searching for studies, collecting data from included

This chapter should be cited as: Thomas J, Kneale D, McKenzie JE, Brennan SE, Bhaumik S. Chapter 2: Determining the scope of the review and the questions it will address. In: Higgins JPT, Thomas J, Chandler J, Cumpston M, Li T, Page MJ, Welch VA (editors). *Cochrane Handbook for Systematic Reviews of Interventions*. 2nd Edition. Chichester (UK): John Wiley & Sons, 2019: 13–32.

MECIR Box 2.1.a Relevant expectations for conduct of intervention reviews	
C1: Formulating review questions (**Mandatory**)	
Ensure that the review question and particularly the outcomes of interest, address issues that are important to review users such as consumers, health professionals and policy makers.	Cochrane Reviews are intended to support clinical practice and policy, not just scientific curiosity. The needs of consumers play a central role in Cochrane Reviews and they can play an important role in defining the review question. Qualitative research, i.e. studies that explore the experience of those involved in providing and receiving interventions, and studies evaluating factors that shape the implementation of interventions, might be used in the same way.
C3: Considering potential adverse effects (**Mandatory**)	
Consider any important potential adverse effects of the intervention(s) and ensure that they are addressed.	It is important that adverse effects are addressed in order to avoid one-sided summaries of the evidence. At a minimum, the review will need to highlight the extent to which potential adverse effects have been evaluated in any included studies. Sometimes data on adverse effects are best obtained from non-randomized studies, or qualitative research studies. This does not mean however that all reviews must include non-randomized studies.

studies, structuring the syntheses and presenting findings (Cooper 1984, Hedges 1994, Oliver et al 2017). In Cochrane Reviews, questions are stated broadly as review 'Objectives', and operationalized in terms of the studies that will be eligible to answer those questions as 'Criteria for considering studies for this review'. As well as focusing review conduct, the contents of these sections are used by readers in their initial assessments of whether the review is likely to be directly relevant to the issues they face.

The FINER criteria have been proposed as encapsulating the issues that should be addressed when developing research questions. These state that questions should be **F**easible, **I**nteresting, **N**ovel, **E**thical, and **R**elevant (Cummings et al 2007). All of these criteria raise important issues for consideration at the outset of a review and should be borne in mind when questions are formulated.

A *feasible* review is one that asks a question that the author team is capable of addressing using the evidence available. Issues concerning the breadth of a review are discussed in Section 2.3.1, but in terms of feasibility it is important not to ask a question that will result in retrieving unmanageable quantities of information; up-front scoping work will help authors to define sensible boundaries for their reviews. Likewise, while it can be useful to identify gaps in the evidence base, review authors and stakeholders should be aware of the possibility of asking a question that may not be answerable using the existing evidence (i.e. that will result in an 'empty' review, see also Section 2.5.3).

Embarking on a review that authors are *interested* in is important because reviews are a significant undertaking and review authors need sufficient commitment to see the work through to its conclusion.

A *novel* review will address a genuine gap in knowledge, so review authors should be aware of any related or overlapping reviews. This reduces duplication of effort, and also ensures that authors understand the wider research context to which their review will contribute. Authors should check for pre-existing syntheses in the published research literature and also for ongoing reviews in the PROSPERO register of systematic reviews before beginning their own review.

Given the opportunity cost involved in undertaking an activity as demanding as a systematic review, authors should ensure that their work is *relevant* by: (i) involving relevant stakeholders in defining its focus and the questions it will address; and (ii) writing up the review in such a way as to facilitate the translation of its findings to inform decisions. The GRADE framework aims to achieve this, and should be considered throughout the review process, not only when it is being written up (see Chapters 14 and 15).

Consideration of opportunity costs is also relevant in terms of the *ethics* of conducting a review, though ethical issues should also be considered primarily in terms of the questions that are prioritized for answering and the way that they are framed. Research questions are often not value-neutral, and the way that a given problem is approached can have political implications which can result in, for example, the widening of health inequalities (whether intentional or not). These issues are explored in Section 2.4.3 and Chapter 16.

2.2 Aims of reviews of interventions

Systematic reviews can address any question that can be answered by a primary research study. This *Handbook* focuses on a subset of all possible review questions: the impact of intervention(s) implemented within a specified human population. Even within these limits, systematic reviews examining the effects of intervention(s) can vary quite markedly in their aims. Some will focus specifically on evidence of an effect of an intervention compared with a specific alternative, whereas others may examine a range of different interventions. Reviews that examine multiple interventions and aim to identify which might be the most effective can be broader and more challenging than those looking at single interventions. These can also be the most useful for end users, where decision making involves selecting from a number of intervention options. The incorporation of network meta-analysis as a core method in this edition of the *Handbook* (see Chapter 11) reflects the growing importance of these types of reviews.

As well as looking at the balance of benefit and harm that can be attributed to a given intervention, reviews within the ambit of this *Handbook* might also aim to investigate the relationship between the size of an intervention effect and other characteristics, such as aspects of the population, the intervention itself, how the outcome is measured, or the methodology of the primary research studies included. Such approaches might be used to investigate which components of multi-component interventions are more or less important or essential (and when). While it is not always necessary to know how an intervention achieves its effect for it to be useful, many reviews will aim to articulate an intervention's mechanisms of action (see Section 2.5.1), either by making this an explicit aim of the review itself (see Chapters 17 and 21), or when describing the scope of the review. Understanding how an intervention works (or is intended to work) can be an important aid to decision makers in assessing the applicability of the review to their situation. These investigations can be assisted by the incorporation of results from process evaluations conducted alongside trials (see Chapter 21). Further, many decisions in policy and practice are at least partially constrained by the resource available, so review authors often need to consider the economic context of interventions (see Chapter 20).

2.3 Defining the scope of a review question

Studies comparing healthcare interventions, notably randomized trials, use the outcomes of participants to compare the effects of different interventions. Statistical syntheses (e.g. meta-analysis) focus on comparisons of interventions, such as a new intervention versus a control intervention (which may represent conditions of usual practice or care), or the comparison of two competing interventions. Throughout the *Handbook* we use the terminology **experimental** intervention versus **comparator** intervention. This implies a need to identify one of the interventions as experimental, and is used only for convenience since all methods apply to both controlled and head-to-head comparisons. The contrast between the outcomes of two groups treated differently is known as the 'effect', the 'treatment effect' or the 'intervention effect'; we generally use the last of these throughout the *Handbook*.

A statement of the review's objectives should begin with a precise statement of the primary objective, ideally in a single sentence (MECIR Box 2.3.a). Where possible the style should be of the form 'To assess the effects of [*intervention or comparison*] for [*health problem*] in [*types of people, disease or problem and setting if specified*]'. This

MECIR Box 2.3.a Relevant expectations for conduct of intervention reviews	
C2: Predefining objectives (**Mandatory**)	
Define in advance the objectives of the review, including population, interventions, comparators and outcomes (PICO).	Objectives give the review focus and must be clear before appropriate eligibility criteria can be developed. If the review will address multiple interventions, clarity is required on how these will be addressed (e.g. summarized separately, combined or explicitly compared).

might be followed by one or more secondary objectives, for example relating to different participant groups, different comparisons of interventions or different outcome measures. The detailed specification of the review question(s) requires consideration of several key components (Richardson et al 1995, Counsell 1997) which can often be encapsulated by the 'PICO' mnemonic, an acronym for **P**opulation, **I**ntervention, **C**omparison(s) and **O**utcome. Equal emphasis in addressing, and equal precision in defining, each PICO component is not necessary. For example, a review might concentrate on competing interventions for a particular stage of breast cancer, with stage and severity of the disease being defined very precisely; or alternately focus on a particular drug for any stage of breast cancer, with the treatment formulation being defined very precisely.

Throughout the *Handbook* we make a distinction between three different stages in the review at which the PICO construct might be used. This division is helpful for understanding the decisions that need to be made:

- The **review PICO** (planned at the protocol stage) is the PICO on which eligibility of studies is based (what will be included and what excluded from the review).
- The **PICO for each synthesis** (also planned at the protocol stage) defines the question that each specific synthesis aims to answer, determining how the synthesis will be structured, specifying planned comparisons (including intervention and comparator groups, any grouping of outcome and population subgroups).
- The **PICO of the included studies** (determined at the review stage) is what was actually investigated in the included studies.

Reaching the point where it is possible to articulate the review's objectives in the above form – the review PICO – requires time and detailed discussion between potential authors and users of the review. It is important that those involved in developing the review's scope and questions have a good knowledge of the practical issues that the review will address as well as the research field to be synthesized. Developing the questions is a critical part of the research process. As such, there are methodological issues to bear in mind, including: how to determine which questions are most important to answer; how to engage stakeholders in question formulation; how to account for changes in focus as the review progresses; and considerations about how broad (or narrow) a review should be.

2.3.1 Broad versus narrow reviews

The questions addressed by a review may be broad or narrow in scope. For example, a review might address a broad question regarding whether antiplatelet agents in general are effective in preventing all thrombotic events in humans. Alternatively, a review might address whether a particular antiplatelet agent, such as aspirin, is effective in decreasing the risks of a particular thrombotic event, stroke, in elderly persons with a previous history of stroke. Increasingly, reviews are becoming broader, aiming, for example, to identify which intervention – out of a range of treatment options – is most effective, or to investigate how an intervention varies depending on implementation and participant characteristics.

Overviews of reviews (online Chapter V), in which multiple reviews are summarized, can be one way of addressing the need for breadth when synthesizing the evidence base, since they can summarize multiple reviews of different interventions for the same condition, or multiple reviews of the same intervention for different types of participants. It may be considered desirable to plan a series of reviews with a relatively narrow scope, alongside an Overview to summarize their findings. Alternatively, it may be more useful – particularly given the growth in support for network meta-analysis – to combine comparisons of different treatment options within the same review (see Chapter 11). When deciding whether or not an overview might be the most appropriate approach, review authors should take account of the breadth of the question being asked and the resources available. Some questions are simply too broad for a review of all relevant primary research to be practicable, and if a field has sufficient high-quality reviews, then the production of another review of primary research that duplicates the others might not be a sensible use of resources.

Some of the advantages and disadvantages of broad and narrow reviews are summarized in Table 2.3.a. While having a broad scope in terms of the range of participants has the potential to increase generalizability, the extent to which findings are ultimately applicable to broader (or different) populations will depend on the participants who have

Table 2.3.a Some advantages and disadvantages of broad versus narrow reviews

	Broad scope	Narrow scope
Choice of population e.g. corticosteroid injection for shoulder tendonitis (narrow) or corticosteroid injection for any tendonitis (broad)	*Advantages:* Comprehensive summary of the evidence. Opportunity to explore consistency of findings (and therefore generalizability) across different types of participants.	*Advantages:* Manageability for review team. Ease of reading.
	Disadvantages: Searching, data collection, analysis and writing may require more resources. Interpretation may be difficult for readers if the review is large and lacks a clear rationale (such as examining consistency of findings) for including diverse types of participants.	*Disadvantages:* Evidence may be sparse. Unable to explore whether an intervention operates differently in other settings or populations (e.g. inability to explore differential effects that could lead to inequity). Increased burden for decision makers if multiple reviews must be accessed (e.g. if evidence is sparse for the population of interest). Scope could be chosen by review authors to produce a desired result.
Mode of intervention e.g. supervised running for depression (narrow) or any exercise for depression (broad)	*Advantages:* Comprehensive summary of the evidence. Opportunity to explore consistency of findings across different implementations of the intervention.	*Advantages:* Manageability for review team. Ease of reading.

Table 2.3.a (Continued)

	Broad scope	**Narrow scope**
	Disadvantages: Searching, data collection, analysis and writing may require more resources. Interpretation may be difficult for readers if the review is large and lacks a clear rationale (such as examining consistency of findings) for including different modes of an intervention.	*Disadvantages:* Evidence may be sparse. Unable to explore whether different modes of an intervention modify the intervention effects. Increased burden for decision makers if multiple reviews must be accessed (e.g. if evidence is sparse for a specific mode). Scope could be chosen by review authors to produce a desired result.
Choice of interventions and comparators e.g. oxybutynin compared with desmopressin for preventing bed-wetting (narrow) or interventions for preventing bed-wetting (broad)	*Advantages:* Comprehensive summary of the evidence. Opportunity to compare the effectiveness of a range of different intervention options.	*Advantages:* Manageability for review team. Relative simplicity of objectives and ease of reading.
	Disadvantages: Searching, data collection, analysis and writing may require more resources. May be unwieldy, and more appropriate to present as an Overview of reviews (see online Chapter V).	*Disadvantages:* Increased burden for decision makers if not included in an Overview since multiple reviews may need to be accessed.

actually been recruited into research studies. Likewise, heterogeneity can be a disadvantage when the expectation is for homogeneity of effects between studies, but an advantage when the review question seeks to understand differential effects (see Chapter 10).

A distinction should be drawn between the scope of a review and the precise questions within, since it is possible to have a broad review that addresses quite narrow questions. In the antiplatelet agents for preventing thrombotic events example, a systematic review with a broad scope might include all available treatments. Rather than combining all the studies into one comparison though, specific treatments would be compared with one another in separate comparisons, thus breaking a heterogeneous set of treatments into narrower, more homogenous groups. This relates to the three levels of PICO, outlined in Section 2.3. The *review PICO* defines the broad scope of the review, and the *PICO for comparison* defines the specific treatments that will be compared with one another; Chapter 3 elaborates on the use of PICOs.

In practice, a Cochrane Review may start (or have started) with a broad scope, and be divided up into narrower reviews as evidence accumulates and the original review becomes unwieldy. This may be done for practical and logistical reasons, for example to make updating easier as well as to make it easier for readers to see which parts of the evidence base are changing. Individual review authors must decide if there are instances where splitting a broader focused review into a series of more narrowly focused reviews is appropriate and implement appropriate methods to achieve this. If a major change is to be undertaken, such as splitting a broad review into a series of more narrowly focused reviews, a new protocol must be written for each of the component reviews that documents the eligibility criteria for each one.

Ultimately, the selected breadth of a review depends upon multiple factors including perspectives regarding a question's relevance and potential impact; supporting theoretical, biologic and epidemiological information; the potential generalizability and validity of answers to the questions; and available resources. As outlined in Section 2.4.2, authors should consider carefully the needs of users of the review and the context(s) in which they expect the review to be used when determining the most optimal scope for their review.

2.3.2 'Lumping' versus 'splitting'

It is important not to confuse the issue of the breadth of the review (determined by the review PICO) with concerns about between-study heterogeneity and the legitimacy of combining results from diverse studies in the same analysis (determined by the PICOs for comparison).

Broad reviews have been criticized as 'mixing apples and oranges', and one of the inventors of meta-analysis, Gene Glass, has responded "Of course it mixes apples and oranges… comparing apples and oranges is the only endeavour worthy of true scientists; comparing apples to apples is trivial" (Glass 2015). In fact, the two concepts ('broad reviews' and 'mixing apples and oranges') are different issues. Glass argues that broad reviews, with diverse studies, provide the opportunity to ask interesting questions about the *reasons for* differential intervention effects.

The 'apples and oranges' critique refers to the inappropriate mixing of studies within a single comparison, where the purpose is to estimate an average effect. In situations where good biologic or sociological evidence suggests that various formulations of an intervention behave very differently or that various definitions of the condition of interest are associated with markedly different effects of the intervention, the uncritical aggregation of results from quite different interventions or populations/settings may well be questionable.

Unfortunately, determining the situations where studies are similar enough to combine with one another is not always straightforward, and it can depend, to some extent, on the question being asked. While the decision is sometimes characterized as 'lumping' (where studies are combined in the same analysis) or 'splitting' (where they are not) (Squires et al 2013), it is better to consider these issues on a continuum, with reviews that have greater variation in the types of included interventions, settings and populations, and study designs being towards the 'lumped' end, and those that include little variation in these elements being towards the 'split' end (Petticrew and Roberts 2006).

While specification of the review PICO sets the boundary for the inclusion and exclusion of studies, decisions also need to be made when planning the *PICO for the comparisons* to be made in the analysis as to whether they aim to address broader ('lumped') or narrower ('split') questions (Caldwell and Welton 2016). The degree of 'lumping' in the comparisons will be primarily driven by the review's objectives, but will sometimes be dictated by the availability of studies (and data) for a particular comparison (see Chapter 9 for discussion of the latter). The former is illustrated by a Cochrane Review that examined the effects of newer-generation antidepressants for depressive disorders in children and adolescents (Hetrick et al 2012).

Newer-generation antidepressants include multiple different compounds (e.g. paroxetine, fluoxetine). The objectives of this review were to (i) estimate the overall effect of newer-generation antidepressants on depression, (ii) estimate the effect of each compound, and (iii) examine whether the compound type and age of the participants (children versus adolescents) is associated with the intervention effect. Objective (i) addresses a broad, 'in principle' (Caldwell and Welton 2016), question of whether newer-generation antidepressants improve depression, where the different compounds are 'lumped' into a single comparison. Objective (ii) seeks to address narrower, 'split', questions that investigate the effect of each compound on depression separately. Answers to both questions can be identified by setting up separate comparisons for each compound, or by subgrouping the 'lumped' comparison by compound (Chapter 10, Section 10.11.2). Objective (iii) seeks to explore factors that explain heterogeneity among the intervention effects, or equivalently, whether the intervention effect varies by the factor. This can be examined using subgroup analysis or meta-regression (Chapter 10, Section 10.11) but, in the case of intervention types, is best achieved using network meta-analysis (see Chapter 11).

There are various advantages and disadvantages to bear in mind when defining the *PICO for the comparison* and considering whether 'lumping' or 'splitting' is appropriate. Lumping allows for the investigation of factors that may explain heterogeneity. Results from these investigations may provide important leads as to whether an intervention operates differently in, for example, different populations (such as in children and adolescents in the example above). Ultimately, this type of knowledge is useful for clinical decision making. However, lumping is likely to introduce heterogeneity, which will not always be explained by a priori specified factors, and this may lead to a combined effect that is clinically difficult to interpret and implement. For example, when multiple intervention types are 'lumped' in one comparison (as in objective (i) above), and there is unexplained heterogeneity, the combined intervention effect would not enable a clinical decision as to which intervention should be selected. Splitting comparisons carries its own risk of there being too few studies to yield a useful synthesis. Inevitably, some degree of aggregation across the PICO elements is required for a meta-analysis to be undertaken (Caldwell and Welton 2016).

2.4 Ensuring the review addresses the right questions

Since systematic reviews are intended for use in healthcare decision making, review teams should ensure not only the application of robust methodology, but also that the review question is meaningful for healthcare decision making. Two approaches are discussed below:

- Using results from existing research priority-setting exercises to define the review question.
- In the absence of, or in addition to, existing research priority-setting exercises, engaging with stakeholders to define review questions and establish their relevance to policy and practice.

2.4.1 Using priority-setting exercises to define review questions

A research priority-setting exercise is a "collective activity for deciding which uncertainties are most worth trying to resolve through research; uncertainties considered may be problems to be understood or solutions to be developed or tested; across broad or narrow areas" (Sandy Oliver, referenced in Nasser 2018). Using research priority-setting exercises to define the scope of a review helps to prevent the waste of scarce resources for research by making the review more relevant to stakeholders (Chalmers et al 2014).

Research priority setting is always conducted in a specific context, setting and population with specific principles, values and preferences (which should be articulated). Different stakeholders' interpretation of the scope and purpose of a 'research question' might vary, resulting in priorities that might be difficult to interpret. Researchers or review teams might find it necessary to translate the research priorities into an answerable PICO research question format, and may find it useful to recheck the question with the stakeholder groups to determine whether they have accurately reflected their intentions.

While Cochrane Review teams are in most cases reviewing the effects of an intervention with a global scope, they may find that the priorities identified by important stakeholders (such as the World Health Organization or other organizations or individuals in a representative health system) are informative in planning the review. Review authors may find that differences between different stakeholder groups' views on priorities and the reasons for these differences can help them to define the scope of the review. This is particularly important for making decisions about excluding specific populations or settings, or being inclusive and potentially conducting subgroup analyses.

Whenever feasible, systematic reviews should be based on priorities identified by key stakeholders such as decision makers, patients/public, and practitioners. Cochrane has developed a list of priorities for reviews led by review groups and networks, in consultation with key stakeholders, which is available on the Cochrane website. Issues relating to equity (see Chapter 16 and Section 2.4.3) need to be taken into account when conducting and interpreting the results from priority-setting exercises. Examples of materials to support these processes are available (Viergever et al 2010, Nasser et al 2013, Tong et al 2017).

The results of research priority-setting exercises can be searched for in electronic databases and via websites of relevant organizations. Examples are: James Lind Alliance, World Health Organization, organizations of health professionals including research disciplines, and ministries of health in different countries (Viergever 2010). Examples of search strategies for identifying research priority-setting exercises are available (Bryant et al 2014, Tong et al 2015).

Other sources of questions are often found in 'implications for future research' sections of articles in journals and clinical practice guidelines. Some guideline developers have prioritized questions identified through the guideline development process (Sharma et al 2018), although these priorities will be influenced by the needs of health systems in which different guideline development teams are working.

2.4.2 Engaging stakeholders to help define the review questions

In the absence of a relevant research priority-setting exercise, or when a systematic review is being conducted for a very specific purpose (for example, commissioned to inform the development of a guideline), researchers should work with relevant stakeholders to define the review question. This practice is especially important when developing review questions for studying the effectiveness of health systems and policies, because of the variability between countries and regions; the significance of these differences may only become apparent through discussion with the stakeholders.

The stakeholders for a review could include consumers or patients, carers, health professionals of different kinds, policy decision makers and others (Chapter 1, Section 1.3.1). Identifying the stakeholders who are critical to a particular question will depend on the question, who the answer is likely to affect, and who will be expected to implement the intervention if it is found to be effective (or to discontinue it if not).

Stakeholder engagement should, optimally, be an ongoing process throughout the life of the systematic review, from defining the question to dissemination of results (Keown et al 2008). Engaging stakeholders increases relevance, promotes mutual learning, improves uptake and decreases research waste (see Chapter 1, Sections 1.3.1 and 1.3.2). However, because such engagement can be challenging and resource intensive, a one-off engagement process to define the review question might only be possible. Review questions that are conceptualized and refined by multiple stakeholders can capture much of the complexity that should be addressed in a systematic review.

2.4.3 Considering issues relating to equity when defining review questions

Deciding what should be investigated, who the participants should be, and how the analysis will be carried out can be considered political activities, with the potential for increasing or decreasing inequalities in health. For example, we now know that well-intended interventions can actually widen inequalities in health outcomes since researchers have chosen to investigate this issue (Lorenc et al 2013). Decision makers can now take account of this knowledge when planning service provision. Authors should therefore consider the potential impact on disadvantaged groups of the intervention(s) that they are investigating, and whether socio-economic inequalities in health might be affected depending on whether or how they are implemented.

Health equity is the absence of avoidable and unfair differences in health (Whitehead 1992). Health inequity may be experienced across characteristics defined by PROGRESS-Plus (Place of residence, Race/ethnicity/culture/language, Occupation, Gender/sex, Religion, Education, Socio-economic status, Social capital, and other characteristics ('Plus') such as sexual orientation, age, and disability) (O'Neill et al 2014). Issues relating to health equity should be considered when review questions are developed (MECIR Box 2.4.a). Chapter 16 presents detailed guidance on this issue for review authors.

MECIR Box 2.4.a Relevant expectations for conduct of intervention reviews	
C4: Considering equity and specific populations (**Highly desirable**)	
Consider in advance whether issues of equity and relevance of evidence to specific populations are important to the review, and plan for appropriate methods to address them if they are. Attention should be paid to the relevance of the review question to populations such as low socio-economic groups, low- or middle-income regions, women, children and older people.	Where possible reviews should include explicit descriptions of the effect of the interventions not only upon the whole population, but also on the disadvantaged, and/or the ability of the interventions to reduce socio-economic inequalities in health, and to promote use of the interventions to the community.

2.5 Methods and tools for structuring the review

It is important for authors to develop the scope of their review with care: without a clear understanding of where the review will contribute to existing knowledge – and how it will be used – it may be at risk of conceptual incoherence. It may mis-specify critical elements of how the intervention(s) interact with the context(s) within which they operate to produce specific outcomes, and become either irrelevant or possibly misleading. For example, in a systematic review about smoking cessation interventions in pregnancy, it was essential for authors to take account of the way that health service provision has changed over time. The type and intensity of 'usual care' in more recent evaluations was equivalent to the interventions being evaluated in older studies, and the analysis needed to take this into account. This review also found that the same intervention can have different effects in different settings depending on whether its materials are culturally appropriate in each context (Chamberlain et al 2017).

In order to protect the review against conceptual incoherence and irrelevance, review authors need to spend time at the outset developing definitions for key concepts and ensuring that they are clear about the prior assumptions on which the review depends. These prior assumptions include, for example, why particular populations should be considered inside or outside the review's scope; how the intervention is thought to achieve its effect; and why specific outcomes are selected for evaluation. Being clear about these prior assumptions also requires review authors to consider the evidential basis for these assumptions and decide for themselves which they can place more or less reliance on. When considered as a whole, this initial conceptual and definitional work states the review's **conceptual framework**. Each element of the review's PICO raises its own definitional challenges, which are discussed in detail in the Chapter 3.

In this section we consider tools that may help to define the scope of the review and the relationships between its key concepts; in particular, articulating how the intervention gives rise to the outcomes selected. In some situations, long sequences of events are expected to occur between an intervention being implemented and an outcome being observed. For example, a systematic review examining the effects of asthma education interventions in schools on children's health and well-being needed to consider:

the interplay between core intervention components and their introduction into differing school environments; different child-level effect modifiers; how the intervention then had an impact on the knowledge of the child (and their family); the child's self-efficacy and adherence to their treatment regime; the severity of their asthma; the number of days of restricted activity; how this affected their attendance at school; and finally, the distal outcomes of education attainment and indicators of child health and well-being (Kneale et al 2015).

Several specific tools can help authors to consider issues raised when defining review questions and planning their review; these are also helpful when developing eligibility criteria and classifying included studies. These include the following.

1) Taxonomies: hierarchical structures that can be used to categorize (or group) related interventions, outcomes or populations.
2) Generic frameworks for examining and structuring the description of intervention characteristics (e.g. TIDieR for the description of interventions (Hoffmann et al 2014), iCAT_SR for describing multiple aspects of complexity in systematic reviews (Lewin et al 2017)).
3) Core outcome sets for identifying and defining agreed outcomes that should be measured for specific health conditions (described in more detail in Chapter 3).

Unlike these tools, which focus on particular aspects of a review, logic models provide a framework for planning and guiding synthesis at the review level (see Section 2.5.1).

2.5.1 Logic models

Logic models (sometimes referred to as conceptual frameworks or theories of change) are graphical representations of theories about how interventions work. They depict intervention components, mechanisms (pathways of action), outputs, and outcomes as sequential (although not necessarily linear) chains of events. Among systematic review authors, they were originally proposed as a useful tool when working with evaluations of complex social and population health programmes and interventions, to conceptualize the pathways through which interventions are intended to change outcomes (Anderson et al 2011).

In reviews where intervention complexity is a key consideration (see Chapter 17), logic models can be particularly helpful. For example, in a review of psychosocial group interventions for those with HIV, a logic model was used to show how the intervention might work (van der Heijden et al 2017). The review authors depicted proximal outcomes, such as self-esteem, but chose only to include psychological health outcomes in their review. In contrast, Bailey and colleagues included proximal outcomes in their review of computer-based interventions for sexual health promotion using a logic model to show how outcomes were grouped (Bailey et al 2010). Finally, in a review of slum upgrading, a logic model showed the broad range of interventions and their interlinkages with health and socio-economic outcomes (Turley et al 2013), and enabled the review authors to select a specific intervention category (physical upgrading) on which to focus the review. Further resources provide further examples of logic models, and can help review authors develop and use logic models (Anderson et al 2011, Baxter et al 2014, Kneale et al 2015, Pfadenhauer et al 2017, Rohwer et al 2017).

Logic models can vary in their emphasis, with a distinction sometimes made between system-based and process-oriented logic models (Rehfuess et al 2018). System-based logic models have particular value in examining the complexity of the system (e.g. the geographical, epidemiological, political, socio-cultural and socio-economic features of a system), and the interactions between contextual features, participants and the intervention (see Chapter 17). Process-oriented logic models aim to capture the complexity of causal pathways by which the intervention leads to outcomes, and any factors that may modify intervention effects. However, this is not a crisp distinction; the two types are interrelated; with some logic models depicting elements of both systems and process models simultaneously.

The way that logic models can be represented diagrammatically (see Chapter 17 for an example) provides a valuable visual summary for readers and can be a communication tool for decision makers and practitioners. They can aid initially in the development of a shared understanding between different stakeholders of the scope of the review and its PICO, helping to support decisions taken throughout the review process, from developing the research question and setting the review parameters, to structuring and interpreting the results. They can be used in planning the PICO elements of a review as well as for determining how the synthesis will be structured (i.e. planned comparisons, including intervention and comparator groups, and any grouping of outcome and population subgroups). These models may help review authors specify the link between the intervention, proximal and distal outcomes, and mediating factors. In other words, they depict the intervention theory underpinning the synthesis plan.

Anderson and colleagues note the main value of logic models in systematic review as (Anderson et al 2011):

- refining review questions;
- deciding on 'lumping' or 'splitting' a review topic;
- identifying intervention components;
- defining and conducting the review;
- identifying relevant study eligibility criteria;
- guiding the literature search strategy;
- explaining the rationale behind surrogate outcomes used in the review;
- justifying the need for subgroup analyses (e.g. age, sex/gender, socio-economic status);
- making the review relevant to policy and practice;
- structuring the reporting of results;
- illustrating how harms and feasibility are connected with interventions; and
- interpreting results based on intervention theory and systems thinking (see Chapter 17).

Logic models can be useful in systematic reviews when considering whether failure to find a beneficial effect of an intervention is due to a theory failure, an implementation failure, or both (see Chapter 17 and Cargo et al 2018). Making a distinction between implementation and intervention theory can help to determine whether and how the intervention interacts with (and potentially changes) its context (see Chapters 3 and 17 for further discussion of context). This helps to elucidate situations in which variations in how the intervention is implemented have the potential to affect the integrity of the intervention and intended outcomes.

Given their potential value in conceptualizing and structuring a review, logic models are increasingly published in review protocols. Logic models may be specified a priori and remain unchanged throughout the review; it might be expected, however, that the findings of reviews produce evidence and new understandings that could be used to update the logic model in some way (Kneale et al 2015). Some reviews take a more staged approach, pre-specifying points in the review process where the model may be revised on the basis of (new) evidence (Rehfuess et al 2018) and a staged logic model can provide an efficient way to report revisions to the synthesis plan. For example, in a review of portion, package and tableware size for changing selection or consumption of food and other products, the authors presented a logic model that clearly showed changes to their original synthesis plan (Hollands et al 2015).

It is preferable to seek out existing logic models for the intervention and revise or adapt these models in line with the review focus, although this may not always be possible. More commonly, new models are developed starting with the identification of outcomes and theorizing the necessary pre-conditions to reach those outcomes. This process of theorizing and identifying the steps and necessary pre-conditions continues, working backwards from the intended outcomes, until the intervention itself is represented. As many mechanisms of action are invisible and can only be 'known' through theory, this process is invaluable in exposing assumptions as to how interventions are thought to work; assumptions that might then be tested in the review. Logic models can be developed with stakeholders (see Section 2.5.2) and it is considered good practice to obtain stakeholder input in their development.

Logic models are representations of how interventions are intended to 'work', but they can also provide a useful basis for thinking through the unintended consequences of interventions and identifying potential adverse effects that may need to be captured in the review (Bonell et al 2015). While logic models provide a guiding theory of how interventions are intended to work, critiques exist around their use, including their potential to oversimplify complex intervention processes (Rohwer et al 2017). Here, contributions from different stakeholders to the development of a logic model may be able to articulate where complex processes may occur; theorizing unintended intervention impacts; and the explicit representation of ambiguity within certain parts of the causal chain where new theory/explanation is most valuable.

2.5.2 Changing review questions

While questions should be posed in the protocol before initiating the full review, these questions should not prevent exploration of unexpected issues. Reviews are analyses of existing data that are constrained by previously chosen study populations, settings, intervention formulations, outcome measures and study designs. It is generally not possible to formulate an answerable question for a review without knowing some of the studies relevant to the question, and it may become clear that the questions a review addresses need to be modified in light of evidence accumulated in the process of conducting the review.

Although a certain fluidity and refinement of questions is to be expected in reviews as a fuller understanding of the evidence is gained, it is important to guard against bias in modifying questions. Data-driven questions can generate false conclusions based on spurious results. Any changes to the protocol that result from revising the question for the review should be documented in the section 'Differences between the protocol and the review'. Sensitivity analyses may be used to assess the impact of changes on the review findings (see Chapter 10, Section 10.14). When refining questions it is useful to ask the following questions.

- What is the motivation for the refinement?
- Could the refinement have been influenced by results from any of the included studies?
- Does the refined question require a modification to the search strategy and/or reassessment of any decisions regarding study eligibility?
- Are data collection methods appropriate to the refined question?
- Does the refined question still meet the FINER criteria discussed in Section 2.1?

2.5.3 Building in contingencies to deal with sparse data

The ability to address the review questions will depend on the maturity and validity of the evidence base. When few studies are identified, there will be limited opportunity to address the question through an informative synthesis. In anticipation of this scenario, review authors may build contingencies into their protocol analysis plan that specify grouping (any or multiple) PICO elements at a broader level; thus potentially enabling synthesis of a larger number of studies. Broader groupings will generally address a less specific question, for example:

- 'the effect of *any antioxidant supplement* on …' instead of 'the effect of *vitamin C* on …';
- 'the effect of sexual health promotion on *biological outcomes*' instead of 'the effect of sexual health promotion on *sexually transmitted infections*'; or
- 'the effect of cognitive behavioural therapy in *children and adolescents* on …' instead of 'the effect of cognitive behavioural therapy in *children* on …'.

However, such broader questions may be useful for identifying important leads in areas that lack effective interventions and for guiding future research. Changes in the grouping may affect the assessment of the certainty of the evidence (see Chapter 14).

2.5.4 Economic data

Decision makers need to consider the economic aspects of an intervention, such as whether its adoption will lead to a more efficient use of resources. Economic data such as resource use, costs or cost-effectiveness (or a combination of these) may therefore be included as outcomes in a review. It is useful to break down measures of resource use and costs to the level of specific items or categories. It is helpful to consider an international perspective in the discussion of costs. Economics issues are discussed in detail in Chapter 20.

2.6 Chapter information

Authors: James Thomas, Dylan Kneale, Joanne E McKenzie, Sue E Brennan, Soumyadeep Bhaumik

Acknowledgements: This chapter builds on earlier versions of the *Handbook*. Mona Nasser, Dan Fox and Sally Crowe contributed to Section 2.4; Hilary J Thomson contributed to Section 2.5.1.

Funding: JT and DK are supported by the National Institute for Health Research (NIHR) Collaboration for Leadership in Applied Health Research and Care North Thames at Barts Health NHS Trust. JEM is supported by an Australian National Health and Medical Research Council (NHMRC) Career Development Fellowship (1143429). SEB's position is supported by the NHMRC Cochrane Collaboration Funding Program. The views expressed are those of the authors and not necessarily those of the NHS, the NIHR, the Department of Health or the NHMRC.

2.7 References

Anderson L, Petticrew M, Rehfuess E, Armstrong R, Ueffing E, Baker P, Francis D, Tugwell P. Using logic models to capture complexity in systematic reviews. *Research Synthesis Methods* 2011; **2**: 33–42.

Bailey JV, Murray E, Rait G, Mercer CH, Morris RW, Peacock R, Cassell J, Nazareth I. Interactive computer-based interventions for sexual health promotion. *Cochrane Database of Systematic Reviews* 2010; **9**: CD006483.

Baxter SK, Blank L, Woods HB, Payne N, Rimmer M, Goyder E. Using logic model methods in systematic review synthesis: describing complex pathways in referral management interventions. *BMC Medical Research Methodology* 2014; **14**: 62.

Bonell C, Jamal F, Melendez-Torres GJ, Cummins S. 'Dark logic': theorising the harmful consequences of public health interventions. *Journal of Epidemiology and Community Health* 2015; **69**: 95–98.

Bryant J, Sanson-Fisher R, Walsh J, Stewart J. Health research priority setting in selected high income countries: a narrative review of methods used and recommendations for future practice. *Cost Effectiveness and Resource Allocation* 2014; **12**: 23.

Caldwell DM, Welton NJ. Approaches for synthesising complex mental health interventions in meta-analysis. *Evidence-Based Mental Health* 2016; **19**: 16–21.

Cargo M, Harris J, Pantoja T, Booth A, Harden A, Hannes K, Thomas J, Flemming K, Garside R, Noyes J. Cochrane Qualitative and Implementation Methods Group guidance series-paper 4: methods for assessing evidence on intervention implementation. *Journal of Clinical Epidemiology* 2018; **97**: 59–69.

Chalmers I, Bracken MB, Djulbegovic B, Garattini S, Grant J, Gülmezoglu AM, Howells DW, Ioannidis JPA, Oliver S. How to increase value and reduce waste when research priorities are set. *Lancet* 2014; **383**: 156–165.

Chamberlain C, O'Mara-Eves A, Porter J, Coleman T, Perlen S, Thomas J, McKenzie J. Psychosocial interventions for supporting women to stop smoking in pregnancy. *Cochrane Database of Systematic Reviews* 2017; **2**: CD001055.

Cooper H. The problem formulation stage. In: Cooper H, editor. *Integrating Research: A Guide for Literature Reviews*. Newbury Park (CA) USA: Sage Publications; 1984.

Counsell C. Formulating questions and locating primary studies for inclusion in systematic reviews. *Annals of Internal Medicine* 1997; **127**: 380–387.

Cummings SR, Browner WS, Hulley SB. Conceiving the research question and developing the study plan. In: Hulley SB, Cummings SR, Browner WS, editors. *Designing Clinical Research: An Epidemiological Approach*. 4th ed. Philadelphia (PA): Lippincott Williams & Wilkins; 2007. p. 14–22.

Glass GV. Meta-analysis at middle age: a personal history. *Research Synthesis Methods* 2015; **6**: 221–231.

Hedges LV. Statistical considerations. In: Cooper H, Hedges LV, editors. *The Handbook of Research Synthesis*. New York (NY): USA: Russell Sage Foundation; 1994.

Hetrick SE, McKenzie JE, Cox GR, Simmons MB, Merry SN. Newer generation antidepressants for depressive disorders in children and adolescents. *Cochrane Database of Systematic Reviews* 2012; **11**: CD004851.

Hoffmann T, Glasziou P, Boutron I. Better reporting of interventions: template for intervention description and replication (TIDieR) checklist and guide. *BMJ* 2014; **348**: g1687.

Hollands GJ, Shemilt I, Marteau TM, Jebb SA, Lewis HB, Wei Y, Higgins JPT, Ogilvie D. Portion, package or tableware size for changing selection and consumption of food, alcohol and tobacco. *Cochrane Database of Systematic Reviews* 2015; **9**: CD011045.

Keown K, Van Eerd D, Irvin E. Stakeholder engagement opportunities in systematic reviews: Knowledge transfer for policy and practice. *Journal of Continuing Education in the Health Professions* 2008; **28**: 67–72.

Kneale D, Thomas J, Harris K. Developing and optimising the use of logic models in systematic reviews: exploring practice and good practice in the use of programme theory in reviews. *PloS One* 2015; **10**: e0142187.

Lewin S, Hendry M, Chandler J, Oxman AD, Michie S, Shepperd S, Reeves BC, Tugwell P, Hannes K, Rehfuess EA, Welch V, McKenzie JE, Burford B, Petkovic J, Anderson LM, Harris J, Noyes J. Assessing the complexity of interventions within systematic reviews: development, content and use of a new tool (iCAT_SR). *BMC Medical Research Methodology* 2017; **17**: 76.

Lorenc T, Petticrew M, Welch V, Tugwell P. What types of interventions generate inequalities? Evidence from systematic reviews. *Journal of Epidemiology and Community Health* 2013; **67**: 190–193.

Nasser M, Ueffing E, Welch V, Tugwell P. An equity lens can ensure an equity-oriented approach to agenda setting and priority setting of Cochrane Reviews. *Journal of Clinical Epidemiology* 2013; **66**: 511–521.

Nasser M. Setting priorities for conducting and updating systematic reviews [PhD Thesis]: University of Plymouth; 2018.

O'Neill J, Tabish H, Welch V, Petticrew M, Pottie K, Clarke M, Evans T, Pardo Pardo J, Waters E, White H, Tugwell P. Applying an equity lens to interventions: using PROGRESS ensures consideration of socially stratifying factors to illuminate inequities in health. *Journal of Clinical Epidemiology* 2014; **67**: 56–64.

Oliver S, Dickson K, Bangpan M, Newman M. Getting started with a review. In: Gough D, Oliver S, Thomas J, editors. *An Introduction to Systematic Reviews*. London (UK): Sage Publications Ltd.; 2017.

Petticrew M, Roberts H. *Systematic Reviews in the Social Sciences: A Practical Guide*. Oxford (UK): Blackwell; 2006.

Pfadenhauer L, Gerhardus A, Mozygemba K, Lysdahl KB, Booth A, Hofmann B, Wahlster P, Polus S, Burns J, Brereton L, Rehfuess E. Making sense of complexity in context and implementation: the Context and Implementation of Complex Interventions (CICI) framework. *Implementation Science* 2017; **12**: 21.

Rehfuess EA, Booth A, Brereton L, Burns J, Gerhardus A, Mozygemba K, Oortwijn W, Pfadenhauer LM, Tummers M, van der Wilt GJ, Rohwer A. Towards a taxonomy of logic models in systematic reviews and health technology assessments: a priori, staged, and iterative approaches. *Research Synthesis Methods* 2018; **9**: 13–24.

Richardson WS, Wilson MC, Nishikawa J, Hayward RS. The well-built clinical question: a key to evidence-based decisions. *ACP Journal Club* 1995; **123**: A12–13.

Rohwer A, Pfadenhauer L, Burns J, Brereton L, Gerhardus A, Booth A, Oortwijn W, Rehfuess E. Series: Clinical epidemiology in South Africa. Paper 3: Logic models help make sense of complexity in systematic reviews and health technology assessments. *Journal of Clinical Epidemiology* 2017; **83**: 37–47.

Sharma T, Choudhury M, Rejón-Parrilla JC, Jonsson P, Garner S. Using HTA and guideline development as a tool for research priority setting the NICE way: reducing research waste by identifying the right research to fund. *BMJ Open* 2018; **8**: e019777.

Squires J, Valentine J, Grimshaw J. Systematic reviews of complex interventions: framing the review question. *Journal of Clinical Epidemiology* 2013; **66**: 1215–1222.

Tong A, Chando S, Crowe S, Manns B, Winkelmayer WC, Hemmelgarn B, Craig JC. Research priority setting in kidney disease: a systematic review. *American Journal of Kidney Diseases* 2015; **65**: 674–683.

Tong A, Sautenet B, Chapman JR, Harper C, MacDonald P, Shackel N, Crowe S, Hanson C, Hill S, Synnot A, Craig JC. Research priority setting in organ transplantation: a systematic review. *Transplant International* 2017; **30**: 327–343.

Turley R, Saith R, Bhan N, Rehfuess E, Carter B. Slum upgrading strategies involving physical environment and infrastructure interventions and their effects on health and socio-economic outcomes. *Cochrane Database of Systematic Reviews* 2013; **1**: CD010067.

van der Heijden I, Abrahams N, Sinclair D. Psychosocial group interventions to improve psychological well-being in adults living with HIV. *Cochrane Database of Systematic Reviews* 2017; **3**: CD010806.

Viergever RF. *Health Research Prioritization at WHO: An Overview of Methodology and High Level Analysis of WHO Led Health Research Priority Setting Exercises*. Geneva (Switzerland): World Health Organization; 2010.

Viergever RF, Olifson S, Ghaffar A, Terry RF. A checklist for health research priority setting: nine common themes of good practice. *Health Research Policy and Systems* 2010; **8**: 36.

Whitehead M. The concepts and principles of equity and health. *International Journal of Health Services* 1992; **22**: 429–25.

3

Defining the criteria for including studies and how they will be grouped for the synthesis

Joanne E McKenzie, Sue E Brennan, Rebecca E Ryan, Hilary J Thomson, Renea V Johnston, James Thomas

KEY POINTS

- The scope of a review is defined by the types of population (participants), types of interventions (and comparisons), and the types of outcomes that are of interest. The acronym PICO (population, interventions, comparators and outcomes) helps to serve as a reminder of these.
- The population, intervention and comparison components of the question, with the additional specification of types of study that will be included, form the basis of the pre-specified eligibility criteria for the review. It is rare to use outcomes as eligibility criteria: studies should be included irrespective of whether they *report* outcome data, but may legitimately be excluded if they do not *measure* outcomes of interest, or if they explicitly aim to prevent a particular outcome.
- Cochrane Reviews should include all outcomes that are likely to be meaningful and not include trivial outcomes. Critical and important outcomes should be limited in number and include adverse as well as beneficial outcomes.
- Review authors should plan at the protocol stage how the different populations, interventions, outcomes and study designs within the scope of the review will be grouped for analysis.

3.1 Introduction

One of the features that distinguishes a systematic review from a narrative review is that systematic review authors should pre-specify criteria for including and excluding studies in the review (eligibility criteria, see MECIR Box 3.2.a).

When developing the protocol, one of the first steps is to determine the elements of the review question (including the population, intervention(s), comparator(s) and

This chapter should be cited as: McKenzie JE, Brennan SE, Ryan RE, Thomson HJ, Johnston RV, Thomas J. Chapter 3: Defining the criteria for including studies and how they will be grouped for the synthesis. In: Higgins JPT, Thomas J, Chandler J, Cumpston M, Li T, Page MJ, Welch VA (editors). *Cochrane Handbook for Systematic Reviews of Interventions*. 2nd Edition. Chichester (UK): John Wiley & Sons, 2019: 33–66.

outcomes, or PICO elements) and how the intervention, in the specified population, produces the expected outcomes (see Chapter 2, Section 2.5.1 and Chapter 17, Section 17.2.1). Eligibility criteria are based on the PICO elements of the review question plus a specification of the types of studies that have addressed these questions. The population, interventions and comparators in the review question usually translate directly into eligibility criteria for the review, though this is not always a straightforward process and requires a thoughtful approach, as this chapter shows. Outcomes usually are not part of the criteria for including studies, and a Cochrane Review would typically seek all sufficiently rigorous studies (most commonly randomized trials) of a particular comparison of interventions in a particular population of participants, irrespective of the outcomes measured or reported. It should be noted that some reviews do legitimately restrict eligibility to specific outcomes. For example, the same intervention may be studied in the same population for different purposes; or a review may specifically address the adverse effects of an intervention used for several conditions (see Chapter 19).

Eligibility criteria do not exist in isolation, but should be specified with the synthesis of the studies they describe in mind. This will involve making plans for how to group variants of the PICO elements for synthesis. This chapter describes the processes by which the structure of the synthesis can be mapped out at the beginning of the review, and the interplay between the review question, considerations for the analysis and their operationalization in terms of eligibility criteria. Decisions about which studies to include (and exclude), and how they will be combined in the review's synthesis, should be documented and justified in the review protocol.

A distinction between three different stages in the review at which the PICO construct might be used is helpful for understanding the decisions that need to be made. In Chapter 2 (Section 2.3) we introduced the ideas of a **review PICO** (on which eligibility of studies is based), the **PICO for each synthesis** (defining the question that each specific synthesis aims to answer) and the **PICO of the included studies** (what was actually investigated in the included studies). In this chapter, we focus on the **review PICO** and the **PICO for each synthesis** as a basis for specifying which studies should be included in the review and planning its syntheses. These PICOs should relate clearly and directly to the questions or hypotheses that are posed when the review is formulated (see Chapter 2) and will involve specifying the population in question, and a set of comparisons between the intervention groups.

An integral part of the process of setting up the review is to specify which characteristics of the interventions (e.g. individual compounds of a drug), populations (e.g. acute and chronic conditions), outcomes (e.g. different depression measurement scales) and study designs, will be grouped together. Such decisions should be made independent of knowing which studies will be included and the methods of synthesis that will be used (e.g. meta-analysis). There may be a need to modify the comparisons and even add new ones at the review stage in light of the data that are collected. For example, important variations in the intervention may be discovered only after data are collected, or modifying the comparison may facilitate the possibility of synthesis when only one or few studies meet the comparison PICO. Planning for the latter scenario at the protocol stage may lead to less post-hoc decision making (Chapter 2, Section 2.5.3) and, of course, any changes made during the conduct of the review should be recorded and documented in the final report.

3.2 Articulating the review and comparison PICO

3.2.1 Defining types of participants: which people and populations?

The criteria for considering types of people included in studies in a review should be sufficiently broad to encompass the likely diversity of studies and the likely scenarios in which the interventions will be used, but sufficiently narrow to ensure that a meaningful answer can be obtained when studies are considered together; they should be specified in advance (see MECIR Box 3.2.a). As discussed in Chapter 2 (Section 2.3.1), the degree of breadth will vary, depending on the question being asked and the analytical approach to be employed. A range of evidence may inform the choice of population characteristics to examine, including theoretical considerations, evidence from other interventions that have a similar mechanism of action, and in vitro or animal studies. Consideration should be given to whether the population characteristic is at the level of the participant (e.g. age, severity of disease) or the study (e.g. care setting, geographical

MECIR Box 3.2.a Relevant expectations for conduct of intervention reviews	
C5: Predefining unambiguous criteria for participants (**Mandatory**)	
Define in advance the eligibility criteria for participants in the studies.	Predefined, unambiguous eligibility criteria are a fundamental prerequisite for a systematic review. The criteria for considering types of people included in studies in a review should be sufficiently broad to encompass the likely diversity of studies, but sufficiently narrow to ensure that a meaningful answer can be obtained when studies are considered in aggregate. Considerations when specifying participants include setting, diagnosis or definition of condition and demographic factors. Any restrictions to study populations must be based on a sound rationale, since it is important that Cochrane Reviews are widely relevant.
C6: Predefining a strategy for studies with a subset of eligible participants (**Highly desirable**)	
Define in advance how studies that include only a subset of relevant participants will be addressed.	Sometimes a study includes some 'eligible' participants and some 'ineligible' participants, for example when an age cut-off is used in the review's eligibility criteria. If data from the eligible participants cannot be retrieved, a mechanism for dealing with this situation should be pre-specified.

location), since this has implications for grouping studies and for the method of synthesis (Chapter 10, Section 10.11.5). It is often helpful to consider the types of people that are of interest in three steps.

First, the **diseases or conditions of interest should be defined** using explicit criteria for establishing their presence (or absence). Criteria that will force the unnecessary exclusion of studies should be avoided. For example, diagnostic criteria that were developed more recently – which may be viewed as the current gold standard for diagnosing the condition of interest – will not have been used in earlier studies. Expensive or recent diagnostic tests may not be available in many countries or settings, and time-consuming tests may not be practical in routine healthcare settings.

Second, the **broad population and setting of interest should be defined**. This involves deciding whether a specific population group is within scope, determined by factors such as age, sex, race, educational status or the presence of a particular condition such as angina or shortness of breath. Interest may focus on a particular setting such as a community, hospital, nursing home, chronic care institution, or outpatient setting. Box 3.2.a outlines some factors to consider when developing population criteria.

Whichever criteria are used for defining the population and setting of interest, it is common to encounter studies that only partially overlap with the review's population. For example, in a review focusing on children, a cut-point of less than 16 years might be desirable, but studies may be identified with participants aged from 12 to 18. Unless the study reports separate data from the eligible section of the population (in which case data from the eligible participants can be included in the review), review authors will need a strategy for dealing with these studies (see MECIR Box 3.2.a). This will involve balancing concerns about reduced applicability by including participants who do not meet the eligibility criteria, against the loss of data when studies are excluded. Arbitrary rules (such as including a study if more than 80% of the participants are under 16) will not be practical if detailed information is not available from the study. A less stringent rule, such as 'the majority of participants are under 16' may be sufficient. Although there is a risk of review authors' biases affecting post-hoc inclusion decisions (which is why many authors endeavour to pre-specify these rules), this may be outweighed by a common-sense strategy in which eligibility decisions keep faith with the objectives of the review rather than with arbitrary rules. Difficult decisions should be documented in the review, checked with the advisory group (if available, see Chapter 1), and

Box 3.2.a Factors to consider when developing criteria for 'Types of participants'

- How is the disease/condition defined?
- What are the most important characteristics that describe these people (participants)?
- Are there any relevant demographic factors (e.g. age, sex, ethnicity)?
- What is the setting (e.g. hospital, community, etc)?
- Who should make the diagnosis?
- Are there other types of people who should be excluded from the review (because they are likely to react to the intervention in a different way)?
- How will studies involving only a subset of relevant participants be handled?

MECIR Box 3.2.b Relevant expectations for conduct of intervention reviews	
C13: Changing eligibility criteria (**Mandatory**)	
Justify any changes to eligibility criteria or outcomes studied. In particular, post-hoc decisions about inclusion or exclusion of studies should keep faith with the objectives of the review rather than with arbitrary rules.	Following pre-specified eligibility criteria is a fundamental attribute of a systematic review. However, unanticipated issues may arise. Review authors should make sensible post-hoc decisions about exclusion of studies, and these should be documented in the review, possibly accompanied by sensitivity analyses. Changes to the protocol must not be made on the basis of the findings of the studies or the synthesis, as this can introduce bias.

sensitivity analyses can assess the impact of these decisions on the review's findings (see Chapter 10, Section 10.14 and MECIR Box 3.2.b).

Third, there should be consideration of whether there are **population characteristics that might be expected to modify the size of the intervention effects** (e.g. different severities of heart failure). Identifying subpopulations may be important for implementation of the intervention. If relevant subpopulations are identified, two courses of action are possible: limiting the scope of the review to exclude certain subpopulations; or maintaining the breadth of the review and addressing subpopulations in the analysis.

Restricting the review with respect to specific population characteristics or settings should be based on a sound rationale. It is important that Cochrane Reviews are globally relevant, so the rationale for the exclusion of studies based on population characteristics should be justified. For example, focusing a review of the effectiveness of mammographic screening on women between 40 and 50 years old may be justified based on biological plausibility, previously published systematic reviews and existing controversy. On the other hand, focusing a review on a particular subgroup of people on the basis of their age, sex or ethnicity simply because of personal interests, when there is no underlying biologic or sociological justification for doing so, should be avoided, as these reviews will be less useful to decision makers and readers of the review.

Maintaining the breadth of the review may be best when it is uncertain whether there are important differences in effects among various subgroups of people, since this allows investigation of these differences (see Chapter 10, Section 10.11.5). Review authors may combine the results from different subpopulations in the same synthesis, examining whether a given subdivision explains variation (heterogeneity) among the intervention effects. Alternatively, the results may be synthesized in separate comparisons representing different subpopulations. Splitting by subpopulation risks there being too few studies to yield a useful synthesis (see Table 3.2.a and Chapter 2, Section 2.3.2). Consideration needs to be given to the subgroup analysis method,

Table 3.2.a Examples of population attributes and characteristics

Population attributes	Examples of population characteristics (and their subpopulations)	Examples of examination of population characteristics in Cochrane Reviews
Intended recipient of intervention	Patient, carer, healthcare provider (general practitioners, nurses, allied health professionals), health system, policy maker, community	In a review of e-learning programmes for health professionals, a subgroup analysis was planned to examine if the effects were modified by the *type of healthcare provider* (doctors, nurses or physiotherapists). The authors hypothesized that e-learning programmes for doctors would be more effective than for other health professionals, but did not provide a rationale (Vaona et al 2018).
Disease/condition (to be treated or prevented)	Type and severity of a condition	In a review of platelet-rich therapies for musculoskeletal soft tissue injuries, a subgroup analysis was undertaken to examine if the effects of platelet-rich therapies were modified by the *type of condition* (e.g. rotator cuff tear, anterior cruciate ligament reconstruction, chronic Achilles tendinopathy) (Moraes et al 2014). In planning a review of beta-blockers for heart failure, subgroup analyses were specified to examine if the effects of beta-blockers are modified by the *underlying cause of heart failure* (e.g. idiopathic dilated cardiomyopathy, ischaemic heart disease, valvular heart disease, hypertension) and the *severity of heart failure* ('reduced left ventricular ejection fraction (LVEF)' ≤ 40%, 'mid-range LVEF' > 40% and < 50%, 'preserved LVEF' ≥ 50%, mixed, not-specified). Studies have shown that patient characteristics and comorbidities differ by heart failure severity, and that therapies have been shown to reduce morbidity in 'reduced LVEF' patients, but the benefits in the other groups are uncertain (Safi et al 2017).
Participant characteristics	Age (neonate, child, adolescent, adult, older adult) Race/ethnicity Sex/gender PROGRESS-Plus equity characteristics (e.g. place of residence, socio-economic status, education) (O'Neill et al 2014)	In a review of newer-generation antidepressants for depressive disorders in children and adolescents, a subgroup analysis was undertaken to examine if the effects of the antidepressants were modified by *age*. The rationale was based on the findings of another review that suggested that children and adolescents may respond differently to antidepressants. The age groups were defined as 'children' (aged approximately 6 to 12 years), 'adolescents' (aged approximately 13 to 18 years), and 'children and adolescents' (when the study included both children and adolescents, and results could not be obtained separately by these subpopulations) (Hetrick et al 2012).
Setting	Setting of care (primary care, hospital, community) Rurality (urban, rural, remote) Socio-economic setting (low and middle-income countries, high-income countries) Hospital ward (e.g. intensive care unit, general medical ward, outpatient)	In a review of hip protectors for preventing hip fractures in older people, separate comparisons were specified based on *setting* (institutional care or community-dwelling) for the critical outcome of hip fracture (Santesso et al 2014).

particularly for population characteristics measured at the participant level (see Chapters 10 and 26, Fisher et al 2017). All subgroup analyses should ideally be planned a priori and stated as a secondary objective in the protocol, and not driven by the availability of data.

In practice, it may be difficult to assign included studies to defined subpopulations because of missing information about the population characteristic, variability in how the population characteristic is measured across studies (e.g. variation in the method used to define the severity of heart failure), or because the study does not wholly fall within (or report the results separately by) the defined subpopulation. The latter issue mainly applies for participant characteristics but can also arise for settings or geographic locations where these vary within studies. Review authors should consider planning for these scenarios (see example reviews Hetrick et al 2012, Safi et al 2017; Table 3.2.b, column 3).

3.2.2 Defining interventions and how they will be grouped

In some reviews, predefining the intervention (MECIR Box 3.2.c) may be straightforward. For example, in a review of the effect of a given anticoagulant on deep vein thrombosis, the intervention can be defined precisely. A more complicated definition might be required for a multi-component intervention composed of dietary advice, training and support groups to reduce rates of obesity in a given population.

The inherent complexity present when defining an intervention often comes to light when considering how it is thought to achieve its intended effect and whether the effect is likely to differ when variants of the intervention are used. In the first example, the anticoagulant warfarin is thought to reduce blood clots by blocking an enzyme that depends on vitamin K to generate clotting factors. In the second, the behavioural intervention is thought to increase individuals' self-efficacy in their ability to prepare healthy food. In both examples, we cannot assume that all forms of the intervention will work in the same way. When defining drug interventions, such as anticoagulants, factors such as the drug preparation, route of administration, dose, duration, and frequency should be considered. For multi-component interventions (such as interventions to reduce rates of obesity), the common or core features of the interventions must be defined, so that the review authors can clearly differentiate them from other interventions not included in the review.

In general, it is useful to consider **exactly what is delivered, who delivers it, how it is delivered, where it is delivered, when and how much is delivered, and whether the intervention can be adapted or tailored**, and to consider this for each type of intervention included in the review (see the TIDieR checklist (Hoffmann et al 2014)). As argued in Chapter 17, separating interventions into 'simple' and 'complex' is a false dichotomy; all interventions can be complex in some ways. The critical issue for review authors is to identify the most important factors to be considered in a specific review. Box 3.2.b outlines some factors to consider when developing broad criteria for the 'Types of interventions' (and comparisons).

Once interventions eligible for the review have been broadly defined, decisions should be made about how variants of the intervention will be handled in the synthesis. Differences in intervention characteristics across studies occur in all reviews. If these reflect minor differences in the form of the intervention used in practice (such as small differences in the duration or content of brief alcohol counselling interventions), then

Table 3.2.b A process for planning intervention groups for synthesis

Step	Considerations	Examples
1. Identify intervention characteristics that may modify the effect of the intervention.	Consider whether differences in interventions characteristics might modify the size of the intervention effect importantly. Content-specific research literature and expertise should inform this step. The TIDieR checklist – a tool for describing interventions – outlines the characteristics across which an intervention might differ (Hoffmann et al 2014). These include 'what' materials and procedures are used, 'who' provides the intervention, 'when and how much' intervention is delivered. The iCAT-SR tool provides equivalent guidance for complex interventions (Lewin et al 2017).	***Exercise interventions*** differ across multiple characteristics, which vary in importance depending on the review. In a review of exercise for osteoporosis, whether the exercise is weight-bearing or non-weight-bearing may be a key characteristic, since the mechanism by which exercise is thought to work is by placing stress or mechanical load on bones (Howe et al 2011). Different mechanisms apply in reviews of exercise for knee osteoarthritis (muscle strengthening), falls prevention (gait and balance), cognitive function (cardiovascular fitness). The differing mechanisms might suggest different ways of grouping interventions (e.g. by intensity, mode of delivery) according to potential modifiers of the intervention effects.
2a. Label and define intervention groups to be considered in the synthesis.	For each intervention group, provide a short label (e.g. supportive psychotherapy) and describe the core characteristics (criteria) that will be used to assign each intervention from an included study to a group. Groups are often defined by intervention content (especially the active components), such as materials, procedures or techniques (e.g. a specific drug, an information leaflet, a behaviour change technique). Other characteristics may also be used, although some are more commonly used to define subgroups (see Chapter 10, Section 10.11.5): the purpose or theoretical underpinning, mode of delivery, provider, dose or intensity, duration or timing of the intervention (Hoffmann et al 2014). In specifying groups: • focus on 'clinically' meaningful groups that will inform selection and implementation of an intervention in practice;	In a review of psychological therapies for coronary heart disease, a single group was specified for meta-analysis that included all types of therapy. Subgroups were defined to examine whether intervention effects were modified by intervention components (e.g. cognitive techniques, stress management) or mode of delivery (e.g. individual, group) (Richards et al 2017). In a review of psychological therapies for panic disorder (Pompoli et al 2016), eight types of therapy were specified: 1) psychoeducation; 2) supportive psychotherapy (with or without a psychoeducational component); 3) physiological therapies; 4) behaviour therapy; 5) cognitive therapy; 6) cognitive behaviour therapy (CBT); 7) 7. third-wave CBT; and

	• consider whether a system exists for defining interventions (see Step 3); • for hard-to-describe groups, provide brief examples of interventions in each group; and • pilot the criteria to ensure that groups are sufficiently distinct to enable categorization, but not so narrow that interventions are split into many groups, making synthesis impossible (see also Step 4). Logic models may help structure the synthesis (see Chapter 2, Section 2.4.1 and Chapter 17, Section 17.2.1).	8) psychodynamic therapies. Groups were defined by the theoretical basis of each therapy (e.g. CBT aims to modify maladaptive thoughts through cognitive restructuring) and the component techniques used.
2b. Define levels for groups based on dose or intensity.	For groups based on 'how much' of an intervention is used (e.g. dose or intensity), criteria are needed to quantify each group. This may be straightforward for easy-to-quantify characteristics, but more complex for characteristics that are hard to quantify (e.g. duration or intensity of rehabilitation or psychological therapy). The levels should be based on how the intervention is used in practice (e.g. cut-offs for low and high doses of a supplement based on recommended nutrient intake), or on a rationale for how the intervention might work.	In reviews of exercise, intensity may be defined by training time (session length, frequency, program duration), amount of work (e.g. repetitions), and effort/energy expenditure (exertion, heart rate) (Regnaux et al 2015). In a review of organized inpatient care for stroke, acute stroke units were categorized as 'intensive', 'semi-intensive' or 'non-intensive' based on whether the unit had continuous monitoring, high nurse staffing, and life support facilities (Stroke Unit Trialists Collaboration 2013).
3. Determine whether there is an existing system for grouping interventions. *Consider this step with step 2a.*	In some fields, intervention taxonomies and frameworks have been developed for labelling and describing interventions, and these can make it easier for those using a review to interpret and apply findings. Using an agreed system is preferable to developing new groupings. Existing systems should be assessed for relevance and usefulness. The most useful systems:	***Generic systems*** The *behaviour change technique* (BCT) *taxonomy* (Michie et al 2013) categorizes intervention elements such as goal setting, self-monitoring and social support. A protocol for a review of social media interventions used this taxonomy to describe interventions and examine different BCTs as potential effect modifiers (Welch et al 2018).

(*Continued*)

Table 3.2.b (Continued)

Step	Considerations	Examples
	• use terminology that is understood by those using or implementing the intervention; • are developed systematically and based on consensus, preferably with stakeholders including clinicians, patients, policy makers, and researchers; and • have been validated through successful use in a range of applications (ideally, including in systematic reviews). Systems for grouping interventions may be generic, widely applicable across clinical areas, or specific to a condition or intervention type. Some Cochrane Groups recommend specific taxonomies.	The *behaviour change wheel* has been used to group interventions (or components) by function (e.g. to educate, persuade, enable) (Michie et al 2011). This system was used to describe the components of dietary advice interventions (Desroches et al 2013). ***Specific systems*** Multiple reviews have used the consensus-based taxonomy developed by the Prevention of Falls Network Europe (ProFaNE) (e.g. Verheyden et al 2013, Kendrick et al 2014). The taxonomy specifies broad groups (e.g. exercise, medication, environment/assistive technology) within which are more specific groups (e.g. exercise: gait, balance and functional training; flexibility; strength and resistance) (Lamb et al 2011).
4. Plan how the specified groups will be used in synthesis and reporting.	Decide whether it is useful to pool all interventions in a single meta-analysis ('lumping'), within which specific characteristics can be explored as effect modifiers (e.g. in subgroups). Alternatively, if pooling all interventions is unlikely to address a useful question, separate synthesis of specific interventions may be more appropriate ('splitting'). Determining the right analytic approach is discussed further in Chapter 2, Section 2.3.2.	In a review of exercise for knee osteoarthritis, the different categories of exercise were combined in a single meta-analysis, addressing the question 'what is the effect of exercise on knee osteoarthritis?'. The categories were also analysed as subgroups within the meta-analysis to explore whether the effect size varied by type of exercise (Fransen et al 2015). Other subgroup analyses examined mode of delivery and dose.
5. Decide how to group interventions with multiple components or co-interventions.	Some interventions, especially those considered 'complex', include multiple components that could also be implemented independently (Guise et al 2014, Lewin et al 2017). These components might be eligible for inclusion in the review alone, or eligible only if used alongside an eligible intervention. Options for considering multi-component interventions may include the following. • Identifying intervention components for meta-regression or a components-based network meta-analysis (see Chapter 11 and Welton et al 2009, Caldwell and Welton 2016, Higgins et al 2019).	**Grouping by main component:** In a review of psychological therapies for panic disorder, two of the eight eligible therapies (psychoeducation and supportive psychotherapy) could be used alone or as part of a multi-component therapy. When accompanied by another eligible therapy, the intervention was categorized as the other therapy (i.e. psychoeducation + cognitive behavioural therapy was categorized as cognitive behavioural therapy) (Pompoli et al 2016). **Separate group:** In a review of psychosocial interventions for smoking cessation in pregnancy, two approaches were used. All intervention types were included in a single meta-analysis

	• Grouping based on the 'main' intervention component (Caldwell and Welton 2016). • Specifying a separate group ('multi-component interventions'). 'Lumping' multi-component interventions together may provide information about their effects in general; however, this approach may lead to unexplained heterogeneity and/or inability to identify which components are effective (Caldwell and Welton 2016). • Reporting results study by study. An option if components are expected to be so diverse that synthesis will not be interpretable. • Excluding multi-component interventions. An option if the effect of the intervention of interest cannot be discerned. This approach may reduce the relevance of the review. The first two approaches may be challenging but are likely to be most useful (Caldwell and Welton 2016). See Section 3.2.3.1. for the special case of when a co-intervention is administered in both treatment arms.	with subgroups for multi-component, single and tailored interventions. Separate meta-analyses were also performed for each intervention type, with categorization of multi-component interventions based on the 'main' component (Chamberlain et al 2017).
6. Build in contingencies by specifying both specific and broader intervention groups.	Consider grouping interventions at more than one level, so that studies of a broader group of interventions can be synthesized if too few studies are identified for synthesis in more specific groups. This will provide flexibility where review authors anticipate few studies contributing to specific groups (e.g. in reviews with diverse interventions, additional diversity in other PICO elements, or few studies overall, see also Chapter 2, Section 2.5.3.	In a review of psychosocial interventions for smoking cessation, the authors planned to group any psychosocial intervention in a single comparison (addressing the higher level question of whether, on average, psychosocial interventions are effective). Given that sufficient data were available, they also presented separate meta-analyses to examine the effects of specific types of psychosocial interventions (e.g. counselling, health education, incentives, social support) (Chamberlain et al 2017).

MECIR Box 3.2.c Relevant expectations for conduct of intervention reviews	
C7: Predefining unambiguous criteria for interventions and comparators (**Mandatory**)	
Define in advance the eligible interventions and the interventions against which these can be compared in the included studies.	Predefined, unambiguous eligibility criteria are a fundamental prerequisite for a systematic review. Specification of comparator interventions requires particular clarity: are the experimental interventions to be compared with an inactive control intervention (e.g. placebo, no treatment, standard care, or a waiting list control), or with an active control intervention (e.g. a different variant of the same intervention, a different drug, a different kind of therapy)? Any restrictions on interventions and comparators, for example, regarding delivery, dose, duration, intensity, co-interventions and features of complex interventions should also be predefined and explained.

Box 3.2.b Factors to consider when developing criteria for 'Types of interventions'

- What are the experimental and control (comparator) interventions of interest?
- Does the intervention have variations (e.g. dosage/intensity, mode of delivery, personnel who deliver it, frequency, duration or timing of delivery)?
- Are all variations to be included (for example, is there a dose below which the intervention may not be clinically appropriate, will all providers be included)?
- Will studies including only part of the intervention be included?
- Will studies including the intervention of interest combined with another intervention (co-intervention) be included?
- Have the different meanings of phrases such as 'control', 'placebo', 'no intervention' or 'usual care' been considered?

an overall synthesis can provide useful information for decision makers. Where differences in intervention characteristics are more substantial (such as delivery of brief alcohol counselling by nurses versus doctors), and are expected to have a substantial impact on the size of intervention effects, these differences should be examined in the synthesis. What constitutes an important difference requires judgement, but in general differences that alter decisions about how an intervention is implemented or whether the intervention is used or not are likely to be important. In such circumstances, review authors should consider specifying separate groups (or subgroups) to examine in their synthesis.

Clearly defined intervention groups serve two main purposes in the synthesis. First, the way in which interventions are grouped for synthesis (meta-analysis or other synthesis) is likely to influence review findings. Careful planning of intervention groups makes best use of the available data, avoids decisions that are influenced by study findings (which may introduce bias), and produces a review focused on questions relevant to decision makers. Second, the intervention groups specified in a protocol provide a standardized terminology for describing the interventions throughout the review, overcoming the varied descriptions used by study authors (e.g. where different labels are used for the same intervention, or similar labels used for different techniques) (Michie et al 2013). This standardization enables comparison and synthesis of information about intervention characteristics across studies (common characteristics and differences) and provides a consistent language for reporting that supports interpretation of review findings.

Table 3.2.b outlines a process for planning intervention groups as a basis for/precursor to synthesis, and the decision points and considerations at each step. The table is intended to guide, rather than to be prescriptive and, although it is presented as a sequence of steps, the process is likely to be iterative, and some steps may be done concurrently or in a different sequence. The process aims to minimize data-driven approaches that can arise once review authors have knowledge of the findings of the included studies. It also includes principles for developing a flexible plan that maximizes the potential to synthesize in circumstances where there are few studies, many variants of an intervention, or where the variants are difficult to anticipate. In all stages, review authors should consider how to categorize studies whose reports contain insufficient detail.

3.2.3 Defining which comparisons will be made

When articulating the PICO for each synthesis, defining the intervention groups alone is not sufficient for complete specification of the planned syntheses. The next step is to define the comparisons that will be made between the intervention groups. Setting aside for a moment more complex analyses such as network meta-analyses, which can simultaneously compare many groups (Chapter 11), standard meta-analysis (Chapter 10) aims to draw conclusions about the comparative effects of two groups at a time (i.e. which of two intervention groups is more effective?). These comparisons form the basis for the syntheses that will be undertaken if data are available. Cochrane Reviews sometimes include one comparison, but most often include multiple comparisons. Three commonly identified types of comparisons include the following (Davey et al 2011).

- Intervention versus placebo (e.g. placebo drug, sham surgical procedure, psychological placebo). Placebos are most commonly used in the evaluation of pharmacological interventions, but may be also be used in some non-pharmacological evaluations. For example:
  - newer generation antidepressants versus placebo (Hetrick et al 2012); and
  - vertebroplasty for osteoporotic vertebral compression fractures versus placebo (sham procedure) (Buchbinder et al 2018).
- Intervention versus control (e.g. no intervention, wait-list control, usual care). Both intervention arms may also receive standard therapy. For example:

  - chemotherapy or targeted therapy plus best supportive care (BSC) versus BSC for palliative treatment of esophageal and gastroesophageal-junction carcinoma (Janmaat et al 2017); and
  - personalized care planning versus usual care for people with long-term conditions (Coulter et al 2015).
- Intervention A versus intervention B. A comparison of active interventions may include comparison of the same intervention delivered at different time points, for different lengths of time or different doses, or two different interventions. For example:
  - early (commenced at less than two weeks of age) versus late (two weeks of age or more) parenteral zinc supplementation in term and preterm infants (Taylor et al 2017);
  - high intensity versus low intensity physical activity or exercise in people with hip or knee osteoarthritis (Regnaux et al 2015);
  - multimedia education versus other education for consumers about prescribed and over the counter medications (Ciciriello et al 2013).

The first two types of comparisons aim to establish the effectiveness of an intervention, while the last aims to compare the effectiveness of two interventions. However, the distinction between the placebo and control is often arbitrary, since any differences in the care provided between trials with a control arm and those with a placebo arm may be unimportant, especially where 'usual care' is provided to both. Therefore, placebo and control groups may be determined to be similar enough to be combined for synthesis.

In reviews including multiple intervention groups, many comparisons are possible. In some of these reviews, authors seek to synthesize evidence on the comparative effectiveness of all their included interventions, including where there may be only indirect comparison of some interventions across the included studies (Chapter 11, Section 11.2.1). However, in many reviews including multiple intervention groups, a limited subset of the possible comparisons will be selected. The chosen subset of comparisons should address the most important clinical and research questions. For example, if an established intervention (or dose of an intervention) is used in practice, then the synthesis would ideally compare novel or alternative interventions to this established intervention, and not, for example, to no intervention.

3.2.3.1 Dealing with co-interventions

Planning is needed for the special case where the *same* supplementary intervention is delivered to both the intervention and comparator groups. A supplementary intervention is an additional intervention delivered alongside the intervention of interest, such as massage in a review examining the effects of aromatherapy (i.e. aromatherapy plus massage versus massage alone). In many cases, the supplementary intervention will be unimportant and can be ignored. In other situations, the effect of the intervention of interest may differ according to whether participants receive the supplementary therapy. For example, the effect of aromatherapy among people who receive a massage may differ from the effect of the aromatherapy given alone. This will be the case if the intervention of interest interacts with the supplementary intervention leading to larger (synergistic) or smaller (dysynergistic/antagonistic) effects than the intervention of interest alone (Squires et al 2013). While qualitative interactions are rare (where the effect of the intervention is in the opposite direction when combined with the supplementary intervention), it is possible that there will be more variation in the intervention effects (heterogeneity) when supplementary interventions are involved, and it is important to plan for this. Approaches for dealing with this in the statistical synthesis may include fitting a random-effects meta-analysis model that encompasses heterogeneity (Chapter 10, Section 10.10.4), or investigating whether the intervention effect is modified by the addition of the supplementary intervention through subgroup analysis (Chapter 10, Section 10.11.2).

3.2.4 Selecting, prioritizing and grouping review outcomes

3.2.4.1 Selecting review outcomes

Broad outcome domains are decided at the time of setting up the review PICO (see Chapter 2). Once the broad domains are agreed, further specification is required to define the domains to facilitate reporting and synthesis (i.e. the PICO for each synthesis) (see Chapter 2, Section 2.3). The process for specifying and grouping outcomes largely parallels that used for specifying intervention groups.

Reporting of outcomes should rarely determine study eligibility for a review. In particular, studies should not be excluded because they do not report results of an outcome they may have measured, or provide 'no usable data' (MECIR Box 3.2.d). This is essential to avoid bias arising from selective reporting of findings by the study authors (see Chapter 13). However, in some circumstances, the measurement of certain outcomes may be a study eligibility criterion. This may be the case, for example, when the review addresses the

MECIR Box 3.2.d Relevant expectations for conduct of intervention reviews	
C8: Clarifying role of outcomes (**Mandatory**)	
Clarify in advance whether outcomes listed under 'Criteria for considering studies for this review' are used as criteria for including studies (rather than as a list of the outcomes of interest within whichever studies are included).	Outcome measures should not always form part of the criteria for including studies in a review. However, some reviews do legitimately restrict eligibility to specific outcomes. For example, the same intervention may be studied in the same population for different purposes (e.g. hormone replacement therapy, or aspirin); or a review may address specifically the adverse effects of an intervention used for several conditions. If authors do exclude studies on the basis of outcomes, care should be taken to ascertain that relevant outcomes are not available because they have not been measured rather than simply not reported.

C14: Predefining outcome domains (**Mandatory**)	
Define in advance outcomes that are critical to the review, and any additional important outcomes.	Full specification of the outcomes includes consideration of outcome domains (e.g. quality of life) and outcome measures (e.g. SF-36). Predefinition of outcome reduces the risk of selective outcome reporting. The *critical outcomes* should be as few as possible and should normally reflect at least one potential benefit and at least one potential area of harm. It is expected that the review should be able to synthesize these outcomes if eligible studies are identified, and that the conclusions of the review will be based largely on the effects of the interventions on these outcomes. Additional important outcomes may also be specified. Up to seven critical and important outcomes will form the basis of the GRADE assessment and summarized in the review's abstract and other summary formats, although the review may measure more than seven outcomes.
C15: Choosing outcomes (**Mandatory**)	
Choose only outcomes that are critical or important to users of the review such as healthcare consumers, health professionals and policy makers.	Cochrane Reviews are intended to support clinical practice and policy, and should address outcomes that are critical or important to consumers. These should be specified at protocol stage. Where available, established sets of core outcomes should be used. Patient-reported outcomes should be included where possible. It is also important to judge whether evidence of resource use and costs might be an important component of decisions to adopt the intervention or alternative management strategies around the world. Large numbers of outcomes, while sometimes necessary, can make reviews unfocused, unmanageable for the user, and prone to selective outcome reporting bias.

	Biochemical, interim and process outcomes should be considered where they are important to decision makers. Any outcomes that would not be described as critical or important can be left out of the review.
C16: Predefining outcome measures (**Highly desirable**)	
Define in advance details of what will constitute acceptable outcome measures (e.g. diagnostic criteria, scales, composite outcomes).	Having decided what outcomes are of interest to the review, authors should clarify acceptable ways in which these outcomes can be measured. It may be difficult, however, to predefine adverse effects.

potential for an intervention to *prevent* a particular outcome, or when the review addresses a specific purpose of an intervention that can be used in the same population for different purposes (such as hormone replacement therapy, or aspirin).

In general, systematic reviews should aim to **include outcomes that are likely to be meaningful to the intended users and recipients of the reviewed evidence.** This may include clinicians, patients (consumers), the general public, administrators and policy makers. Outcomes may include survival (mortality), clinical events (e.g. strokes or myocardial infarction), behavioural outcomes (e.g. changes in diet, use of services), patient-reported outcomes (e.g. symptoms, quality of life), adverse events, burdens (e.g. demands on caregivers, frequency of tests, restrictions on lifestyle) and economic outcomes (e.g. cost and resource use). It is critical that outcomes used to assess adverse effects as well as outcomes used to assess beneficial effects are among those addressed by a review (see Chapter 19).

Outcomes that are trivial or meaningless to decision makers should not be included in Cochrane Reviews. Inclusion of outcomes that are of little or no importance risks overwhelming and potentially misleading readers. Interim or surrogate outcomes measures, such as laboratory results or radiologic results (e.g. loss of bone mineral content as a surrogate for fractures in hormone replacement therapy), while potentially helpful in explaining effects or determining intervention integrity (see Chapter 5, Section 5.3.4.1), can also be misleading since they may not predict clinically important outcomes accurately. Many interventions reduce the risk for a surrogate outcome but have no effect or have harmful effects on clinically relevant outcomes, and some interventions have no effect on surrogate measures but improve clinical outcomes.

Various sources can be used to develop a list of relevant outcomes, including input from consumers and advisory groups (see Chapter 2), the clinical experiences of the review authors, and evidence from the literature (including qualitative research about outcomes important to those affected (see Chapter 21)). A further driver of outcome selection is consideration of outcomes used in related reviews. Harmonization of outcomes across reviews addressing related questions facilitates broader evidence synthesis questions being addressed through the use of Overviews of reviews (see online Chapter V).

Outcomes considered to be meaningful, and therefore addressed in a review, may not have been reported in the primary studies. For example, quality of life is an important outcome, perhaps the most important outcome, for people considering whether or not to use chemotherapy for advanced cancer, even if the available studies are found to report only survival (see Chapter 18). A further example arises with timing of the outcome measurement, where time points determined as clinically meaningful in a review are not measured in the primary studies. Including and discussing all important outcomes in a review will highlight gaps in the primary research and encourage researchers to address these gaps in future studies.

3.2.4.2 Prioritizing review outcomes

Once a full list of relevant outcomes has been compiled for the review, authors should prioritize the outcomes and select the outcomes of most relevance to the review question. The GRADE approach to assessing the certainty of evidence (see Chapter 14) suggests that review authors separate outcomes into those that are 'critical', 'important' and 'not important' for decision making.

The critical outcomes are the essential outcomes for decision making, and are those that would form the basis of a 'Summary of findings' table or other summary versions of the review, such as the Abstract or Plain Language Summary. 'Summary of findings' tables provide key information about the amount of evidence for important comparisons and outcomes, the quality of the evidence and the magnitude of effect (see Chapter 14, Section 14.1). There should be no more than seven outcomes included in a 'Summary of findings' table, and those outcomes that will be included in summaries should be specified at the protocol stage. They should generally not include surrogate or interim outcomes. They should not be chosen on the basis of any anticipated or observed magnitude of effect, or because they are likely to have been addressed in the studies to be reviewed. Box 3.2.c summarizes the principal factors to consider when selecting and prioritizing review outcomes.

Box 3.2.c Factors to consider when selecting and prioritizing review outcomes

- Consider outcomes relevant to all potential decision makers.
- Critical outcomes are those that are essential for decision making, and should usually have an emphasis on patient-important outcomes and be determined by core outcomes sets.
- Additional outcomes important to decision makers may also be included in the review. Any outcomes not considered important to decision makers should be excluded from the review.
- Up to seven critical and important outcomes should be selected for inclusion in summary versions of the review, including 'Summary of findings' tables, Abstracts and Plain Language Summaries. Remember that summaries may be read alone, and should include the most important outcomes for decision makers.
- Ensure that outcomes cover potential as well as actual adverse effects.

3.2.4.3 Defining and grouping outcomes for synthesis

Table 3.2.c outlines a process for planning for the diversity in outcome measurement that may be encountered in the studies included in a review and which can complicate, and sometimes prevent, synthesis. Research has repeatedly documented inconsistency in the outcomes measured across trials in the same clinical areas (Harrison et al 2016, Williamson et al 2017). This inconsistency occurs across all aspects of outcome measurement, including the broad domains considered, the outcomes measured, the way these outcomes are labelled and defined, and the methods and timing of measurement. For example, a review of outcome measures used in 563 studies of interventions for dementia and mild cognitive impairment found that 321 unique measurement methods were used for 1278 assessments of cognitive outcomes (Harrison et al 2016). Initiatives like COMET (Core Outcome Measures in Effectiveness Trials) aim to encourage standardization of outcome measurement across trials (Williamson et al 2017), but these initiatives are comparatively new and review authors will inevitably encounter diversity in outcomes across studies.

The process begins by describing the scope of each outcome domain in sufficient detail to enable outcomes from included studies to be categorized (Table 3.2.c Step 1). This step may be straightforward in areas for which core outcome sets (or equivalent systems) exist (Table 3.2.c Step 2). The methods and timing of outcome measurement also need to be specified, giving consideration to how differences across studies will be handled (Table 3.2.c Steps 3 and 4). Subsequent steps consider options for dealing with studies that report multiple measures within an outcome domain (Table 3.2.c Step 5), planning how outcome domains will be used in synthesis (Table 3.2.c Step 6), and building in contingencies to maximize potential to synthesize (Table 3.2.c Step 7).

3.3 Determining which study designs to include

Some study designs are more appropriate than others for answering particular questions. Authors need to consider a priori what study designs are likely to provide reliable data with which to address the objectives of their review (MECIR Box 3.3.a). Sections 3.3.1 and 3.3.2 cover randomized and non-randomized designs for assessing treatment effects; Chapter 17 (Section 17.2.5) discusses other study designs in the context of addressing intervention complexity.

3.3.1 Including randomized trials

Because Cochrane Reviews address questions about the effects of health care, they focus primarily on randomized trials and randomized trials should be included if they are feasible for the interventions of interest (MECIR Box 3.3.b). Randomization is the only way to prevent systematic differences between baseline characteristics of participants in different intervention groups in terms of both known and unknown (or unmeasured) confounders (see Chapter 8), and claims about cause and effect can be based on their findings with far more confidence than almost any other type of study. For clinical interventions, deciding who receives an intervention and who does not is influenced by many factors, including prognostic factors. Empirical evidence

Table 3.2.c A process for planning outcome groups for synthesis

Step	Considerations	Examples
1. Fully specify outcome domains.	For each outcome domain, provide a short label (e.g. cognition, consumer evaluation of care) and describe the domain in sufficient detail to enable eligible outcomes from each included study to be categorized. The definition should be based on the concept (or construct) measured, that is 'what' is measured. 'When' and 'how' the outcome is measured will be considered in subsequent steps. Outcomes can be defined hierarchically, starting with very broad groups (e.g. physiological/clinical outcomes, life impact, adverse events), then outcome domains (e.g. functioning and perceived health status are domains within 'life impact'). Within these may be narrower domains (e.g. physical function, cognitive function), and then specific outcome measures (Dodd et al 2018). The level at which outcomes are grouped for synthesis alters the question addressed, and so decisions should be guided by the review objectives. In specifying outcome domains: • definitions should reflect existing systems if available, or relevant literature and terminology understood by decision makers; • where outcomes are likely to be inconsistently labelled and described, listing examples may convey the scope of the domain; • consider the level at which domains will be defined (broad versus narrow) and the implications for reporting and synthesis: combining diverse outcomes may lead to unexplained heterogeneity whereas narrowly specified outcomes may prevent synthesis when few studies report specific measures;	In a review of computer-based interventions for sexual health promotion, three broad outcome domains were defined (cognitions, behaviours, biological) based on a conceptual model of how the intervention might work. Each domain comprised more specific domains and outcomes (e.g. condom use, seeking health services such as STI testing); listing these helped define the broad domains and guided categorization of the diverse outcomes reported in included studies (Bailey et al 2010). In a protocol for a review of social media interventions for improving health, the rationale for synthesizing broad groupings of outcomes (e.g. health behaviours, physical health) was based on prediction of a common underlying mechanism by which the intervention would work, and the review objective, which focused on overall health rather than specific outcomes (Welch et al 2018).

	• a causal path or logic model may help identify logical groupings of related outcomes for reporting and analysis, and alternative levels at which to synthesize.	
2. Determine whether there is an existing system for identifying and grouping important outcomes.	Systems for categorizing outcomes include core outcome sets including the COMET and ICHOM initiatives, and outcome taxonomies (Dodd et al 2018). These systems define agreed outcomes that should be measured for specific conditions (Williamson et al 2017).These systems can be used to standardize the varied outcome labels used across studies and enable grouping and comparison (Kirkham et al 2013). Agreed terminology may help decision makers interpret review findings. The COMET website provides a database of core outcome sets agreed or in development. Some Cochrane Groups have developed their own outcome sets. While the availability of outcome sets and taxonomies varies across clinical areas, several taxonomies exist for specifying broad outcome domains (e.g. Dodd et al 2018, ICHOM 2018).	In a review of combined diet and exercise for preventing gestational diabetes mellitus, a core outcome set agreed by the Cochrane Pregnancy and Childbirth group was used (Shepherd et al 2017). In a review of decision aids for people facing health treatment or screening decisions (Stacey et al 2017), outcome domains were based on criteria for evaluating decision aids agreed in the International Patient Decision Aids Standards (IPDAS). Doing so helped to assess the use of aids across diverse clinical decisions. The Cochrane Consumers and Communication Group has an agreed taxonomy to guide specification of outcomes of importance in evaluating communication interventions (Cochrane Consumers & Communication Group).
3. Define the outcome time points.	A key attribute of defining an outcome is specifying the time of measurement. In reviews, time frames, and not specific time points, are often specified to handle the likely diversity in timing of outcome measurement across studies (e.g. a 'medium-term' time frame might be defined as including outcomes measured between 6 and 12 months). In specifying outcome timing: • focus on 'clinically meaningful' time points (e.g. considering the course of the condition over time and duration of the intervention may determine whether	In a review of psychological therapies for panic disorder, the main outcomes were 'short-term' (≤ 6 months from treatment commencement). 'Long-term' outcomes (> 6 months from treatment commencement) were considered important, but not specified as critical because of concerns of participant attrition (Pompoli et al 2018). In contrast, in a review of antidepressants, a clinically meaningful time frame of 6 to 12 months might be specified for the critical outcome 'depression', since this is the recommended treatment duration. However, it may be anticipated that many studies will be of shorter

(*Continued*)

Table 3.2.c (Continued)

Step	Considerations	Examples
	short-term or long-term outcomes are important); • consider whether there are agreed or accepted outcome time points (e.g. standards in a clinical area such as an NIH task force suggestion for at least 6 to 12 months follow-up for chronic low back pain (Deyo et al 2014), or core outcome sets (Williamson et al 2017); • consider carefully the width of the time frame (e.g. what constitutes 'short term' for this review?). Narrow time frames may lead to few studies in the synthesis. Broad time frames may lead to multiplicity (see Step 5) and difficulties with interpretation if the timing is very diverse across studies.	duration with short-term follow-up, so an additional important outcome of 'depression (< 3 months)' might also be specified.
4. Specify the measurement tool or measurement method.	For each outcome domain, specify: • measurement methods or tools that provide an appropriate assessment of the domain or specific outcome (e.g. including clinical assessment, laboratory tests, objective measures, and patient-reported outcome measures (PROMs)); • whether different methods or tools are comparable measures of a domain, which has implications for synthesis (Step 6). Minimum criteria for inclusion of a measure may include: • adequate evidence of *reliability* (e.g. consistent scores across time and raters when the outcome is unchanged), and *validity* (e.g. comparable results to similar measures, including a gold standard if available); and	In a review of interventions to support women to stop smoking, objective (biochemically validated) and subjective (self-report) measures of smoking cessation were specified separately to examine bias due to the method used to measure the outcome (Step 6) (Chamberlain et al 2017). In a review of high-intensity versus low-intensity exercise for osteoarthritis, measures of pain were selected based on relevance of the content and properties of the measurement tool (i.e. evidence of validity and reliability) (Regnaux et al 2015).

<table>
<tr><td></td><td>• for self-reported measures, items that cover the outcome/domain and are developed using theory, empirical evidence and consumer involvement.

Measures may be identified from core outcome sets (e.g. Williamson et al 2017, ICHOM 2018) or systematic reviews of instruments (see COnsensus-based Standards for the selection of health Measurement INstruments (COSMIN) initiative for a database of examples).</td><td></td></tr>
<tr><td>5. Specify how multiplicity of outcomes will be handled.</td><td>For a particular domain, multiple outcomes within a study may be available for inclusion. This may arise from:

• multiple outcomes measured within a domain (e.g. ‘anxiety’ and ‘depression’ in a ‘mental health’ domain);
• multiple methods to measure the outcome (e.g. self-reported depression, clinician-rated depression), or tools/instruments (e.g. Hamilton Depression Rating Scale, Beck Depression Inventory), as well as their subscales;
• multiple time points measured within a time frame.

Effects of the intervention calculated from these different sources of multiplicity are statistically dependent, since they have been calculated using the same participants. To deal with this dependency, select only one outcome per study for a particular comparison, or use a meta-analysis method that accounts for the dependency (see Step 6).

Pre-specify the method of selection from multiple outcomes or measures in the protocol, using an approach that is independent of the result (see Chapter 9, Table 9.3.c) (López-López et al 2018). Document all eligible outcomes or measures in the ‘Characteristics of included studies’ table, noting which was selected and why.</td><td>The following hierarchy was specified to select one outcome per domain in a review examining the effects of portion, package or tableware size (Hollands et al 2015):

• the study’s primary outcome;
• the outcome that was most proximal to the health outcome in the context of the specific intervention;
• the outcome that provided the largest-scale measure of the domain (e.g. total amount of food consumed selected ahead of amount of vegetables consumed).

Selection of the outcome was made blinded to the results. All available outcome measures were documented in the ‘Characteristics of included studies’ table.

In a review of audit and feedback for healthcare providers, the outcome domains were ‘provider performance’ (e.g. compliance with recommended use of a laboratory test) and ‘patient health outcomes’ (e.g. smoking status, blood pressure) (Ivers et al 2012). For each domain, outcomes were selected using the following hierarchy:

• the study’s primary outcome;
• the outcome used in the sample size calculation; and
• the outcome with the median effect.</td></tr>
</table>

(*Continued*)

Table 3.2.c (Continued)

Step	Considerations	Examples
	Multiplicity can arise from the reporting of multiple analyses of the same outcome (e.g. analyses that do and do not adjust for prognostic factors; intention-to-treat and per-protocol analyses) and multiple reports of the same study (e.g. journal articles, conference abstracts). Approaches for dealing with this type of multiplicity should also be specified in the protocol (López-López et al 2018). It may be difficult to anticipate all forms of multiplicity when developing a protocol. Any post-hoc approaches used to select outcomes or results should be noted in the 'Differences between protocol and review' section.	
6. Plan how the specified outcome domains will be used in the synthesis.	When different measurement methods or tools have been used across studies, consideration must be given to how these will be synthesized. Options include the following. • Synthesize different measures of the same outcome (or outcome domain) together. This approach is likely to maximize the potential to synthesize. A subgroup or sensitivity analysis might be undertaken to examine if the effects are modified by, or robust to, the type of measurement method or tool (Chapter 10, Sections 10.11.2 and 10.14). There may be increased heterogeneity, warranting use of a random-effects model (Chapter 10, Section 10.10.4). • Synthesize each outcome measure separately (e.g. separate meta-analyses of Beck's Depression Inventory and Hamilton Depression Rating Scale). However, when the measurement methods all provide a measure of the same domain, multiple meta-analyses	In a review of interventions to support women to stop smoking, separate outcome domains were specified for biochemically validated measures of smoking and self-report measures. The two domains were meta-analysed together, but sensitivity analyses were undertaken restricting the meta-analyses to studies with only biochemically validated outcomes, to examine if the results were robust to the method of measurement (Chamberlain et al 2017). In a review of psychological therapies for youth internalizing and externalizing disorders, most studies contributed multiple effects (e.g. in one meta-analysis of 443 studies, there were 5139 included measures). The authors used multilevel modelling to address the dependency among multiple effects contributed from each study (Weisz et al 2017).

	can lead to difficulties in interpretation and an increase in the type I error rate (Bender et al 2008, López-López et al 2018). • Include all the available effect estimates, using a meta-analysis method that models or accounts for the dependency. This option has the advantage of using all information which may lead to greater precision in estimating the intervention effects (López-López et al 2018). Options include multivariate meta-analysis (Mavridis and Salanti 2013), multilevel models (Konstantopoulos 2011) or robust variance estimation (Hedges et al 2010) (see López-López et al 2018 for further discussion).	
7. Where possible, build in contingencies by specifying both specific and broader outcome domains.	Consider building in flexibility to group outcomes at different levels or time intervals. Inflexible approaches can undermine the potential to synthesize, especially when few studies are anticipated, or there is likely to be diversity in the way outcomes are defined and measured and the timing of measurement. If insufficient studies report data for meaningful synthesis using the narrower domains, the broader domains can be used (see also Chapter 2, Section 2.5.3).	Consider a hypothetical review aiming to examine the effects of behavioural psychological interventions for the treatment of overweight and obese adults. A specific outcome is body mass index (BMI). However, also specifying a broader outcome domain 'indicator of body mass' will facilitate synthesis in the circumstance where few studies report BMI, but most report an indicator of body mass (such as weight or waist circumference). This is particularly important when few studies may be anticipated or there is expected diversity in the measurement methods or tools.

MECIR Box 3.3.a Relevant expectations for conduct of intervention reviews

C9: Predefining study designs (**Mandatory**)

Define in advance the eligibility criteria for study designs in a clear and unambiguous way, with a focus on features of a study's design rather than design labels.	Predefined, unambiguous eligibility criteria are a fundamental prerequisite for a systematic review. This is particularly important when non-randomized studies are considered. Some labels commonly used to define study designs can be ambiguous. For example a 'double blind' study may not make it clear who was blinded; a 'case-control' study may be nested within a cohort, or be undertaken in a cross-sectional manner; or a 'prospective' study may have only some features defined or undertaken prospectively.

C11: Justifying choice of study designs (**Mandatory**)

Justify the choice of eligible study designs.	It might be difficult to address some interventions or some outcomes in randomized trials. Authors should be able to justify why they have chosen either to restrict the review to randomized trials or to include non-randomized studies. The particular study designs included should be justified with regard to appropriateness to the review question and with regard to potential for bias.

MECIR Box 3.3.b Relevant expectations for conduct of intervention reviews

C10: Including randomized trials (**Mandatory**)

Include randomized trials as eligible for inclusion in the review, if it is feasible to conduct them to evaluate the interventions and outcomes of interest.	Randomized trials are the best study design for evaluating the efficacy of interventions. If it is feasible to conduct them to evaluate questions that are being addressed by the review, they must be considered eligible for the review. However, appropriate exclusion criteria may be put in place, for example regarding length of follow-up.

suggests that, on average, non-randomized studies produce effect estimates that indicate more extreme benefits of the effects of health care than randomized trials. However, the extent, and even the direction, of the bias is difficult to predict. These issues are discussed at length in Chapter 24, which provides guidance on when it might be appropriate to include non-randomized studies in a Cochrane Review.

Practical considerations also motivate the restriction of many Cochrane Reviews to randomized trials. In recent decades there has been considerable investment internationally in establishing infrastructure to index and identify randomized trials. Cochrane has contributed to these efforts, including building up and maintaining a database of randomized trials, developing search filters to aid their identification, working with MEDLINE to improve tagging and identification of randomized trials, and using machine learning and crowdsourcing to reduce author workload in identifying randomized trials (Chapter 4, Section 4.6.6.2). The same scale of organizational investment has not (yet) been matched for the identification of other types of studies. Consequently, identifying and including other types of studies may require additional efforts to identify studies and to keep the review up to date, and might increase the risk that the result of the review will be influenced by publication bias. This issue and other bias-related issues that are important to consider when defining types of studies are discussed in detail in Chapters 7 and 13.

Specific aspects of study design and conduct should be considered when defining eligibility criteria, even if the review is restricted to randomized trials. For example, whether cluster-randomized trials (Chapter 23, Section 23.1) and crossover trials (Chapter 23, Section 23.2) are eligible, as well as other criteria for eligibility such as use of a placebo comparison group, evaluation of outcomes blinded to allocation sequence, or a minimum period of follow-up. There will always be a trade-off between restrictive study design criteria (which might result in the inclusion of studies that are at low risk of bias, but very few in number) and more liberal design criteria (which might result in the inclusion of more studies, but at a higher risk of bias). Furthermore, excessively broad criteria might result in the inclusion of misleading evidence. If, for example, interest focuses on whether a therapy improves survival in patients with a chronic condition, it might be inappropriate to look at studies of very short duration, except to make explicit the point that they cannot address the question of interest.

3.3.2 Including non-randomized studies

The decision of whether non-randomized studies (and what type) will be included is decided alongside the formulation of the review PICO. The main drivers that may lead to the inclusion of non-randomized studies include: (i) when randomized trials are unable to address the effects of the intervention on harm and long-term outcomes or in specific populations or settings; or (ii) for interventions that cannot be randomized (e.g. policy change introduced in a single or small number of jurisdictions) (see Chapter 24). Cochrane, in collaboration with others, has developed guidance for review authors to support their decision about when to look for and include non-randomized studies (Schünemann et al 2013).

Non-randomized designs have the commonality of not using randomization to allocate units to comparison groups, but their different design features mean that they are variable in their susceptibility to bias. Eligibility criteria should be based on explicit study design features, and not the study labels applied by the primary researchers (e.g. case-control, cohort), which are often used inconsistently (Reeves et al 2017; see Chapter 24).

When non-randomized studies are included, review authors should consider how the studies will be grouped and used in the synthesis. The Cochrane Non-randomized Studies Methods Group taxonomy of design features (see Chapter 24) may provide a basis for grouping together studies that are expected to have similar inferential strength and for providing a consistent language for describing the study design.

Once decisions have been made about grouping study designs, planning of how these will be used in the synthesis is required. Review authors need to decide whether it is useful to synthesize results from non-randomized studies and, if so, whether results from randomized trials and non-randomized studies should be included in the same synthesis (for the purpose of examining whether study design explains heterogeneity among the intervention effects), or whether the effects should be synthesized in separate comparisons (Valentine and Thompson 2013). Decisions should be made for each of the different types of non-randomized studies under consideration. Review authors might anticipate increased heterogeneity when non-randomized studies are synthesized, and adoption of a meta-analysis model that encompasses heterogeneity is wise (Valentine and Thompson 2013) (such as a random effects model, see Chapter 10, Section 10.10.4). For further discussion of non-randomized studies, see Chapter 24.

3.4 Eligibility based on publication status and language

Chapter 4 contains detailed guidance on how to identify studies from a range of sources including, but not limited to, those in peer-reviewed journals. In general, a strategy to include studies reported in all types of publication will reduce bias (Chapter 7). There would need to be a compelling argument for the exclusion of studies on the basis of their publication status (MECIR Box 3.4.a), including unpublished studies, partially published studies, and studies published in 'grey' literature sources. Given the additional challenge in obtaining unpublished studies, it is possible that any unpublished studies identified in a given review may be an unrepresentative subset of all the unpublished studies in existence. However, the bias this introduces is of less concern than the bias

MECIR Box 3.4.a Relevant expectations for conduct of intervention reviews	
C12: Excluding studies based on publication status (**Mandatory**)	
Include studies irrespective of their publication status, unless exclusion is explicitly justified.	Obtaining and including data from unpublished studies (including grey literature) can reduce the effects of publication bias. However, the unpublished studies that can be located may be an unrepresentative sample of all unpublished studies.

introduced by excluding all unpublished studies, given what is known about the impact of reporting biases (see Chapter 13 on bias due to missing studies, and Chapter 4, Section 4.3 for a more detailed discussion of searching for unpublished and grey literature).

Likewise, while searching for, and analysing, studies in any language can be extremely resource-intensive, review authors should consider carefully the implications for bias (and equity, see Chapter 16) if they restrict eligible studies to those published in one specific language (usually English). See Chapter 4 (Section 4.4.5) for further discussion of language and other restrictions while searching.

3.5 Chapter information

Authors: Joanne E McKenzie, Sue E Brennan, Rebecca E Ryan, Hilary J Thomson, Renea V Johnston, James Thomas

Acknowledgements: This chapter builds on earlier versions of the *Handbook*. In particular, Chapter 5, edited by Denise O'Connor, Sally Green and Julian Higgins.

Funding: JEM is supported by an Australian National Health and Medical Research Council (NHMRC) Career Development Fellowship (1143429). SEB and RER's positions are supported by the NHMRC Cochrane Collaboration Funding Program. HJT is funded by the UK Medical Research Council (MC_UU_12017-13 and MC_UU_12017-15) and Scottish Government Chief Scientist Office (SPHSU13 and SPHSU15). RVJ's position is supported by the NHMRC Cochrane Collaboration Funding Program and Cabrini Institute. JT is supported by the National Institute for Health Research (NIHR) Collaboration for Leadership in Applied Health Research and Care North Thames at Barts Health NHS Trust. The views expressed are those of the author(s) and not necessarily those of the NHS, the NIHR or the Department of Health.

3.6 References

Bailey JV, Murray E, Rait G, Mercer CH, Morris RW, Peacock R, Cassell J, Nazareth I. Interactive computer-based interventions for sexual health promotion. *Cochrane Database of Systematic Reviews* 2010; **9**: CD006483.

Bender R, Bunce C, Clarke M, Gates S, Lange S, Pace NL, Thorlund K. Attention should be given to multiplicity issues in systematic reviews. *Journal of Clinical Epidemiology* 2008; **61**: 857–865.

Buchbinder R, Johnston RV, Rischin KJ, Homik J, Jones CA, Golmohammadi K, Kallmes DF. Percutaneous vertebroplasty for osteoporotic vertebral compression fracture. *Cochrane Database of Systematic Reviews* 2018; **4**: CD006349.

Caldwell DM, Welton NJ. Approaches for synthesising complex mental health interventions in meta-analysis. *Evidence-Based Mental Health* 2016; **19**: 16–21.

Chamberlain C, O'Mara-Eves A, Porter J, Coleman T, Perlen S, Thomas J, McKenzie J. Psychosocial interventions for supporting women to stop smoking in pregnancy. *Cochrane Database of Systematic Reviews* 2017; **2**: CD001055.

Ciciriello S, Johnston RV, Osborne RH, Wicks I, deKroo T, Clerehan R, O'Neill C, Buchbinder R. Multimedia educational interventions for consumers about prescribed and over-the-counter medications. *Cochrane Database of Systematic Reviews* 2013; **4**: CD008416.

Cochrane Consumers & Communication Group. Outcomes of Interest to the Cochrane Consumers & Communication Group: taxonomy. http://cccrg.cochrane.org/.

COnsensus-based Standards for the selection of health Measurement INstruments (COSMIN) initiative. COSMIN database of systematic reviews of outcome measurement instruments. https://database.cosmin.nl/.

Coulter A, Entwistle VA, Eccles A, Ryan S, Shepperd S, Perera R. Personalised care planning for adults with chronic or long-term health conditions. *Cochrane Database of Systematic Reviews* 2015; **3**: CD010523.

Davey J, Turner RM, Clarke MJ, Higgins JPT. Characteristics of meta-analyses and their component studies in the Cochrane Database of Systematic Reviews: a cross-sectional, descriptive analysis. *BMC Medical Research Methodology* 2011; **11**: 160.

Desroches S, Lapointe A, Ratte S, Gravel K, Legare F, Turcotte S. Interventions to enhance adherence to dietary advice for preventing and managing chronic diseases in adults. *Cochrane Database of Systematic Reviews* 2013; **2**: CD008722.

Deyo RA, Dworkin SF, Amtmann D, Andersson G, Borenstein D, Carragee E, Carrino J, Chou R, Cook K, DeLitto A, Goertz C, Khalsa P, Loeser J, Mackey S, Panagis J, Rainville J, Tosteson T, Turk D, Von Korff M, Weiner DK. Report of the NIH Task Force on research standards for chronic low back pain. *Journal of Pain* 2014; **15**: 569–585.

Dodd S, Clarke M, Becker L, Mavergames C, Fish R, Williamson PR. A taxonomy has been developed for outcomes in medical research to help improve knowledge discovery. *Journal of Clinical Epidemiology* 2018; **96**: 84–92.

Fisher DJ, Carpenter JR, Morris TP, Freeman SC, Tierney JF. Meta-analytical methods to identify who benefits most from treatments: daft, deluded, or deft approach? *BMJ* 2017; **356**: j573.

Fransen M, McConnell S, Harmer AR, Van der Esch M, Simic M, Bennell KL. Exercise for osteoarthritis of the knee. *Cochrane Database of Systematic Reviews* 2015; **1**: CD004376.

Guise JM, Chang C, Viswanathan M, Glick S, Treadwell J, Umscheid CA. *Systematic reviews of complex multicomponent health care interventions. Report No. 14-EHC003-EF*. Rockville, MD: Agency for Healthcare Research and Quality; 2014.

Harrison JK, Noel-Storr AH, Demeyere N, Reynish EL, Quinn TJ. Outcomes measures in a decade of dementia and mild cognitive impairment trials. *Alzheimer's Research and Therapy* 2016; **8**: 48.

Hedges LV, Tipton E, Johnson M, C. Robust variance estimation in meta-regression with dependent effect size estimates. *Research Synthesis Methods* 2010; **1**: 39–65.

Hetrick SE, McKenzie JE, Cox GR, Simmons MB, Merry SN. Newer generation antidepressants for depressive disorders in children and adolescents. *Cochrane Database of Systematic Reviews* 2012; **11**: CD004851.

Higgins JPT, López-López JA, Becker BJ, Davies SR, Dawson S, Grimshaw JM, McGuinness LA, Moore THM, Rehfuess E, Thomas J, Caldwell DM. Synthesizing quantitative evidence in systematic reviews of complex health interventions. *BMJ Global Health* 2019; **4**: e000858.

Hoffmann T, Glasziou P, Barbour V, Macdonald H. Better reporting of interventions: template for intervention description and replication (TIDieR) checklist and guide. *BMJ* 2014; **1687**: 1–13.

Hollands GJ, Shemilt I, Marteau TM, Jebb SA, Lewis HB, Wei Y, Higgins JPT, Ogilvie D. Portion, package or tableware size for changing selection and consumption of food, alcohol and tobacco. *Cochrane Database of Systematic Reviews* 2015; **9**: CD011045.

Howe TE, Shea B, Dawson LJ, Downie F, Murray A, Ross C, Harbour RT, Caldwell LM, Creed G. Exercise for preventing and treating osteoporosis in postmenopausal women. *Cochrane Database of Systematic Reviews* 2011; **7**: CD000333.

ICHOM. The International Consortium for Health Outcomes Measurement 2018. http://www.ichom.org/.

IPDAS. International Patient Decision Aid Standards Collaboration (IPDAS) standards. www.ipdas.ohri.ca.

Ivers N, Jamtvedt G, Flottorp S, Young JM, Odgaard-Jensen J, French SD, O'Brien MA, Johansen M, Grimshaw J, Oxman AD. Audit and feedback: effects on professional practice and healthcare outcomes. *Cochrane Database of Systematic Reviews* 2012; **6**: CD000259.

Janmaat VT, Steyerberg EW, van der Gaast A, Mathijssen RH, Bruno MJ, Peppelenbosch MP, Kuipers EJ, Spaander MC. Palliative chemotherapy and targeted therapies for esophageal and gastroesophageal junction cancer. *Cochrane Database of Systematic Reviews* 2017; **11**: CD004063.

Kendrick D, Kumar A, Carpenter H, Zijlstra GAR, Skelton DA, Cook JR, Stevens Z, Belcher CM, Haworth D, Gawler SJ, Gage H, Masud T, Bowling A, Pearl M, Morris RW, Iliffe S, Delbaere K. Exercise for reducing fear of falling in older people living in the community. *Cochrane Database of Systematic Reviews* 2014; **11**: CD009848.

Kirkham JJ, Gargon E, Clarke M, Williamson PR. Can a core outcome set improve the quality of systematic reviews? A survey of the Co-ordinating Editors of Cochrane Review Groups. *Trials* 2013; **14**: 21.

Konstantopoulos S. Fixed effects and variance components estimation in three-level meta-analysis. *Research Synthesis Methods* 2011; **2**: 61–76.

Lamb SE, Becker C, Gillespie LD, Smith JL, Finnegan S, Potter R, Pfeiffer K. Reporting of complex interventions in clinical trials: development of a taxonomy to classify and describe fall-prevention interventions. *Trials* 2011; **12**: 125.

Lewin S, Hendry M, Chandler J, Oxman AD, Michie S, Shepperd S, Reeves BC, Tugwell P, Hannes K, Rehfuess EA, Welch V, Mckenzie JE, Burford B, Petkovic J, Anderson LM, Harris J, Noyes J. Assessing the complexity of interventions within systematic reviews: development, content and use of a new tool (iCAT_SR). *BMC Medical Research Methodology* 2017; **17**: 76.

López-López JA, Page MJ, Lipsey MW, Higgins JPT. Dealing with multiplicity of effect sizes in systematic reviews and meta-analyses. *Research Synthesis Methods* 2018; **9**: 336–351.

Mavridis D, Salanti G. A practical introduction to multivariate meta-analysis. *Statistical Methods in Medical Research* 2013; **22**: 133–158.

Michie S, van Stralen M, West R. The Behaviour Change Wheel: a new method for characterising and designing behaviour change interventions. *Implementation Science* 2011; **6**: 42.

Michie S, Richardson M, Johnston M, Abraham C, Francis J, Hardeman W, Eccles MP, Cane J, Wood CE. The behavior change technique taxonomy (v1) of 93 hierarchically clustered techniques: building an international consensus for the reporting of behavior change interventions. *Annals of Behavioral Medicine* 2013; **46**: 81–95.

Moraes VY, Lenza M, Tamaoki MJ, Faloppa F, Belloti JC. Platelet-rich therapies for musculoskeletal soft tissue injuries. *Cochrane Database of Systematic Reviews* 2014; **4**: CD010071.

O'Neill J, Tabish H, Welch V, Petticrew M, Pottie K, Clarke M, Evans T, Pardo Pardo J, Waters E, White H, Tugwell P. Applying an equity lens to interventions: using PROGRESS ensures consideration of socially stratifying factors to illuminate inequities in health. *Journal of Clinical Epidemiology* 2014; **67**: 56–64.

Pompoli A, Furukawa TA, Imai H, Tajika A, Efthimiou O, Salanti G. Psychological therapies for panic disorder with or without agoraphobia in adults: a network meta-analysis. *Cochrane Database of Systematic Reviews* 2016; **4**: CD011004.

Pompoli A, Furukawa TA, Efthimiou O, Imai H, Tajika A, Salanti G. Dismantling cognitive-behaviour therapy for panic disorder: a systematic review and component network meta-analysis. *Psychological Medicine* 2018; **48**: 1–9.

Reeves BC, Wells GA, Waddington H. Quasi-experimental study designs series-paper 5: a checklist for classifying studies evaluating the effects on health interventions – a taxonomy without labels. *Journal of Clinical Epidemiology* 2017; **89**: 30–42.

Regnaux J-P, Lefevre-Colau M-M, Trinquart L, Nguyen C, Boutron I, Brosseau L, Ravaud P. High-intensity versus low-intensity physical activity or exercise in people with hip or knee osteoarthritis. *Cochrane Database of Systematic Reviews* 2015; **10**: CD010203.

Richards SH, Anderson L, Jenkinson CE, Whalley B, Rees K, Davies P, Bennett P, Liu Z, West R, Thompson DR, Taylor RS. Psychological interventions for coronary heart disease. *Cochrane Database of Systematic Reviews* 2017; **4**: CD002902.

Safi S, Korang SK, Nielsen EE, Sethi NJ, Feinberg J, Gluud C, Jakobsen JC. Beta-blockers for heart failure. *Cochrane Database of Systematic Reviews* 2017; **12**: CD012897.

Santesso N, Carrasco-Labra A, Brignardello-Petersen R. Hip protectors for preventing hip fractures in older people. *Cochrane Database of Systematic Reviews* 2014; **3**: CD001255.

Shepherd E, Gomersall JC, Tieu J, Han S, Crowther CA, Middleton P. Combined diet and exercise interventions for preventing gestational diabetes mellitus. *Cochrane Database of Systematic Reviews* 2017; **11**: CD010443.

Squires J, Valentine J, Grimshaw J. Systematic reviews of complex interventions: framing the review question. *Journal of Clinical Epidemiology* 2013; **66**: 1215–1222.

Stacey D, Légaré F, Lewis K, Barry MJ, Bennett CL, Eden KB, Holmes-Rovner M, Llewellyn-Thomas H, Lyddiatt A, Thomson R, Trevena L. Decision aids for people facing health treatment or screening decisions. *Cochrane Database of Systematic Reviews* 2017; **4**: CD001431.

Stroke Unit Trialists Collaboration. Organised inpatient (stroke unit) care for stroke. *Cochrane Database of Systematic Reviews* 2013; **9**: CD000197.

Taylor AJ, Jones LJ, Osborn DA. Zinc supplementation of parenteral nutrition in newborn infants. *Cochrane Database of Systematic Reviews* 2017; **2**: CD012561.

Valentine JC, Thompson SG. Issues relating to confounding and meta-analysis when including non-randomized studies in systematic reviews on the effects of interventions. *Research Synthesis Methods* 2013; **4**: 26–35.

Vaona A, Banzi R, Kwag KH, Rigon G, Cereda D, Pecoraro V, Tramacere I, Moja L. E-learning for health professionals. *Cochrane Database of Systematic Reviews* 2018; **1**: CD011736.

Verheyden GSAF, Weerdesteyn V, Pickering RM, Kunkel D, Lennon S, Geurts ACH, Ashburn A. Interventions for preventing falls in people after stroke. *Cochrane Database of Systematic Reviews* 2013; **5**: CD008728.

Weisz JR, Kuppens S, Ng MY, Eckshtain D, Ugueto AM, Vaughn-Coaxum R, Jensen-Doss A, Hawley KM, Krumholz Marchette LS, Chu BC, Weersing VR, Fordwood SR. What five decades of research tells us about the effects of youth psychological therapy: a multilevel meta-analysis and implications for science and practice. *American Psychologist* 2017; **72**: 79–117.

Welch V, Petkovic J, Simeon R, Presseau J, Gagnon D, Hossain A, Pardo Pardo J, Pottie K, Rader T, Sokolovski A, Yoganathan M, Tugwell P, DesMeules M. Interactive social media interventions for health behaviour change, health outcomes, and health equity in the adult population. *Cochrane Database of Systematic Reviews* 2018; **2**: CD012932.

Welton NJ, Caldwell DM, Adamopoulos E, Vedhara K. Mixed treatment comparison meta-analysis of complex interventions: psychological interventions in coronary heart disease. *American Journal of Epidemiology* 2009; **169**: 1158–1165.

Williamson PR, Altman DG, Bagley H, Barnes KL, Blazeby JM, Brookes ST, Clarke M, Gargon E, Gorst S, Harman N, Kirkham JJ, McNair A, Prinsen CAC, Schmitt J, Terwee CB, Young B. The COMET Handbook: version 1.0. *Trials* 2017; **18**: 280.

4

Searching for and selecting studies

Carol Lefebvre, Julie Glanville, Simon Briscoe, Anne Littlewood, Chris Marshall, Maria-Inti Metzendorf, Anna Noel-Storr, Tamara Rader, Farhad Shokraneh, James Thomas, L. Susan Wieland; on behalf of the Cochrane Information Retrieval Methods Group

KEY POINTS

- Review authors should work closely, from the start of the protocol, with an experienced medical/healthcare librarian or information specialist.
- Studies (not reports of studies) are included in Cochrane Reviews but identifying reports of studies is currently the most convenient approach to identifying the majority of studies and obtaining information about them and their results.
- The Cochrane Central Register of Controlled Trials (CENTRAL) and MEDLINE, together with Embase (if access to Embase is available to the review team) should be searched for all Cochrane Reviews.
- Additionally, for all Cochrane Reviews, the Specialized Register of the relevant Cochrane Review Groups should be searched, either internally within the Review Group or via CENTRAL.
- Trials registers should be searched for all Cochrane Reviews and other sources such as regulatory agencies and clinical study reports (CSRs) are an increasingly important source of information for study results.
- Searches should aim for high sensitivity, which may result in relatively low precision.
- Search strategies should avoid using too many *different* search concepts but a wide variety of search terms should be combined with OR within *each* included concept.
- Both free-text and subject headings (e.g. Medical Subject Headings (MeSH) and Emtree) should be used.
- Published, highly sensitive, validated search strategies (filters) to identify randomized trials should be considered, such as the Cochrane Highly Sensitive Search Strategies for identifying randomized trials in MEDLINE (but do not apply these randomized trial or human filters in CENTRAL).

This chapter should be cited as: Lefebvre C, Glanville J, Briscoe S, Littlewood A, Marshall C, Metzendorf M-I, Noel-Storr A, Rader T, Shokraneh F, Thomas J, Wieland LS. Chapter 4: Searching for and selecting studies. In: Higgins JPT, Thomas J, Chandler J, Cumpston M, Li T, Page MJ, Welch VA (editors). *Cochrane Handbook for Systematic Reviews of Interventions*. 2nd Edition. Chichester (UK): John Wiley & Sons, 2019: 67–108.

4.1 Introduction

Cochrane Reviews take a systematic and comprehensive approach to identifying studies that meet the eligibility criteria for the review. This chapter outlines some general issues in searching for studies; describes the main sources of potential studies; and discusses how to plan the search process, design and carry out search strategies, manage references found during the search process, correctly document the search process and select studies from the search results.

This chapter aims to provide review authors with background information on all aspects of searching for studies so that they can better understand the search process. All authors of systematic reviews should, however, identify an experienced medical/healthcare librarian or information specialist to provide support for the search process. The chapter also aims to provide advice and guidance for medical/healthcare librarians and information specialists (within and beyond Cochrane) involved in the search process to identify studies for inclusion in systematic reviews.

This chapter focuses on searching for randomized trials. Many of the search principles discussed, however, will also apply to other study designs. Considerations for searching for non-randomized studies are discussed in Chapter 24 (see also Chapter 19 when these are specifically for adverse effects). Other discussion of searching for specific types of evidence appears in chapters dedicated to these types of evidence, such as Chapter 17 on complex and public health interventions, Chapter 20 on economics evidence and Chapter 21 on qualitative research.

An online Technical Supplement to this chapter provides more detail on searching methods and is available from Cochrane Training.

4.2 General issues

4.2.1 Role of the information specialist/librarian

Medical/healthcare librarians and information specialists have an integral role in the production of Cochrane Reviews. There is increasing evidence to support the involvement of an information specialist in the review to improve the quality of various aspects of the search process (Rethlefsen et al 2015, Meert et al 2016, Metzendorf 2016).

Most Cochrane Review Groups (CRGs) employ an information specialist to support authors. The range of services, however, offered by CRGs and/or their information specialists varies according to the resources available. Cochrane Review authors should, therefore, contact their Cochrane Information Specialist at the earliest stage to find out what advice and support is available to them. Authors conducting their own searches should seek advice from their Cochrane Information Specialist not only on which sources to search, but also with respect to the exact strategies to be run (see Section 4.4). If the CRG does not provide this service or employ an information specialist, we recommend that review authors seek guidance from a medical/healthcare librarian or information specialist, preferably one with experience in supporting systematic reviews.

Cochrane Information Specialists are responsible for providing assistance to authors with searching for studies for inclusion in their reviews, and for keeping up to date with Cochrane methodological developments in information retrieval (Littlewood et al 2017).

A key element of the role is the maintenance of a Specialized Register for their Review Group, containing reports of trials relating to the group's scope. Within the limits of licensing restrictions, the content of these group registers is shared with users worldwide via the Cochrane Central Register of Controlled Trials (CENTRAL), part of the Cochrane Library (see Section 4.3.3).

Most CRGs offer support to authors in study identification from the early planning stage to the final write-up of the review, and the support available may include some or all of the following:

- advising authors on which databases and other sources to search;
- designing, or providing guidance on designing, search strategies for the main bibliographic databases and/or trials registers;
- running searches in databases and/or registers available to the information specialist;
- saving and collating search results, and sharing them with authors in appropriate formats;
- advising authors on how to run searches in other sources and how to download results;
- drafting, or assisting authors in drafting, the search methods sections of a Cochrane Protocol and Review and/or Update;
- ensuring that Cochrane Protocols, Reviews and Updates meet the requirements set out in the Methodological Expectations of Cochrane Intervention Reviews (MECIR) relating to searching activities for reviews;
- organizing translations, or at least data extraction, of papers where required to enable authors to assess papers for inclusion/exclusion in their reviews;
- obtaining copies of trial reports for review teams when required (within copyright legislation);
- providing advice and support to author teams on the use of reference management tools, and other software used in review production, including review production tools such as RevMan, Covidence and EPPI-Reviewer; and
- checking and formatting the references to included and/or excluded studies in line with the Cochrane Style Manual.

The Cochrane Information Specialists' Handbook (Chapter 6, Author support) contains further information about how Cochrane Information Specialists can support authors (Littlewood et al 2017).

4.2.2 Minimizing bias

Systematic reviews require a thorough, objective and reproducible search of a range of sources to identify as many eligible studies as possible (within resource limits). This is a major factor distinguishing systematic reviews from traditional narrative reviews, which helps to minimize bias and achieve more reliable estimates of effects and uncertainties. A search of MEDLINE alone is not considered adequate. Research evidence indicates that not all known published randomized trials are available in MEDLINE and that even if relevant records are in MEDLINE, it can be difficult to retrieve them (see Section 4.3.2).

Going beyond MEDLINE is important not only for ensuring that as many relevant studies as possible are identified, but also to minimize selection bias for those that are found. Relying exclusively on a MEDLINE search may retrieve a set of reports unrepresentative of all reports that would have been identified through a wider or more extensive search of several sources.

Time and budget restraints require the review team to balance the thoroughness of the search with efficiency in the use of time and funds. The best way of achieving this balance is to be aware of, and try to minimize, the biases such as publication bias and language bias that can result from restricting searches in different ways (see Chapters 8 and 13 for further guidance on assessing these biases). Unlike for tasks such as study selection or data extraction, it is not considered necessary (or even desirable) for two people to conduct independent searches in parallel. It is strongly recommended, however, that all search strategies should be peer reviewed by a suitably qualified and experienced medical/healthcare librarian or information specialist (see Section 4.4.8).

4.2.3 Studies versus reports of studies

Systematic reviews have studies as the primary units of interest and analysis. A single study may have more than one report about it, and each of these reports may contribute useful information for the review (see Section 4.6.1). For most of the sources listed in Section 4.3, the search process will retrieve individual reports of studies, so that multiple reports of the same study will need to be identified and associated with each other manually by the review authors. There is, however, an increasing number of *study-based* sources, which link multiple records of the same study together, such as the Cochrane Register of Studies and the Specialized Registers of a number of CRGs and Fields (see online Technical Supplement), and some other trials registers and regulatory and industry sources. Processes and software to select and group publications by study are discussed in Section 4.6.

4.2.4 Copyright and licensing

It is Cochrane policy that all review authors and others involved in Cochrane should adhere to copyright legislation and the terms of database licensing agreements. With respect to searching for studies, this refers in particular to adhering to the terms and conditions of use when searching databases and other sources and downloading records, as well as adhering to copyright legislation when obtaining copies of publications. Review authors should seek guidance on this from their medical/healthcare librarian or information specialist, as copyright legislation varies across jurisdictions and licensing agreements vary across organizations.

4.3 Sources to search

4.3.1 Bibliographic databases

4.3.1.1 Introduction to bibliographic databases

The search for studies in a Cochrane Review should be as extensive as possible in order to reduce the risk of reporting bias and to identify as much relevant evidence as possible (see MECIR Box 4.3.a). Searches of health-related bibliographic databases are

MECIR Box 4.3.a Relevant expectations for conduct of intervention reviews	
C19: Planning the search (**Mandatory**)	
Plan in advance the methods to be used for identifying studies. Design searches to capture as many studies as possible that meet the eligibility criteria, ensuring that relevant time periods and sources are covered and not restricted by language or publication status.	Searches should be motivated directly by the eligibility criteria for the review, and it is important that all types of eligible studies are considered when planning the search. If searches are restricted by publication status or by language of publication, there is a possibility of publication bias, or language bias (whereby the language of publication is selected in a way that depends on the findings of the study), or both. Removing language restrictions in English language databases is not a good substitute for searching non-English language journals and databases.
C24: Searching general bibliographic databases and CENTRAL (**Mandatory**)	
Search the Cochrane Review Group's (CRG's) Specialized Register (internally, e.g. via the Cochrane Register of Studies, or externally via CENTRAL). Ensure that CENTRAL, MEDLINE and Embase (if Embase is available to either the CRG or the review author), have been searched (either for the review or for the Review Group's Specialized Register).	Searches for studies should be as extensive as possible in order to reduce the risk of publication bias and to identify as much relevant evidence as possible. The minimum databases to be covered are the CRG's Specialized Register (if it exists and was designed to support reviews in this way), CENTRAL, MEDLINE and Embase (if Embase is available to either the CRG or the review author). Expertise may be required to avoid unnecessary duplication of effort. Some, but not all, reports of eligible studies from MEDLINE, Embase and the CRGs' Specialized Registers are already included in CENTRAL.

generally the most efficient way to identify an initial set of relevant reports of studies (EUnetHTA 2017). Database selection should be guided by the review topic (Suarez-Almazor et al 2000, Stevinson and Lawlor 2004, Lorenzetti et al 2014). When topics are specialized, cross-disciplinary, or involve emerging technologies (Rice et al 2016), additional databases may need to be identified and searched (Wallace et al 1997, Stevinson and Lawlor 2004).

The three bibliographic databases generally considered to be the most important sources to search for reports of trials are CENTRAL, MEDLINE (Halladay et al 2015,

Sampson et al 2016) and Embase (Woods and Trewheellar 1998, Sampson et al 2003, Bai et al 2007). These databases are described in more detail in Sections 4.3.1.2 and 4.3.1.3 and in the online Technical Supplement. For Cochrane Reviews, CENTRAL, MEDLINE and Embase (if access to Embase is available to the review team) should be searched (see MECIR Box 4.3.a). These searches may be undertaken specifically for the review, or indirectly by searching the CRG's Specialized Register.

Some bibliographic databases, such as MEDLINE and Embase, include abstracts for the majority of recent records. A key advantage of such databases is that they can be searched electronically both for words in the title or abstract and by using the standardized indexing terms, or controlled vocabulary, assigned to each record (see Section 4.3.1.2). Cochrane has developed a database of reports of randomized trials called the Cochrane Central Register of Controlled Trials (CENTRAL), which is published within the Cochrane Library (see Section 4.3.1.3).

Bibliographic databases are available to individuals for a fee (by subscription or on a 'pay-as-you-go' basis) or free at the point of use. They may be available through national provisions, site-wide licences at institutions such as universities or hospitals, through professional organizations as part of their membership packages or free-of-charge on the internet. Some international initiatives provide free or low-cost online access to databases (and full-text journals) over the internet. The Health InterNetwork Access to Research Initiative (HINARI) programme, set up by the World Health Organization (WHO) together with major publishers, provides access to a wide range of databases including the Cochrane Library for healthcare professionals in local, not-for-profit institutions in more than 115 countries, areas and territories. The International Network for the Availability of Scientific Publications (INASP) also provides access to a wide range of databases (and journals) including the Cochrane Library. Electronic Information for Libraries (EIFL) is a similar initiative based on library consortia to support affordable licensing of journals and other sources in more than 60 low-income and transition countries in central, eastern and south-east Europe, the former Soviet Union, Africa, the Middle East and South-east Asia.

The online Technical Supplement provides more detailed information about how to search these sources and other databases. It also provides a list of general healthcare databases by region and healthcare databases by subject area. Further evidence-based information about sources to search can be found on the SuRe Info portal, which is updated twice per year.

4.3.1.2 MEDLINE and Embase

Cochrane Reviews of interventions should include a search of MEDLINE (see MECIR Box 4.3.a). MEDLINE (as of August 2018) contains over 25 million references to journal articles in biomedicine and health from 1946 onwards. More than 5200 journals in about 40 languages are indexed for MEDLINE (US National Library of Medicine 2019).

PubMed provides access to a free version of MEDLINE that also includes up-to-date citations not yet indexed for MEDLINE (US National Library of Medicine 2018). Additionally, PubMed includes records from journals that are not indexed for MEDLINE and records considered 'out-of-scope' from journals that are partially indexed for MEDLINE (US National Library of Medicine no date).

MEDLINE is also available on subscription from a number of other database vendors, such as EBSCO, Ovid, ProQuest and STN. Access is usually 'free at-the-point-of-use' to members of the institutions paying the subscriptions (e.g. hospitals and universities). Ovid MEDLINE (segment name 'medall') covers all of the available content and metadata in PubMed with a delay of one day (except during the annual reload, at the end of each year, when Ovid MEDLINE will not match the PubMed baseline). Aside from the MEDLINE records, Ovid includes all content types available in PubMed including; Epub Ahead of Print, PubMed-not-MEDLINE, In-process citations and citations for books available on the NCBI Bookshelf.

When searching MEDLINE via service providers or interfaces other than Ovid or PubMed, we recommend verification of the exact coverage of the database in relation to PubMed, where no explicit information on this is readily available.

Cochrane Reviews of interventions should include a search of Embase (if access to Embase is available to the review team) (see MECIR Box 4.3.a). Embase (as of June 2018) contains over 30 million records from more than 8000 currently published journals. Embase now includes all MEDLINE records, thus, technically, allowing both databases to be searched simultaneously. Further details on the implications of this for searching are available in the online Technical Supplement. There are more than 6 million records in Embase, from more than 2900 journals that are not indexed in MEDLINE (Elsevier 2016a). Embase includes articles from about 90 countries. Embase Classic provides access to almost 2 million records digitized from the Excerpta Medica print journals (the original print indexes from which Embase was created) from 1947 to 1973 (Elsevier 2016b).

Embase is only available by subscription, either directly via Elsevier (as Embase.com) or from other database vendors, such as Ovid, ProQuest or STN. It is mandatory for Cochrane intervention reviews to include a search of Embase if access is available to the review team (see MECIR Box 4.3.a). Note that Embase is searched regularly by Cochrane for reports of trials. These records are included in CENTRAL (see online Technical Supplement).

The online Technical Supplement provides guidance on how to search MEDLINE and Embase for reports of trials. The actual degree of reference overlap between MEDLINE and Embase varies widely according to the topic, but studies comparing searches of the two databases have generally concluded that a comprehensive search requires that both databases be searched (Lefebvre et al 2008) (see MECIR Box 4.3.a).

Conversely, two recent studies examined different samples of Cochrane Reviews and identified the databases from which the included studies of these reviews originated (Halladay et al 2015, Hartling et al 2016). Halladay showed that the majority of included studies could be identified via PubMed (range 75% to 92%) and Hartling showed that the majority of included studies could be identified by using a combination of two databases, but the two databases were different in each case. Both studies, one across all healthcare areas (Halladay et al 2015) and the other on child health (Hartling et al 2016), report a minimal extent to which the inclusion of studies not indexed in PubMed altered the meta-analyses. Hence, the current recommendation of searching multiple databases needs to be evaluated further, so as to confirm under which circumstances more comprehensive searches of multiple databases is warranted.

4.3.1.3 The Cochrane Central Register of Controlled Trials (CENTRAL)

Since its inception, the Cochrane Central Register of Controlled Trials (CENTRAL) has been recognized as the most comprehensive source of reports of randomized trials (Egger and Smith 1998). CENTRAL is published as part of the Cochrane Library and is updated monthly. As of June 2018, CENTRAL contains over 1,275,000 records of reports of trials/trials registry records potentially eligible for inclusion in Cochrane Reviews, by far the majority of which are randomized trials.

Many of the records in CENTRAL have been identified through systematic searches of MEDLINE and Embase (see online Technical Supplement). CENTRAL, however, also includes citations to reports of randomized trials that are not indexed in MEDLINE, Embase or other bibliographic databases; citations published in many languages; and citations that are available only in conference proceedings or other sources that are difficult to access. It also includes records from trials registers and trials results registers.

These additional records are, for the most part, identified by Cochrane Information Specialists, many of whom conduct comprehensive searches to populate CRG Specialized Registers, collecting records of trials eligible for Cochrane Reviews in their field. These Specialized Registers are included in CENTRAL. Where a Specialized Register is available, for which sufficiently comprehensive searching has been conducted, a search of the Specialized Register may be conducted instead of separately searching CENTRAL, MEDLINE and Embase for a specific review. In these cases, the search will be more precise, but an equivalent number of included studies will be identified with lower numbers of records to screen. There will, however, be a time-lag between records appearing in databases such as MEDLINE or Embase and their inclusion in a Specialized Register.

CENTRAL is available through the Cochrane Library. Many review authors have access free-of-charge at the point-of-use through national provisions and other similar arrangements, or as part of a paid subscription to the Cochrane Library. All Cochrane Information Specialists have access to CENTRAL.

The online Technical Supplement provides information on what is in CENTRAL from MEDLINE, Embase and other sources, as well as guidance on searching CENTRAL.

4.3.1.4 Other bibliographic databases

Many countries and regions produce bibliographic databases that focus on the literature produced in those regions and which often include journals and other literature not indexed elsewhere. There are also subject-specific bibliographic databases, such as AMED (alternative therapies), CINAHL (nursing and allied health) and PsycINFO (psychology and psychiatry). It is highly desirable that searches be conducted of appropriate national, regional and subject specific bibliographic databases (see MECIR Box 4.3.b). Further details are provided in the online Technical Supplement.

Citation indexes are bibliographic databases that record instances where a particular reference is cited, in addition to the standard bibliographic content. Citation indexes can be used to identify studies that are similar to a study report of interest, as it is probable that other reports citing or cited by a study will contain similar or related content.

<table>
<tr><th colspan="2">MECIR Box 4.3.b Relevant expectations for conduct of intervention reviews</th></tr>
<tr><td colspan="2">C25: Searching specialist bibliographic databases (Highly desirable)</td></tr>
<tr><td>Search appropriate national, regional and subject-specific bibliographic databases.</td><td>Searches for studies should be as extensive as possible in order to reduce the risk of publication bias and to identify as much relevant evidence as possible. Databases relevant to the review topic should be covered (e.g. CINAHL for nursing-related topics, PsycINFO for psychological interventions), and regional databases (e.g. LILACS) should be considered.</td></tr>
</table>

4.3.2 Ongoing studies and unpublished data sources

Initiatives to provide access to ongoing studies and unpublished data constitute a fast-moving field (Isojarvi et al 2018). Review authors should therefore consult their medical/healthcare librarian or information specialist for current advice.

It is important to identify ongoing studies, so that when a review is updated these can be assessed for possible inclusion. Awareness of the existence of a possibly relevant ongoing study and its expected completion date might affect not only decisions with respect to when to update a specific review, but also when to aim to complete a review. Information about possibly relevant ongoing studies should be included in the review in the 'Characteristics of ongoing studies' table.

Even when studies are completed, some are never published. An association between 'statistically significant' results and publication has been documented across a number of studies, as summarized in Chapter 13. Finding out about unpublished studies, and including their results in a systematic review when eligible and appropriate (Cook et al 1993), is important for minimizing bias. Several studies and other articles addressing issues around identifying unpublished studies have been published (Easterbrook et al 1991, Weber et al 1998, Manheimer and Anderson 2002, MacLean et al 2003, Lee et al 2008, Chan 2012, Bero 2013, Schroll et al 2013, Chapman et al 2014, Kreis et al 2014, Scherer et al 2015, Hwang et al 2016, Lampert et al 2016).

There is no easy and reliable single way to obtain information about studies that have been completed but never published. There have, however, been several important initiatives resulting in better access to studies and their results from sources other than the main bibliographic databases and journals. These include trials registers and trials results registers (see Section 4.3.3), regulatory agency sources and clinical study reports (CSRs); (the very detailed reports prepared by industry for regulatory approval) (see Section 4.3.4). A recent study (Halfpenny et al 2016) assessed the value and usability for systematic reviews and network meta-analyses of data from trials registers, CSRs and regulatory authorities, and concluded that data from these sources have the potential to influence systematic review results. Two earlier studies showed that a considerably higher proportion of CSRs prepared for regulatory approval of drugs provided complete information on study methods and results than did trials register records or journal publications (Wieseler et al 2012) and that conventional, publicly available sources (European Public Assessment Reports, journal publications, and trials register records) provide insufficient information on new drugs, especially on patient relevant outcomes in approved subpopulations (Köhler et al 2015).

A Cochrane Methodology Review examined studies assessing methods for obtaining unpublished data and concluded that those carrying out systematic reviews should continue to contact authors for missing data and that email contact was more successful than other methods (Young and Hopewell 2011). An annotated bibliography of published studies addressing searching for unpublished studies and obtaining access to unpublished data is also available (Arber et al 2013). One particular study focused on the contribution of unpublished studies, including dissertations, and studies in languages other than English, to the results of meta-analyses in reviews relevant to children (Hartling et al 2017). They found that, in their sample, unpublished studies and studies in languages other than English rarely had any impact on the results and conclusions of the review. They did, however, concede that inclusion of these study types may have an impact in situations where there are few relevant studies, or where there are 'questionable vested interests' in the published literature.

Correspondence can be an important source of information about unpublished studies. It is highly desirable for authors of Cochrane Reviews of interventions to contact relevant individuals and organizations for information about unpublished or ongoing studies (see MECIR Box 4.3.c). Letters of request for information can be used to identify completed but unpublished studies. One way of doing this is to send a comprehensive list of relevant articles along with the eligibility criteria for the review to the first author of reports of included studies, asking if they know of any additional studies (ongoing or completed; published or unpublished) that might be relevant. This approach may be especially useful in areas where there are few trials or a limited number of active research groups. It may also be desirable to send the same letter to other experts and pharmaceutical companies or others with an interest in the area. Some review teams set up websites for systematic review projects, listing the studies identified to date and inviting submission of information on studies not already listed.

MECIR Box 4.3.c Relevant expectations for conduct of intervention reviews	
C31: Searching by contacting relevant individuals and organizations (**Highly desirable**)	
Contact relevant individuals and organizations for information about unpublished or ongoing studies.	Searches for studies should be as extensive as possible in order to reduce the risk of publication bias and to identify as much relevant evidence as possible. It is important to identify ongoing studies, so that these can be assessed for possible inclusion when a review is updated.

Asking researchers for information about completed but never published studies has not always been found to be fruitful (Hetherington et al 1989, Horton 1997) though some researchers have reported that this is an important method for retrieving studies for systematic reviews (Royle and Milne 2003, Greenhalgh and Peacock 2005, Reveiz et al 2006). The RIAT (Restoring Invisible and Abandoned Trials) initiative (Doshi et al 2013) aims to address these problems by offering a methodology that allows others to re-publish mis-reported and to publish unreported trials. Anyone who can access the trial data and document trial abandonment can use this methodology. The RIAT Support Centre offers free-of-charge support and competitive funding to researchers interested in this approach. It has been suggested that legislation such as Freedom of Information Acts in various countries might be used to gain access to information about unpublished trials (Bennett and Jull 2003, MacLean et al 2003).

4.3.3 Trials registers and trials results registers

A recent study suggested that trials registers are an important source for identifying additional randomized trials (Baudard et al 2017). Cochrane Reviews of interventions should search relevant trials registers and repositories of results (see MECIR Box 4.3.d). Although there are many other trials registers, ClinicalTrials.gov and the WHO International Clinical Trials Registry Platform (ICTRP) portal (Pansieri et al 2017) are considered to be the most important for searching to identify studies for a systematic review. Research has shown that even though ClinicalTrials.gov is included in the WHO ICTRP Search Portal, not all ClinicalTrials.gov records can be successfully retrieved via searches of the ICTRP Search Portal (Glanville et al 2014, Knelangen et al 2018). Therefore, it is not sufficient to search the ICTRP alone. Guidance for searching these and other trials registers is provided in the online Technical Supplement.

In addition to Cochrane, other organizations such as the Agency for Healthcare Research and Quality (AHRQ) (Agency for Healthcare Research and Quality 2014) and the US Institute of Medicine (Institute of Medicine 2011) also advocate searching trials registers.

MECIR Box 4.3.d Relevant expectations for conduct of intervention reviews

C27: Searching trials registers (**Mandatory**)

Search trials registers and repositories of results, where relevant to the topic, through ClinicalTrials.gov, the WHO International Clinical Trials Registry Platform (ICTRP) portal and other sources as appropriate.	Searches for studies should be as extensive as possible in order to reduce the risk of publication bias and to identify as much relevant evidence as possible. Although ClinicalTrials.gov is included as one of the registers within the WHO ICTRP portal, it is recommended that both ClinicalTrials.gov and the ICTRP portal are searched separately due to additional features in ClinicalTrials.gov.

There has been an increasing acceptance by investigators of the importance of registering trials at inception and providing access to their trials results. Despite perceptions and even assertions to the contrary, however, there is no global, universal legal requirement to register clinical trials at inception or at any other stage in the process, although some countries are beginning to introduce such legislation (Viergever and Li 2015).

Efforts have been made by a number of organizations, including organizations representing the pharmaceutical industry and individual pharmaceutical companies, to begin to provide central access to ongoing trials and in some cases trial results on completion, either on a national or international basis. A recent audit of pharmaceutical companies' policies on access to trial data, results and methods, however, showed that the commitments made by companies to transparency of trials were highly variable (Goldacre et al 2017). Increasingly, as already noted, trials registers such as ClinicalTrials.gov also contain the results of completed trials, not just simply listing the details of the trial.

4.3.4 Regulatory agency sources and clinical study reports

Potentially relevant regulatory agency sources include the EU Clinical Trials Register, Drugs@FDA and OpenTrialsFDA. Details of these are provided in the online Technical Supplement. Clinical study reports (CSRs) are the reports of clinical trials providing detailed information on the methods and results of clinical trials submitted in support of marketing authorization applications. In late 2010, the European Medicines Agency (EMA) began releasing CSRs (on request) under their Policy 0043. In October 2016, they began to release CSRs under their Policy 0070. The policy applies only to documents received since 1 January 2015. The terms of use for access are based on the purposes to which the clinical data will be put.

A recent study by Jefferson and colleagues (Jefferson et al 2018) that looked at use of regulatory documents in Cochrane Reviews, found that understanding within the Cochrane community was limited and guidance and support would be required if review authors were to engage with regulatory documents as a source of evidence. Specifically, guidance on how to use data from regulatory sources is needed. For more information about using CSRs, see the online Technical Supplement. Further guidance on collecting data from CSRs is provided in Chapter 5, Section 5.5.6.

4.3.5 Other sources

The online Technical Supplement describes several other important sources of reports of studies. The term 'grey literature' is often used to refer to reports published outside of traditional commercial publishing. Review authors should generally search sources such as dissertations and conference abstracts (see MECIR Box 4.3.e).

Review authors may also consider searching the internet, handsearching of journals and searching full texts of journals electronically where available (see online Technical Supplement for details). They should examine previous reviews on the same topic and check reference lists of included studies and relevant systematic reviews (see MECIR Box 4.3.e).

MECIR Box 4.3.e Relevant expectations for conduct of intervention reviews

C28: Searching for grey literature (**Highly desirable**)

Search relevant grey literature sources such as reports, dissertations, theses, databases and databases of conference abstracts.	Searches for studies should be as extensive as possible in order to reduce the risk of publication bias and to identify as much relevant evidence as possible.

C29: Searching within other reviews (**Highly desirable**)

Search within previous reviews on the same topic.	Searches for studies should be as extensive as possible in order to reduce the risk of publication bias and to identify as much relevant evidence as possible.

C30: Searching reference lists (**Mandatory**)

Check reference lists in included studies and any relevant systematic reviews identified.	Searches for studies should be as extensive as possible in order to reduce the risk of publication bias and to identify as much relevant evidence as possible.

4.4 Designing search strategies

4.4.1 Introduction to search strategies

This section highlights some of the issues to consider when designing search strategies. Designing search strategies can be complex and the section does not fully address the many complexities in this area. Review teams will benefit from the skills and expertise of a medical/healthcare librarian or information specialist. Many of the issues highlighted relate to both the subject aspects of the search (e.g. the PICO elements) and to the study method (e.g. randomized trials). For a search to be robust, both aspects require attention to be sure that relevant records are not missed.

Issues to consider in planning a search include:

- the nature or type of the intervention(s) being assessed;
- the complexity of the review question and the need to consider additional conceptual frameworks (see Chapters 3 and 17);
- the time period when any evaluations of the interventions may have taken place (as specified in the review protocol) (see Section 4.4.5);
- any geographic considerations, such as the need to search the African Index Medicus for studies relating to African populations or the Chinese literature for studies in Chinese herbal medicine (see online Technical Supplement);
- whether the review is limited to randomized trials or other study designs are eligible (see Chapter 24);
- whether a validated methodological search filter (for specific study designs) is available (see Section 4.4.7);
- whether unpublished data are to be sought specifically (see Sections 4.3.2, 4.3.3 and 4.3.4); and

MECIR Box 4.4.a Relevant expectations for conduct of intervention reviews	
C26: Searching for different types of evidence (**Mandatory**)	
If the review has specific eligibility criteria around study design to address adverse effects, economic issues or qualitative research questions, undertake searches to address them.	Sometimes different searches will be conducted for different types of evidence, such as for non-randomized studies for addressing adverse effects, or for economic evaluation studies.

- whether the review has specific eligibility criteria around study design to address adverse effects (see Chapter 19), economic issues (see Chapter 20) or qualitative research questions (see Chapter 21), in which case searches to address these criteria should be undertaken (see MECIR Box 4.4.a).

Further evidence-based information about designing search strategies can be found on the SuRe Info portal, which is updated twice per year.

4.4.2 Structure of a search strategy

The starting point for developing a search strategy is to consider the main concepts being examined in a review. This is often referred to as PICO – that is Patient (or Participant or Population or Problem), Intervention, Comparison and Outcomes (Richardson et al 1995): see also Chapters 2 and 3 for guidance on developing and refining PICO definitions that will be operationalized in the search strategy. Examples are provided in the appendices to the Cochrane Information Specialists' Handbook (Littlewood et al 2017). For a Cochrane Review, the review objective should provide the PICO concepts, and the eligibility criteria for studies to be included will further assist in the selection of appropriate subject headings and text words for the search strategy.

The structure of search strategies in bibliographic databases should be informed by the main concepts of the review (see Chapter 3), using appropriate elements from PICO and study design (see MECIR Box 4.4.b). It is usually unnecessary, however, and may even be undesirable, to search on every aspect of the review's clinical question. Although a research question may specify particular comparators or outcomes, these concepts may not be well described in the title or abstract of an article and are often not well indexed with controlled vocabulary terms. Therefore, in general databases, such as MEDLINE, a search strategy will typically have three sets of terms: (i) terms to search for the health condition of interest, i.e. the population; (ii) terms to search for the intervention(s) evaluated; and (iii) terms to search for the types of study design to be included. Typically, a broad set of search terms will be gathered for each concept, and combined with the OR Boolean operator to achieve sensitivity within concepts. The results for each concept are then combined using the AND Boolean operator, to ensure each concept is represented in the final search results.

It is important to consider the structure of the search strategy on a question-by-question basis. In some cases it is possible and reasonable to search for the

MECIR Box 4.4.b Relevant expectations for conduct of intervention reviews	
C32: Structuring search strategies for bibliographic databases (**Mandatory**)	
Inform the structure of search strategies in bibliographic databases around the main concepts of the review, using appropriate elements from PICO and study design. In structuring the search, maximize sensitivity whilst striving for reasonable precision. Ensure correct use of the 'AND' and 'OR' operators.	Inappropriate or inadequate search strategies may fail to identify records that are included in bibliographic databases. Expertise may need to be sought, in particular from the CRG's Information Specialist. The structure of a search strategy should be based on the main concepts being examined in a review. In general databases, such as MEDLINE, a search strategy to identify studies for a Cochrane Review will typically have three sets of terms: (i) terms to search for the health condition of interest, i.e. the population; (ii) terms to search for the intervention(s) evaluated; and (iii) terms to search for the types of study design to be included (typically a 'filter' for randomized trials). There are exceptions, however. For instance, for reviews of complex interventions, it may be necessary to search only for the population or the intervention. Within each concept, terms are joined together with the Boolean 'OR' operator, and the concepts are combined with the Boolean 'AND' operator. The 'NOT' operator should be avoided where possible to avoid the danger of inadvertently removing records that are relevant from the search set.

comparator, for example if the comparator is explicitly placebo; in other cases the outcomes may be particularly well defined and consistently reported in abstracts. The advice on whether or not to search for outcomes for adverse effects differs from the advice given earlier (see Chapter 19).

Some search strategies may not easily divide into the structure suggested, particularly for reviews addressing complex or unknown interventions, or diagnostic tests (Huang et al 2006, Irvin and Hayden 2006, Petticrew and Roberts 2006, de Vet et al 2008, Booth 2016). Cochrane Reviews of public health interventions and of qualitative data may adopt very different search approaches to those described here (Lorenc et al 2014, Booth 2016) (see Chapter 17 on complex and public health interventions, and Chapter 21 on qualitative research). Some options to explore for such situations include:

- use a single concept such as searching for the intervention alone (European Food Safety Authority 2010);
- break a concept into two or more subconcepts;
- use a multi-stranded or multi-faceted approach that uses a series of searches, with different combinations of concepts, to capture a complex research question (Lefebvre et al 2013);
- use a variety of different search approaches to compensate for when a specific concept is difficult to define (Shemilt et al 2014); or
- use citation searching on key papers in addition to a database search (Haddaway et al 2015, Hinde and Spackman 2015) (see online Technical Supplement).

4.4.3 Sensitivity versus precision

Searches for systematic reviews aim to be as extensive as possible in order to ensure that as many of the relevant studies as possible are included in the review. It is, however, necessary to strike a balance between striving for comprehensiveness and maintaining relevance when developing a search strategy.

The properties of searches are often quantified using 'sensitivity' (also called 'recall') and 'precision' (see Table 4.4.a). Sensitivity is defined as the number of relevant reports identified divided by the total number of relevant reports in the resource. Precision is defined as the number of relevant reports identified divided by the total number of reports identified. Increasing the comprehensiveness (or sensitivity) of a search will reduce its precision and will usually retrieve more non-relevant reports.

Searches for Cochrane Reviews should seek to maximize sensitivity whilst striving for reasonable precision (see MECIR Box 4.4.b). Article abstracts identified through a database search can usually be screened very quickly to ascertain potential relevance. At a conservatively estimated reading rate of one or two abstracts per minute, the results of a database search can be screened at the rate of 60–120 per hour (or approximately 500–1000 over an 8-hour period), so the high yield and low precision associated with systematic review searching may not be as daunting as it might at first appear in comparison with the total time to be invested in the review.

Table 4.4.a Sensitivity and precision of a search

	Reports retrieved	Reports not retrieved
Relevant reports	Relevant reports retrieved (a)	Relevant reports not retrieved (b)
Irrelevant reports	Irrelevant reports retrieved (c)	Irrelevant reports not retrieved (d)

Sensitivity: fraction of relevant reports retrieved from all relevant reports (a/(a+b))
Precision: fraction of relevant reports retrieved from all reports retrieved (a/(a+c))

4.4.4 Controlled vocabulary and text words

MEDLINE and Embase (and many other databases) can be searched using a combination of two retrieval approaches. One is based on text words, that is terms occurring in the title, abstract or other relevant fields available in the database. The other is based on standardized subject terms assigned to the references by indexers (specialists who appraise the articles and describe their topics by assigning terms from a specific thesaurus or controlled vocabulary). Searches for Cochrane Reviews should use an appropriate combination of these two approaches (see MECIR Box 4.4.c). Approaches for identifying text words and controlled vocabulary to combine appropriately within a search strategy, including text mining approaches, are presented in the online Technical Supplement.

4.4.5 Language, date and document format restrictions

Searches should capture as many studies as possible that meet the eligibility criteria, ensuring that relevant time periods and sources are covered and not restricted by language or publication status (see MECIR Box 4.3.a). Review authors should justify the use of any restrictions in the search strategy on publication date and publication format

MECIR Box 4.4.c Relevant expectations for conduct of intervention reviews	
C33: Developing search strategies for bibliographic databases (**Mandatory**)	
Identify appropriate controlled vocabulary (e.g. MeSH, Emtree, including 'exploded' terms) and free-text terms (considering, for example, spelling variants, synonyms, acronyms, truncation and proximity operators).	Inappropriate or inadequate search strategies may fail to identify records that are included in bibliographic databases. Search strategies need to be customized for each database. It is important that MeSH terms are 'exploded' wherever appropriate, in order not to miss relevant articles. The same principle applies to Emtree when searching Embase and also to a number of other databases. The controlled vocabulary search terms for MEDLINE and Embase are not identical, and neither is the approach to indexing. In order to be as comprehensive as possible, it is necessary to include a wide range of free-text terms for each of the concepts selected. This might include the use of truncation and wildcards. Developing a search strategy is an iterative process in which the terms that are used are modified, based on what has already been retrieved.

MECIR Box 4.4.d Relevant expectations for conduct of intervention reviews	
C35: Restricting database searches (**Mandatory**)	
Justify the use of any restrictions in the search strategy on publication date and publication format.	Date restrictions in the search should only be used when there are date restrictions in the eligibility criteria for studies. They should be applied only if it is known that relevant studies could only have been reported during a specific time period, for example if the intervention was only available after a certain time point. Searches for updates to reviews might naturally be restricted by date of entry into the database (rather than date of publication) to avoid duplication of effort. Publication format restrictions (e.g. exclusion of letters) should generally not be used in Cochrane Reviews, since any information about an eligible study may be of value.

(see MECIR Box 4.4.d). For example, excluding letters is not recommended because letters may contain important additional information relating to an earlier trial report or new information about a trial not reported elsewhere (Iansavichene et al 2008). In addition, articles indexed as 'Comments' should not be routinely excluded without further examination as these may contain early warnings of suspected fraud (see Section 4.4.6).

Evidence indicates that excluding non-English studies does not change the conclusions of most systematic reviews (Morrison et al 2012, Jiao et al 2013, Hartling et al 2017), although exceptions have been observed for complementary and alternative medicine (Moher et al 2003, Pham et al 2005, Wu et al 2013). There is, however, also research related to language bias that supports the inclusion of non-English studies in systematic reviews (Egger et al 1997). For further discussion of these issues see Chapter 13.

Inclusion of non-English studies may also increase the precision of the result and the generalizability and applicability of the findings. There may be differences in therapeutic response to pharmaceutical agents according to ethnicity, either because of phenotype and pathogenesis of disease due to environmental factors or because of population pharmacogenomics and pharmacogenetics (Brusselle and Blasi 2015). The inclusion of non-English studies also makes it possible to perform sensitivity analyses to find out if there is any geographical bias in reporting the positive findings (Vickers et al 1998, Kaptchuk 1999). It also could be an indicator of quality of systematic reviews (Wang et al 2015).

Limiting searching to databases containing predominantly English-language records, even if no language restrictions are applied, may result in missed relevant studies

(Pilkington et al 2005). Review authors should, therefore, attempt to identify and assess for eligibility all possibly relevant reports of trials irrespective of language of publication. If a Cochrane Review team requires help with translation of and/or data extraction from non-English language reports of studies, they should seek assistance to do so (this is a common task for which volunteer assistance can be sought via Cochrane's TaskExchange platform, accessible to both Cochrane and non-Cochrane review teams). Where it is not possible to extract the relevant information and data from non-English language reports, the review team should file the study in 'Studies Awaiting Classification' rather than 'Excluded Studies', to inform readers of the review of the availability of other possibly relevant reports and reflect this information in the PRISMA flow diagram (or, if there is no flow diagram, then in the text of the review) as 'Studies Awaiting Classification'.

4.4.6 Identifying fraudulent studies, other retracted publications, errata and comments

When considering the eligibility of studies for inclusion in a Cochrane Review, it is important to be aware that some studies may have been found to contain errors or to be fraudulent or may, for other reasons, have been corrected or retracted since publication. Review authors should examine any relevant retraction statements and errata for information (MECIR Box 4.4.e). This applies both to 'new' studies identified for inclusion in a review and to studies that are already included in a review when the review is updated. For review updates, it is important to search MEDLINE and Embase for the latest version of the citations to the records for the (previously) included studies, in case they have since been corrected or retracted.

Errata are published to correct unintended errors (accepted as errors by the author(s)). Retraction notices are published (usually by the journal editor) where data have been found to be fraudulent, for example in the case of plagiarism. Comments are published under a range of circumstances including when errors are suggested by others and also for early concerns regarding fraud.

MECIR Box 4.4.e Relevant expectations for conduct of intervention reviews	
C48: Examining errata (**Mandatory**)	
Examine any relevant retraction statements and errata for information.	Some studies may have been found to be fraudulent or may have been retracted since publication for other reasons. Errata can reveal important limitations, or even fatal flaws, in included studies. All of these may lead to the potential exclusion of a study from a review or meta-analysis. Care should be taken to ensure that this information is retrieved in all database searches by downloading the appropriate fields, together with the citation data.

Including data from studies that are fraudulent or studies that include errors can have an impact on the overall estimates in systematic reviews. Details of how to identify fraudulent studies, other retracted publications, errata and comments are described in the online Technical Supplement.

4.4.7 Search filters

Search filters are search strategies that are designed to retrieve specific types of records, such as those of a particular methodological design. When searching for randomized trials in humans, a validated filter should be used to identify studies with the appropriate design (see MECIR Box 4.4.f). Filters to identify randomized trials have been developed specifically for MEDLINE and Embase: see the online Technical Supplement for details. CENTRAL, however, aims to contain only reports with study designs possibly relevant for inclusion in Cochrane Reviews, so searches of CENTRAL should not use a trials 'filter' or be limited to human studies.

The InterTASC Information Specialists' Subgroup Search Filter Resource offers a collection of search filters, focusing predominantly on methodological search filters and providing critical appraisals of some of these filters. The site includes, amongst others, filters for identifying systematic reviews, randomized and non-randomized studies and qualitative research in a range of databases and across a range of service providers (Glanville et al 2019). For further discussion around the design and use of search filters, see the online Technical Supplement.

4.4.8 Peer review of search strategies

It is strongly recommended that search strategies should be peer reviewed. Peer review of search strategies is increasingly recognized as a necessary step in designing and executing high-quality search strategies to identify studies for possible inclusion in systematic reviews. Studies have shown that errors occur in the search strategies

MECIR Box 4.4.f Relevant expectations for conduct of intervention reviews	
C34: Using search filters (**Highly desirable**)	
Use specially designed and tested search filters where appropriate including the Cochrane Highly Sensitive Search Strategies for identifying randomized trials in MEDLINE, but do not use filters in pre-filtered databases e.g. do not use a randomized trial filter in CENTRAL or a systematic review filter in DARE.	Inappropriate or inadequate search strategies may fail to identify records that are included in bibliographic databases. Search filters should be used with caution. They should be assessed not only for the reliability of their development and reported performance, but also for their current accuracy, relevance and effectiveness given the frequent interface and indexing changes affecting databases.

underpinning systematic reviews (Sampson and McGowan 2006) and that search strategies are not always conducted or reported to a high standard (Mullins et al 2014, Layton 2017). An evidence-based checklist such as the PRESS Evidence-Based Checklist should be used to assess which elements are important in peer review of electronic search strategies (McGowan et al 2016a, McGowan et al 2016b). The checklist covers not only the technical accuracy of the strategy (line numbers, spellings, etc), but also that the search strategy covers all relevant aspects of the protocol and has interpreted the research question appropriately. Research has shown that peer review using a specially designed checklist can improve the quality of searches (Relevo and Paynter 2012, Spry et al 2013). The names, credentials and institutions of the peer reviewers of the search strategies should be noted in the review (with their permission) in the Acknowledgements section.

4.4.9 Alerts

Alerts, also called literature surveillance services, 'push' services or SDIs (selective dissemination of information), are an excellent method of staying up to date with the medical literature currently being published, as a supplement to designing and running specific searches for specific reviews. In practice, alerts are based on a previously developed search strategy, which is saved in a personal account on the database platform (e.g. 'My EBSCOhost – search alerts' on EBSCO, 'My searches & alerts' on Ovid and 'MyNCBI – saved searches' on PubMed). These saved strategies filter the content as the database is being updated with new information. The account owner is notified (usually via email) when new publications meeting their specified search parameters are added to the database. In the case of PubMed, the alert can be set up to be delivered weekly or monthly, or in real-time and can comprise email or RSS feeds.

For review authors, alerts are a useful tool to help monitor what is being published in their review topic after the original search has been conducted. By following the alert, authors can become aware of a new study that meets the review's eligibility criteria, and decide either to include it in the review immediately or mention it as a 'study awaiting assessment' for inclusion during the next review update (see online Chapter IV). Authors should consider setting up alerts so that the review can be as current as possible at the time of publication.

Another way of attempting to stay current with the literature as it emerges is by using alerts based on journal tables of contents (TOCs). These usually cannot be specifically tailored to the information needs in the same way as search strategies developed to cover a specific topic. They can, however, be a good way of trying to keep up to date on a more general level by monitoring what is currently being published in journals of interest. Many journals, even those that are available by subscription only, offer TOC alert services free of charge. In addition, a number of publishers and organizations offer TOC services (see online Technical Supplement). Use of TOCs is not proposed as a single alternative to the various other methods of study identification necessary for undertaking systematic reviews, rather as a supplementary method. (See also Chapter 22, Section 22.2 for a discussion of new technologies to support evidence surveillance in the context of 'living' systematic reviews.)

4.4.10 Timing of searches

The published review should be as up to date as possible. Searches for all the relevant databases should be rerun prior to publication, if the initial search date is more than 12 months (preferably six months) from the intended publication date (see MECIR Box 4.4.g). This is also good practice for searches of non-database sources. The results should also be screened to identify potentially eligible studies. Ideally, the studies should be incorporated fully in the review. If not, then the potentially eligible studies will need to be reported as references under 'Studies awaiting classification' (or under 'Ongoing studies' if they are not yet completed).

4.4.11 When to stop searching

Developing a search is often an iterative and exploratory process. It involves exploring trade-offs between search terms and assessing their overall impact on the sensitivity and precision of the search. It is often difficult to decide in a scientific or objective way when a search is complete and search strategy development can stop. The ability to decide when to stop typically develops through experience of developing many strategies. Suggestions for stopping rules have been made around the retrieval of new records, for example to stop if adding in a series of new terms to a database search strategy yields no new relevant records, or if precision falls below a particular

MECIR Box 4.4.g Relevant expectations for conduct of intervention reviews	
C37: Rerunning searches (**Mandatory**)	
Rerun or update searches for all relevant databases within 12 months before publication of the review or review update, and screen the results for potentially eligible studies.	The published review should be as up to date as possible. The search must be rerun close to publication, if the initial search date is more than 12 months (preferably six months) from the intended publication date, and the results screened for potentially eligible studies. Ideally, the studies should be incorporated fully in the review. If not, then the potentially eligible studies will need to be reported, at a minimum as a reference under 'Studies awaiting classification' (or 'Ongoing studies' if they have not yet completed).
C38: Incorporating findings from rerun searches (**Highly desirable**)	
Fully incorporate any studies identified in the rerun or update of the search within 12 months before publication of the review or review update.	The published review should be as up to date as possible. After the rerun of the search, the decision whether to incorporate any new studies fully into the review will need to be balanced against the delay in publication.

cut-off (Chilcott et al 2003). Stopping might also be appropriate when the removal of terms or concepts results in missing relevant records. Another consideration is the amount of evidence that has already accrued: in topics where evidence is scarce, authors might need to be more cautious about deciding when to stop searching. Although many methods have been described to assist with deciding when to stop developing the search, there has been little formal evaluation of the approaches (Booth 2010, Wood and Arber 2019).

At a basic level, investigation is needed as to whether a strategy is performing adequately. One simple test is to check whether the search is finding the publications that have been recommended as key publications or that have been included in other similar reviews (EUnetHTA 2017). It is not enough, however, for the strategy to find only those records, otherwise this might be a sign that the strategy is biased towards known studies and other relevant records might be being missed. In addition, citation searches and reference checking are useful checks of strategy performance. If those additional methods are finding documents that the searches have already retrieved, but that the team did not necessarily know about in advance, then this is one sign that the strategy might be performing adequately. Also, an evidence-based checklist such as the PRESS Evidence-Based Checklist (McGowan et al 2016b) should be used to assess whether the search strategy is adequate (see Section 4.4.8). If some of the PRESS dimensions seem to be missing without adequate explanation or arouse concerns, then the search may not yet be complete.

Statistical techniques can be used to assess performance, such as capture-recapture (Spoor et al 1996) (also known as capture-mark-recapture; Kastner et al 2009), or the relative recall technique (Sampson et al 2006, Sampson and McGowan 2011). Kastner suggests the capture-mark-recapture technique merits further investigation since it could be used to estimate the number of studies in a literature prospectively and to determine where to stop searches once suitable cut-off levels have been identified. Kastner's approach involves searching databases, conducting record selection, calculating capture-mark-recapture and then making decisions about whether further searches are necessary. This would entail potentially an iterative search and selection process. Capture-recapture needs results from at least two searches to estimate the number of missed studies. Further investigation of published prospective techniques seems warranted to learn more about the potential benefits.

Relative recall (Sampson et al 2006, Sampson and McGowan 2011) requires a range of searches to have been conducted so that the relevant studies have been built up by a set of sensitive searches. The performance of the individual searches can then be assessed in each individual database by determining how many of the studies that were deemed eligible for the evidence synthesis and were indexed within a database, can be found by the database search used to populate the synthesis. If a search in a database did not perform well and missed many studies, then that search strategy is likely to have been suboptimal. If the search strategy found most of the studies that were available to be found in the database then it was likely to have been a sensitive strategy. Assessments of precision could also be made, but these mostly inform future search approaches since they cannot affect the searches and record assessment already undertaken. Relative recall may be most useful at the end of the search process since it relies on the achievement of several searches to make judgements about the overall performance of strategies.

In evidence synthesis involving qualitative data, searching is often more organic and intertwined with the analysis such that the searching stops when new information ceases to be identified (Booth 2016). The reasons for stopping need to be documented and it is suggested that explanations or justifications for stopping may centre around saturation (Booth 2016). Further information on searches for qualitative evidence can be found in Chapter 21.

4.5 Documenting and reporting the search process

Review authors should document the search process in enough detail to ensure that it can be reported correctly in the review (see MECIR Box 4.5.a). The searches of all the databases should be reproducible to the extent that this is possible. By documenting the search process, we refer to internal record-keeping, which is distinct from reporting the search process in the review (discussed in online Chapter III).

Medical/healthcare librarians and information specialists involved with the review should draft, or at least comment on, the search strategy sections of the review prior to publication.

There is currently no clear consensus regarding optimum reporting of systematic review search methods, although suboptimal reporting of commonly recommended items has been observed (Sampson et al 2008, Roundtree et al 2009, Niederstadt and Droste 2010). Research has also shown a lack of compliance with guidance in the *Handbook* with respect to search strategy description in published Cochrane Reviews (Sampson and McGowan 2006, Yoshii et al 2009, Franco et al 2018). The PRISMA-Search (PRISMA-S) Extension, an extension to the PRISMA Statement, addressing the reporting of search strategies in systematic reviews, should go some way to addressing this, as should the major revision of PRISMA itself, which is due to report in 2019.

It is recommended that review authors seek guidance from their medical/healthcare librarian or information specialist at the earliest opportunity with respect to documenting the search process. For Cochrane Reviews, the bibliographic database search strategies should be copied and pasted into an appendix exactly as run and in full, together with the search set numbers and the total number of records retrieved by each search

MECIR Box 4.5.a Relevant expectations for conduct of intervention reviews	
C36: Documenting the search process (**Mandatory**)	
Document the search process in enough detail to ensure that it can be reported correctly in the review.	The search process (including the sources searched, when, by whom, and using which terms) needs to be documented in enough detail throughout the process to ensure that it can be reported correctly in the review, to the extent that all the searches of all the databases are reproducible.

strategy. The search strategies should not be re-typed, because this can introduce errors. The same process is also good practice for searches of trials registers and other sources, where the interface used, such as introductory or advanced, should also be specified. Creating a report of the search process can be accomplished through methodical documentation of the steps taken by the searcher. This need not be onerous if suitable record keeping is performed during the process of the search, but it can be nearly impossible to recreate post hoc. Many database interfaces have facilities for search strategies to be saved online or to be emailed; an offline copy in text format should also be saved. For some databases, taking and saving a screenshot of the search may be the most practical approach (Rader et al 2014).

Documenting the searching of sources other than databases, including the search terms used, is also required if searches are to be reproducible (Atkinson et al 2015, Chow 2015, Witkowski and Aldhouse 2015). Details about contacting experts or manufacturers, searching reference lists, scanning websites, and decisions about search iterations can be kept internally for future updates or external requests and can be reproduced as an appendix in the final document. Since the purpose of search documentation is to support transparency, internal assessment, and reference for any future update, it is important to plan how to record searching of sources other than databases since some activities (contacting experts, reference list searching, and forward citation searching) will occur later on in the review process after the database results have been screened (Rader et al 2014). The searcher should record any correspondence on key decisions and report a summary of this correspondence alongside the search strategy. The narrative describes the major decisions that shaped the strategy and can give a peer reviewer an insight into the rationale for the search approach (Craven and Levay 2011).

It is particularly important to save locally or file print copies of any information found on the internet, such as information about ongoing and/or unpublished trials, as this information may no longer be accessible at the time the review is written. Local copies should be stored in a structured way to allow retrieval when needed. There are also web-based tools which archive webpage content for future reference, such as WebCite (Eysenbach and Trudel 2005). The results of web searches will not be reproducible to the same extent as bibliographic database searches because web content and search engine algorithms frequently change, and search results can differ between users due to a general move towards localization and personalization. It is still important, however, to document the search process to ensure that the methods used can be transparently reported (Briscoe 2018). In cases where a search engine retrieves more results than it is practical to screen in full (it is rarely practical to search thousands of web results, as the precision of web searches is likely to be relatively low), the number of results that are documented and reported should be the number that were screened rather than the total number (Dellavalle et al 2003, Bramer 2016).

Decisions should be documented for all records identified by the search. Details of the flow of studies from the number(s) of references identified in the search to the number of studies included in the review will need to be reported in the final review, ideally using a flow diagram such as that proposed by PRISMA (see online Chapter III); these can be generated using software including Covidence, DistillerSR, EPPI-Reviewer, the METAGEAR package for R, the PRISMA Flow Diagram Generator, and RevMan. A table of 'Characteristics of excluded studies' will also need to be presented (see Section 4.6.5). Numbers of records are sufficient for exclusions based on initial screening of titles and abstracts. Broad categorizations are sufficient for records classed as potentially eligible during an initial screen of the full text. Authors will need to decide for each review when to map records to studies (if multiple records refer to one study). The flow diagram records initially the total number of records retrieved from various sources, then the total number of studies to which these records relate. Review authors need to match the various records to the various studies in order to complete the flow diagram correctly. Lists of included and excluded studies must be based on studies rather than records (see also Section 4.6.1).

4.6 Selecting studies

4.6.1 Studies (not reports) as the unit of interest

A Cochrane Review is a review of studies that meet pre-specified eligibility criteria. Since each study may have been reported in several articles, abstracts or other reports, an extensive search for studies for the review may identify many reports for each potentially relevant study. Two distinct processes are therefore required to determine which studies can be included in the review. One is to link together multiple reports of the same study; and the other is to use the information available in the various reports to determine which studies are eligible for inclusion. Although sometimes there is a single report for each study, it should never be assumed that this is the case.

As well as the studies that inform the systematic review, other studies will also be identified and these should be recorded or tagged as they are encountered, so that they can be listed in the relevant tables in the review:

- records of ongoing trials for which results (either published or unpublished) are not (yet) available; and
- records of studies which seem to be eligible but for which data are incomplete or the publication related to the record could not be obtained.

4.6.2 Identifying multiple reports from the same study

Duplicate publication can introduce substantial biases if studies are inadvertently included more than once in a meta-analysis (Tramèr et al 1997). Duplicate publication can take various forms, ranging from identical manuscripts to reports describing different outcomes of the study or results at different time points (von Elm et al 2004). The number of participants may differ in the different publications. It can be difficult to detect duplicate publication and some 'detective work' by the review authors may be required.

Some of the most useful criteria for comparing reports are:

- trial identification numbers (e.g. ClinicalTrials.gov Identifier (NCT number); ISRCTN; Universal Trial Number (UTN) (assigned by the ICTRP); other identifiers such as those from the sponsor);
- author names (most duplicate reports have one or more authors in common, although this is not always the case);

MECIR Box 4.6.a Relevant expectations for conduct of intervention reviews	
C42: Collating multiple reports (**Mandatory**)	
Collate multiple reports of the same study, so that each study, rather than each report, is the unit of interest in the review.	It is wrong to consider multiple reports of the same study as if they are multiple studies. Secondary reports of a study should not be discarded, however, since they may contain valuable information about the design and conduct. Review authors must choose and justify which report to use as a source for study results.

- location and setting (particularly if institutions, such as hospitals, are named);
- specific details of the interventions (e.g. dose, frequency);
- numbers of participants and baseline data; and
- date and duration of the study (which can also clarify whether different sample sizes are due to different periods of recruitment).

Where uncertainties remain after considering these and other factors, it may be necessary to correspond with the authors of the reports.

Multiple reports of the same study should be collated, so that each study, rather than each report, is the unit of interest in the review (see MECIR Box 4.6.a). Review authors will need to choose and justify which report (the primary report) to use as a source for study results, particularly if two reports include conflicting results. They should not discard other (secondary) reports, since they may contain additional outcome measures and valuable information about the design and conduct of the study.

4.6.3 A typical process for selecting studies

A typical process for selecting studies for inclusion in a review is as follows (the process should be detailed in the protocol for the review):

1) Merge search results from different sources using reference management software, and remove duplicate records of the same report (i.e. records reporting the same journal title, volume and pages).
2) **Examine titles and abstracts** to remove obviously irrelevant reports (authors should generally be over-inclusive at this stage).
3) Retrieve the full text of the potentially relevant reports.
4) Link together multiple reports of the same study (see Section 4.6.2).
5) **Examine full-text reports** for compliance of studies with eligibility criteria.
6) Correspond with investigators, where appropriate, to clarify study eligibility (it may be appropriate to request further information, such as missing methods information or results, at the same time). If studies remain incomplete/unobtainable they should be tagged/recorded as incomplete, and should be listed in the table of 'Studies awaiting assessment' in the review.
7) Make final decisions on study inclusion and proceed to data collection.

MECIR Box 4.6.b Relevant expectations for conduct of intervention reviews	
C40: Excluding studies without useable data (**Mandatory**)	
Include studies in the review irrespective of whether measured outcome data are reported in a 'usable' way.	Systematic reviews typically should seek to include all relevant participants who have been included in eligible study designs of the relevant interventions and had the outcomes of interest measured. Reviews must not exclude studies solely on the basis of reporting of the outcome data, since this may introduce bias due to selective outcome reporting and risk undermining the systematic review process. While such studies cannot be included in meta-analyses, the implications of their omission should be considered. Note that studies may legitimately be excluded because outcomes were not measured. Furthermore, issues may be different for adverse effects outcomes, since the pool of studies may be much larger and it can be difficult to assess whether such outcomes were measured.

8) Tag or record any ongoing trials which have not yet been reported so that they can be added to the ongoing studies table.

Note that studies should not be omitted from a review solely on the basis of measured outcome data not being reported (see MECIR Box 4.6.b and Chapter 13).

4.6.4 Implementation of the selection process

Decisions about which studies to include in a review are among the most influential decisions that are made in the review process and they involve judgement.

Use (at least) two people working independently to determine whether each study meets the eligibility criteria.

Ideally, screening of titles and abstracts to remove irrelevant reports should be done in duplicate by two people working independently (although it is acceptable that this initial screening of titles and abstracts is undertaken by only one person). It is essential, however, that two people working independently are used to make a final determination as to whether each study considered possibly eligible after title/abstract screening meets the eligibility criteria based on the full text of the study report(s) (see MECIR Box 4.6.c).

It has been shown that using at least two authors may reduce the possibility that relevant reports will be discarded (Edwards et al 2002) although other case reports

MECIR Box 4.6.c Relevant expectations for conduct of intervention reviews	
C39: Making inclusion decisions (**Mandatory**)	
Use (at least) two people working independently to determine whether each study meets the eligibility criteria, and define in advance the process for resolving disagreements.	Duplicating the study selection process reduces both the risk of making mistakes and the possibility that selection is influenced by a single person's biases. The inclusion decisions should be based on the full texts of potentially eligible studies when possible, usually after an initial screen of titles and abstracts. It is desirable, but not mandatory, that two people undertake this initial screening, working independently.

have suggested single screening approaches may be adequate (Doust et al 2005, Shemilt et al 2016). Opportunities for screening efficiencies seem likely to become available through promising developments in single human screening in combination with machine learning approaches (O'Mara-Eves et al 2015).

Experts in a particular area frequently have pre-formed opinions that can bias their assessment of both the relevance and validity of articles (Cooper and Ribble 1989, Oxman and Guyatt 1993). Thus, while it is important that at least one author is knowledgeable in the area under review, it may be an advantage to have a second author who is not a content expert.

Disagreements about whether a study should be included can generally be resolved by discussion. Often the cause of disagreement is a simple oversight on the part of one of the review authors. When the disagreement is due to a difference in interpretation, this may require arbitration by another person. Occasionally, it will not be possible to resolve disagreements about whether to include a study without additional information. In these cases, authors may choose to categorize the study in their review as one that is awaiting assessment until the additional information is obtained from the study authors.

A single failed eligibility criterion is sufficient for a study to be excluded from a review. In practice, therefore, eligibility criteria for each study should be assessed in order of importance, so that the first 'no' response can be used as the primary reason for exclusion of the study, and the remaining criteria need not be assessed. The eligibility criteria order may be different in different reviews and they do not always need to be the same.

For most reviews it will be worthwhile to pilot test the eligibility criteria on a sample of reports (say six to eight articles, including ones that are thought to be definitely eligible, definitely not eligible and doubtful). The pilot test can be used to refine and clarify the eligibility criteria, train the people who will be applying them and ensure that the criteria can be applied consistently by more than one person.

For Cochrane Reviews the selection process must be documented in sufficient detail to be able to complete a flow diagram and a table of 'Characteristics of excluded studies' (see MECIR Box 4.6.d). During the selection process it is crucial to keep track of the

MECIR Box 4.6.d Relevant expectations for conduct of intervention reviews	
C41: Documenting decisions about records identified (**Mandatory**)	
Document the selection process in sufficient detail to be able to complete a flow diagram and a table of 'Characteristics of excluded studies'.	Decisions should be documented for all records identified by the search. Numbers of records are sufficient for exclusions based on initial screening of titles and abstracts. Broad categorizations are sufficient for records classed as potentially eligible during an initial screen. Studies listed in the table of 'Characteristics of excluded studies' should be those that a user might reasonably expect to find in the review. At least one explicit reason for their exclusion must be documented. Authors will need to decide for each review when to map records to studies (if multiple records refer to one study). Lists of included and excluded studies must be based on studies rather than records.

number of references and subsequently the number of studies so that a flow diagram can be constructed. The decision and reasons for exclusion can be tracked using reference software, a simple document or spreadsheet, or using specialist systematic review software (see Section 4.6.6.1).

4.6.5 Selecting 'excluded studies'

A Cochrane Review includes a list of excluded studies called 'Characteristics of excluded studies', detailing the specific reason for exclusion for any studies that a reader might plausibly expect to see among the included studies. This covers all studies that may, on the surface, appear to meet the eligibility criteria but which, on further inspection, do not. It also covers those that do not meet all of the criteria but are well known and likely to be thought relevant by some readers. By listing such studies as excluded and giving the primary reason for exclusion, the review authors can show that consideration has been given to these studies. The list of excluded studies should be as brief as possible. It should not list all of the reports that were identified by an extensive search. It should not list studies that obviously do not fulfil the eligibility criteria for the review, such as 'Types of studies', 'Types of participants', and 'Types of interventions'. In particular, it should not list studies that are obviously not randomized if the review includes only randomized trials. Based on a (recent) sample of approximately 60% of the intervention reviews in The Cochrane Library which included randomized trials (only), the average number of studies listed in the 'excluded studies' table is 30.

4.6.6 Software support for selecting studies

An extensive search for eligible studies in a systematic review can often identify thousands of records that need to be manually screened. Selecting studies from within these records can be a particularly time-consuming, laborious and logistically challenging aspect of conducting a systematic review. These and other challenges have led to the development of various software tools and packages that offer support for the selection process.

Broadly, software to support selecting studies can be classified as:

- systems that support the study selection process, typically involving multiple reviewers (see Section 4.6.6.1); and
- tools and techniques based on text mining and/or machine learning, which aim to semi- or fully-automate the selection process (see Section 4.6.6.2).

Software to support the selection process, along with other stages of a systematic review, including text mining tools, can be identified using the Systematic Review Toolbox. The SR Toolbox is a community driven, web-based catalogue of tools that provide support for systematic reviews (Marshall and Brereton 2015).

4.6.6.1 Software for managing the selection process

Managing the selection process can be challenging, particularly in a large-scale systematic review that involves multiple reviewers. Basic productivity tools can help (such as word processors, spreadsheets and reference management software), and several purpose-built systems are also available that offer support for the study selection process.

Examples of tools that support selecting studies include:

- **Abstrackr** – a free web-based screening tool that can prioritize the screening of records using machine learning techniques.
- **Covidence** – a web-based software platform for conducting systematic reviews, which includes support for collaborative title and abstract screening, full-text review, risk-of-bias assessment and data extraction. Full access to this system normally requires a paid subscription but is free for authors of Cochrane Reviews. A free trial for non-Cochrane review authors is also available.
- **DistillerSR** – a web-based software application for undertaking bibliographic record screening and data extraction. It has a number of management features to track progress, assess interrater reliability and export data for further analysis. Reduced pricing for Cochrane and Campbell reviews is available.
- **EPPI-Reviewer** – web-based software designed to support all stages of the systematic review process, including reference management, screening, risk of bias assessment, data extraction and synthesis. The system is free to use for Cochrane and Campbell reviews, otherwise it requires a paid subscription. A free trial is available.
- **Rayyan** – a web-based application for collaborative citation screening and full-text selection. The system is currently available free of charge (June 2018).

Compatibility with other software tools used in the review process (such as RevMan) may be a consideration when selecting a tool to support study selection.

Covidence and EPPI-Reviewer are Cochrane-preferred tools, and are likely to have the strongest integration with RevMan.

4.6.6.2 Automating the selection process

Research into automating the study selection process through machine learning and text mining has received considerable attention over recent years, resulting in the development of various tools and techniques for reviewers to consider. The use of automated tools has the potential to reduce the workload involved with selecting studies significantly (Thomas et al 2017). For example, research suggests that adopting automation can reduce the need for manual screening by at least 30% and possibly more than 90%, although sometimes at the cost of up to a 5% reduction in sensitivity (O'Mara-Eves et al 2015).

Machine learning models (or 'classifiers') can be built where sufficient data are available. Of particular practical use to Cochrane Review authors is a classifier (the 'RCT Classifier') that can identify reports of randomized trials based on titles and abstracts. The classifier is highly accurate because it is built on a large dataset of hundreds of thousands of records screened by Cochrane Crowd, Cochrane's citizen science platform, where contributors help to identify and describe health research (Marshall et al 2018). Guidance on using the RCT Classifier in Cochrane Reviews, for example to exclude studies already flagged as not being randomized trials, or to access Cochrane Crowd to assist with screening, is available from the Cochrane Information Specialists' handbook (Littlewood et al 2017).

In addition to learning from large datasets such as those generated by Cochrane Crowd, it is also possible for machine learning models to learn how to apply eligibility criteria for individual reviews. This approach uses a process called 'active learning' and it is able to semi-automate study selection by continuously promoting records most likely to be relevant to the top of the results list (O'Mara-Eves et al 2015). It is difficult for authors to determine in advance when it is safe to stop screening and allow some records to be eliminated automatically without manual assessment. The automatic elimination of records using this approach has not been recommended for use in Cochrane Reviews at the time of writing. This active learning process can still be useful, however, since by prioritizing records for screening in order of relevance, it enables authors to identify the studies that are most likely to be included much earlier in the screening process than would otherwise be possible. A number of software tools support 'active learning' including:

- Abstrackr (http://abstrackr.cebm.brown.edu/);
- Colandr (https://www.colandrapp.com/);
- EPPI-Reviewer (http://eppi.ioe.ac.uk/);
- Rayyan (http://rayyan.qcri.org/);
- RobotAnalyst (http://nactem.ac.uk/robotanalyst/); and
- Swift-review (http://swift.sciome.com/swift-review/).

Finally, tools are available that use natural language processing to highlight sentences and key phrases automatically (e.g. PICO elements, trial characteristics, details of randomization) to support the reviewer whilst screening (Tsafnat et al 2014).

4.7 Chapter information

Authors: Carol Lefebvre, Julie Glanville, Simon Briscoe, Anne Littlewood, Chris Marshall, Maria-Inti Metzendorf, Anna Noel-Storr, Tamara Rader, Farhad Shokraneh, James Thomas, L. Susan Wieland; on behalf of the Cochrane Information Retrieval Methods Group

Acknowledgements: This chapter has been developed from sections of previous editions of the Cochrane Handbook co-authored since 1995 by Kay Dickersin, Julie Glanville, Kristen Larson, Carol Lefebvre and Eric Manheimer. Many of the sources listed in this chapter and the accompanying online Technical Supplement have been brought to our attention by a variety of people over the years and we should like to acknowledge this. We should like to acknowledge: Ruth Foxlee, (formerly) Information Specialist, Cochrane Editorial Unit; Miranda Cumpston, (formerly) Head of Learning & Support, Cochrane Central Executive; Colleen Finley, Product Manager, John Wiley and Sons, for checking sections relating to searching the Cochrane Library; the (UK) National Institute for Health and Care Excellence and the German Institute for Quality and Efficiency in Health Care (IQWiG) for support in identifying some of the references; the (US) Agency for Healthcare Research and Quality (AHRQ) Effective Healthcare Program Scientific Resource Center Article Alert service; Tianjing Li, Co-Convenor, Comparing Multiple Interventions Methods Group, for text and references that formed the basis of the re-drafting of parts of Section 4.6 Selecting studies; Lesley Gillespie, Cochrane author and former Editor and Trials Search Co-ordinator of the Cochrane Bone, Joint and Muscle Trauma Group, for copy-editing an early draft; the Cochrane Information Specialist Executive, the Cochrane Information Specialists' Support Team, Cochrane Information Specialists and members of the Cochrane Information Retrieval Methods Group for comments on drafts; Su Golder, Co-Convenor, Adverse Effects Methods Group and Steve McDonald, Co-Director, Cochrane Australia for peer review.

4.8 References

Agency for Healthcare Research and Quality. Methods guide for effectiveness and comparative effectiveness reviews: AHRQ publication no. 10(14)-EHC063-EF. 2014. https://effectivehealthcare.ahrq.gov/topics/cer-methods-guide/overview.

Arber M, Cikalo M, Glanville J, Lefebvre C, Varley D, Wood H. Annotated bibliography of published studies addressing searching for unpublished studies and obtaining access to unpublished data. 2013. https://methods.cochrane.org/sites/methods.cochrane.org.irmg/files/public/uploads/Annotatedbibliographtifyingunpublishedstudies.pdf.

Atkinson KM, Koenka AC, Sanchez CE, Moshontz H, Cooper H. Reporting standards for literature searches and report inclusion criteria: making research syntheses more transparent and easy to replicate. *Research Synthesis Methods* 2015; **6**: 87–95.

Bai Y, Gao J, Zou D, Li Z. Is MEDLINE alone enough for a meta-analysis? *Alimentary Pharmacology and Therapeutics* 2007; **26**: 125–126; author reply 126.

Baudard M, Yavchitz A, Ravaud P, Perrodeau E, Boutron I. Impact of searching clinical trial registries in systematic reviews of pharmaceutical treatments: methodological systematic review and reanalysis of meta-analyses. *BMJ* 2017; **356**: j448.

Bennett DA, Jull A. FDA: untapped source of unpublished trials. *Lancet* 2003; **361**: 1402–1403.

Bero L. Searching for unpublished trials using trials registers and trials web sites and obtaining unpublished trial data and corresponding trial protocols from regulatory agencies. 2013. http://web.archive.org/web/20150108071243/http://methods.cochrane.org:80/projects-developments/searching-unpublished-trials-using-trials-registers-and-trials-web-sites-and-o.

Booth A. How much searching is enough? Comprehensive versus optimal retrieval for technology assessments. *International Journal of Technology Assessment in Health Care* 2010; **26**: 431–435.

Booth A. Searching for qualitative research for inclusion in systematic reviews: a structured methodological review. *Systematic Reviews* 2016; **5**: 74.

Bramer WM. Variation in number of hits for complex searches in Google Scholar. *Journal of the Medical Library Association* 2016; **104**: 143–145.

Briscoe S. A review of the reporting of web searching to identify studies for Cochrane systematic reviews. *Research Synthesis Methods* 2018; **9**: 89–99.

Brusselle GG, Blasi F. Risk of a biased assessment of the evidence when limiting literature searches to the English language: macrolides in asthma as an illustrative example. *Pulmonary Pharmacology and Therapeutics* 2015; **31**: 109–110.

Chan AW. Out of sight but not out of mind: how to search for unpublished clinical trial evidence. *BMJ* 2012; **344**: d8013.

Chapman SJ, Shelton B, Mahmood H, Fitzgerald JE, Harrison EM, Bhangu A. Discontinuation and non-publication of surgical randomised controlled trials: observational study. *BMJ* 2014; **349**: g6870.

Chilcott J, Brennan A, Booth A, Karnon J, Tappenden P. The role of modelling in prioritising and planning clinical trials. *Health Technology Assessment* 2003; **7**: iii, 1–125.

Chow TK. Electronic search strategies should be repeatable. *European Journal of Pain* 2015; **19**: 1562–1563.

Cook DJ, Guyatt GH, Ryan G, Clifton J, Buckingham L, Willan A, McIlroy W, Oxman AD. Should unpublished data be included in meta-analyses? Current convictions and controversies. *JAMA* 1993; **269**: 2749–2753.

Cooper H, Ribble RG. Influences on the outcome of literature searches for integrative research reviews. *Science Communication* 1989; **10**: 179–201.

Craven J, Levay P. Recording database searches for systematic reviews – what is the value of adding a narrative to peer-review checklists? A case study of NICE interventional procedures guidance. *Evidence Based Library and Information Practice* 2011; **6**: 72–87.

de Vet H, Eisinga A, Riphagen I, Aertgeerts B, Pewsner D. Chapter 7: Searching for studies. In: Deeks J, Bossuyt P, Gatsonis C, editors. *Cochrane Handbook for Systematic Reviews of Diagnostic Test Accuracy Version 04 (updated September 2008)*: The Cochrane Collaboration; 2008. https://methods.cochrane.org/sites/methods.cochrane.org.sdt/files/public/uploads/Chapter07-Searching-%28September-2008%29.pdf.

Dellavalle RP, Hester EJ, Heilig LF, Drake AL, Kuntzman JW, Graber M, Schilling LM. Information science. Going, going, gone: lost Internet references. *Science* 2003; **302**: 787–788.

Doshi P, Dickersin K, Healy D, Vedula SS, Jefferson T. Restoring invisible and abandoned trials: a call for people to publish the findings. *BMJ* 2013; **346**: f2865.

Doust JA, Pietrzak E, Sanders S, Glasziou PP. Identifying studies for systematic reviews of diagnostic tests was difficult due to the poor sensitivity and precision of methodologic filters and the lack of information in the abstract. *Journal of Clinical Epidemiology* 2005; **58**: 444–449.

Easterbrook PJ, Berlin JA, Gopalan R, Matthews DR. Publication bias in clinical research. *Lancet* 1991; **337**: 867–872.

Edwards P, Clarke M, DiGuiseppi C, Pratap S, Roberts I, Wentz R. Identification of randomized controlled trials in systematic reviews: accuracy and reliability of screening records. *Statistics in Medicine* 2002; **21**: 1635–1640.

Egger M, Zellweger-Zähner T, Schneider M, Junker C, Lengeler C, Antes G. Language bias in randomised controlled trials published in English and German. *Lancet* 1997; **350**: 326–329.

Egger M, Smith GD. Bias in location and selection of studies. *BMJ* 1998; **316**: 61–66.

Elsevier. Embase content 2016a. https://www.elsevier.com/solutions/embase-biomedical-research/embase-coverage-and-content.

Elsevier. Embase classic fact sheet 2016b. https://www.elsevier.com/__data/assets/pdf_file/0005/58982/R_D-Solutions_Embase_Fact-Sheet_Classic-DIGITAL.pdf.

EUnetHTA. Process of information retrieval for systematic reviews and health technology assessments on clinical effectiveness (Version 1.2). Germany: European network for Health Technology Assessment; 2017. https://www.eunethta.eu/wp-content/uploads/2018/01/Guideline_Information_Retrieval_V1-2_2017.pdf.

European Food Safety Authority. Application of systematic review methodology to food and feed safety assessments to support decision making. *EFSA Journal* 2010; **8**: 1637. doi:10.2903/j.efsa.2010.1637. www.efsa.europa.eu.

Eysenbach G, Trudel M. Going, going, still there: using the WebCite service to permanently archive cited web pages. *Journal of Medical Internet Research* 2005; **7**: e60.

Franco JVA, Garrote VL, Escobar Liquitay CM, Vietto V. Identification of problems in search strategies in Cochrane Reviews. *Research Synthesis Methods* 2018; **9**: 408–416.

Glanville J, Lefebvre C, Wright Ke, editors. ISSG search filter resource York (UK): The InterTASC Information Specialists' Sub-Group 2019. https://sites.google.com/a/york.ac.uk/issg-search-filters-resource/home.

Glanville JM, Duffy S, McCool R, Varley D. Searching ClinicalTrials.gov and the International Clinical Trials Registry Platform to inform systematic reviews: what are the optimal search approaches? *Journal of the Medical Library Association* 2014; **102**: 177–183.

Goldacre B, Lane S, Mahtani KR, Heneghan C, Onakpoya I, Bushfield I, Smeeth L. Pharmaceutical companies' policies on access to trial data, results, and methods: audit study. *BMJ* 2017; **358**: j3334.

Greenhalgh T, Peacock R. Effectiveness and efficiency of search methods in systematic reviews of complex evidence: audit of primary sources. *BMJ* 2005; **331**: 1064–1065.

Haddaway NR, Collins AM, Coughlin D, Kirk S. The role of Google Scholar in evidence reviews and its applicability to grey literature searching. *PloS One* 2015; **10**: e0138237.

Halfpenny NJ, Quigley JM, Thompson JC, Scott DA. Value and usability of unpublished data sources for systematic reviews and network meta-analyses. *Evidence-Based Medicine* 2016; **21**: 208–213.

Halladay CW, Trikalinos TA, Schmid IT, Schmid CH, Dahabreh IJ. Using data sources beyond PubMed has a modest impact on the results of systematic reviews of therapeutic interventions. *Journal of Clinical Epidemiology* 2015; **68**: 1076–1084.

Hartling L, Featherstone R, Nuspl M, Shave K, Dryden DM, Vandermeer B. The contribution of databases to the results of systematic reviews: a cross-sectional study. *BMC Medical Research Methodology* 2016; **16**: 127.

Hartling L, Featherstone R, Nuspl M, Shave K, Dryden DM, Vandermeer B. Grey literature in systematic reviews: a cross-sectional study of the contribution of non-English reports, unpublished studies and dissertations to the results of meta-analyses in child-relevant reviews. *BMC Medical Research Methodology* 2017; **17**: 64.

Hetherington J, Dickersin K, Chalmers I, Meinert CL. Retrospective and prospective identification of unpublished controlled trials: lessons from a survey of obstetricians and pediatricians. *Pediatrics* 1989; **84**: 374–380.

Hinde S, Spackman E. Bidirectional citation searching to completion: an exploration of literature searching methods. *Pharmacoeconomics* 2015; **33**: 5–11.

Horton R. Medical editors trial amnesty. *Lancet* 1997; **350**: 756.

Huang X, Lin J, Demner-Fushman D. Evaluation of PICO as a knowledge representation for clinical questions. *AMIA Annual Symposium Proceedings/AMIA Symposium* 2006: 359–363.

Hwang TJ, Carpenter D, Lauffenburger JC, Wang B, Franklin JM, Kesselheim AS. Failure of investigational drugs in late-stage clinical development and publication of trial results. *JAMA Internal Medicine* 2016; **176**: 1826–1833.

Iansavichene AE, Sampson M, McGowan J, Ajiferuke IS. Should systematic reviewers search for randomized, controlled trials published as letters? *Annals of Internal Medicine* 2008; **148**: 714–715.

Institute of Medicine. Finding what works in health care: standards for systematic reviews. Washington, DC: The National Academies Press; 2011. http://books.nap.edu/openbook.php?record_id=13059

Irvin E, Hayden J. Developing and testing an optimal search strategy for identifying studies of prognosis [Poster]. 14th Cochrane Colloquium; 2006 October 23–26; Dublin, Ireland; 2006. https://abstracts.cochrane.org/2006-dublin/developing-and-testing-optimal-search-strategy-identifying-studies-prognosis.

Isojarvi J, Wood H, Lefebvre C, Glanville J. Challenges of identifying unpublished data from clinical trials: getting the best out of clinical trials registers and other novel sources. *Research Synthesis Methods* 2018; **9**: 561–578.

Jefferson T, Doshi P, Boutron I, Golder S, Heneghan C, Hodkinson A, Jones M, Lefebvre C, Stewart LA. When to include clinical study reports and regulatory documents in systematic reviews. *BMJ Evidence-Based Medicine* 2018; **23**: 210–217.

Jiao S, Tsutani K, Haga N. Review of Cochrane reviews on acupuncture: how Chinese resources contribute to Cochrane reviews. *Journal of Alternative and Complementary Medicine* 2013; **19**: 613–621.

Kaptchuk T. Certain countries produce only positive trial results. *Focus on Alternative and Complementary Therapies* 1999; **4**: 86–87.

Kastner M, Straus SE, McKibbon KA, Goldsmith CH. The capture-mark-recapture technique can be used as a stopping rule when searching in systematic reviews. *Journal of Clinical Epidemiology* 2009; **62**: 149–157.

Knelangen M, Hausner E, Metzendorf M-I, Sturtz S, Waffenschmidt S. Trial registry searches for randomized controlled trials of new drugs required registry-specific adaptation to achieve adequate sensitivity. *Journal of Clinical Epidemiology* 2018; **94**: 69–75.

Köhler M, Haag S, Biester K, Brockhaus AC, McGauran N, Grouven U, Kölsch H, Seay U, Hörn H, Moritz G, Staeck K, Wieseler B. Information on new drugs at market entry: retrospective analysis of health technology assessment reports versus regulatory reports, journal publications, and registry reports. *BMJ* 2015; **350**: h796.

Kreis J, Panteli D, Busse R. How health technology assessment agencies address the issue of unpublished data. *International Journal of Technology Assessment in Health Care* 2014; **30**: 34–43.

Lampert A, Hoffmann GF, Ries M. Ten years after the International Committee of Medical Journal Editors' clinical trial registration initiative, one quarter of phase 3 pediatric epilepsy clinical trials still remain unpublished: a cross sectional analysis. *PloS One* 2016; **11**: e0144973.

Layton D. A critical review of search strategies used in recent systematic reviews published in selected prosthodontic and implant-related journals: are systematic reviews actually systematic? *International Journal of Prosthodontics* 2017; **30**: 13–21.

Lee K, Bacchetti P, Sim I. Publication of clinical trials supporting successful new drug applications: a literature analysis. *PLoS Medicine* 2008; **5**: e191.

Lefebvre C, Eisinga A, McDonald S, Paul N. Enhancing access to reports of randomized trials published world-wide – the contribution of EMBASE records to the Cochrane Central Register of Controlled Trials (CENTRAL) in The Cochrane Library. *Emerging Themes in Epidemiology* 2008; **5**: 13.

Lefebvre C, Glanville J, Wieland LS, Coles B, Weightman AL. Methodological developments in searching for studies for systematic reviews: past, present and future? *Systematic Reviews* 2013; **2**: 78.

Littlewood A, Bridges C, for the Cochrane Information Specialist Support Team. Cochrane Information Specialists' Handbook Oslo: The Cochrane Collaboration; 2017. http://training.cochrane.org/resource/cochrane-information-specialists-handbook.

Lorenc T, Tyner EF, Petticrew M, Duffy S, Martineau FP, Phillips G, Lock K. Cultures of evidence across policy sectors: systematic review of qualitative evidence. *European Journal of Public Health* 2014; **24**: 1041–1047.

Lorenzetti DL, Topfer LA, Dennett L, Clement F. Value of databases other than MEDLINE for rapid health technology assessments. *International Journal of Technology Assessment in Health Care* 2014; **30**: 173–178.

MacLean CH, Morton SC, Ofman JJ, Roth EA, Shekelle PG; Southern California Evidence-Based Practice Center. How useful are unpublished data from the Food and Drug Administration in meta-analysis? *Journal of Clinical Epidemiology* 2003; **56**: 44–51.

Manheimer E, Anderson D. Survey of public information about ongoing clinical trials funded by industry: evaluation of completeness and accessibility. *BMJ* 2002; **325**: 528–531.

Marshall C, Brereton P. Systematic review toolbox: a catalogue of tools to support systematic reviews. *Proceedings of the 19th International Conference on Evaluation and Assessment in Software Engineering (EASE)* 2015: Article no. 23.

Marshall I, Noel-Storr A, Kuiper J, Thomas J, Wallace BC. Machine learning for identifying randomized controlled trials: an evaluation and practitioner's guide. *Research Synthesis Methods* 2018; **9**: 602–614.

McGowan J, Sampson M, Salzwedel D, Cogo E, Foerster V, Lefebvre C. PRESS Peer Review of Electronic Search Strategies: 2015 Guideline Explanation and Elaboration (PRESS E&E). Ottawa: CADTH; 2016a. https://www.cadth.ca/sites/default/files/pdf/CP0015_PRESS_Update_Report_2016.pdf.

McGowan J, Sampson M, Salzwedel DM, Cogo E, Foerster V, Lefebvre C. PRESS Peer Review of Electronic Search Strategies: 2015 Guideline Statement. *Journal of Clinical Epidemiology* 2016b; **75**: 40–46.

Meert D, Torabi N, Costella J. Impact of librarians on reporting of the literature searching component of pediatric systematic reviews. *Journal of the Medical Library Association* 2016; **104**: 267–277.

Metzendorf M-I. Why medical information specialists should routinely form part of teams producing high quality systematic reviews – a Cochrane perspective. *Journal of the European Association for Health Information and Libraries* 2016; **12**(4): 6–9.

Moher D, Pham B, Lawson ML, Klassen TP. The inclusion of reports of randomised trials published in languages other than English in systematic reviews. *Health Technology Assessment* 2003; **7**: 1–90.

Morrison A, Polisena J, Husereau D, Moulton K, Clark M, Fiander M, Mierzwinski-Urban M, Clifford T, Hutton B, Rabb D. The effect of English-language restriction on systematic review-based meta-analyses: a systematic review of empirical studies. *International Journal of Technology Assessment in Health Care* 2012; **28**: 138–144.

Mullins MM, DeLuca JB, Crepaz N, Lyles CM. Reporting quality of search methods in systematic reviews of HIV behavioral interventions (2000–2010): are the searches clearly explained, systematic and reproducible? *Research Synthesis Methods* 2014; **5**: 116–130.

Niederstadt C, Droste S. Reporting and presenting information retrieval processes: the need for optimizing common practice in health technology assessment. *International Journal of Technology Assessment in Health Care* 2010; **26**: 450–457.

O'Mara-Eves A, Thomas J, McNaught J, Miwa M, Ananiadou S. Using text mining for study identification in systematic reviews: a systematic review of current approaches. *Systematic Reviews* 2015; **4**: 5. (Erratum in: *Systematic Reviews* 2015; **4**: 59).

Oxman AD, Guyatt GH. The science of reviewing research. *Annals of the New York Academy of Sciences* 1993; **703**: 125–133; discussion 133–134.

Pansieri C, Pandolfini C, Bonati M. Clinical trial registries: more international, converging efforts are needed. *Trials* 2017; **18**: 86.

Petticrew M, Roberts H. *Systematic Reviews in the Social Sciences: a Practical Guide*. Oxford (UK): Blackwell; 2006.

Pham B, Klassen TP, Lawson ML, Moher D. Language of publication restrictions in systematic reviews gave different results depending on whether the intervention was conventional or complementary. *Journal of Clinical Epidemiology* 2005; **58**: 769–776.

Pilkington K, Boshnakova A, Clarke M, Richardson J. 'No language restrictions' in database searches: what does this really mean? *Journal of Alternative and Complementary Medicine* 2005; **11**: 205–207.

Rader T, Mann M, Stansfield C, Cooper C, Sampson M. Methods for documenting systematic review searches: a discussion of common issues. *Research Synthesis Methods* 2014; **5**: 98–115.

Relevo R, Paynter R. Peer Review of Search Strategies. Rockville (MD): Agency for Healthcare Research and Quality (US); 2012. https://www.ncbi.nlm.nih.gov/books/NBK98353/.

Rethlefsen ML, Farrell AM, Osterhaus Trzasko LC, Brigham TJ. Librarian co-authors correlated with higher quality reported search strategies in general internal medicine systematic reviews. *Journal of Clinical Epidemiology* 2015; **68**: 617–626.

Reveiz L, Cardona AF, Ospina EG, de Agular S. An e-mail survey identified unpublished studies for systematic reviews. *Journal of Clinical Epidemiology* 2006; **59**: 755–758.

Rice DB, Kloda LA, Levis B, Qi B, Kingsland E, Thombs BD. Are MEDLINE searches sufficient for systematic reviews and meta-analyses of the diagnostic accuracy of depression screening tools? A review of meta-analyses. *Journal of Psychosomatic Research* 2016; **87**: 7–13.

Richardson WS, Wilson MC, Nishikawa J, Hayward RS. The well-built clinical question: a key to evidence-based decisions. *ACP Journal Club* 1995; **123**: A12–13.

Roundtree AK, Kallen MA, Lopez-Olivo MA, Kimmel B, Skidmore B, Ortiz Z, Cox V, Suarez-Almazor ME. Poor reporting of search strategy and conflict of interest in over 250 narrative and systematic reviews of two biologic agents in arthritis: a systematic review. *Journal of Clinical Epidemiology* 2009; **62**: 128–137.

Royle P, Milne R. Literature searching for randomized controlled trials used in Cochrane reviews: rapid versus exhaustive searches. *International Journal of Technology Assessment in Health Care* 2003; **19**: 591–603.

Sampson M, Barrowman NJ, Moher D, Klassen TP, Pham B, Platt R, St John PD, Viola R, Raina P. Should meta-analysts search Embase in addition to Medline? *Journal of Clinical Epidemiology* 2003; **56**: 943–955.

Sampson M, Zhang L, Morrison A, Barrowman NJ, Clifford TJ, Platt RW, Klassen TP, Moher D. An alternative to the hand searching gold standard: validating methodological search filters using relative recall. *BMC Medical Research Methodology* 2006; **6**: 33.

Sampson M, McGowan J. Errors in search strategies were identified by type and frequency. *Journal of Clinical Epidemiology* 2006; **59**: 1057–1063.

Sampson M, McGowan J, Tetzlaff J, Cogo E, Moher D. No consensus exists on search reporting methods for systematic reviews. *Journal of Clinical Epidemiology* 2008; **61**: 748–754.

Sampson M, McGowan J. Inquisitio validus Index Medicus: a simple method of validating MEDLINE systematic review searches. *Research Synthesis Methods* 2011; **2**: 103–109.

Sampson M, de Bruijn B, Urquhart C, Shojania K. Complementary approaches to searching MEDLINE may be sufficient for updating systematic reviews. *Journal of Clinical Epidemiology* 2016; **78**: 108–115.

Scherer RW, Ugarte-Gil C, Schmucker C, Meerpohl JJ. Authors report lack of time as main reason for unpublished research presented at biomedical conferences: a systematic review. *Journal of Clinical Epidemiology* 2015; **68**: 803–810.

Schroll JB, Bero L, Gøtzsche PC. Searching for unpublished data for Cochrane reviews: cross sectional study. *BMJ* 2013; **346**: f2231.

Shemilt I, Simon A, Hollands GJ, Marteau TM, Ogilvie D, O'Mara-Eves A, Kelly MP, Thomas J. Pinpointing needles in giant haystacks: use of text mining to reduce impractical screening workload in extremely large scoping reviews. *Research Synthesis Methods* 2014; **5**: 31–49.

Shemilt I, Khan N, Park S, Thomas J. Use of cost-effectiveness analysis to compare the efficiency of study identification methods in systematic reviews. *Systematic Reviews* 2016; **5**: 140.

Spoor P, Airey M, Bennett C, Greensill J, Williams R. Use of the capture-recapture technique to evaluate the completeness of systematic literature searches. *BMJ* 1996; **313**: 342–343.

Spry C, Mierzwinski-Urban M, Rabb D. Peer review of literature search strategies: does it make a difference? 21st Cochrane Colloquium; 2013; Quebec City, Canada. https://abstracts.cochrane.org/2013-québec-city/peer-review-literature-search-strategies-does-it-make-difference.

Stevinson C, Lawlor DA. Searching multiple databases for systematic reviews: added value or diminishing returns? *Complementary Therapies in Medicine* 2004; **12**: 228–232.

Suarez-Almazor ME, Belseck E, Homik J, Dorgan M, Ramos-Remus C. Identifying clinical trials in the medical literature with electronic databases: MEDLINE alone is not enough. *Controlled Clinical Trials* 2000; **21**: 476–487.

Thomas J, Noel-Storr A, Marshall I, Wallace B, McDonald S, Mavergames C, Glasziou P, Shemilt I, Synnot A, Turner T, Elliott J; Living Systematic Review Network. Living systematic reviews: 2. Combining human and machine effort. *Journal of Clinical Epidemiology* 2017; **91**: 31–37.

Tramèr MR, Reynolds DJ, Moore RA, McQuay HJ. Impact of covert duplicate publication on meta-analysis: a case study. *BMJ* 1997; **315**: 635–640.

Tsafnat G, Glasziou P, Choong MK, Dunn A, Galgani F, Coiera E. Systematic review automation technologies. *Systematic Reviews* 2014; **3**: 74.

US National Library of Medicine. PubMed. 2018. https://www.nlm.nih.gov/bsd/pubmed.html.

US National Library of Medicine. MEDLINE®: Description of the Database. 2019. https://www.nlm.nih.gov/bsd/medline.html.

US National Library of Medicine. Fact Sheet: MEDLINE, PubMed, and PMC (PubMed Central): How are they different? no date. https://www.nlm.nih.gov/bsd/difference.html.

Vickers A, Goyal N, Harland R, Rees R. Do certain countries produce only positive results? A systematic review of controlled trials. *Controlled Clinical Trials* 1998; **19**: 159–166.

Viergever RF, Li K. Trends in global clinical trial registration: an analysis of numbers of registered clinical trials in different parts of the world from 2004 to 2013. *BMJ Open* 2015; **5**: e008932.

von Elm E, Poglia G, Walder B, Tramèr MR. Different patterns of duplicate publication: an analysis of articles used in systematic reviews. *JAMA* 2004; **291**: 974–980.

Wallace S, Daly C, Campbell M, Cody J, Grant A, Vale L, Donaldson C, Khan I, Lawrence P, MacLeod A. After MEDLINE? Dividend from other potential sources of randomised controlled trials. Second International Conference Scientific Basis of Health Services & Fifth Annual Cochrane Colloquium; 1997; Amsterdam, The Netherlands.

Wang Z, Brito JP, Tsapas A, Griebeler ML, Alahdab F, Murad MH. Systematic reviews with language restrictions and no author contact have lower overall credibility: a methodology study. *Clinical Epidemiology* 2015; **7**: 243–247.

Weber EJ, Callaham ML, Wears RL, Barton C, Young G. Unpublished research from a medical specialty meeting: why investigators fail to publish. *JAMA* 1998; **280**: 257–259.

Wieseler B, Kerekes MF, Vervoelgyi V, McGauran N, Kaiser T. Impact of document type on reporting quality of clinical drug trials: a comparison of registry reports, clinical study reports, and journal publications. *BMJ* 2012; **344**: d8141.

Witkowski MA, Aldhouse N. Transparency and reproducibility of supplementary search methods in NICE single technology appraisal manufacturer submissions. *Value in Health* 2015; **18**: A721–722.

Wood H, Arber M. Search strategy development [webpage]. In: Summarized Research in Information Retrieval for HTA (SuRe Info) 2009. Last updated 2019. http://www.htai.org/vortal/?q=node/790.

Woods D, Trewheellar K. Medline and Embase complement each other in literature searches. *BMJ* 1998; **316**: 1166.

Wu XY, Tang JL, Mao C, Yuan JQ, Qin Y, Chung VC. Systematic reviews and meta-analyses of traditional Chinese medicine must search Chinese databases to reduce language bias. *Evidence-Based Complementary and Alternative Medicine* 2013: 812179.

Yoshii A, Plaut DA, McGraw KA, Anderson MJ, Wellik KE. Analysis of the reporting of search strategies in Cochrane systematic reviews. *Journal of the Medical Library Association* 2009; **97**: 21–29.

Young T, Hopewell S. Methods for obtaining unpublished data. *Cochrane Database of Systematic Reviews* 2011; **11**: MR000027.

Wieseler B, Kerekes MF, Vervolgyi V, McGauran N, Kaiser T. Impact of document type on reporting quality of clinical drug trials: a comparison of registry reports, clinical study reports, and journal publications. *BMJ* 2012; 344: d8141.

Witkowski MA, Aldhouse N. Transparency and reproducibility of supplementary search methods in NICE single technology appraisal manufacturer submissions. *Value in Health* 2015; 18: A721–722.

Wood H, Arber M. Search strategy development [webpage]. In: Summarized Research in Information Retrieval for HTA (SuRe Info) 2009. Last updated 2019. http://www.htai.org/vortal/?q=node/790.

[illegible]

[illegible]

[illegible] 2015; 32: [illegible].

Yoshii A, Plaut DA, McGraw KA, Anderson MJ, Wellik KE. Analysis of the reporting of search strategies in Cochrane systematic reviews. *Journal of the Medical Library Association* 2009; 97: 21–29.

Young T, Hopewell S. Methods for obtaining unpublished data. *Cochrane Database of Systematic Reviews* 2011; 11: MR000027.

5

Collecting data

Tianjing Li, Julian PT Higgins, Jonathan J Deeks

KEY POINTS

- Systematic reviews have studies, rather than reports, as the unit of interest, and so multiple reports of the same study need to be identified and linked together before or after data extraction.
- Because of the increasing availability of data sources (e.g. trials registers, regulatory documents, clinical study reports), review authors should decide on which sources may contain the most useful information for the review, and have a plan to resolve discrepancies if information is inconsistent across sources.
- Review authors are encouraged to develop outlines of tables and figures that will appear in the review to facilitate the design of data collection forms. The key to successful data collection is to construct easy-to-use forms and collect sufficient and unambiguous data that faithfully represent the source in a structured and organized manner.
- Effort should be made to identify data needed for meta-analyses, which often need to be calculated or converted from data reported in diverse formats.
- Data should be collected and archived in a form that allows future access and data sharing.

5.1 Introduction

Systematic reviews aim to identify all studies that are relevant to their research questions and to synthesize data about the design, risk of bias, and results of those studies. Consequently, the findings of a systematic review depend critically on decisions relating to which data from these studies are presented and analysed. Data collected for systematic reviews should be accurate, complete, and accessible for future updates of the review and for data sharing. Methods used for these decisions must be transparent; they should be chosen to minimize biases and human error. Here we describe

This chapter should be cited as: Li T, Higgins JPT, Deeks JJ (editors). Chapter 5: Collecting data. In: Higgins JPT, Thomas J, Chandler J, Cumpston M, Li T, Page MJ, Welch VA (editors). *Cochrane Handbook for Systematic Reviews of Interventions*. 2nd Edition. Chichester (UK): John Wiley & Sons, 2019: 109–142.

approaches that should be used in systematic reviews for collecting data, including extraction of data directly from journal articles and other reports of studies.

5.2 Sources of data

Studies are reported in a range of sources which are detailed later. As discussed in Section 5.2.1, it is important to link together multiple reports of the same study. The relative strengths and weaknesses of each type of source are discussed in Section 5.2.2. For guidance on searching for and selecting reports of studies, refer to Chapter 4.

Journal articles are the source of the majority of data included in systematic reviews. Note that a study can be reported in multiple journal articles, each focusing on some aspect of the study (e.g. design, main results, and other results).

Conference abstracts are commonly available. However, the information presented in conference abstracts is highly variable in reliability, accuracy, and level of detail (Li et al 2017).

Errata and **letters** can be important sources of information about studies, including critical weaknesses and retractions, and review authors should examine these if they are identified (see MECIR Box 5.2.a).

Trials registers (e.g. ClinicalTrials.gov) catalogue trials that have been planned or started, and have become an important data source for identifying trials, for comparing published outcomes and results with those planned, and for obtaining efficacy and safety data that are not available elsewhere (Ross et al 2009, Jones et al 2015, Baudard et al 2017).

Clinical study reports (CSRs) contain unabridged and comprehensive descriptions of the clinical problem, design, conduct and results of clinical trials, following a structure and content guidance prescribed by the International Conference on Harmonisation (ICH 1995). To obtain marketing approval of drugs and biologics for a specific indication, pharmaceutical companies submit CSRs and other required materials to regulatory

MECIR Box 5.2.a Relevant expectations for conduct of intervention reviews	
C48: Examining errata (**Mandatory**)	
Examine any relevant retraction statements and errata for information.	Some studies may have been found to be fraudulent or may for other reasons have been retracted since publication. Errata can reveal important limitations, or even fatal flaws, in included studies. All of these may potentially lead to the exclusion of a study from a review or meta-analysis. Care should be taken to ensure that this information is retrieved in all database searches by downloading the appropriate fields together with the citation data.

authorities. Because CSRs also incorporate tables and figures, with appendices containing the protocol, statistical analysis plan, sample case report forms, and patient data listings (including narratives of all serious adverse events), they can be thousands of pages in length. CSRs often contain more data about trial methods and results than any other single data source (Mayo-Wilson et al 2018). CSRs are often difficult to access, and are usually not publicly available. Review authors could request CSRs from the European Medicines Agency (Davis and Miller 2017). The US Food and Drug and Administration had historically avoided releasing CSRs but launched a pilot programme in 2018 whereby selected portions of CSRs for new drug applications were posted on the agency's website. Many CSRs are obtained through unsealed litigation documents, repositories (e.g. clinicalstudydatarequest.com), and other open data and data-sharing channels (e.g. The Yale University Open Data Access Project) (Doshi et al 2013, Wieland et al 2014, Mayo-Wilson et al 2018)).

Regulatory reviews such as those available from the US Food and Drug Administration or European Medicines Agency provide useful information about trials of drugs, biologics, and medical devices submitted by manufacturers for marketing approval (Turner 2013). These documents are summaries of CSRs and related documents, prepared by agency staff as part of the process of approving the products for marketing, after reanalysing the original trial data. Regulatory reviews often are available only for the first approved use of an intervention and not for later applications (although review authors may request those documents, which are usually brief). Using regulatory reviews from the US Food and Drug Administration as an example, drug approval packages are available on the agency's website for drugs approved since 1997 (Turner 2013); for drugs approved before 1997, information must be requested through a freedom of information request. The drug approval packages contain various documents: approval letter(s), medical review(s), chemistry review(s), clinical pharmacology review(s), and statistical reviews(s).

Individual participant data (IPD) are usually sought directly from the researchers responsible for the study, or may be identified from open data repositories (e.g. www.clinicalstudydatarequest.com). These data typically include variables that represent the characteristics of each participant, intervention (or exposure) group, prognostic factors, and measurements of outcomes (Stewart et al 2015). Access to IPD has the advantage of allowing review authors to reanalyse the data flexibly, in accordance with the preferred analysis methods outlined in the protocol, and can reduce the variation in analysis methods across studies included in the review. IPD reviews are addressed in detail in Chapter 26.

5.2.1 Studies (not reports) as the unit of interest

In a systematic review, *studies* rather than *reports* of studies are the principal unit of interest. Since a study may have been reported in several sources, a comprehensive search for studies for the review may identify many reports from a potentially relevant study (Mayo-Wilson et al 2017a, Mayo-Wilson et al 2018). Conversely, a report may describe more than one study.

Multiple reports of the same study should be linked together (see MECIR Box 5.2.b). Some authors prefer to link reports before they collect data, and collect data from across the reports onto a single form. Other authors prefer to collect data from each

MECIR Box 5.2.b Relevant expectations for conduct of intervention reviews	
C42: Collating multiple reports (**Mandatory**)	
Collate multiple reports of the same study, so that each study rather than each report is the unit of interest in the review.	It is wrong to consider multiple reports of the same study as if they are multiple studies. Secondary reports of a study should not be discarded, however, since they may contain valuable information about the design and conduct. Review authors must choose and justify which report to use as a source for study results.

report and then link together the collected data across reports. Either strategy may be appropriate, depending on the nature of the reports at hand. It may not be clear that two reports relate to the same study until data collection has commenced. Although sometimes there is a single report for each study, it should never be assumed that this is the case.

It can be difficult to link multiple reports from the same study, and review authors may need to do some 'detective work'. Multiple sources about the same trial may not reference each other, do not share common authors (Gøtzsche 1989, Tramèr et al 1997), or report discrepant information about the study design, characteristics, outcomes, and results (von Elm et al 2004, Mayo-Wilson et al 2017a).

Some of the most useful criteria for linking reports are:

- trial registration numbers;
- authors' names;
- sponsor for the study and sponsor identifiers (e.g. grant or contract numbers);
- location and setting (particularly if institutions, such as hospitals, are named);
- specific details of the interventions (e.g. dose, frequency);
- numbers of participants and baseline data; and
- date and duration of the study (which also can clarify whether different sample sizes are due to different periods of recruitment), length of follow-up, or subgroups selected to address secondary goals.

Review authors should use as many trial characteristics as possible to link multiple reports. When uncertainties remain after considering these and other factors, it may be necessary to correspond with the study authors or sponsors for confirmation.

5.2.2 Determining which sources might be most useful

A comprehensive search to identify all eligible studies from all possible sources is resource-intensive but necessary for a high-quality systematic review (see Chapter 4). Because some data sources are more useful than others (Mayo-Wilson et al 2018), review authors should consider which data sources may be available and which may contain the most useful information for the review. These considerations should be described in the protocol. Table 5.2.a summarizes the strengths and

Table 5.2.a Strengths and limitations of different data sources for systematic reviews

Source	Strengths	Limitations
Public sources		
Journal articles	Found easily Data extracted quickly Include useful information about methods and results	Available for some, but not all studies (with a risk of reporting biases: see Chapters 7 and 13) Contain limited study characteristics and methods Can omit outcomes, especially harms
Conference abstracts	Identify unpublished studies	Include little information about study design Include limited and unclear information for meta-analysis May result in double-counting studies in meta-analysis if not correctly linked to other reports of the same study
Trial registrations	Identify otherwise unpublished trials May contain information about design, risk of bias, and results not included in other public sources Link multiple sources about the same trial using unique registration number	Limited to more recent studies that comply with registration requirements Often contain limited information about trial design and quantitative results May report only harms (adverse events) occurring above a threshold (e.g. 5%) May be inaccurate or incomplete for trials whose methods have changed during the conduct of the study, or results not kept up to date
Regulatory information	Identify studies not reported in other public sources Describe details of methods and results not found in other sources	Available only for studies submitted to regulators Available for approved indications, but not 'off-label' uses Not always in a standard format Not often available for old products
Non-public sources		
Clinical study reports (CSRs)	Contain detailed information about study characteristics, methods, and results Can be particularly useful for identifying detailed information about harms Describe aggregate results, which are easy to analyse and sufficient for most reviews	Do not exist or difficult to obtain for most studies Require more time to obtain and analyse than public sources
Individual participant data	Allow review authors to use contemporary statistical methods and to standardize analyses across studies Permit additional analyses that the review authors desire (e.g. subgroup analyses)	Require considerable expertise and time to obtain and analyse May lead to the same results that can be found in aggregate report May not be necessary if one has a CSR

MECIR Box 5.2.c Relevant expectations for conduct of intervention reviews	
C49: Obtaining unpublished data (**Highly desirable**)	
Seek key unpublished information that is missing from reports of included studies.	Contacting study authors to obtain or confirm data makes the review more complete, potentially enhances precision and reduces the impact of reporting biases. Missing information includes details to inform risk of bias assessments, details of interventions and outcomes, and study results (including breakdowns of results by important subgroups).

limitations of different data sources (Mayo-Wilson et al 2018). Gaining access to CSRs and IPD often takes a long time. Review authors should begin searching repositories and contact trial investigators and sponsors as early as possible to negotiate data usage agreements (Mayo-Wilson et al 2015, Mayo-Wilson et al 2018).

5.2.3 Correspondence with investigators

Review authors often find that they are unable to obtain all the information they seek from available reports about the details of the study design, the full range of outcomes measured and the numerical results. In such circumstances, authors are strongly encouraged to contact the original investigators (see MECIR Box 5.2.c). Contact details of study authors, when not available from the study reports, often can be obtained from more recent publications, from university or institutional staff listings, from membership directories of professional societies, or by a general search of the web. If the contact author named in the study report cannot be contacted or does not respond, it is worthwhile attempting to contact other authors.

Review authors should consider the nature of the information they require and make their request accordingly. For descriptive information about the conduct of the trial, it may be most appropriate to ask open-ended questions (e.g. how was the allocation process conducted, or how were missing data handled?). If specific numerical data are required, it may be more helpful to request them specifically, possibly providing a short data collection form (either uncompleted or partially completed). If IPD are required, they should be specifically requested (see also Chapter 26). In some cases, study investigators may find it more convenient to provide IPD rather than conduct additional analyses to obtain the specific statistics requested.

5.3 What data to collect

5.3.1 What are data?

For the purposes of this chapter, we define 'data' to be any information about (or derived from) a study, including details of methods, participants, setting, context, interventions, outcomes, results, publications, and investigators. Review authors should

MECIR Box 5.3.a Relevant expectations for conduct of intervention reviews	
C44: Describing studies (**Mandatory**)	
Collect characteristics of the included studies in sufficient detail to populate a table of 'Characteristics of included studies'.	Basic characteristics of each study will need to be presented as part of the review, including details of participants, interventions and comparators, outcomes and study design.

plan in advance what data will be required for their systematic review, and develop a strategy for obtaining them (see MECIR Box 5.3.a). The involvement of consumers and other stakeholders can be helpful in ensuring that the categories of data collected are sufficiently aligned with the needs of review users (Chapter 1, Section 1.3). The data to be sought should be described in the protocol, with consideration wherever possible of the issues raised in the rest of this chapter.

The data collected for a review should adequately describe the included studies, support the construction of tables and figures, facilitate the risk of bias assessment, and enable syntheses and meta-analyses. Review authors should familiarize themselves with reporting guidelines for systematic reviews (see online Chapter III and the PRISMA statement; Liberati et al 2009) to ensure that relevant elements and sections are incorporated. The following sections review the types of information that should be sought, and these are summarized in Table 5.3.a (Li et al 2015).

5.3.2 Study methods and potential sources of bias

Different research methods can influence study outcomes by introducing different biases into results. Important study design characteristics should be collected to allow the selection of appropriate methods for assessment and analysis, and to enable description of the design of each included study in a table of 'Characteristics of included studies', including whether the study is randomized, whether the study has a cluster or crossover design, and the duration of the study. If the review includes non-randomized studies, appropriate features of the studies should be described (see Chapter 24).

Detailed information should be collected to facilitate assessment of the risk of bias in each included study. Risk-of-bias assessment should be conducted using the tool most appropriate for the design of each study, and the information required to complete the assessment will depend on the tool. Randomized studies should be assessed using the tool described in Chapter 8. The tool covers bias arising from the randomization process, due to deviations from intended interventions, due to missing outcome data, in measurement of the outcome, and in selection of the reported result. For each item in the tool, a description of what happened in the study is required, which may include verbatim quotes from study reports. Information for assessment of bias due to missing outcome data and selection of the reported result may be most conveniently collected alongside information on outcomes and results. Chapter 7 (Section 7.3.1) discusses some issues in the collection of information for

Table 5.3.a Checklist of items to consider in data collection

Information about data extraction from reports

Name of data extractors, date of data extraction, and identification features of each report from which data are being extracted

Eligibility criteria

Confirm eligibility of the study for the review

Reason for exclusion

Study methods

Study design:

- Parallel, factorial, crossover, cluster aspects of design for randomized trials, and/or study design features for non-randomized studies
- Single or multicentre study; if multicentre, number of recruiting centres

Recruitment and sampling procedures used (including at the level of individual participants and clusters/sites if relevant)

Enrolment start and end dates; length of participant follow-up

Details of random sequence generation, allocation sequence concealment, and masking for randomized trials, and methods used to prevent and control for confounding, selection biases, and information biases for non-randomized studies*

Methods used to prevent and address missing data*

Statistical analysis:

Unit of analysis (e.g. individual participant, clinic, village, body part)

Statistical methods used if computed effect estimates are extracted from reports, including any covariates included in the statistical model

Likelihood of reporting and other biases*

Source(s) of funding or other material support for the study

Authors' financial relationship and other potential conflicts of interest

Participants

Setting

Region(s) and country/countries from which study participants were recruited

Study eligibility criteria, including diagnostic criteria

Characteristics of participants at the beginning (or baseline) of the study (e.g. age, sex, comorbidity, socio-economic status)

Intervention

Description of the intervention(s) and comparison intervention(s), ideally with sufficient detail for replication:

- Components, routes of delivery, doses, timing, frequency, intervention protocols, length of intervention
- Factors relevant to implementation (e.g. staff qualifications, equipment requirements)
- Integrity of interventions (i.e. the degree to which specified procedures or components of the intervention were implemented as planned)
- Description of co-interventions
- Definition of 'control' groups (e.g. no intervention, placebo, minimally active comparator, or components of usual care)
- Components, dose, timing, frequency
- For observational studies: description of how intervention status was assessed; length of exposure, cumulative exposure

Table 5.3.a (Continued)

Outcomes
For each pre-specified outcome domain (e.g. anxiety) in the systematic review: • Whether there is evidence that the outcome domain was assessed (especially important if the outcome was assessed but the results not presented; see Chapter 13) • Measurement tool or instrument (including definition of clinical outcomes or endpoints); for a scale, name of the scale (e.g. the Hamilton Anxiety Rating Scale), upper and lower limits, and whether a high or low score is favourable, definitions of any thresholds if appropriate • Specific metric (e.g. post-intervention anxiety, or change in anxiety from baseline to a post-intervention time point, or post-intervention presence of anxiety (yes/no)) • Method of aggregation (e.g. mean and standard deviation of anxiety scores in each group, or proportion of people with anxiety) • Timing of outcome measurements (e.g. assessments at end of eight-week intervention period, events occurring during the eight-week intervention period) • Adverse outcomes need special attention depending on whether they are collected systematically or non-systematically (e.g. by voluntary report)
Results
For each group, and for each outcome at each time point: number of participants randomly assigned and included in the analysis; and number of participants who withdrew, were lost to follow-up or were excluded (with reasons for each)
Summary data for each group (e.g. 2×2 table for dichotomous data; means and standard deviations for continuous data)
Between-group estimates that quantify the effect of the intervention, and their precision (e.g. risk ratio, odds ratio, mean difference)
If subgroup analysis is planned, the same information would need to be extracted for each participant subgroup
Miscellaneous
Key conclusions of the study authors
Reference to other relevant studies
Correspondence required
Miscellaneous comments from the study authors or by the review authors

* Full description required for assessments of risk of bias (see Chapters 8, 23 and 25).

assessments of risk of bias. For non-randomized studies, the most appropriate tool is described in Chapter 25. A separate tool also covers bias due to missing results in meta-analysis (see Chapter 13).

A particularly important piece of information is the funding source of the study and potential conflicts of interest of the study authors.

Some review authors will wish to collect additional information on study characteristics that bear on the quality of the study's conduct but that may not lead directly to risk of bias, such as whether ethical approval was obtained and whether a sample size calculation was performed a priori.

5.3.3 Participants and setting

Details of participants are collected to enable an understanding of the comparability of, and differences between, the participants within and between included studies, and to allow assessment of how directly or completely the participants in the included studies reflect the original review question.

Typically, aspects that should be collected are those that could (or are believed to) affect presence or magnitude of an intervention effect and those that could help review users assess applicability to populations beyond the review. For example, if the review authors suspect important differences in intervention effect between different socio-economic groups, this information should be collected. If intervention effects are thought constant over such groups, and if such information would not be useful to help apply results, it should not be collected. Participant characteristics that are often useful for assessing applicability include age and sex. Summary information about these should always be collected unless they are not obvious from the context. These characteristics are likely to be presented in different formats (e.g. ages as means or medians, with standard deviations or ranges; sex as percentages or counts for the whole study or for each intervention group separately). Review authors should seek consistent quantities where possible, and decide whether it is more relevant to summarize characteristics for the study as a whole or by intervention group. It may not be possible to select the most consistent statistics until data collection is complete across all or most included studies. Other characteristics that are sometimes important include ethnicity, socio-demographic details (e.g. education level) and the presence of comorbid conditions. Clinical characteristics relevant to the review question (e.g. glucose level for reviews on diabetes) also are important for understanding the severity or stage of the disease.

Diagnostic criteria that were used to define the condition of interest can be a particularly important source of diversity across studies and should be collected. For example, in a review of drug therapy for congestive heart failure, it is important to know how the definition and severity of heart failure was determined in each study (e.g. systolic or diastolic dysfunction, severe systolic dysfunction with ejection fractions below 20%). Similarly, in a review of antihypertensive therapy, it is important to describe baseline levels of blood pressure of participants.

If the settings of studies may influence intervention effects or applicability, then information on these should be collected. Typical settings of healthcare intervention studies include acute care hospitals, emergency facilities, general practice, and extended care facilities such as nursing homes, offices, schools, and communities. Sometimes studies are conducted in different geographical regions with important differences that could affect delivery of an intervention and its outcomes, such as cultural characteristics, economic context, or rural versus city settings. Timing of the study may be associated with important technology differences or trends over time. If such information is important for the interpretation of the review, it should be collected.

Important characteristics of the participants in each included study should be summarized for the reader in the table of 'Characteristics of included studies'.

5.3.4 Interventions

Details of all experimental and comparator interventions of relevance to the review should be collected. Again, details are required for aspects that could affect the presence or magnitude of an effect or that could help review users assess applicability to their own circumstances. Where feasible, information should be sought (and presented in the review) that is sufficient for replication of the interventions under study. This includes any co-interventions administered as part of the study, and applies similarly to comparators such as 'usual care'. Review authors may need to request missing information from study authors.

The Template for Intervention Description and Replication (TIDieR) provides a comprehensive framework for full description of interventions and has been proposed for use in systematic reviews as well as reports of primary studies (Hoffmann et al 2014). The checklist includes descriptions of:

- the rationale for the intervention and how it is expected to work;
- any documentation that instructs the recipient on the intervention;
- what the providers do to deliver the intervention (procedures and processes);
- who provides the intervention (including their skill level), how (e.g. face to face, web-based) and in what setting (e.g. home, school, or hospital);
- the timing and intensity;
- whether any variation is permitted or expected, and whether modifications were actually made; and
- any strategies used to ensure or assess fidelity or adherence to the intervention, and the extent to which the intervention was delivered as planned.

For clinical trials of pharmacological interventions, key information to collect will often include routes of delivery (e.g. oral or intravenous delivery), doses (e.g. amount or intensity of each treatment, frequency of delivery), timing (e.g. within 24 hours of diagnosis), and length of treatment. For other interventions, such as those that evaluate psychotherapy, behavioural and educational approaches, or healthcare delivery strategies, the amount of information required to characterize the intervention will typically be greater, including information about multiple elements of the intervention, who delivered it, and the format and timing of delivery. Chapter 17 provides further information on how to manage intervention complexity, and how the intervention Complexity Assessment Tool (iCAT) can facilitate data collection (Lewin et al 2017).

Important characteristics of the interventions in each included study should be summarized for the reader in the table of 'Characteristics of included studies'. Additional tables or diagrams such as logic models (Chapter 2, Section 2.5.1) can assist descriptions of multi-component interventions so that review users can better assess review applicability to their context.

5.3.4.1 Integrity of interventions

The degree to which specified procedures or components of the intervention are implemented as planned can have important consequences for the findings from a study. We describe this as **intervention integrity**; related terms include adherence, compliance and fidelity (Carroll et al 2007). The verification of intervention integrity may be particularly important in reviews of non-pharmacological trials such as behavioural interventions and complex interventions, which are often implemented in conditions that present numerous obstacles to idealized delivery.

It is generally expected that reports of randomized trials provide detailed accounts of intervention implementation (Zwarenstein et al 2008, Moher et al 2010). In assessing whether interventions were implemented as planned, review authors should bear in mind that some interventions are standardized (with no deviations permitted in the intervention protocol), whereas others explicitly allow a degree of tailoring (Zwarenstein et al 2008).

In addition, the growing field of implementation science has led to an increased awareness of the impact of setting and context on delivery of interventions (Damschroder et al 2009). (See Chapter 17, Section 17.1.2.1 for further information and discussion about how an intervention may be tailored to local conditions in order to preserve its integrity.)

Information about integrity can help determine whether unpromising results are due to a poorly conceptualized intervention or to an incomplete delivery of the prescribed components. It can also reveal important information about the feasibility of implementing a given intervention in real life settings. If it is difficult to achieve full implementation in practice, the intervention will have low feasibility (Dusenbury et al 2003).

Whether a lack of intervention integrity leads to a risk of bias in the estimate of its effect depends on whether review authors and users are interested in the effect of assignment to intervention or the effect of adhering to intervention, as discussed in more detail in Chapter 8, Section 8.2.2. Assessment of deviations from intended interventions is important for assessing risk of bias in the latter, but not the former (see Chapter 8, Section 8.4), but both may be of interest to decision makers in different ways.

An example of a Cochrane Review evaluating intervention integrity is provided by a review of smoking cessation in pregnancy (Chamberlain et al 2017). The authors found that process evaluation of the intervention occurred in only some trials and that the implementation was less than ideal in others, including some of the largest trials. The review highlighted how the transfer of an intervention from one setting to another may reduce its effectiveness when elements are changed, or aspects of the materials are culturally inappropriate.

5.3.4.2 Process evaluations

Process evaluations seek to evaluate the process (and mechanisms) between the intervention's intended implementation and the actual effect on the outcome (Moore et al 2015). Process evaluation studies are characterized by a flexible approach to data collection and the use of numerous methods to generate a range of different types of data, encompassing both quantitative and qualitative methods. Guidance for including process evaluations in systematic reviews is provided in Chapter 21. When it is considered important, review authors should aim to collect information on whether the trial accounted for, or measured, key process factors and whether the trials that thoroughly addressed integrity showed a greater impact. Process evaluations can be a useful source of factors that potentially influence the effectiveness of an intervention.

5.3.5 Outcomes

An outcome is an event or a measurement value observed or recorded for a particular person or intervention unit in a study during or following an intervention, and that is used to assess the efficacy and safety of the studied intervention (Meinert 2012). Review authors should indicate in advance whether they plan to collect information about all outcomes measured in a study or only those outcomes of (pre-specified) interest in the review. Research has shown that trials addressing the same condition and intervention seldom agree on which outcomes are the most important, and consequently report on numerous different outcomes (Dwan et al 2014, Ismail et al 2014,

Denniston et al 2015, Saldanha et al 2017a). The selection of outcomes across systematic reviews of the same condition is also inconsistent (Page et al 2014, Saldanha et al 2014, Saldanha et al 2016, Liu et al 2017). Outcomes used in trials and in systematic reviews of the same condition have limited overlap (Saldanha et al 2017a, Saldanha et al 2017b).

We recommend that only the outcomes defined in the protocol be described in detail. However, a complete list of the names of all outcomes measured may allow a more detailed assessment of the risk of bias due to missing outcome data (see Chapter 13).

Review authors should collect all five elements of an outcome (Zarin et al 2011, Saldanha et al 2014):

1) outcome domain or title (e.g. anxiety);
2) measurement tool or instrument (including definition of clinical outcomes or endpoints); for a scale, name of the scale (e.g. the Hamilton Anxiety Rating Scale), upper and lower limits, and whether a high or low score is favourable, definitions of any thresholds if appropriate;
3) specific metric used to characterize each participant's results (e.g. post-intervention anxiety, or change in anxiety from baseline to a post-intervention time point, or post-intervention presence of anxiety (yes/no));
4) method of aggregation (e.g. mean and standard deviation of anxiety scores in each group, or proportion of people with anxiety);
5) timing of outcome measurements (e.g. assessments at end of eight-week intervention period, events occurring during eight-week intervention period).

Further considerations for economics outcomes are discussed in Chapter 20, and for patient-reported outcomes in Chapter 18.

5.3.5.1 Adverse effects

Collection of information about the harmful effects of an intervention can pose particular difficulties, discussed in detail in Chapter 19. These outcomes may be described using multiple terms, including 'adverse event', 'adverse effect', 'adverse drug reaction', 'side effect' and 'complication'. Many of these terminologies are used interchangeably in the literature, although some are technically different. Harms might additionally be interpreted to include undesirable changes in other outcomes measured during a study, such as a decrease in quality of life where an improvement may have been anticipated.

In clinical trials, adverse events can be collected either systematically or non-systematically. Systematic collection refers to collecting adverse events in the same manner for each participant using defined methods such as a questionnaire or a laboratory test. For systematically collected outcomes representing harm, data can be collected by review authors in the same way as efficacy outcomes (see Section 5.3.5).

Non-systematic collection refers to collection of information on adverse events using methods such as open-ended questions (e.g. 'Have you noticed any symptoms since your last visit?'), or reported by participants spontaneously. In either case, adverse events may be selectively reported based on their severity, and whether the participant suspected that the effect may have been caused by the intervention, which could lead to bias in the available data. Unfortunately, most adverse events are collected non-systematically rather than systematically, creating a challenge for review authors. The following pieces of information are useful and worth collecting (Nicole Fusco, personal communication):

- any coding system or standard medical terminology used (e.g. COSTART, MedDRA), including version number;
- name of the adverse events (e.g. dizziness);
- reported intensity of the adverse event (e.g. mild, moderate, severe);
- whether the trial investigators categorized the adverse event as 'serious';
- whether the trial investigators identified the adverse event as being related to the intervention;
- time point (most commonly measured as a count over the duration of the study);
- any reported methods for how adverse events were selected for inclusion in the publication (e.g. 'We reported all adverse events that occurred in at least 5% of participants'); and
- associated results.

Different collection methods lead to very different accounting of adverse events (Safer 2002, Bent et al 2006, Ioannidis et al 2006, Carvajal et al 2011, Allen et al 2013). Non-systematic collection methods tend to underestimate how frequently an adverse event occurs. It is particularly problematic when the adverse event of interest to the review is collected systematically in some studies but non-systematically in other studies. Different collection methods introduce an important source of heterogeneity. In addition, when non-systematic adverse events are reported based on quantitative selection criteria (e.g. only adverse events that occurred in at least 5% of participants were included in the publication), use of reported data alone may bias the results of meta-analyses. Review authors should be cautious of (or refrain from) synthesizing adverse events that are collected differently.

Regardless of the collection methods, precise definitions of adverse effect outcomes and their intensity should be recorded, since they may vary between studies. For example, in a review of aspirin and gastrointestinal haemorrhage, some trials simply reported gastrointestinal bleeds, while others reported specific categories of bleeding, such as haematemesis, melaena, and proctorrhagia (Derry and Loke 2000). The definition and reporting of severity of the haemorrhages (e.g. major, severe, requiring hospital admission) also varied considerably among the trials (Zanchetti and Hansson 1999). Moreover, a particular adverse effect may be described or measured in different ways among the studies. For example, the terms 'tiredness', 'fatigue' or 'lethargy' may all be used in reporting of adverse effects. Study authors also may use different thresholds for 'abnormal' results (e.g. hypokalaemia diagnosed at a serum potassium concentration of 3.0 mmol/L or 3.5 mmol/L).

No mention of adverse events in trial reports does not necessarily mean that no adverse events occurred. It is usually safest to assume that they were not reported. Quality of life measures are sometimes used as a measure of the participants' experience during the study, but these are usually general measures that do not look specifically at particular adverse effects of the intervention. While quality of life measures are important and can be used to gauge overall participant well-being, they should not be regarded as substitutes for a detailed evaluation of safety and tolerability.

5.3.6 Results

Results data arise from the measurement or ascertainment of outcomes for individual participants in an intervention study. Results data may be available for each individual in a study (i.e. individual participant data; see Chapter 26), or summarized at arm level, or summarized at study level into an intervention effect by comparing two intervention arms. Results data should be collected only for the intervention groups and outcomes specified to be of interest in the protocol (see MECIR Box 5.3.b). Results for other outcomes should not be collected unless the protocol is modified to add them. Any modification should be reported in the review. However, review authors should be alert to the possibility of important, unexpected findings, particularly serious adverse effects.

Reports of studies often include several results for the same outcome. For example, different measurement scales might be used, results may be presented separately for different subgroups, and outcomes may have been measured at different follow-up time points. Variation in the results can be very large, depending on which data are selected (Gøtzsche et al 2007, Mayo-Wilson et al 2017a). Review protocols should be as specific as possible about which outcome domains, measurement tools, time points, and summary statistics (e.g. final values versus change from baseline) are to be collected (Mayo-Wilson et al 2017b). A framework should be pre-specified in the protocol to facilitate making choices between multiple eligible measures or results. For example, a hierarchy of preferred measures might be created, or plans articulated to select the result with the median effect size, or to average across all eligible results for a particular outcome domain (see also Chapter 9, Section 9.3.3). Any additional decisions or changes to this framework made once the data are collected should be reported in the review as changes to the protocol.

Section 5.6 describes the numbers that will be required to perform meta-analysis, if appropriate. The unit of analysis (e.g. participant, cluster, body part, treatment period) should be recorded for each result when it is not obvious (see Chapter 6, Section 6.2). The type of outcome data determines the nature of the numbers that will be sought for each outcome. For example, for a dichotomous ('yes' or 'no') outcome, the number of participants and the number who experienced the outcome will be sought for each

MECIR Box 5.3.b Relevant expectations for conduct of intervention reviews	
C50: Choosing intervention groups in multi-arm studies (**Mandatory**)	
If a study is included with more than two intervention arms, include in the review only interventions that meet the eligibility criteria.	There is no point including irrelevant interventions in the review. Authors should, however, make it clear in the table of 'Characteristics of included studies' that these interventions were present in the study.

group. It is important to collect the sample size relevant to each result, although this is not always obvious. A flow diagram as recommended in the CONSORT Statement (Moher et al 2001) can help to determine the flow of participants through a study. If one is not available in a published report, review authors can consider drawing one (available from www.consort-statement.org).

The numbers required for meta-analysis are not always available. Often, other statistics can be collected and converted into the required format. For example, for a continuous outcome, it is usually most convenient to seek the number of participants, the mean and the standard deviation for each intervention group. These are often not available directly, especially the standard deviation. Alternative statistics enable calculation or estimation of the missing standard deviation (such as a standard error, a confidence interval, a test statistic (e.g. from a t-test or F-test) or a P value). These should be extracted if they provide potentially useful information (see MECIR Box 5.3.c). Details of recalculation are provided in Section 5.6. Further considerations for dealing with missing data are discussed in Chapter 10 (Section 10.12).

5.3.7 Other information to collect

We recommend that review authors collect the key conclusions of the included study as reported by its authors. It is not necessary to report these conclusions in the review, but they should be used to verify the results of analyses undertaken by the review authors,

MECIR Box 5.3.c Relevant expectations for conduct of intervention reviews	
C47: Making maximal use of data (**Mandatory**)	
Collect and utilize the most detailed numerical data that might facilitate similar analyses of included studies. Where 2×2 tables or means and standard deviations are not available, this might include effect estimates (e.g. odds ratios, regression coefficients), confidence intervals, test statistics (e.g. t, F, Z, Chi^2) or P values, or even data for individual participants.	Data entry into RevMan is easiest when 2×2 tables are reported for dichotomous outcomes, and when means and standard deviations are presented for continuous outcomes. Sometimes these statistics are not reported but some manipulations of the reported data can be performed to obtain them. For instance, 2×2 tables can often be derived from sample sizes and percentages, while standard deviations can often be computed using confidence intervals or P values. Furthermore, the inverse-variance data entry format can be used even if the detailed data required for dichotomous or continuous data are not available, for instance if only odds ratios and their confidence intervals are presented. The RevMan calculator facilitates many of these manipulations.

particularly in relation to the direction of effect. Further comments by the study authors, for example any explanations they provide for unexpected findings, may be noted. References to other studies that are cited in the study report may be useful, although review authors should be aware of the possibility of citation bias (see Chapter 7, Section 7.2.3.2). Documentation of any correspondence with the study authors is important for review transparency.

5.4 Data collection tools

5.4.1 Rationale for data collection forms

Data collection for systematic reviews should be performed using structured data collection forms (see MECIR Box 5.4.a). These can be paper forms, electronic forms (e.g. Google Form), or commercially or custom-built data systems (e.g. Covidence, EPPI-Reviewer, Systematic Review Data Repository (SRDR)) that allow online form building, data entry by several users, data sharing, and efficient data management (Li et al 2015). All different means of data collection require data collection forms.

The data collection form is a bridge between what is reported by the original investigators (e.g. in journal articles, abstracts, personal correspondence) and what is ultimately reported by the review authors. The data collection form serves several important functions (Meade and Richardson 1997). First, the form is linked directly to the review question and criteria for assessing eligibility of studies, and provides a clear summary of these that can be used to identify and structure the data to be extracted from study reports. Second, the data collection form is the historical record of the provenance of the data used in the review, as well as the multitude of decisions (and changes to decisions) that occur throughout the review process. Third, the form is the source of data for inclusion in an analysis.

Given the important functions of data collection forms, ample time and thought should be invested in their design. Because each review is different, data collection forms will vary across reviews. However, there are many similarities in the types of

MECIR Box 5.4.a Relevant expectations for conduct of intervention reviews	
C43: Using data collection forms (**Mandatory**)	
Use a data collection form, which has been piloted.	Review authors often have different backgrounds and level of systematic review experience. Using a data collection form ensures some consistency in the process of data extraction, and is necessary for comparing data extracted in duplicate. The completed data collection forms should be available to the CRG on request. Piloting the form within the review team is highly desirable. At minimum, the data collection form (or a very close variant of it) must have been assessed for usability.

information that are important. Thus, forms can be adapted from one review to the next. Although we use the term 'data collection form' in the singular, in practice it may be a series of forms used for different purposes: for example, a separate form could be used to assess the eligibility of studies for inclusion in the review to assist in the quick identification of studies to be excluded from or included in the review.

5.4.2 Considerations in selecting data collection tools

The choice of data collection tool is largely dependent on review authors' preferences, the size of the review, and resources available to the author team. Potential advantages and considerations of selecting one data collection tool over another are outlined in Table 5.4.a (Li et al 2015). A significant advantage that data systems have is in data management (Chapter 1, Section 1.6) and re-use. They make review updates more efficient, and also facilitate methodological research across reviews. Numerous 'meta-epidemiological' studies have been carried out using Cochrane Review data, resulting in methodological advances which would not have been possible if thousands of studies had not all been described using the same data structures in the same system.

Table 5.4.a Considerations in selecting data collection tools

	Paper forms	Electronic forms	Data systems
Examples	Forms developed using word processing software	Microsoft Access Google Forms	Covidence EPPI-Reviewer Systematic Review Data Repository (SRDR) DistillerSR (Evidence Partners) Doctor Evidence
Suitable review type and team sizes	Small-scale reviews (< 10 included studies) Small team with 2 to 3 data extractors in the same physical location	Small- to medium-scale reviews (10 to 20 studies) Small to moderate-sized team with 4 to 6 data extractors	For small-, medium-, and especially large-scale reviews (> 20 studies), as well as reviews that need constant updating All team sizes, especially large teams (i.e. > 6 data extractors)
Resource needs	Low	Low to medium	Low (open-access tools such as Covidence or SRDR, or tools for which authors have institutional licences) High (commercial data systems with no access via an institutional licence)
Advantages	Do not rely on access to computer and network or internet connectivity	Allow extracted data to be processed electronically for	Specifically designed for data collection for systematic reviews

Table 5.4.a (Continued)

	Paper forms	Electronic forms	Data systems
	Can record notes and explanations easily Require minimal software skills	editing and analysis Allow electronic data storage, sharing and collation Easy to expand or edit forms as required Can automate data comparison with additional programming Can copy data to analysis software without manual re-entry, reducing errors	Allow online data storage, linking, and sharing Easy to expand or edit forms as required Can be integrated with title/abstract, full-text screening and other functions Can link data items to locations in the report to facilitate checking Can readily automate data comparison between independent data collection for the same study Allow easy monitoring of progress and performance of the author team Facilitate coordination among data collectors such as allocation of studies for collection and monitoring team progress Allow simultaneous data entry by multiple authors Can export data directly to analysis software In some cases, improve public accessibility through open data sharing
Disadvantages	Inefficient and potentially unreliable because data must be entered into software for analysis and reporting Susceptible to errors Data collected by multiple authors must be manually collated Difficult to amend as the review progresses If the papers are lost, all data will need to be re-created	Require familiarity with software packages to design and use forms Susceptible to changes in software versions	Upfront investment of resources to set up the form and train data extractors Structured templates may not be as flexible as electronic forms Cost of commercial data systems Require familiarity with data systems Susceptible to changes in software versions

5.4.3 Design of a data collection form

Regardless of whether data are collected using a paper or electronic form, or a data system, the key to successful data collection is to construct easy-to-use forms and collect sufficient and unambiguous data that faithfully represent the source in a structured and organized manner (Li et al 2015). In most cases, a document format should be developed for the form before building an electronic form or a data system. This can be distributed to others, including programmers and data analysts, and as a guide for creating an electronic form and any guidance or codebook to be used by data extractors. Review authors also should consider compatibility of any electronic form or data system with analytical software, as well as mechanisms for recording, assessing and correcting data entry errors.

Data described in multiple reports (or even within a single report) of a study may not be consistent. Review authors will need to describe how they work with multiple reports in the protocol, for example, by pre-specifying which report will be used when sources contain conflicting data that cannot be resolved by contacting the investigators. Likewise, when there is only one report identified for a study, review authors should specify the section within the report (e.g. abstract, methods, results, tables, and figures) for use in case of inconsistent information.

A good data collection form should minimize the need to go back to the source documents. When designing a data collection form, review authors should involve all members of the team, that is, content area experts, authors with experience in systematic review methods and data collection form design, statisticians, and persons who will perform data extraction. Here are suggested steps and some tips for designing a data collection form, based on the informal collation of experiences from numerous review authors (Li et al 2015).

Step 1. Develop outlines of tables and figures expected to appear in the systematic review, considering the comparisons to be made between different interventions within the review, and the various outcomes to be measured. This step will help review authors decide the right amount of data to collect (not too much or too little). Collecting too much information can lead to forms that are longer than original study reports, and can be very wasteful of time. Collection of too little information, or omission of key data, can lead to the need to return to study reports later in the review process.

Step 2. Assemble and group data elements to facilitate form development. Review authors should consult Table 5.3.a, in which the data elements are grouped to facilitate form development and data collection. Note that it may be more efficient to group data elements in the order in which they are usually found in study reports (e.g. starting with reference information, followed by eligibility criteria, intervention description, statistical methods, baseline characteristics and results).

Step 3. Identify the optimal way of framing the data items. Much has been written about how to frame data items for developing robust data collection forms in primary research studies. We summarize a few key points and highlight issues that are pertinent to systematic reviews.

- Ask closed-ended questions (i.e. questions that define a list of permissible responses) as much as possible. Closed-ended questions do not require post hoc coding and provide better control over data quality than open-ended questions. When setting up a closed-ended question, one must anticipate and structure possible responses and include an 'other, specify' category because the anticipated list may not be exhaustive. Avoid asking data extractors to summarize data into uncoded text, no matter how short it is.

- Avoid asking a question in a way that the response may be left blank. Include 'not applicable', 'not reported' and 'cannot tell' options as needed. The 'cannot tell' option tags uncertain items that may promote review authors to contact study authors for clarification, especially on data items critical to reach conclusions.
- Remember that the form will focus on what is reported in the article rather what has been done in the study. The study report may not fully reflect how the study was actually conducted. For example, a question 'Did the article report that the participants were masked to the intervention?' is more appropriate than 'Were participants masked to the intervention?'
- Where a judgement is required, record the raw data (i.e. quote directly from the source document) used to make the judgement. It is also important to record the source of information collected, including where it was found in a report or whether information was obtained from unpublished sources or personal communications. As much as possible, questions should be asked in a way that minimizes subjective interpretation and judgement to facilitate data comparison and adjudication.
- Incorporate flexibility to allow for variation in how data are reported. It is strongly recommended that outcome data be collected in the format in which they were reported and transformed in a subsequent step if required. Review authors also should consider the software they will use for analysis and for publishing the review (e.g. RevMan).

Step 4. Develop and pilot-test data collection forms, ensuring that they provide data in the right format and structure for subsequent analysis. In addition to data items described in Step 2, data collection forms should record the title of the review as well as the person who is completing the form and the date of completion. Forms occasionally need revision; forms should therefore include the version number and version date to reduce the chances of using an outdated form by mistake. Because a study may be associated with multiple reports, it is important to record the study ID as well as the report ID. Definitions and instructions helpful for answering a question should appear next to the question to improve quality and consistency across data extractors (Stock 1994). Provide space for notes, regardless of whether paper or electronic forms are used.

All data collection forms and data systems should be thoroughly pilot-tested before launch (see MECIR Box 5.4.a). Testing should involve several people extracting data from at least a few articles. The initial testing focuses on the clarity and completeness of questions. Users of the form may provide feedback that certain coding instructions are confusing or incomplete (e.g. a list of options may not cover all situations). The testing may identify data that are missing from the form, or likely to be superfluous. After initial testing, accuracy of the extracted data should be checked against the source document or verified data to identify problematic areas. It is wise to draft entries for the table of 'Characteristics of included studies' and complete a risk of bias assessment (Chapter 8) using these pilot reports to ensure all necessary information is collected. A consensus between review authors may be required before the form is modified to avoid any misunderstandings or later disagreements. It may be necessary to repeat the pilot testing on a new set of reports if major changes are needed after the first pilot test.

Problems with the data collection form may surface after pilot testing has been completed, and the form may need to be revised after data extraction has started. When changes are made to the form or coding instructions, it may be necessary to return to reports that have already undergone data extraction. In some situations, it may be necessary to clarify only coding instructions without modifying the actual data collection form.

5.5 Extracting data from reports

5.5.1 Introduction

In most systematic reviews, the primary source of information about each study is published reports of studies, usually in the form of journal articles. Despite recent developments in machine learning models to automate data extraction in systematic reviews (see Section 5.5.9), data extraction is still largely a manual process. Electronic searches for text can provide a useful aid to locating information within a report. Examples include using search facilities in PDF viewers, internet browsers and word processing software. However, text searching should not be considered a replacement for reading the report, since information may be presented using variable terminology and presented in multiple formats.

5.5.2 Who should extract data?

Data extractors should have at least a basic understanding of the topic, and have knowledge of study design, data analysis and statistics. They should pay attention to detail while following instructions on the forms. Because errors that occur at the data extraction stage are rarely detected by peer reviewers, editors, or users of systematic reviews, it is recommended that more than one person extract data from every report to minimize errors and reduce introduction of potential biases by review authors (see MECIR Box 5.5.a). As a minimum, information that involves subjective interpretation and information that is critical to the interpretation of results (e.g. outcome data) should be extracted independently by at least two people (see MECIR Box 5.5.a). In common with implementation of the selection process (Chapter 4, Section 4.6), it is preferable that data extractors are from complementary disciplines, for example a methodologist and a topic area specialist. It is important that everyone involved in data extraction has practice using the form and, if the form was designed by someone else, receives appropriate training.

Evidence in support of duplicate data extraction comes from several indirect sources. One study observed that independent data extraction by two authors resulted in fewer errors than data extraction by a single author followed by verification by a second (Buscemi et al 2006). A high prevalence of data extraction errors (errors in 20 out of 34 reviews) has been observed (Jones et al 2005). A further study of data extraction to compute standardized mean differences found that a minimum of seven out of 27 reviews had substantial errors (Gøtzsche et al 2007).

5.5.3 Training data extractors

Training of data extractors is intended to familiarize them with the review topic and methods, the data collection form or data system, and issues that may arise during data

MECIR Box 5.5.a Relevant expectations for conduct of intervention reviews

C45: Extracting study characteristics in duplicate (**Highly desirable**)	
Use (at least) two people working independently to extract study characteristics from reports of each study, and define in advance the process for resolving disagreements.	Duplicating the data extraction process reduces both the risk of making mistakes and the possibility that data selection is influenced by a single person's biases. Dual data extraction may be less important for study characteristics than it is for outcome data, so it is not a mandatory standard for the former.
C46: Extracting outcome data in duplicate (**Mandatory**)	
Use (at least) two people working independently to extract outcome data from reports of each study, and define in advance the process for resolving disagreements.	Duplicating the data extraction process reduces both the risk of making mistakes and the possibility that data selection is influenced by a single person's biases. Dual data extraction is particularly important for outcome data, which feed directly into syntheses of the evidence and hence to conclusions of the review.

extraction. Results of the pilot testing of the form should prompt discussion among review authors and extractors of ambiguous questions or responses to establish consistency. Training should take place at the onset of the data extraction process and periodically over the course of the project (Li et al 2015). For example, when data related to a single item on the form are present in multiple locations within a report (e.g. abstract, main body of text, tables, and figures) or in several sources (e.g. publications, ClinicalTrials.gov, or CSRs), the development and documentation of instructions to follow an agreed algorithm are critical and should be reinforced during the training sessions.

Some have proposed that some information in a report, such as its authors, be blinded to the review author prior to data extraction and assessment of risk of bias (Jadad et al 1996). However, blinding of review authors to aspects of study reports generally is not recommended for Cochrane Reviews as there is little evidence that it alters the decisions made (Berlin 1997).

5.5.4 Extracting data from multiple reports of the same study

Studies frequently are reported in more than one publication or in more than one source (Tramèr et al 1997, von Elm et al 2004). A single source rarely provides complete information about a study; on the other hand, multiple sources may contain conflicting information about the same study (Mayo-Wilson et al 2017a, Mayo-Wilson et al 2017b, Mayo-Wilson et al 2018). Because the unit of interest in a systematic review is the study and not the report, information from multiple reports often needs to be collated and reconciled. It is not appropriate to discard any report of an included study without careful examination, since it may contain valuable information not included in the primary report. Review authors will need to decide between two strategies:

- Extract data from each report separately, then combine information across multiple data collection forms.
- Extract data from all reports directly into a single data collection form.

The choice of which strategy to use will depend on the nature of the reports and may vary across studies and across reports. For example, when a full journal article and multiple conference abstracts are available, it is likely that the majority of information will be obtained from the journal article; completing a new data collection form for each conference abstract may be a waste of time. Conversely, when there are two or more detailed journal articles, perhaps relating to different periods of follow-up, then it is likely to be easier to perform data extraction separately for these articles and collate information from the data collection forms afterwards. When data from all reports are extracted into a single data collection form, review authors should identify the 'main' data source for each study when sources include conflicting data and these differences cannot be resolved by contacting authors (Mayo-Wilson et al 2018). Flow diagrams such as those modified from the PRISMA statement can be particularly helpful when collating and documenting information from multiple reports (Mayo-Wilson 2018).

5.5.5 Reliability and reaching consensus

When more than one author extracts data from the same reports, there is potential for disagreement. After data have been extracted independently by two or more extractors, responses must be compared to assure agreement or to identify discrepancies. An explicit procedure or decision rule should be specified in the protocol for identifying and resolving disagreements. Most often, the source of the disagreement is an error by one of the extractors and is easily resolved. Thus, discussion among the authors is a sensible first step. More rarely, a disagreement may require arbitration by another person. Any disagreement that cannot be resolved should be addressed by contacting the study authors; if this is unsuccessful, the disagreement should be reported in the review.

The presence and resolution of disagreements should be carefully recorded. Maintaining a copy of the data 'as extracted' (in addition to the consensus data) allows assessment of reliability of coding. Examples of ways in which this can be achieved include the following:

- Use one author's (paper) data collection form and record changes after consensus in a different ink colour.
- Enter consensus data onto an electronic form.
- Record original data extracted and consensus data in separate forms (some online tools do this automatically).

Agreement of coded items before reaching consensus can be quantified, for example using kappa statistics (Orwin 1994), although this is not routinely done in Cochrane Reviews. If agreement is assessed, this should be done only for the most important data (e.g. key risk of bias assessments, or availability of key outcomes).

Throughout the review process informal consideration should be given to the reliability of data extraction. For example, if after reaching consensus on the first few studies, the authors note a frequent disagreement for specific data, then coding instructions may need modification. Furthermore, an author's coding strategy may change over time, as the coding rules are forgotten, indicating a need for retraining and, possibly, some recoding.

5.5.6 Extracting data from clinical study reports

Clinical study reports (CSRs) obtained for a systematic review are likely to be in PDF format. Although CSRs can be thousands of pages in length and very time-consuming to review, they typically follow the content and format required by the International Conference on Harmonisation (ICH 1995). Information in CSRs is usually presented in a structured and logical way. For example, numerical data pertaining to important demographic, efficacy, and safety variables are placed within the main text in tables and figures. Because of the clarity and completeness of information provided in CSRs, data extraction from CSRs may be clearer and conducted more confidently than from journal articles or other short reports.

To extract data from CSRs efficiently, review authors should familiarize themselves with the structure of the CSRs. In practice, review authors may want to browse or create 'bookmarks' within a PDF document that record section headers and subheaders and search key words related to the data extraction (e.g. randomization). In addition, it may be useful to utilize optical character recognition software to convert tables of data in the PDF to an analysable format when additional analyses are required, saving time and minimizing transcription errors.

CSRs may contain many outcomes and present many results for a single outcome (due to different analyses) (Mayo-Wilson et al 2017b). We recommend review authors extract results only for outcomes of interest to the review (Section 5.3.6). With regard to different methods of analysis, review authors should have a plan and pre-specify preferred metrics in their protocol for extracting results pertaining to different populations (e.g. 'all randomized', 'all participants taking at least one dose of medication'), methods for handling missing data (e.g. 'complete case analysis', 'multiple imputation'), and adjustment (e.g. unadjusted, adjusted for baseline covariates). It may be important to record the range of analysis options available, even if not all are extracted in detail. In some cases it may be preferable to use metrics that are comparable across multiple included studies, which may not be clear until data collection for all studies is complete.

CSRs are particularly useful for identifying outcomes assessed but not presented to the public. For efficacy outcomes and systematically collected adverse events, review authors can compare what is described in the CSRs with what is reported in published reports to assess the risk of bias due to missing outcome data (Chapter 8, Section 8.6) and in selection of reported result (Chapter 8, Section 8.8). Note that non-systematically collected adverse events are not amenable to such comparisons because these adverse events may not be known ahead of time and thus not pre-specified in the protocol.

5.5.7 Extracting data from regulatory reviews

Data most relevant to systematic reviews can be found in the medical and statistical review sections of a regulatory review. Both of these are substantially longer than journal articles (Turner 2013). A list of all trials on a drug usually can be found in the medical review. Because trials are referenced by a combination of numbers and letters, it may be difficult for the review authors to link the trial with other reports of the same trial (Section 5.2.1).

Many of the documents downloaded from the US Food and Drug Administration's website for older drugs are scanned copies and are not searchable because of redaction of confidential information (Turner 2013). Optical character recognition software can convert most of the text. Reviews for newer drugs have been redacted electronically; documents remain searchable as a result.

Compared to CSRs, regulatory reviews contain less information about trial design, execution, and results. They provide limited information for assessing the risk of bias. In terms of extracting outcomes and results, review authors should follow the guidance provided for CSRs (Section 5.5.6).

5.5.8 Extracting data from figures with software

Sometimes numerical data needed for systematic reviews are only presented in figures. Review authors may request the data from the study investigators, or alternatively, extract the data from the figures either manually (e.g. with a ruler) or by using software. Numerous tools are available, many of which are free. Those available at the time of writing include tools called Plot Digitizer, WebPlotDigitizer, Engauge, Dexter, ycasd, GetData Graph Digitizer. The software works by taking an image of a figure and then digitizing the data points off the figure using the axes and scales set by the users. The numbers exported can be used for systematic reviews, although additional calculations may be needed to obtain the summary statistics, such as calculation of means and standard deviations from individual-level data points (or conversion of time-to-event data presented on Kaplan-Meier plots to hazard ratios; see Chapter 6, Section 6.8.2).

It has been demonstrated that software is more convenient and accurate than visual estimation or use of a ruler (Gross et al 2014, Jelicic Kadic et al 2016). Review authors should consider using software for extracting numerical data from figures when the data are not available elsewhere.

5.5.9 Automating data extraction in systematic reviews

Because data extraction is time-consuming and error-prone, automating or semi-automating this step may make the extraction process more efficient and accurate. The state of science relevant to automating data extraction is summarized here (Jonnalagadda et al 2015).

- At least 26 studies have tested various natural language processing and machine learning approaches for facilitating data extraction for systematic reviews.
- Each tool focuses on only a limited number of data elements (ranges from one to seven). Most of the existing tools focus on the PICO information (e.g. number of participants, their age, sex, country, recruiting centres, intervention groups, outcomes, and time points). A few are able to extract study design and results (e.g. objectives, study duration, participant flow), and two extract risk of bias information (Marshall et al 2016, Millard et al 2016). To date, well over half of the data elements needed for systematic reviews have not been explored for automated extraction.

- Most tools highlight the sentence(s) that may contain the data elements as opposed to directly recording these data elements into a data collection form or a data system.
- There is no gold standard or common dataset to evaluate the performance of these tools, limiting our ability to interpret the significance of the reported accuracy measures.

At the time of writing, we cannot recommend a specific tool for automating data extraction for routine systematic review production. There is a need for review authors to work with experts in informatics to refine these tools and evaluate them rigorously. Such investigations should address how the tool will fit into existing workflows. For example, the automated or semi-automated data extraction approaches may first act as checks for manual data extraction before they can replace it.

5.5.10 Suspicions of scientific misconduct

Systematic review authors can uncover suspected misconduct in the published literature. Misconduct includes fabrication or falsification of data or results, plagiarism, and research that does not adhere to ethical norms. Review authors need to be aware of scientific misconduct because the inclusion of fraudulent material could undermine the reliability of a review's findings. Plagiarism of results data in the form of duplicated publication (either by the same or by different authors) may, if undetected, lead to study participants being double counted in a synthesis.

It is preferable to identify potential problems before, rather than after, publication of the systematic review, so that readers are not misled. However, empirical evidence indicates that the extent to which systematic review authors explore misconduct varies widely (Elia et al 2016). Text-matching software and systems such as CrossCheck may be helpful for detecting plagiarism, but they can detect only matching text, so data tables or figures need to be inspected by hand or using other systems (e.g. to detect image manipulation). Lists of data such as in a meta-analysis can be a useful means of detecting duplicated studies. Furthermore, examination of baseline data can lead to suspicions of misconduct for an individual randomized trial (Carlisle et al 2015). For example, Al-Marzouki and colleagues concluded that a trial report was fabricated or falsified on the basis of highly unlikely baseline differences between two randomized groups (Al-Marzouki et al 2005).

Cochrane Review authors are advised to consult with their Cochrane Review Group editors if cases of suspected misconduct are identified. Searching for comments, letters or retractions may uncover additional information. Sensitivity analyses can be used to determine whether the studies arousing suspicion are influential in the conclusions of the review. Guidance for editors for addressing suspected misconduct will be available from Cochrane's Editorial Publishing and Policy Resource (see community.cochrane.org). Further information is available from the Committee on Publication Ethics (COPE; publicationethics.org), including a series of flowcharts on how to proceed if various types of misconduct are suspected. Cases should be followed up, typically including an approach to the editors of the journals in which suspect reports were published. It may be useful to write first to the primary investigators to request clarification of apparent inconsistencies or unusual observations.

Because investigations may take time, and institutions may not always be responsive (Wager 2011), articles suspected of being fraudulent should be classified as 'awaiting assessment'. If a misconduct investigation indicates that the publication is unreliable, or if a publication is retracted, it should not be included in the systematic review, and the reason should be noted in the 'excluded studies' section.

5.5.11 Key points in planning and reporting data extraction

In summary, the methods section of both the protocol and the review should detail:

- the data categories that are to be extracted;
- how extracted data from each report will be verified (e.g. extraction by two review authors, independently);
- whether data extraction is undertaken by content area experts, methodologists, or both;
- pilot testing, training and existence of coding instructions for the data collection form;
- how data are extracted from multiple reports from the same study; and
- how disagreements are handled when more than one author extracts data from each report.

5.6 Extracting study results and converting to the desired format

In most cases, it is desirable to collect summary data separately for each intervention group of interest and to enter these into software in which effect estimates can be calculated, such as RevMan. Sometimes the required data may be obtained only indirectly, and the relevant results may not be obvious. Chapter 6 provides many useful tips and techniques to deal with common situations. When summary data cannot be obtained from each intervention group, or where it is important to use results of adjusted analyses (for example to account for correlations in crossover or cluster-randomized trials) effect estimates may be available directly.

5.7 Managing and sharing data

When data have been collected for each individual study, it is helpful to organize them into a comprehensive electronic format, such as a database or spreadsheet, before entering data into a meta-analysis or other synthesis. When data are collated electronically, all or a subset of them can easily be exported for cleaning, consistency checks and analysis.

Tabulation of collected information about studies can facilitate classification of studies into appropriate comparisons and subgroups. It also allows identification of comparable outcome measures and statistics across studies. It will often be necessary to perform calculations to obtain the required statistics for presentation or synthesis. It is important through this process to retain clear information on the provenance of the data, with a clear distinction between data from a source document and data obtained through calculations. Statistical conversions, for example from standard errors to standard deviations, ideally should be undertaken with a computer rather than using a hand calculator to maintain a permanent record of the original and calculated numbers as well as the actual calculations used.

Ideally, data only need to be extracted once and should be stored in a secure and stable location for future updates of the review, regardless of whether the original review authors or a different group of authors update the review (Ip et al 2012). Standardizing and sharing data collection tools as well as data management systems among review authors working in similar topic areas can streamline systematic review production. Review authors have the opportunity to work with trialists, journal editors, funders, regulators, and other stakeholders to make study data (e.g. CSRs, IPD, and any other form of study data) publicly available, increasing the transparency of research. When legal and ethical to do so, we encourage review authors to share the data used in their systematic reviews to reduce waste and to allow verification and reanalysis because data will not have to be extracted again for future use (Mayo-Wilson et al 2018).

5.8 Chapter information

Editors: Tianjing Li, Julian PT Higgins, Jonathan J Deeks

Acknowledgements: This chapter builds on earlier versions of the *Handbook*. For details of previous authors and editors of the *Handbook*, see Preface. Andrew Herxheimer, Nicki Jackson, Yoon Loke, Deirdre Price and Helen Thomas contributed text. Stephanie Taylor and Sonja Hood contributed suggestions for designing data collection forms. We are grateful to Judith Anzures, Mike Clarke, Miranda Cumpston and Peter Gøtzsche for helpful comments.

Funding: JPTH is a member of the National Institute for Health Research (NIHR) Biomedical Research Centre at University Hospitals Bristol NHS Foundation Trust and the University of Bristol. JJD received support from the NIHR Birmingham Biomedical Research Centre at the University Hospitals Birmingham NHS Foundation Trust and the University of Birmingham. JPTH received funding from National Institute for Health Research Senior Investigator award NF-SI-0617-10145. The views expressed are those of the author(s) and not necessarily those of the NHS, the NIHR or the Department of Health.

5.9 References

Al-Marzouki S, Evans S, Marshall T, Roberts I. Are these data real? Statistical methods for the detection of data fabrication in clinical trials. *BMJ* 2005; **331**: 267–270.

Allen EN, Mushi AK, Massawe IS, Vestergaard LS, Lemnge M, Staedke SG, Mehta U, Barnes KI, Chandler CI. How experiences become data: the process of eliciting adverse event, medical history and concomitant medication reports in antimalarial and antiretroviral interaction trials. *BMC Medical Research Methodology* 2013; **13**: 140.

Baudard M, Yavchitz A, Ravaud P, Perrodeau E, Boutron I. Impact of searching clinical trial registries in systematic reviews of pharmaceutical treatments: methodological systematic review and reanalysis of meta-analyses. *BMJ* 2017; **356**: j448.

Bent S, Padula A, Avins AL. Better ways to question patients about adverse medical events: a randomized, controlled trial. *Annals of Internal Medicine* 2006; **144**: 257–261.

Berlin JA. Does blinding of readers affect the results of meta-analyses? University of Pennsylvania Meta-analysis Blinding Study Group. *Lancet* 1997; **350**: 185–186.

Buscemi N, Hartling L, Vandermeer B, Tjosvold L, Klassen TP. Single data extraction generated more errors than double data extraction in systematic reviews. *Journal of Clinical Epidemiology* 2006; **59**: 697–703.

Carlisle JB, Dexter F, Pandit JJ, Shafer SL, Yentis SM. Calculating the probability of random sampling for continuous variables in submitted or published randomised controlled trials. *Anaesthesia* 2015; **70**: 848–858.

Carroll C, Patterson M, Wood S, Booth A, Rick J, Balain S. A conceptual framework for implementation fidelity. *Implementation Science* 2007; **2**: 40.

Carvajal A, Ortega PG, Sainz M, Velasco V, Salado I, Arias LHM, Eiros JM, Rubio AP, Castrodeza J. Adverse events associated with pandemic influenza vaccines: comparison of the results of a follow-up study with those coming from spontaneous reporting. *Vaccine* 2011; **29**: 519–522.

Chamberlain C, O'Mara-Eves A, Porter J, Coleman T, Perlen SM, Thomas J, McKenzie JE. Psychosocial interventions for supporting women to stop smoking in pregnancy. *Cochrane Database of Systematic Reviews* 2017; **2**: CD001055.

Damschroder LJ, Aron DC, Keith RE, Kirsh SR, Alexander JA, Lowery JC. Fostering implementation of health services research findings into practice: a consolidated framework for advancing implementation science. *Implementation Science* 2009; **4**: 50.

Davis AL, Miller JD. The European Medicines Agency and publication of clinical study reports: a challenge for the US FDA. *JAMA* 2017; **317**: 905–906.

Denniston AK, Holland GN, Kidess A, Nussenblatt RB, Okada AA, Rosenbaum JT, Dick AD. Heterogeneity of primary outcome measures used in clinical trials of treatments for intermediate, posterior, and panuveitis. *Orphanet Journal of Rare Diseases* 2015; **10**: 97.

Derry S, Loke YK. Risk of gastrointestinal haemorrhage with long term use of aspirin: meta-analysis. *BMJ* 2000; **321**: 1183–1187.

Doshi P, Dickersin K, Healy D, Vedula SS, Jefferson T. Restoring invisible and abandoned trials: a call for people to publish the findings. *BMJ* 2013; **346**: f2865.

Dusenbury L, Brannigan R, Falco M, Hansen WB. A review of research on fidelity of implementation: implications for drug abuse prevention in school settings. *Health Education Research* 2003; **18**: 237–256.

Dwan K, Altman DG, Clarke M, Gamble C, Higgins JPT, Sterne JAC, Williamson PR, Kirkham JJ. Evidence for the selective reporting of analyses and discrepancies in clinical trials: a systematic review of cohort studies of clinical trials. *PLoS Medicine* 2014; **11**: e1001666.

Elia N, von Elm E, Chatagner A, Popping DM, Tramèr MR. How do authors of systematic reviews deal with research malpractice and misconduct in original studies? A cross-sectional analysis of systematic reviews and survey of their authors. *BMJ Open* 2016; **6**: e010442.

Gøtzsche PC. Multiple publication of reports of drug trials. *European Journal of Clinical Pharmacology* 1989; **36**: 429–432.

Gøtzsche PC, Hróbjartsson A, Maric K, Tendal B. Data extraction errors in meta-analyses that use standardized mean differences. *JAMA* 2007; **298**: 430–437.

Gross A, Schirm S, Scholz M. Ycasd – a tool for capturing and scaling data from graphical representations. *BMC Bioinformatics* 2014; **15**: 219.

Hoffmann TC, Glasziou PP, Boutron I, Milne R, Perera R, Moher D, Altman DG, Barbour V, Macdonald H, Johnston M, Lamb SE, Dixon-Woods M, McCulloch P, Wyatt JC, Chan AW, Michie S. Better reporting of interventions: template for intervention description and replication (TIDieR) checklist and guide. *BMJ* 2014; **348**: g1687.

ICH. ICH Harmonised tripartite guideline: Struture and content of clinical study reports E31995. ICH1995. www.ich.org/fileadmin/Public_Web_Site/ICH_Products/Guidelines/Efficacy/E3/E3_Guideline.pdf.

Ioannidis JPA, Mulrow CD, Goodman SN. Adverse events: the more you search, the more you find. *Annals of Internal Medicine* 2006; **144**: 298–300.

Ip S, Hadar N, Keefe S, Parkin C, Iovin R, Balk EM, Lau J. A web-based archive of systematic review data. *Systematic Reviews* 2012; **1**: 15.

Ismail R, Azuara-Blanco A, Ramsay CR. Variation of clinical outcomes used in glaucoma randomised controlled trials: a systematic review. *British Journal of Ophthalmology* 2014; **98**: 464–468.

Jadad AR, Moore RA, Carroll D, Jenkinson C, Reynolds DJM, Gavaghan DJ, McQuay H. Assessing the quality of reports of randomized clinical trials: is blinding necessary? *Controlled Clinical Trials* 1996; **17**: 1–12.

Jelicic Kadic A, Vucic K, Dosenovic S, Sapunar D, Puljak L. Extracting data from figures with software was faster, with higher interrater reliability than manual extraction. *Journal of Clinical Epidemiology* 2016; **74**: 119–123.

Jones AP, Remmington T, Williamson PR, Ashby D, Smyth RL. High prevalence but low impact of data extraction and reporting errors were found in Cochrane systematic reviews. *Journal of Clinical Epidemiology* 2005; **58**: 741–742.

Jones CW, Keil LG, Holland WC, Caughey MC, Platts-Mills TF. Comparison of registered and published outcomes in randomized controlled trials: a systematic review. *BMC Medicine* 2015; **13**: 282.

Jonnalagadda SR, Goyal P, Huffman MD. Automating data extraction in systematic reviews: a systematic review. *Systematic Reviews* 2015; **4**: 78.

Lewin S, Hendry M, Chandler J, Oxman AD, Michie S, Shepperd S, Reeves BC, Tugwell P, Hannes K, Rehfuess EA, Welch V, McKenzie JE, Burford B, Petkovic J, Anderson LM, Harris J, Noyes J. Assessing the complexity of interventions within systematic reviews: development, content and use of a new tool (iCAT_SR). *BMC Medical Research Methodology* 2017; **17**: 76.

Li G, Abbade LPF, Nwosu I, Jin Y, Leenus A, Maaz M, Wang M, Bhatt M, Zielinski L, Sanger N, Bantoto B, Luo C, Shams I, Shahid H, Chang Y, Sun G, Mbuagbaw L, Samaan Z, Levine MAH, Adachi JD, Thabane L. A scoping review of comparisons between abstracts and full reports in primary biomedical research. *BMC Medical Research Methodology* 2017; **17**: 181.

Li TJ, Vedula SS, Hadar N, Parkin C, Lau J, Dickersin K. Innovations in data collection, management, and archiving for systematic reviews. *Annals of Internal Medicine* 2015; **162**: 287–294.

Liberati A, Altman DG, Tetzlaff J, Mulrow C, Gøtzsche PC, Ioannidis JPA, Clarke M, Devereaux PJ, Kleijnen J, Moher D. The PRISMA statement for reporting systematic reviews and meta-analyses of studies that evaluate health care interventions: explanation and elaboration. *PLoS Medicine* 2009; **6**: e1000100.

Liu ZM, Saldanha IJ, Margolis D, Dumville JC, Cullum NA. Outcomes in Cochrane systematic reviews related to wound care: an investigation into prespecification. *Wound Repair and Regeneration* 2017; **25**: 292–308.

Marshall IJ, Kuiper J, Wallace BC. RobotReviewer: evaluation of a system for automatically assessing bias in clinical trials. *Journal of the American Medical Informatics Association* 2016; **23**: 193–201.

Mayo-Wilson E, Doshi P, Dickersin K. Are manufacturers sharing data as promised? *BMJ* 2015; **351**: h4169.

Mayo-Wilson E, Li TJ, Fusco N, Bertizzolo L, Canner JK, Cowley T, Doshi P, Ehmsen J, Gresham G, Guo N, Haythomthwaite JA, Heyward J, Hong H, Pham D, Payne JL, Rosman L, Stuart EA, Suarez-Cuervo C, Tolbert E, Twose C, Vedula S, Dickersin K. Cherry-picking by trialists and meta-analysts can drive conclusions about intervention efficacy. *Journal of Clinical Epidemiology* 2017a; **91**: 95–110.

Mayo-Wilson E, Fusco N, Li TJ, Hong H, Canner JK, Dickersin K, MUDS Investigators. Multiple outcomes and analyses in clinical trials create challenges for interpretation and research synthesis. *Journal of Clinical Epidemiology* 2017b; **86**: 39–50.

Mayo-Wilson E, Li T, Fusco N, Dickersin K. Practical guidance for using multiple data sources in systematic reviews and meta-analyses (with examples from the MUDS study). *Research Synthesis Methods* 2018; **9**: 2–12.

Meade MO, Richardson WS. Selecting and appraising studies for a systematic review. *Annals of Internal Medicine* 1997; **127**: 531–537.

Meinert CL. *Clinical Trials Dictionary: Terminology and Usage Recommendations*. Hoboken (NJ): Wiley; 2012.

Millard LAC, Flach PA, Higgins JPT. Machine learning to assist risk-of-bias assessments in systematic reviews. *International Journal of Epidemiology* 2016; **45**: 266–277.

Moher D, Schulz KF, Altman DG. The CONSORT Statement: revised recommendations for improving the quality of reports of parallel-group randomised trials. *Lancet* 2001; **357**: 1191–1194.

Moher D, Hopewell S, Schulz KF, Montori V, Gøtzsche PC, Devereaux PJ, Elbourne D, Egger M, Altman DG. CONSORT 2010 explanation and elaboration: updated guidelines for reporting parallel group randomised trials. *BMJ* 2010; **340**: c869.

Moore GF, Audrey S, Barker M, Bond L, Bonell C, Hardeman W, Moore L, O'Cathain A, Tinati T, Wight D, Baird J. Process evaluation of complex interventions: Medical Research Council guidance. *BMJ* 2015; **350**: h1258.

Orwin RG. Evaluating coding decisions. In: Cooper H, Hedges LV, editors. *The Handbook of Research Synthesis*. New York (NY): Russell Sage Foundation; 1994. pp. 139–162.

Page MJ, McKenzie JE, Kirkham J, Dwan K, Kramer S, Green S, Forbes A. Bias due to selective inclusion and reporting of outcomes and analyses in systematic reviews of randomised trials of healthcare interventions. *Cochrane Database of Systematic Reviews* 2014; **10**: MR000035.

Ross JS, Mulvey GK, Hines EM, Nissen SE, Krumholz HM. Trial publication after registration in ClinicalTrials.Gov: a cross-sectional analysis. *PLoS Medicine* 2009; **6**: e1000144.

Safer DJ. Design and reporting modifications in industry-sponsored comparative psychopharmacology trials. *Journal of Nervous and Mental Disease* 2002; **190**: 583–592.

Saldanha IJ, Dickersin K, Wang X, Li TJ. Outcomes in Cochrane systematic reviews addressing four common eye conditions: an evaluation of completeness and comparability. *PloS One* 2014; **9**: e109400.

Saldanha IJ, Li T, Yang C, Ugarte-Gil C, Rutherford GW, Dickersin K. Social network analysis identified central outcomes for core outcome sets using systematic reviews of HIV/AIDS. *Journal of Clinical Epidemiology* 2016; **70**: 164–175.

Saldanha IJ, Lindsley K, Do DV, Chuck RS, Meyerle C, Jones LS, Coleman AL, Jampel HD, Dickersin K, Virgili G. Comparison of clinical trial and systematic review outcomes for the 4 most prevalent eye diseases. *JAMA Ophthalmology* 2017a; **135**: 933–940.

Saldanha IJ, Li TJ, Yang C, Owczarzak J, Williamson PR, Dickersin K. Clinical trials and systematic reviews addressing similar interventions for the same condition do not consider similar outcomes to be important: a case study in HIV/AIDS. *Journal of Clinical Epidemiology* 2017b; **84**: 85–94.

Stewart LA, Clarke M, Rovers M, Riley RD, Simmonds M, Stewart G, Tierney JF, PRISMA-IPD Development Group. Preferred reporting items for a systematic review and meta-analysis of individual participant data: the PRISMA-IPD statement. *JAMA* 2015; **313**: 1657–1665.

Stock WA. Systematic coding for research synthesis. In: Cooper H, Hedges LV, editors. *The Handbook of Research Synthesis*. New York (NY): Russell Sage Foundation; 1994. pp. 125–138.

Tramèr MR, Reynolds DJ, Moore RA, McQuay HJ. Impact of covert duplicate publication on meta-analysis: a case study. *BMJ* 1997; **315**: 635–640.

Turner EH. How to access and process FDA drug approval packages for use in research. *BMJ* 2013; **347**.

von Elm E, Poglia G, Walder B, Tramèr MR. Different patterns of duplicate publication: an analysis of articles used in systematic reviews. *JAMA* 2004; **291**: 974–980.

Wager E. Coping with scientific misconduct. *BMJ* 2011; **343**: d6586.

Wieland LS, Rutkow L, Vedula SS, Kaufmann CN, Rosman LM, Twose C, Mahendraratnam N, Dickersin K. Who has used internal company documents for biomedical and public health research and where did they find them? *PloS One* 2014; **9**: e94709.

Zanchetti A, Hansson L. Risk of major gastrointestinal bleeding with aspirin (Authors' reply). *Lancet* 1999; **353**: 149–150.

Zarin DA, Tse T, Williams RJ, Califf RM, Ide NC. The ClinicalTrials.gov results database: update and key issues. *New England Journal of Medicine* 2011; **364**: 852–860.

Zwarenstein M, Treweek S, Gagnier JJ, Altman DG, Tunis S, Haynes B, Oxman AD, Moher D. Improving the reporting of pragmatic trials: an extension of the CONSORT statement. *BMJ* 2008; **337**: a2390.

Saldanha IJ, Dickersin K, Wang X, Li T. Outcomes in Cochrane systematic reviews addressing four common eye conditions: an evaluation of completeness and comparability. PLoS One 2014; 9: e109400.

Saldanha IJ, Li T, Yang C, Ugarte-Gil C, Rutherford GW, Dickersin K. Social network analysis identified central outcomes for core outcome sets using systematic reviews of HIV/AIDS. J Clin Epidemiol 2016; 70: 164–175.

6

Choosing effect measures and computing estimates of effect

Julian PT Higgins, Tianjing Li, Jonathan J Deeks

KEY POINTS
• The types of outcome data that review authors are likely to encounter are dichotomous data, continuous data, ordinal data, count or rate data and time-to-event data. • There are several different ways of comparing outcome data between two intervention groups ('effect measures') for each data type. For example, dichotomous outcomes can be compared between intervention groups using a risk ratio, an odds ratio, a risk difference or a number needed to treat. Continuous outcomes can be compared between intervention groups using a mean difference or a standardized mean difference. • Effect measures are either ratio measures (e.g. risk ratio, odds ratio) or difference measures (e.g. mean difference, risk difference). Ratio measures are typically analysed on a logarithmic scale. • Results extracted from study reports may need to be converted to a consistent, or usable, format for analysis.

6.1 Types of data and effect measures

6.1.1 Types of data

A key early step in analysing results of studies of effectiveness is identifying the data type for the outcome measurements. Throughout this chapter we consider outcome data of five common types:

1) dichotomous (or binary) data, where each individual's outcome is one of only two possible categorical responses;
2) continuous data, where each individual's outcome is a measurement of a numerical quantity;

This chapter should be cited as: Higgins JPT, Li T, Deeks JJ (editors). Chapter 6: Choosing effect measures and computing estimates of effect. In: Higgins JPT, Thomas J, Chandler J, Cumpston M, Li T, Page MJ, Welch VA (editors). *Cochrane Handbook for Systematic Reviews of Interventions*. 2nd Edition. Chichester (UK): John Wiley & Sons, 2019: 143–176.

3) ordinal data (including measurement scales), where each individual's outcome is one of several ordered categories, or generated by scoring and summing categorical responses;
4) counts and rates calculated from counting the number of events experienced by each individual; and
5) time-to-event (typically survival) data that analyse the time until an event occurs, but where not all individuals in the study experience the event (censored data).

The ways in which the effect of an intervention can be assessed depend on the nature of the data being collected. In this chapter, for each of the above types of data, we review definitions, properties and interpretation of standard measures of intervention effect, and provide tips on how effect estimates may be computed from data likely to be reported in sources such as journal articles. Formulae to estimate effects (and their standard errors) for the commonly used effect measures are provided in a supplementary document Statistical algorithms in Review Manager, as well as other standard textbooks (Deeks et al 2001). Chapter 10 discusses issues in the selection of one of these measures for a particular meta-analysis.

6.1.2 Effect measures

By **effect measures**, we refer to statistical constructs that compare outcome data between two intervention groups. Examples include odds ratios (which compare the odds of an event between two groups) and mean differences (which compare mean values between two groups). Effect measures can broadly be divided into ratio measures and difference measures (sometimes also called relative and absolute measures, respectively). For example, the odds ratio is a ratio measure and the mean differences is a difference measure.

Estimates of effect describe the magnitude of the **intervention effect** in terms of how different the outcome data were between the two groups. For ratio effect measures, a value of 1 represents no difference between the groups. For difference measures, a value of 0 represents no difference between the groups. Values higher and lower than these 'null' values may indicate either benefit or harm of an experimental intervention, depending both on how the interventions are ordered in the comparison (e.g. A versus B or B versus A), and on the nature of the outcome.

The true effects of interventions are never known with certainty, and can only be estimated by the studies available. Every estimate should always be expressed with a measure of that uncertainty, such as a confidence interval or standard error (SE).

6.1.2.1 A note on ratio measures of intervention effect: the use of log scales

The values of ratio measures of intervention effect (such as the odds ratio, risk ratio, rate ratio and hazard ratio) usually undergo log transformations before being analysed, and they may occasionally be referred to in terms of their log transformed values (e.g. log odds ratio). Typically the *natural* log transformation (log base *e*, written 'ln') is used.

Ratio summary statistics all have the common features that the lowest value that they can take is 0, that the value 1 corresponds to no intervention effect, and that the highest value that they can take is infinity. This number scale is not symmetric. For example, whilst an odds ratio (OR) of 0.5 (a halving) and an OR of 2 (a doubling) are opposites such that they should average to no effect, the average of 0.5 and 2 is not an OR of 1 but an OR of 1.25. The log transformation makes the scale symmetric: the log of 0 is minus infinity, the log of 1 is zero, and the log of infinity is infinity. In the example, the log of the above OR of 0.5 is −0.69 and the log of the OR of 2 is 0.69. The average of −0.69 and 0.69 is 0 which is the log transformed value of an OR of 1, correctly implying no intervention effect on average.

Graphical displays for meta-analyses performed on ratio scales usually use a log scale. This has the effect of making the confidence intervals appear symmetric, for the same reasons.

6.1.2.2 A note on effects of interest

Review authors should not confuse *effect measures* with *effects of interest*. The effect of interest in any particular analysis of a randomized trial is usually either the effect of assignment to intervention (the 'intention-to-treat' effect) or the effect of adhering to intervention (the 'per-protocol' effect). These effects are discussed in Chapter 8 (Section 8.2.2). The data collected for inclusion in a systematic review, and the computations performed to produce effect estimates, will differ according to the effect of interest to the review authors. Most often in Cochrane Reviews the effect of interest will be the effect of assignment to intervention, for which an intention-to-treat analysis will be sought. Most of this chapter relates to this situation. However, specific analyses that have estimated the effect of adherence to intervention may be encountered.

6.2 Study designs and identifying the unit of analysis

6.2.1 Unit-of-analysis issues

An important principle in randomized trials is that the analysis must take into account the level at which randomization occurred. In most circumstances the number of observations in the analysis should match the number of 'units' that were randomized. In a simple parallel group design for a clinical trial, participants are individually randomized to one of two intervention groups, and a single measurement for each outcome from each participant is collected and analysed. However, there are numerous variations on this design. Authors should consider whether in each study:

1) groups of individuals were randomized together to the same intervention (i.e. cluster-randomized trials);
2) individuals underwent more than one intervention (e.g. in a crossover trial, or simultaneous treatment of multiple sites on each individual); and
3) there were multiple observations for the same outcome (e.g. repeated measurements, recurring events, measurements on different body parts).

Review authors should consider the impact on the analysis of any such clustering, matching or other non-standard design features of the included studies (see MECIR Box 6.2.a). A more detailed list of situations in which unit-of-analysis issues commonly arise follows, together with directions to relevant discussions elsewhere in this *Handbook*.

MECIR Box 6.2.a Relevant expectations for conduct of intervention reviews	
C70: Addressing non-standard designs (**Mandatory**)	
Consider the impact on the analysis of clustering, matching or other non- standard design features of the included studies.	Cluster-randomized studies, crossover studies, studies involving measurements on multiple body parts, and other designs need to be addressed specifically, since a naive analysis might underestimate or overestimate the precision of the study. Failure to account for clustering is likely to overestimate the precision of the study, that is, to give it confidence intervals that are too narrow and a weight that is too large. Failure to account for correlation is likely to underestimate the precision of the study, that is, to give it confidence intervals that are too wide and a weight that is too small.

6.2.2 Cluster-randomized trials

In a cluster-randomized trial, groups of participants are randomized to different interventions. For example, the groups may be schools, villages, medical practices, patients of a single doctor or families (see Chapter 23, Section 23.1).

6.2.3 Crossover trials

In a crossover trial, all participants receive all interventions in sequence: they are randomized to an ordering of interventions, and participants act as their own control (see Chapter 23, Section 23.2).

6.2.4 Repeated observations on participants

In studies of long duration, results may be presented for several periods of follow-up (for example, at 6 months, 1 year and 2 years). Results from more than one time point for each study cannot be combined in a standard meta-analysis without a unit-of-analysis error. Some options in selecting and computing effect estimates are as follows.

1) Obtain individual participant data and perform an analysis (such as time-to-event analysis) that uses the whole follow-up for each participant. Alternatively, compute an effect measure for each individual participant that incorporates all time points, such as total number of events, an overall mean, or a trend over time. Occasionally, such analyses are available in published reports.
2) Define several different outcomes, based on different periods of follow-up, and plan separate analyses. For example, time frames might be defined to reflect short-term, medium-term and long-term follow-up.

3) Select a single time point and analyse only data at this time for studies in which it is presented. Ideally this should be a clinically important time point. Sometimes it might be chosen to maximize the data available, although authors should be aware of the possibility of reporting biases.
4) Select the longest follow-up from each study. This may induce a lack of consistency across studies, giving rise to heterogeneity.

6.2.5 Events that may re-occur

If the outcome of interest is an event that can occur more than once, then care must be taken to avoid a unit-of-analysis error. Count data should not be treated as if they are dichotomous data (see Section 6.7).

6.2.6 Multiple treatment attempts

Similarly, multiple treatment attempts per participant can cause a unit-of-analysis error. Care must be taken to ensure that the number of participants randomized, and not the number of treatment attempts, is used to calculate confidence intervals. For example, in subfertility studies, women may undergo multiple cycles, and authors might erroneously use cycles as the denominator rather than women. This is similar to the situation in cluster-randomized trials, except that each participant is the 'cluster' (see methods described in Chapter 23, Section 23.1).

6.2.7 Multiple body parts I: body parts receive the same intervention

In some studies, people are randomized, but multiple parts (or sites) of the body receive the same intervention, a separate outcome judgement being made for each body part, and the number of body parts is used as the denominator in the analysis. For example, eyes may be mistakenly used as the denominator without adjustment for the non-independence between eyes. This is similar to the situation in cluster-randomized studies, except that participants are the 'clusters' (see methods described in Chapter 23, Section 23.1).

6.2.8 Multiple body parts II: body parts receive different interventions

A different situation is that in which different parts of the body are randomized to *different* interventions. 'Split-mouth' designs in oral health are of this sort, in which different areas of the mouth are assigned different interventions. These trials have similarities to crossover trials: whereas in crossover studies individuals receive multiple interventions at different times, in these trials they receive multiple interventions at different sites. See methods described in Chapter 23 (Section 23.2). It is important to distinguish these trials from those in which participants receive the same intervention at multiple sites (Section 6.2.7).

6.2.9 Multiple intervention groups

Studies that compare more than two intervention groups need to be treated with care. Such studies are often included in meta-analysis by making multiple pair-wise comparisons between all possible pairs of intervention groups. A serious unit-of-analysis

<table>
<tr><th colspan="2">MECIR Box 6.2.b Relevant expectations for conduct of intervention reviews</th></tr>
<tr><td colspan="2">C66: Addressing studies with more than two groups (Mandatory)</td></tr>
<tr><td>If multi-arm studies are included, analyse multiple intervention groups in an appropriate way that avoids arbitrary omission of relevant groups and double-counting of participants.</td><td>Excluding relevant groups decreases precision and double-counting increases precision spuriously; both are inappropriate and unnecessary. Alternative strategies include combining intervention groups, separating comparisons into different forest plots and using multiple treatments meta-analysis.</td></tr>
</table>

problem arises if the same group of participants is included twice in the same meta-analysis (for example, if 'Dose 1 vs Placebo' and 'Dose 2 vs Placebo' are both included in the same meta-analysis, with the same placebo patients in both comparisons). Review authors should approach multiple intervention groups in an appropriate way that avoids arbitrary omission of relevant groups and double-counting of participants (see MECIR Box 6.2.b) (see Chapter 23, Section 23.3). One option is network meta-analysis, as discussed in Chapter 11.

6.3 Extracting estimates of effect directly

In reviews of randomized trials, it is generally recommended that summary data from each intervention group are collected as described in Sections 6.4.2 and 6.5.2, so that effects can be estimated by the review authors in a consistent way across studies. On occasion, however, it is necessary or appropriate to extract an estimate of effect directly from a study report (some might refer to this as 'contrast-based' data extraction rather than 'arm-based' data extraction). Some situations in which this is the case include:

1) *For specific types of randomized trials:* analyses of cluster-randomized trials and crossover trials should account for clustering or matching of individuals, and it is often preferable to extract effect estimates from analyses undertaken by the trial authors (see Chapter 23).
2) *For specific analyses of randomized trials:* there may be other reasons to extract effect estimates directly, such as when analyses have been performed to adjust for variables used in stratified randomization or minimization, or when analysis of covariance has been used to adjust for baseline measures of an outcome. Other examples of sophisticated analyses include those undertaken to reduce risk of bias, to handle missing data or to estimate a 'per-protocol' effect using instrumental variables analysis (see also Chapter 8).
3) *For specific types of outcomes:* time-to-event data are not conveniently summarized by summary statistics from each intervention group, and it is usually more

convenient to extract hazard ratios (see Section 6.8.2). Similarly, for ordinal data and rate data it may be convenient to extract effect estimates (see Sections 6.6.2 and 6.7.2).

4) *For non-randomized studies:* when extracting data from non-randomized studies, adjusted effect estimates may be available (e.g. adjusted odds ratios from logistic regression analyses, or adjusted rate ratios from Poisson regression analyses). These are generally preferable to analyses based on summary statistics, because they usually reduce the impact of confounding. The variables that have been used for adjustment should be recorded (see Chapter 24).
5) *When summary data for each group are not available:* on occasion, summary data for each intervention group may be sought, but cannot be extracted. In such situations it may still be possible to include the study in a meta-analysis (using the generic inverse variance method) if an effect estimate is extracted directly from the study report.

An estimate of effect may be presented along with a confidence interval or a P value. It is usually necessary to obtain a SE from these numbers, since software procedures for performing meta-analyses using generic inverse-variance weighted averages mostly take input data in the form of an effect estimate and its SE from each study (see Chapter 10, Section 10.3). The procedure for obtaining a SE depends on whether the effect measure is an absolute measure (e.g. mean difference, standardized mean difference, risk difference) or a ratio measure (e.g. odds ratio, risk ratio, hazard ratio, rate ratio). We describe these procedures in Sections 6.3.1 and 6.3.2, respectively. However, for continuous outcome data, the special cases of extracting results for a mean from one intervention arm, and extracting results for the difference between two means, are addressed in Section 6.5.2.

A limitation of this approach is that estimates and SEs of the same effect measure must be calculated for all the other studies in the same meta-analysis, even if they provide the summary data by intervention group. For example, when numbers in each outcome category by intervention group are known for some studies, but only ORs are available for other studies, then ORs would need to be calculated for the first set of studies to enable meta-analysis with the second set of studies. Statistical software such as RevMan may be used to calculate these ORs (in this example, by first analysing them as dichotomous data), and the confidence intervals calculated may be transformed to SEs using the methods in Section 6.3.2.

6.3.1 Obtaining standard errors from confidence intervals and P values: absolute (difference) measures

When a 95% confidence interval (CI) is available for an absolute effect measure (e.g. standardized mean difference, risk difference, rate difference), then the SE can be calculated as

$$(\text{upper limit} - \text{lower limit})/3.92.$$

For 90% confidence intervals 3.92 should be replaced by 3.29, and for 99% confidence intervals it should be replaced by 5.15. Specific considerations are required for continuous outcome data when extracting mean differences. This is because confidence intervals should have been computed using t distributions, especially when the sample sizes are small: see Section 6.5.2.3 for details.

Where exact P values are quoted alongside estimates of intervention effect, it is possible to derive SEs. While all tests of statistical significance produce P values, different tests use different mathematical approaches. The method here assumes P values have been obtained through a particularly simple approach of dividing the effect estimate by its SE and comparing the result (denoted Z) with a standard normal distribution (statisticians often refer to this as a Wald test).

The first step is to obtain the Z value corresponding to the reported P value from a table of the standard normal distribution. A SE may then be calculated as

$$\text{SE} = \text{intervention effect estimate}/Z.$$

As an example, suppose a conference abstract presents an estimate of a risk difference of 0.03 (P = 0.008). The Z value that corresponds to a P value of 0.008 is Z = 2.652. This can be obtained from a table of the standard normal distribution or a computer program (for example, by entering **=abs(normsinv(0.008/2))** into any cell in a Microsoft Excel spreadsheet). The SE of the risk difference is obtained by dividing the risk difference (0.03) by the Z value (2.652), which gives 0.011.

Where significance tests have used other mathematical approaches, the estimated SEs may not coincide exactly with the true SEs. For P values that are obtained from t-tests for continuous outcome data, refer instead to Section 6.5.2.3.

6.3.2 Obtaining standard errors from confidence intervals and P values: ratio measures

The process of obtaining SE for ratio measures is similar to that for absolute measures, but with an additional first step. Analyses of ratio measures are performed on the natural log scale (see Section 6.1.2.1). For a ratio measure, such as a risk ratio, odds ratio or hazard ratio (which we denote generically as RR here), first calculate

$$\text{lower limit} = \ln\left(\text{lower confidence limit given for RR}\right)$$
$$\text{upper limit} = \ln\left(\text{upper confidence limit given for RR}\right)$$
$$\text{intervention effect estimate} = \ln\text{RR}.$$

Then the formulae in Section 6.3.1 can be used. Note that the SE refers to the log of the ratio measure. When using the generic inverse variance method in RevMan, the data should be entered on the natural log scale, that is as lnRR and the SE of lnRR, as calculated here (see Chapter 10, Section 10.3).

6.4 Dichotomous outcome data

6.4.1 Effect measures for dichotomous outcomes

Dichotomous (binary) outcome data arise when the outcome for every participant is one of two possibilities, for example, dead or alive, or clinical improvement or no clinical improvement. This section considers the possible summary statistics to use when the outcome of interest has such a binary form. The most commonly encountered effect measures used in randomized trials with dichotomous data are:

1) the risk ratio (RR; also called the relative risk);
2) the odds ratio (OR);
3) the risk difference (RD; also called the absolute risk reduction); and
4) the number needed to treat for an additional beneficial or harmful outcome (NNT).

Details of the calculations of the first three of these measures are given in Box 6.4.a. Numbers needed to treat are discussed in detail in Chapter 15 (Section 15.4), as they are primarily used for the communication and interpretation of results.

Methods for meta-analysis of dichotomous outcome data are covered in Chapter 10 (Section 10.4).

Aside: as events of interest may be desirable rather than undesirable, it would be preferable to use a more neutral term than risk (such as probability), but for the sake of convention we use the terms risk ratio and risk difference throughout. We also use the term 'risk ratio' in preference to 'relative risk' for consistency with other terminology. The two are interchangeable and both conveniently abbreviate to 'RR'. Note also that we have been careful with the use of the words 'risk' and 'rates'. These words are often treated synonymously. However, we have tried to reserve use of the word 'rate' for the data type 'counts and rates' where it describes the frequency of events in a measured period of time.

Box 6.4.a Calculation of risk ratio (RR), odds ratio (OR) and risk difference (RD) from a 2×2 table

The results of a two-group randomized trial with a dichotomous outcome can be displayed as a 2×2 table:

	Event ('**S**uccess')	No event ('**F**ail')	Total
Experimental intervention	S_E	F_E	N_E
Comparator intervention	S_C	F_C	N_C

where S_E, S_C, F_E and F_C are the numbers of participants with each outcome ('S' or 'F') in each group ('E' or 'C'). The following summary statistics can be calculated:

$$\text{RR} = \frac{\text{risk of event in experimental group}}{\text{risk of event in comparator group}} = \frac{S_E/N_E}{S_C/N_C}$$

$$\text{OR} = \frac{\text{odds of event in experimental group}}{\text{odds of event in comparator group}} = \frac{S_E/F_E}{S_C/F_C} = \frac{S_E F_C}{F_E S_C}$$

$$\text{RD} = \text{risk of event in experimental group} - \text{risk of event in comparator group}$$
$$= \frac{S_E}{N_E} - \frac{S_C}{N_C}$$

6.4.1.1 Risk and odds

In general conversation the terms 'risk' and 'odds' are used interchangeably (and also with the terms 'chance', 'probability' and 'likelihood') as if they describe the same quantity. In statistics, however, risk and odds have particular meanings and are calculated in different ways. When the difference between them is ignored, the results of a systematic review may be misinterpreted.

Risk is the concept more familiar to health professionals and the general public. Risk describes the probability with which a health outcome will occur. In research, risk is commonly expressed as a decimal number between 0 and 1, although it is occasionally converted into a percentage. In 'Summary of findings' tables in Cochrane Reviews, it is often expressed as a number of individuals per 1000 (see Chapter 14, Section 14.1.4). It is simple to grasp the relationship between a risk and the likely occurrence of events: in a sample of 100 people the number of events observed will on average be the risk multiplied by 100. For example, when the risk is 0.1, about 10 people out of every 100 will have the event; when the risk is 0.5, about 50 people out of every 100 will have the event. In a sample of 1000 people, these numbers are 100 and 500 respectively.

Odds is a concept that may be more familiar to gamblers. The 'odds' refers to the ratio of the probability that a particular event will occur to the probability that it will not occur, and can be any number between zero and infinity. In gambling, the odds describes the ratio of the size of the potential winnings to the gambling stake; in health care it is the ratio of the number of people with the event to the number without. It is commonly expressed as a ratio of two integers. For example, an odds of 0.01 is often written as 1 : 100, odds of 0.33 as 1 : 3, and odds of 3 as 3 : 1. Odds can be converted to risks, and risks to odds, using the formulae:

$$\text{risk} = \frac{\text{odds}}{1+\text{odds}};\ \text{odds} = \frac{\text{risk}}{1-\text{risk}}.$$

The interpretation of odds is more complicated than for a risk. The simplest way to ensure that the interpretation is correct is first to convert the odds into a risk. For example, when the odds are 1 : 10, or 0.1, one person will have the event for every 10 who do not, and, using the formula, the risk of the event is $0.1/(1 + 0.1) = 0.091$. In a sample of 100, about 9 individuals will have the event and 91 will not. When the odds are equal to 1, one person will have the event for every person who does not, so in a sample of 100, $100 \times 1/(1 + 1) = 50$ will have the event and 50 will not.

The difference between odds and risk is small when the event is rare (as illustrated in the example above where a risk of 0.091 was seen to be similar to an odds of 0.1). When events are common, as is often the case in clinical trials, the differences between odds and risks are large. For example, a risk of 0.5 is equivalent to an odds of 1; and a risk of 0.95 is equivalent to odds of 19.

Effect measures for randomized trials with dichotomous outcomes involve comparing either risks or odds from two intervention groups. To compare them we can look at their ratio (risk ratio or odds ratio) or the difference in risk (risk difference).

6.4.1.2 Measures of relative effect: the risk ratio and odds ratio

Measures of relative effect express the expected outcome in one group relative to that in the other. The **risk ratio** (RR, or relative risk) is the ratio of the risk of an event in the two groups, whereas the **odds ratio** (OR) is the ratio of the odds of an event (see Box 6.4.a). For both measures a value of 1 indicates that the estimated effects are the same for both interventions.

Neither the risk ratio nor the odds ratio can be calculated for a study if there are no events in the comparator group. This is because, as can be seen from the formulae in Box 6.4.a, we would be trying to divide by zero. The odds ratio also cannot be calculated if everybody in the intervention group experiences an event. In these situations, and others where SEs cannot be computed, it is customary to add ½ to each cell of the 2×2 table (for example, RevMan automatically makes this correction when necessary). In the case where no events (or all events) are observed in both groups the study provides no information about relative probability of the event and is omitted from the meta-analysis. This is entirely appropriate. Zeros arise particularly when the event of interest is rare, such as unintended adverse outcomes. For further discussion of choice of effect measures for such sparse data (often with lots of zeros) see Chapter 10 (Section 10.4.4).

Risk ratios describe the multiplication of the risk that occurs with use of the experimental intervention. For example, a risk ratio of 3 for an intervention implies that events with intervention are three times more likely than events without intervention. Alternatively we can say that intervention increases the risk of events by $100 \times (\text{RR} - 1)\% = 200\%$. Similarly, a risk ratio of 0.25 is interpreted as the probability of an event with intervention being one-quarter of that without intervention. This may be expressed alternatively by saying that intervention decreases the risk of events by $100 \times (1 - \text{RR})\% = 75\%$. This is known as the **relative risk reduction** (see also Chapter 15, Section 15.4.1). The interpretation of the clinical importance of a given risk ratio cannot be made without knowledge of the typical risk of events without intervention: a risk ratio of 0.75 could correspond to a clinically important reduction in events from 80% to 60%, or a small, less clinically important reduction from 4% to 3%. What constitutes clinically important will depend on the outcome and the values and preferences of the person or population.

The numerical value of the observed risk ratio must always lie somewhere between 0 and 1/CGR, where CGR (abbreviation of 'comparator group risk', sometimes referred to as the control group risk or the control event rate) is the observed risk of the event in the comparator group expressed as a number between 0 and 1. This means that for common events large values of risk ratio are impossible. For example, when the observed risk of events in the comparator group is 0.66 (or 66%) then the observed risk ratio cannot exceed 1.5. This boundary applies only for increases in risk, and can cause problems when the results of an analysis are extrapolated to a different population in which the comparator group risks are above those observed in the study.

Odds ratios, like odds, are more difficult to interpret (Sinclair and Bracken 1994, Sackett et al 1996). Odds ratios describe the multiplication of the odds of the outcome that occur with use of the intervention. To understand what an odds ratio means in terms of changes in numbers of events it is simplest to convert it first into a risk ratio, and then interpret the risk ratio in the context of a typical comparator group risk, as outlined here. The formula for converting an odds ratio to a risk ratio is provided in Chapter 15 (Section 15.4.4). Sometimes it may be sensible to calculate the RR for more than one assumed comparator group risk.

6.4.1.3 Warning: OR and RR are not the same

Since risk and odds are different when events are common, the risk ratio and the odds ratio also differ when events are common. This non-equivalence does not indicate that either is wrong: both are entirely valid ways of describing an intervention effect. Problems may arise, however, if the odds ratio is misinterpreted as a risk ratio. For interventions that increase the chances of events, the odds ratio will be larger than the risk ratio, so the misinterpretation will tend to overestimate the intervention effect, especially when events are common (with, say, risks of events more than 20%). For interventions that reduce the chances of events, the odds ratio will be smaller than the risk ratio, so that, again, misinterpretation overestimates the effect of the intervention. This error in interpretation is unfortunately quite common in published reports of individual studies and systematic reviews.

6.4.1.4 Measure of absolute effect: the risk difference

The **risk difference** is the difference between the observed risks (proportions of individuals with the outcome of interest) in the two groups (see Box 6.4.a). The risk difference can be calculated for any study, even when there are no events in either group. The risk difference is straightforward to interpret: it describes the difference in the observed risk of events between experimental and comparator interventions; for an individual it describes the estimated difference in the probability of experiencing the event. However, the clinical importance of a risk difference may depend on the underlying risk of events in the population. For example, a risk difference of 0.02 (or 2%) may represent a small, clinically insignificant change from a risk of 58% to 60% or a proportionally much larger and potentially important change from 1% to 3%. Although the risk difference provides more directly relevant information than relative measures (Laupacis et al 1988, Sackett et al 1997), it is still important to be aware of the underlying risk of events, and consequences of the events, when interpreting a risk difference. Absolute measures, such as the risk difference, are particularly useful when considering trade-offs between likely benefits and likely harms of an intervention.

The risk difference is naturally constrained (like the risk ratio), which may create difficulties when applying results to other patient groups and settings. For example, if a study or meta-analysis estimates a risk difference of –0.1 (or –10%), then for a group with an initial risk of, say, 7% the outcome will have an impossible estimated negative probability of –3%. Similar scenarios for increases in risk occur at the other end of the scale. Such problems can arise only when the results are applied to populations with different risks from those observed in the studies.

The number needed to treat is obtained from the risk difference. Although it is often used to summarize results of clinical trials, NNTs cannot be combined in a meta-analysis (see Chapter 10, Section 10.4.3). However, odds ratios, risk ratios and risk differences may be usefully converted to NNTs and used when interpreting the results of a meta-analysis as discussed in Chapter 15 (Section 15.4).

6.4.1.5 What is the event?

In the context of dichotomous outcomes, healthcare interventions are intended either to reduce the risk of occurrence of an adverse outcome or increase the chance of a good outcome. It is common to use the term ‘event’ to describe whatever the outcome or state of interest is in the analysis of dichotomous data. For example, when participants have particular symptoms at the start of the study the event of interest is usually recovery or cure. If participants are well or, alternatively, at risk of some adverse outcome at the beginning of the study, then the event is the onset of disease or occurrence of the adverse outcome.

It is possible to switch events and non-events and consider instead the proportion of patients not recovering or not experiencing the event. For meta-analyses using risk differences or odds ratios the impact of this switch is of no great consequence: the switch simply changes the sign of a risk difference, indicating an identical effect size in the opposite direction, whilst for odds ratios the new odds ratio is the reciprocal ($1/x$) of the original odds ratio.

In contrast, switching the outcome can make a substantial difference for risk ratios, affecting the effect estimate, its statistical significance, and the consistency of intervention effects across studies. This is because the precision of a risk ratio estimate differs markedly between those situations where risks are low and those where risks are high. In a meta-analysis, the effect of this reversal cannot be predicted easily. The identification, before data analysis, of which risk ratio is more likely to be the most relevant summary statistic is therefore important. It is often convenient to choose to focus on the event that represents a *change* in state. For example, in treatment studies where everyone starts in an adverse state and the intention is to 'cure' this, it may be more natural to focus on 'cure' as the event. Alternatively, in prevention studies where everyone starts in a 'healthy' state and the intention is to prevent an adverse event, it may be more natural to focus on 'adverse event' as the event. A general rule of thumb is to focus on the *less common state* as the event of interest. This reduces the problems associated with extrapolation (see Section 6.4.1.2) and may lead to less heterogeneity across studies. Where interventions aim to reduce the incidence of an adverse event, there is empirical evidence that risk ratios of the adverse event are more consistent than risk ratios of the non-event (Deeks 2002).

6.4.2 Data extraction for dichotomous outcomes

To calculate summary statistics and include the result in a meta-analysis, the only data required for a dichotomous outcome are the numbers of participants in each of the intervention groups who did and did not experience the outcome of interest (the numbers needed to fill in a standard 2×2 table, as in Box 6.4.a). In RevMan, these can be entered as the numbers with the outcome and the total sample sizes for the two groups. Although in theory this is equivalent to collecting the total numbers and the numbers experiencing the outcome, it is not always clear whether the reported total numbers are the whole sample size or only those for whom the outcome was measured or observed. Collecting the numbers of actual observations is preferable, as it avoids assumptions about any participants for whom the outcome was not measured. Occasionally the numbers of participants who experienced the event must be derived from percentages (although it is not always clear which denominator to use, because rounded percentages may be compatible with more than one numerator).

Sometimes the numbers of participants and numbers of events are not available, but an effect estimate such as an odds ratio or risk ratio may be reported. Such data may be included in meta-analyses (using the generic inverse variance method) only when they are accompanied by measures of uncertainty such as a SE, 95% confidence interval or an exact P value (see Section 6.3).

6.5 Continuous outcome data

6.5.1 Effect measures for continuous outcomes

The term 'continuous' in statistics conventionally refers to a variable that can take any value in a specified range. When dealing with numerical data, this means that a number may be measured and reported to an arbitrary number of decimal places. Examples of truly continuous data are weight, area and volume. In practice, we can use the same statistical methods for other types of data, most commonly measurement scales and counts of large numbers of events (see Section 6.6.1).

A common feature of continuous data is that a measurement used to assess the outcome of each participant is also measured at baseline, that is, before interventions are administered. This gives rise to the possibility of computing effects based on **change from baseline** (also called a **change score**). When effect measures are based on change from baseline, a single measurement is created for each participant, obtained either by subtracting the post-intervention measurement from the baseline measurement or by subtracting the baseline measurement from the post-intervention measurement. Analyses then proceed as for any other type of continuous outcome variable.

Two summary statistics are commonly used for meta-analysis of continuous data: the mean difference and the standardized mean difference. These can be calculated whether the data from each individual are post-intervention measurements or change-from-baseline measures. It is also possible to measure effects by taking ratios of means, or to use other alternatives.

Sometimes review authors may consider dichotomizing continuous outcome measures so that the result of the trial can be expressed as an odds ratio, risk ratio or risk difference. This might be done either to improve interpretation of the results (see Chapter 15, Section 15.5), or because the majority of the studies present results after dichotomizing a continuous measure. Results reported as means and SDs can, under some assumptions, be converted to risks (Anzures-Cabrera et al 2011). Typically a normal distribution is assumed for the outcome variable within each intervention group.

Methods for meta-analysis of continuous outcome data are covered in Chapter 10 (Section 10.5).

6.5.1.1 The mean difference (or difference in means)

The **mean difference** (MD, or more correctly, 'difference in means') is a standard statistic that measures the absolute difference between the mean value in two groups of a randomized trial. It estimates the amount by which the experimental intervention changes the outcome on average compared with the comparator intervention. It can be used as a summary statistic in meta-analysis when outcome measurements in all studies are made on the same scale.

Aside: analyses based on this effect measure were historically termed 'weighted mean difference' (WMD) analyses in the *Cochrane Database of Systematic Reviews*. This name is potentially confusing: although the meta-analysis computes a weighted average of these differences in means, no weighting is involved in calculation of a statistical summary of a single study. Furthermore, all meta-analyses involve a weighted combination of estimates, yet we do not use the word 'weighted' when referring to other methods.

6.5.1.2 The standardized mean difference

The **standardized mean difference** (SMD) is used as a summary statistic in meta-analysis when the studies all assess the same outcome, but measure it in a variety of ways (for example, all studies measure depression but they use different psychometric scales). In this circumstance it is necessary to standardize the results of the studies to a uniform scale before they can be combined. The SMD expresses the size of the intervention effect in each study relative to the between-participant variability in outcome measurements observed in that study. (Again in reality the intervention effect is a difference in means and not a mean of differences.)

$$\text{SMD} = \frac{\text{difference in mean outcome between groups}}{\text{standard deviation of outcome among participants}}.$$

Thus, studies for which the difference in means is the same proportion of the standard deviation (SD) will have the same SMD, regardless of the actual scales used to make the measurements.

However, the method assumes that the differences in SDs among studies reflect differences in measurement scales and not real differences in variability among study populations. If in two trials the true effect (as measured by the difference in means) is identical, but the SDs are different, then the SMDs will be different. This may be problematic in some circumstances where real differences in variability between the participants in different studies are expected. For example, where early explanatory trials are combined with later pragmatic trials in the same review, pragmatic trials may include a wider range of participants and may consequently have higher SDs. The overall intervention effect can also be difficult to interpret as it is reported in units of SD rather than in units of any of the measurement scales used in the review, but several options are available to aid interpretation (see Chapter 15, Section 15.6).

The term 'effect size' is frequently used in the social sciences, particularly in the context of meta-analysis. Effect sizes typically, though not always, refer to versions of the SMD. It is recommended that the term 'SMD' be used in Cochrane Reviews in preference to 'effect size' to avoid confusion with the more general plain language use of the latter term as a synonym for 'intervention effect' or 'effect estimate'.

It should be noted that the SMD method does not correct for differences in the direction of the scale. If some scales increase with disease severity (for example, a higher score indicates more severe depression) whilst others decrease (a higher score indicates less severe depression), it is essential to multiply the mean values from one set of studies by –1 (or alternatively to subtract the mean from the maximum possible value for the scale) to ensure that all the scales point in the same direction, before standardization. Any such adjustment should be described in the statistical methods section of the review. The SD does not need to be modified.

Different variations on the SMD are available depending on exactly what choice of SD is chosen for the denominator. The particular definition of SMD used in Cochrane Reviews is the effect size known in social science as Hedges' (adjusted) *g*. This uses a pooled SD in the denominator, which is an estimate of the SD based on outcome data from both intervention groups, assuming that the SDs in the two groups are similar. In contrast, Glass' delta (Δ) uses only the SD from the comparator group, on the basis that if the experimental intervention affects between-person variation, then such an impact of the intervention should not influence the effect estimate.

To overcome problems associated with estimating SDs within small studies, and with real differences across studies in between-person variability, it may sometimes be desirable to standardize using an external estimate of SD. External estimates might be derived, for example, from a cross-sectional analysis of many individuals assessed using the same continuous outcome measure (the sample of individuals might be derived from a large cohort study). Typically the external estimate would be assumed to be known without error, which is likely to be reasonable if it is based on a large number of individuals. Under this assumption, the statistical methods used for MDs would be used, with both the MD and its SE divided by the externally derived SD.

6.5.1.3 The ratio of means

The **ratio of means** (RoM) is a less commonly used statistic that measures the relative difference between the mean value in two groups of a randomized trial (Friedrich et al 2008). It estimates the amount by which the average value of the outcome is multiplied for participants on the experimental intervention compared with the comparator intervention. For example, a RoM of 2 for an intervention implies that the mean score in the participants receiving the experimental intervention is on average twice as high as that of the group without intervention. It can be used as a summary statistic in meta-analysis when outcome measurements can only be positive. Thus it is suitable for single (post-intervention) assessments but not for change-from-baseline measures (which can be negative).

An advantage of the RoM is that it can be used in meta-analysis to combine results from studies that used different measurement scales. However, it is important that these different scales have comparable lower limits. For example, a RoM might meaningfully be used to combine results from a study using a scale ranging from 0 to 10 with results from a study ranging from 1 to 50. However, it is unlikely to be reasonable to combine RoM results from a study using a scale ranging from 0 to 10 with RoM results from a study using a scale ranging from 20 to 30: it is not possible to obtain RoM values outside of the range 0.67 to 1.5 in the latter study, whereas such values are readily obtained in the former study. RoM is not a suitable effect measure for the latter study.

The RoM might be a particularly suitable choice of effect measure when the outcome is a physical measurement that can only take positive values, but when different studies use different measurement approaches that cannot readily be converted from one to another. For example, it was used in a meta-analysis where studies assessed urine output using some measures that did, and some measures that did not, adjust for body weight (Friedrich et al 2005).

6.5.1.4 Other effect measures for continuous outcome data

Other effect measures for continuous outcome data include the following.

- *Standardized difference in terms of the minimal important differences (MID) on each scale*. This expresses the MD as a proportion of the amount of change on a scale that would be considered clinically meaningful (Johnston et al 2010).
- *Prevented fraction*. This expresses the MD in change scores in relation to the comparator group mean change. Thus it describes how much change in the comparator group might have been prevented by the experimental intervention. It has commonly been used in dentistry (Dubey et al 1965).
- *Difference in percentage change from baseline*. This is a version of the MD in which each intervention group is summarized by the mean change divided by the mean baseline level, thus expressing it as a percentage. The measure has often been used, for example, for outcomes such as cholesterol level, blood pressure and glaucoma. Care is needed to ensure that the SE correctly accounts for correlation between baseline and post-intervention values (Vickers 2001).
- *Direct mapping from one scale to another*. If conversion factors are available that map one scale to another (e.g. pounds to kilograms) then these should be used. Methods are also available that allow these conversion factors to be estimated (Ades et al 2015).

6.5.2 Data extraction for continuous outcomes

To perform a meta-analysis of continuous data using MDs, SMDs or ratios of means, review authors should seek:

- the mean value of the outcome measurements in each intervention group;
- the standard deviation of the outcome measurements in each intervention group; and
- the number of participants for whom the outcome was measured in each intervention group.

Due to poor and variable reporting it may be difficult or impossible to obtain these numbers from the data summaries presented. Studies vary in the statistics they use to summarize the average (sometimes using medians rather than means) and variation (sometimes using SEs, confidence intervals, interquartile ranges and ranges rather than SDs). They also vary in the scale chosen to analyse the data (e.g. post-intervention measurements versus change from baseline; raw scale versus logarithmic scale).

A particularly misleading error is to misinterpret a SE as a SD. Unfortunately, it is not always clear which is being reported and some intelligent reasoning, and comparison with other studies, may be required. SDs and SEs are occasionally confused in the reports of studies, and the terminology is used inconsistently.

When needed, missing information and clarification about the statistics presented should always be sought from the authors. However, for several measures of variation there is an approximate or direct algebraic relationship with the SD, so it may be possible to obtain the required statistic even when it is not published in a paper, as explained in Sections 6.5.2.1 to 6.5.2.6. More details and examples are available elsewhere (Deeks 1997a, Deeks 1997b). Section 6.5.2.7 discusses options whenever SDs remain missing after attempts to obtain them.

Sometimes the numbers of participants, means and SDs are not available, but an effect estimate such as a MD or SMD has been reported. Such data may be included in meta-analyses using the generic inverse variance method only when they are accompanied by measures of uncertainty such as a SE, 95% confidence interval or an exact P value. A suitable SE from a confidence interval for a MD should be obtained using the early steps of the process described in Section 6.5.2.3. For SMDs, see Section 6.3.

6.5.2.1 Extracting post-intervention versus change from baseline data

Commonly, studies in a review will have reported a mixture of changes from baseline and post-intervention values (i.e. values at various follow-up time points, including 'final value'). Some studies will report both; others will report only change scores or only post-intervention values. As explained in Chapter 10 (Section 10.5.2), both post-intervention values and change scores can sometimes be combined in the same analysis so this is not necessarily a problem. Authors may wish to extract data on both change from baseline and post-intervention outcomes if the required means and SDs are available (see Section 6.5.2.7 for cases where the applicable SDs are not available). The choice of measure reported in the studies may be associated with the direction and magnitude of results. Review authors should seek evidence of whether such selective reporting may be the case in one or more studies (see Chapter 8, Section 8.7).

A final problem with extracting information on change from baseline measures is that often baseline and post-intervention measurements may have been reported for different numbers of participants due to missed visits and study withdrawals. It may be difficult to identify the subset of participants who report both baseline and post-intervention measurements for whom change scores can be computed.

6.5.2.2 Obtaining standard deviations from standard errors and confidence intervals for group means

A standard deviation can be obtained from the SE of a mean by multiplying by the square root of the sample size:

$$\mathrm{SD} = \mathrm{SE} \times \sqrt{N}.$$

When making this transformation, the SE must be calculated from within a single intervention group, and must not be the SE of the mean difference between two intervention groups.

The confidence interval for a mean can also be used to calculate the SD. Again, the following applies to the confidence interval for a mean value calculated within an intervention group and not for estimates of differences between interventions (for these, see Section 6.5.2.3). Most reported confidence intervals are 95% confidence intervals. If the sample size is large (say larger than 100 in each group), the 95% confidence interval is 3.92 SE wide (3.92 = 2 × 1.96). The SD for each group is obtained by dividing the width of the confidence interval by 3.92, and then multiplying by the square root of the sample size in that group:

$$\mathrm{SD} = \sqrt{N} \times \left(\text{upper limit} - \text{lower limit}\right)/3.92.$$

For 90% confidence intervals, 3.92 should be replaced by 3.29, and for 99% confidence intervals it should be replaced by 5.15.

If the sample size is small (say fewer than 60 participants in each group) then confidence intervals should have been calculated using a value from a t distribution. The numbers 3.92, 3.29 and 5.15 are replaced with slightly larger numbers specific to the t distribution, which can be obtained from tables of the t distribution with degrees of freedom equal to the group sample size minus 1. Relevant details of the t distribution are available as appendices of many statistical textbooks or from standard computer spreadsheet packages. For example the t statistic for a 95% confidence interval from a sample size of 25 can be obtained by typing **=tinv(1-0.95,25-1)** in a cell in a Microsoft Excel spreadsheet (the result is 2.0639). The divisor, 3.92, in the formula above would be replaced by $2 \times 2.0639 = 4.128$.

For moderate sample sizes (say between 60 and 100 in each group), either a t distribution or a standard normal distribution may have been used. Review authors should look for evidence of which one, and use a t distribution when in doubt.

As an example, consider data presented as follows:

Group	Sample size	Mean	95% CI
Experimental intervention	25	32.1	(30.0, 34.2)
Comparator intervention	22	28.3	(26.5, 30.1)

The confidence intervals should have been based on t distributions with 24 and 21 degrees of freedom, respectively. The divisor for the experimental intervention group is 4.128, from above. The SD for this group is $\sqrt{25} \times (34.2 - 30.0)/4.128 = 5.09$. Calculations for the comparator group are performed in a similar way.

It is important to check that the confidence interval is symmetrical about the mean (the distance between the lower limit and the mean is the same as the distance between the mean and the upper limit). If this is not the case, the confidence interval may have been calculated on transformed values (see Section 6.5.2.4).

6.5.2.3 Obtaining standard deviations from standard errors, confidence intervals, t statistics and P values for differences in means

Standard deviations can be obtained from a SE, confidence interval, t statistic or P value that relates to a difference between means in two groups (i.e. the MD). The MD is required in the calculations from the t statistic or the P value. An assumption that the SDs of outcome measurements are the same in both groups is required in all cases. The same SD is then used for both intervention groups. We describe first how a t statistic can be obtained from a P value, then how a SE can be obtained from a t statistic or a confidence interval, and finally how a SD is obtained from the SE. Review authors may select the appropriate steps in this process according to what results are available to them. Related methods can be used to derive SDs from certain F statistics, since taking the square root of an F statistic may produce the same t statistic. Care often is required to ensure that an appropriate F statistic is used. Advice from a knowledgeable statistician is recommended.

1) **From P value to t statistic**

Where actual P values obtained from t-tests are quoted, the corresponding t statistic may be obtained from a table of the t distribution. The degrees of freedom are given by $N_E + N_C - 2$, where N_E and N_C are the sample sizes in the experimental and comparator groups. We will illustrate with an example. Consider a trial of an experimental intervention ($N_E = 25$) versus a comparator intervention ($N_C = 22$), where the MD = 3.8. The P value for the comparison was P = 0.008, obtained using a two-sample t-test.

The t statistic that corresponds with a P value of 0.008 and 25 + 22 – 2 = 45 degrees of freedom is t = 2.78. This can be obtained from a table of the t distribution with 45 degrees of freedom or a computer (for example, by entering =**tinv(0.008, 45)** into any cell in a Microsoft Excel spreadsheet).

Difficulties are encountered when levels of significance are reported (such as P < 0.05 or even P = NS ('not significant', which usually implies P > 0.05) rather than exact P values. A conservative approach would be to take the P value at the upper limit (e.g. for P < 0.05 take P = 0.05, for P < 0.01 take P = 0.01 and for P < 0.001 take P = 0.001). However, this is not a solution for results that are reported as P = NS, or P > 0.05 (see Section 6.5.2.7).

2) **From t statistic to standard error**

The t statistic is the ratio of the MD to the SE of the MD. The SE of the MD can therefore be obtained by dividing it by the t statistic:

$$\mathrm{SE} = \left|\frac{\mathrm{MD}}{\mathrm{t}}\right|,$$

where $|X|$ denotes 'the absolute value of X'. In the example, where MD = 3.8 and t = 2.78, the SE of the MD is obtained by dividing 3.8 by 2.78, which gives 1.37.

3) **From confidence interval to standard error**

If a 95% confidence interval is available for the MD, then the same SE can be calculated as:

$$\mathrm{SE} = (\text{upper limit} - \text{lower limit})/3.92,$$

as long as the trial is large. For 90% confidence intervals divide by 3.29 rather than 3.92; for 99% confidence intervals divide by 5.15. If the sample size is small (say fewer than 60 participants in each group) then confidence intervals should have been calculated using a t distribution. The numbers 3.92, 3.29 and 5.15 are replaced with larger numbers specific to both the t distribution and the sample size, and can be obtained from tables of the t distribution with degrees of freedom equal to $N_E + N_C - 2$, where N_E and N_C are the sample sizes in the two groups. Relevant details of the t distribution are available as appendices of many statistical textbooks or from standard computer spreadsheet packages. For example, the t statistic for a 95% confidence interval from a comparison of a sample size of 25 with a sample size of 22 can be obtained by typing =**tinv(1-0.95, 25+22-2)** in a cell in a Microsoft Excel spreadsheet.

4) **From standard error to standard deviation**

The within-group SD can be obtained from the SE of the MD using the following formula:

$$\mathrm{SD} = \frac{\mathrm{SE}}{\sqrt{\frac{1}{N_E} + \frac{1}{N_C}}}.$$

In the example,

$$\mathrm{SD} = \frac{1.37}{\sqrt{\frac{1}{25} + \frac{1}{22}}} = 4.69.$$

Note that this SD is the average of the SDs of the experimental and comparator arms, and should be entered into RevMan twice (once for each intervention group).

6.5.2.4 Transformations and skewed data

Studies may present summary statistics calculated after a transformation has been applied to the raw data. For example, means and SDs of logarithmic values may be available (or, equivalently, a geometric mean and its confidence interval). Such results should be collected, as they may be included in meta-analyses, or – with certain assumptions – may be transformed back to the raw scale (Higgins et al 2008).

For example, a trial reported meningococcal antibody responses 12 months after vaccination with meningitis C vaccine and a control vaccine (MacLennan et al 2000), as geometric mean titres of 24 and 4.2 with 95% confidence intervals of 17 to 34 and 3.9 to 4.6, respectively. These summaries were obtained by finding the means and confidence intervals of the natural logs of the antibody responses (for vaccine 3.18 (95% CI 2.83 to 3.53), and control 1.44 (1.36 to 1.53)), and taking their exponentials (anti-logs). A meta-analysis may be performed on the scale of these natural log antibody responses, rather than the geometric means. SDs of the log-transformed data may be derived from the latter pair of confidence intervals using methods described in Section 6.5.2.1. For further discussion of meta-analysis with skewed data, see Chapter 10 (Section 10.5.3).

6.5.2.5 Interquartile ranges

Interquartile ranges describe where the central 50% of participants' outcomes lie. When sample sizes are large and the distribution of the outcome is similar to the normal distribution, the width of the interquartile range will be approximately 1.35 SDs. In other situations, and especially when the outcome's distribution is skewed, it is not possible to estimate a SD from an interquartile range. Note that the use of interquartile ranges rather than SDs often can indicate that the outcome's distribution is skewed. Wan and colleagues provided a sample size-dependent extension to the formula for approximating the SD using the interquartile range (Wan et al 2014).

6.5.2.6 Ranges

Ranges are very unstable and, unlike other measures of variation, increase when the sample size increases. They describe the extremes of observed outcomes rather than the average variation. One common approach has been to make use of the fact that, with normally distributed data, 95% of values will lie within 2 × SD either side of the mean. The SD may therefore be estimated to be approximately one-quarter of the typical range of data values. This method is not robust and we recommend that it not be used. Walter and Yao based an imputation method on the minimum and maximum observed values. Their enhancement of the “range' method provided a lookup table, according to sample size, of conversion factors from range to SD (Walter and Yao 2007). Alternative methods have been proposed to estimate SDs from ranges and quantiles (Hozo et al 2005, Wan et al 2014, Bland 2015), although to our knowledge these have not been evaluated using empirical data. As a general rule, we recommend that ranges should not be used to estimate SDs.

6.5.2.7 No information on variability

Missing SDs are a common feature of meta-analyses of continuous outcome data. When none of the above methods allow calculation of the SDs from the trial report (and the information is not available from the trialists) then a review author may be forced to impute (‘fill in') the missing data if they are not to exclude the study from the meta-analysis.

The simplest imputation is to borrow the SD from one or more other studies. Furukawa and colleagues found that imputing SDs either from other studies in the same meta-analysis, or from studies in another meta-analysis, yielded approximately correct results in two case studies (Furukawa et al 2006). If several candidate SDs are available, review authors should decide whether to use their average, the highest, a ‘reasonably high' value, or some other strategy. For meta-analyses of MDs, choosing a higher SD down-weights a study and yields a wider confidence interval. However, for SMD meta-analyses, choosing a higher SD will bias the result towards a lack of effect. More complicated alternatives are available for making use of multiple candidate SDs. For example, Marinho and colleagues implemented a linear regression of log(SD) on log(mean), because of a strong linear relationship between the two (Marinho et al 2003).

All imputation techniques involve making assumptions about unknown statistics, and it is best to avoid using them wherever possible. If the majority of studies in a meta-analysis have missing SDs, these values should not be imputed. A narrative approach might then be needed for the synthesis (see Chapter 12). However, imputation may be reasonable for a small proportion of studies comprising a small proportion of the data if it enables them to be combined with other studies for which full data are available. Sensitivity analyses should be used to assess the impact of changing the assumptions made.

6.5.2.8 Imputing standard deviations for changes from baseline

A special case of missing SDs is for changes from baseline measurements. Often, only the following information is available:

	Baseline	Final	Change
Experimental intervention (sample size)	mean, SD	mean, SD	mean
Comparator intervention (sample size)	mean, SD	mean, SD	mean

Note that the mean change in each group can be obtained by subtracting the post-intervention mean from the baseline mean even if it has not been presented explicitly. However, the information in this table does *not* allow us to calculate the SD of the changes. We cannot know whether the changes were very consistent or very variable across individuals. Some other information in a paper may help us determine the SD of the changes.

When there is not enough information available in a paper to calculate the SDs for the changes, they can be imputed, for example, by using change-from-baseline SDs for the same outcome measure from other studies in the review. However, the appropriateness of using a SD from another study relies on whether the studies used the same measurement scale, had the same degree of measurement error, had the same time interval between baseline and post-intervention measurement, and in a similar population.

When statistical analyses comparing the changes themselves are presented (e.g. confidence intervals, SEs, t statistics, P values, F statistics) then the techniques described in Section 6.5.2.3 may be used. Also note that an alternative to these methods is simply to use a comparison of post-intervention measurements, which in a randomized trial in theory estimates the same quantity as the comparison of changes from baseline.

The following alternative technique may be used for calculating or imputing missing SDs for changes from baseline (Follmann et al 1992, Abrams et al 2005). A typically unreported number known as the correlation coefficient describes how similar the baseline and post-intervention measurements were across participants. Here we describe (1) how to calculate the correlation coefficient from a study that is reported in considerable detail and (2) how to impute a change-from-baseline SD in another study, making use of a calculated or imputed correlation coefficient. Note that the methods in (2) are applicable both to correlation coefficients obtained using (1) and to correlation coefficients obtained in other ways (for example, by reasoned argument). Methods in (2) should be used sparingly because one can never be sure that an imputed correlation is appropriate. This is because correlations between baseline and post-intervention values usually will, for example, decrease with increasing time between baseline and post-intervention measurements, as well as depending on the outcomes, characteristics of the participants and intervention effects.

1) **Calculating a correlation coefficient from a study reported in considerable detail**

Suppose a study presents means and SDs for change as well as for baseline and post-intervention ('Final') measurements, for example:

	Baseline	**Final**	**Change**
Experimental intervention (sample size 129)	mean = 15.2 SD = 6.4	mean = 16.2 SD = 7.1	mean = 1.0 SD = 4.5
Comparator intervention (sample size 135)	mean = 15.7 SD = 7.0	mean = 17.2 SD = 6.9	mean = 1.5 SD = 4.2

An analysis of change from baseline is available from this study, using only the data in the final column. We can use other data in this study to calculate two correlation coefficients, one for each intervention group. Let us use the following notation:

	Baseline	Final	Change
Experimental intervention (sample size N_E)	$M_{E,baseline}$, $SD_{E,baseline}$	$M_{E,final}$, $SD_{E,final}$	$M_{E,change}$, $SD_{E,change}$
Comparator intervention (sample size N_C)	$M_{C,baseline}$, $SD_{C,baseline}$	$M_{C,final}$, $SD_{C,final}$	$M_{C,change}$, $SD_{C,change}$

The correlation coefficient in the experimental group, Corr_E, can be calculated as:

$$\text{Corr}_E = \frac{\text{SD}^2_{E,\text{baseline}} + \text{SD}^2_{E,\text{final}} - \text{SD}^2_{E,\text{change}}}{2 \times \text{SD}_{E,\text{baseline}} \times \text{SD}_{E,\text{final}}}$$

and similarly for the comparator intervention, to obtain Corr_C. In the example, these turn out to be

$$\text{Corr}_E = \frac{6.4^2 + 7.1^2 - 4.5^2}{2 \times 6.4 \times 7.1} = 0.78,$$

$$\text{Corr}_C = \frac{7.0^2 + 6.9^2 - 4.2^2}{2 \times 7.0 \times 6.9} = 0.82.$$

When either the baseline or post-intervention SD is unavailable, then it may be substituted by the other, providing it is reasonable to assume that the intervention does not alter the variability of the outcome measure. Assuming the correlation coefficients from the two intervention groups are reasonably similar to each other, a simple average can be taken as a reasonable measure of the similarity of baseline and final measurements across all individuals in the study (in the example, the average of 0.78 and 0.82 is 0.80). It is recommended that correlation coefficients be computed for many (if not all) studies in the meta-analysis and examined for consistency. If the correlation coefficients differ, then either the sample sizes are too small for reliable estimation, the intervention is affecting the variability in outcome measures, or the intervention effect depends on baseline level, and the use of average is best avoided. In addition, if a value less than 0.5 is obtained (correlation coefficients lie between –1 and 1), then there is little benefit in using change from baseline and an analysis of post-intervention measurements will be more precise.

2) **Imputing a change-from-baseline standard deviation using a correlation coefficient**

Now consider a study for which the SD of changes from baseline is missing. When baseline and post-intervention SDs are known, we can impute the missing SD using an imputed value, Corr, for the correlation coefficient. The value Corr may be calculated from another study in the meta-analysis (using the method in (1)), imputed from elsewhere, or hypothesized based on reasoned argument. In all of these situations, a sensitivity analysis should be undertaken, trying different values of Corr, to determine whether the overall result of the analysis is robust to the use of imputed correlation coefficients.

To impute a SD of the change from baseline for the experimental intervention, use

$$\text{SD}_{E,\text{change}} = \sqrt{\text{SD}^2_{E,\text{baseline}} + \text{SD}^2_{E,\text{final}} - \left(2 \times \text{Corr} \times \text{SD}_{E,\text{baseline}} \times \text{SD}_{E,\text{final}}\right)},$$

and similarly for the comparator intervention. Again, if either of the SDs (at baseline and post-intervention) is unavailable, then one may be substituted by the other as long as it is reasonable to assume that the intervention does not alter the variability of the outcome measure.

As an example, consider the following data:

	Baseline	Final	Change
Experimental intervention (sample size 35)	mean = 12.4 SD = 4.2	mean = 15.2 SD = 3.8	mean = 2.8
Comparator intervention (sample size 38)	mean = 10.7 SD = 4.0	mean = 13.8 SD = 4.4	mean = 3.1

Using the correlation coefficient calculated in step 1 above of 0.80, we can impute the change-from-baseline SD in the comparator group as:

$$SD_{C,\text{change}} = \sqrt{4.0^2 + 4.4^2 - (2 \times 0.80 \times 4.0 \times 4.4)} = 2.68.$$

6.5.2.9 Missing means

Missing mean values sometimes occur for continuous outcome data. If a median is available instead, then this will be very similar to the mean when the distribution of the data is symmetrical, and so occasionally can be used directly in meta-analyses. However, means and medians can be very different from each other when the data are skewed, and medians often are reported because the data are skewed (see Chapter 10, Section 10.5.3). Nevertheless, Hozo and colleagues conclude that the median may often be a reasonable substitute for a mean (Hozo et al 2005).

Wan and colleagues proposed a formula for imputing a missing mean value based on the lower quartile, median and upper quartile summary statistics (Wan et al 2014). Bland derived an approximation for a missing mean using the sample size, the minimum and maximum values, the lower and upper quartile values, and the median (Bland 2015). Both of these approaches assume normally distributed outcomes but have been observed to perform well when analysing skewed outcomes; the same simulation study indicated that the Wan method had better properties (Weir et al 2018). Caveats about imputing values summarized in Section 6.5.2.7 should be observed.

6.5.2.10 Combining groups

Sometimes it is desirable to combine two reported subgroups into a single group. For example, a study may report results separately for men and women in each of the intervention groups. The formulae in Table 6.5.a can be used to combine numbers into a single sample size, mean and SD for each intervention group (i.e. combining across men and women in each intervention group in this example). Note that the rather complex-looking formula for the SD produces the SD of outcome measurements *as if the combined group had never been divided into two*. This SD is different from the usual pooled SD that is used to compute a confidence interval for a MD or as the denominator in computing the SMD. This usual pooled SD provides a within-subgroup SD rather than an SD for the combined group, so provides an underestimate of the desired SD.

Table 6.5.a Formulae for combining summary statistics across two groups: Group 1 (with sample size = N_1, mean = M_1 and SD = SD_1) and Group 2 (with sample size = N_2, mean = M_2 and SD = SD_2)

	Combined groups
Sample size	$N_1 + N_2$
Mean	$\frac{N_1 M_1 + N_2 M_2}{N_1 + N_2}$
SD	$\sqrt{\frac{(N_1 - 1)\mathrm{SD}_1^2 + (N_2 - 1)\mathrm{SD}_2^2 + \frac{N_1 N_2}{N_1 + N_2}\left(M_1^2 + M_2^2 - 2M_1 M_2\right)}{N_1 + N_2 - 1}}$

These formulae are also appropriate for use in studies that compared three or more interventions, two of which represent the same intervention category as defined for the purposes of the review. In that case, it may be appropriate to combine these two groups and consider them as a single intervention (see Chapter 23, Section 23.3). For example, 'Group 1' and 'Group 2' may refer to two slightly different variants of an intervention to which participants were randomized, such as different doses of the same drug.

When there are more than two groups to combine, the simplest strategy is to apply the above formula sequentially (i.e. combine Group 1 and Group 2 to create Group '1+2', then combine Group '1+2' and Group 3 to create Group '1+2+3', and so on).

6.6 Ordinal outcome data and measurement scales

6.6.1 Effect measures for ordinal outcomes and measurement scales

Ordinal outcome data arise when each participant is classified in a category and when the categories have a natural order. For example, a 'trichotomous' outcome such as the classification of disease severity into 'mild', 'moderate' or 'severe', is of ordinal type. As the number of categories increases, ordinal outcomes acquire properties similar to continuous outcomes, and probably will have been analysed as such in a randomized trial.

Measurement scales are one particular type of ordinal outcome frequently used to measure conditions that are difficult to quantify, such as behaviour, depression and cognitive abilities. Measurement scales typically involve a series of questions or tasks, each of which is scored and the scores then summed to yield a total 'score'. If the items are not considered of equal importance a weighted sum may be used.

Methods are available for analysing ordinal outcome data that describe effects in terms of **proportional odds ratios** (Agresti 1996). Suppose that there are three categories, which are ordered in terms of desirability such that 1 is the best and 3 the worst. The data could be dichotomized in two ways: either category 1 constitutes a success and categories 2 and 3 a failure; or categories 1 and 2 constitute a success and category 3 a failure. A proportional odds model assumes that there is an equal odds ratio for both dichotomies of the data. Therefore, the odds ratio calculated from the proportional odds model can be interpreted as the odds of success on the experimental intervention relative to comparator, irrespective of how the ordered categories might be divided into success or failure. Methods (specifically polychotomous logistic regression models) are available for calculating study estimates of the log odds ratio and its SE.

Methods specific to ordinal data become unwieldy (and unnecessary) when the number of categories is large. In practice, longer ordinal scales acquire properties similar to continuous outcomes, and are often analysed as such, whilst shorter ordinal scales are often made into dichotomous data by combining adjacent categories together until only two remain. The latter is especially appropriate if an established, defensible cut-point is available. However, inappropriate choice of a cut-point can induce bias, particularly if it is chosen to maximize the difference between two intervention arms in a randomized trial.

Where ordinal scales are summarized using methods for dichotomous data, one of the two sets of grouped categories is defined as the event and intervention effects are described using risk ratios, odds ratios or risk differences (see Section 6.4.1). When ordinal scales are summarized using methods for continuous data, the mean score is calculated in each group and intervention effect is expressed as a MD or SMD, or possibly a RoM (see Section 6.5.1). Difficulties will be encountered if studies have summarized their results using medians (see Section 6.5.2.5). Methods for meta-analysis of ordinal outcome data are covered in Chapter 10 (Section 10.7).

6.6.2 Data extraction for ordinal outcomes

The data to be extracted for ordinal outcomes depend on whether the ordinal scale will be dichotomized for analysis (see Section 6.4), treated as a continuous outcome (see Section 6.5.2) or analysed directly as ordinal data. This decision, in turn, will be influenced by the way in which study authors analysed and reported their data. It may be impossible to pre-specify whether data extraction will involve calculation of numbers of participants above and below a defined threshold, or mean values and SDs. In practice, it is wise to extract data in all forms in which they are given as it will not be clear which is the most common form until all studies have been reviewed. In some circumstances more than one form of analysis may justifiably be included in a review.

Where ordinal data are to be dichotomized and there are several options for selecting a cut-point (or the choice of cut-point is arbitrary) it is sensible to plan from the outset to investigate the impact of choice of cut-point in a sensitivity analysis (see Chapter 10, Section 10.14). To collect the data that would be used for each alternative dichotomization, it is necessary to record the numbers in each category of short ordinal scales to avoid having to extract data from a paper more than once. This approach of recording all categorizations is also sensible when studies used slightly different short ordinal scales and it is not clear whether there is a cut-point that is common across all the studies which can be used for dichotomization.

It is also necessary to record the numbers in each category of the ordinal scale for each intervention group when the proportional odds ratio method will be used (see Chapter 10, Section 10.7).

6.7 Count and rate data

6.7.1 Effect measures for counts and rates

Some types of event can happen to a person more than once, for example, a myocardial infarction, an adverse reaction or a hospitalization. It may be preferable, or necessary, to address the number of times these events occur rather than simply whether each person experienced an event or not (that is, rather than treating them as dichotomous data). We refer to this type of data as **count data**. For practical purposes, count data may be conveniently divided into counts of rare events and counts of common events.

Counts of rare events are often referred to as 'Poisson data' in statistics. Analyses of rare events often focus on **rates**. Rates relate the counts to the amount of time during which they could have happened. For example, the result of one arm of a clinical trial could be that 18 myocardial infarctions (MIs) were experienced, across all participants in that arm, during a period of 314 person-years of follow-up (that is, the total number of years for which all the participants were collectively followed). The rate is 0.057 per person-year or 5.7 per 100 person-years. The summary statistic usually used in meta-analysis is the **rate ratio** (also abbreviated to RR), which compares the rate of events in the two groups by dividing one by the other.

Suppose E_E events occurred during T_E person-years of follow-up in the experimental intervention group, and E_C events during T_C person-years in the comparator intervention group. The rate ratio is:

$$\text{rate ratio} = \frac{E_E/T_E}{E_C/T_C} = \frac{E_E T_C}{E_C T_E}.$$

As a ratio measure, this rate ratio should then be log transformed for analysis (see Section 6.3.2). An approximate SE of the log rate ratio is given by:

$$\text{SE of ln rate ratio} = \sqrt{\frac{1}{E_E} + \frac{1}{E_C}}.$$

A correction of 0.5 may be added to each count in the case of zero events. Note that the choice of time unit (i.e. patient-months, woman-years, etc) is irrelevant since it is cancelled out of the rate ratio and does not figure in the SE. However, the units should still be displayed when presenting the study results.

It is also possible to use a **rate difference** (or difference in rates) as a summary statistic, although this is much less common:

$$\text{rate difference} = \frac{E_E}{T_E} - \frac{E_C}{T_C}.$$

An approximate SE for the rate difference is:

$$\text{SE of rate difference} = \sqrt{\frac{E_E}{T_E^2} + \frac{E_C}{T_C^2}}.$$

Counts of more common events, such as counts of decayed, missing or filled teeth, may often be treated in the same way as continuous outcome data. The intervention effect used will be the MD which will compare the difference in the mean number of events (possibly standardized to a unit time period) experienced by participants in the intervention group compared with participants in the comparator group.

6.7.2 Data extraction for counts and rates

Data that are inherently counts may have been analysed in several ways. Both primary investigators and review authors will need to decide whether to make the outcome of interest dichotomous, continuous, time-to-event or a rate (see Section 6.8).

Although it is preferable to decide how count data will be analysed in a review in advance, the choice often is determined by the format of the available data, and thus cannot be decided until the majority of studies have been reviewed. Review authors should plan to extract count data in the form in which they are reported.

Sometimes detailed data on events and person-years at risk are not available, but results calculated from them are. For example, an estimate of a rate ratio or rate difference may be presented. Such data may be included in meta-analyses only when they are accompanied by measures of uncertainty such as a 95% confidence interval (see Section 6.3), from which a SE can be obtained and the generic inverse variance method used for meta-analysis.

6.7.2.1 Extracting counts as dichotomous data

A common error is to attempt to treat count data as dichotomous data. Suppose that in the example just presented, the 18 MIs in 314 person-years arose from 157 patients observed on average for 2 years. One may be tempted to quote the results as 18/157, or even 18/314. This is inappropriate if multiple MIs from the same patient could have contributed to the total of 18 (say if the 18 arose through 12 patients having single MIs and 3 patients each having 2 MIs). The total number of events could theoretically exceed the number of patients, making the results nonsensical. For example, over the course of one year, 35 epileptic participants in a study could experience a total of 63 seizures.

To consider the outcome as a dichotomous outcome, the author must determine the number of participants in each intervention group, and the number of participants in each intervention group who experienced *at least one event* (or some other appropriate criterion which classified all participants into one of two possible groups). Any time element in the data is lost through this approach, though it may be possible to create a series of dichotomous outcomes, for example at least one stroke during the first year of follow-up, at least one stroke during the first two years of follow-up, and so on. It may be difficult to derive such data from published reports.

6.7.2.2 Extracting counts as continuous data

To extract counts as continuous data (i.e. the mean number of events per patient), guidance in Section 6.5.2 should be followed, although particular attention should be paid to the likelihood that the data will be highly skewed.

6.7.2.3 Extracting counts as time-to-event data

For rare events that can happen more than once, an author may be faced with studies that treat the data as time-to-first-event. To extract counts as time-to-event data, guidance in Section 6.8.2 should be followed.

6.7.2.4 Extracting counts as rate data

When it is possible to extract the total number of events in each group, and the total amount of person-time at risk in each group, then count data can be analysed as rates (see Chapter 10, Section 10.8). Note that the total number of participants is not required for an analysis of rate data but should be recorded as part of the description of the study.

6.8 Time-to-event data

6.8.1 Effect measures for time-to-event outcomes

Time-to-event data arise when interest is focused on the time elapsing before an event is experienced. They are known generically as **survival data** in the medical statistics literature, since death is often the event of interest, particularly in cancer and heart disease. Time-to-event data consist of pairs of observations for each individual: first, a length of time during which no event was observed, and second, an indicator of whether the end of that time period corresponds to an event or just the end of observation. Participants who contribute some period of time that does not end in an event are said to be 'censored'. Their event-free time contributes information and they are included in the analysis. Time-to-event data may be based on events other than death, such as recurrence of a disease event (for example, time to the end of a period free of epileptic fits) or discharge from hospital.

Time-to-event data can sometimes be analysed as dichotomous data. This requires the status of all patients in a study to be known at a fixed time point. For example, if all patients have been followed for at least 12 months, and the proportion who have incurred the event before 12 months is known for both groups, then a 2×2 table can be constructed (see Box 6.4.a) and intervention effects expressed as risk ratios, odds ratios or risk differences.

It is not appropriate to analyse time-to-event data using methods for continuous outcomes (e.g. using mean times-to-event), as the relevant times are only known for the subset of participants who have had the event. Censored participants must be excluded, which almost certainly will introduce bias.

The most appropriate way of summarizing time-to-event data is to use methods of survival analysis and express the intervention effect as a **hazard ratio**. Hazard is similar in notion to risk, but is subtly different in that it measures instantaneous risk and may change continuously (for example, one's hazard of death changes as one crosses a busy road). A hazard ratio describes how many times more (or less) likely a participant is to suffer the event at a particular point in time if they receive the experimental rather than the comparator intervention. When comparing interventions in a study or meta-analysis, a simplifying assumption is often made that the hazard ratio is constant across the follow-up period, even though hazards themselves may vary continuously. This is known as the proportional hazards assumption.

6.8.2 Data extraction for time-to-event outcomes

Meta-analysis of time-to-event data commonly involves obtaining individual patient data from the original investigators, re-analysing the data to obtain estimates of the hazard ratio and its statistical uncertainty, and then performing a meta-analysis (see Chapter 26). Conducting a meta-analysis using summary information from published papers or trial reports is often problematic as the most appropriate summary statistics often are not presented.

Where summary statistics are presented, three approaches can be used to obtain estimates of hazard ratios and their uncertainty from study reports for inclusion in a meta-analysis using the generic inverse variance methods. For practical guidance, review authors should consult Tierney and colleagues (Tierney et al 2007).

The first approach can be used when trialists have analysed the data using a Cox proportional hazards model (or some other regression models for survival data). Cox models produce direct estimates of the log hazard ratio and its SE, which are sufficient to perform a generic inverse variance meta-analysis. If the hazard ratio is quoted in a report together with a confidence interval or P value, an estimate of the SE can be obtained as described in Section 6.3.

The second approach is to estimate the hazard ratio approximately using statistics computed during a log-rank analysis. Collaboration with a knowledgeable statistician is advised if this approach is followed. The log hazard ratio (experimental relative to comparator) is estimated by $(O - E)/V$, which has $SE = 1/\sqrt{V}$, where O is the observed number of events on the experimental intervention, E is the log-rank expected number of events on the experimental intervention, $O - E$ is the log-rank statistic and V is the variance of the log-rank statistic (Simmonds et al 2011).

These statistics sometimes can be extracted from quoted statistics and survival curves (Parmar et al 1998, Williamson et al 2002). Alternatively, use can sometimes be made of aggregated data for each intervention group in each trial. For example, suppose that the data comprise the number of participants who have the event during the first year, second year, etc, and the number of participants who are event free and still being followed up at the end of each year. A log-rank analysis can be performed on these data, to provide the $O - E$ and V values, although careful thought needs to be given to the handling of censored times. Because of the coarse grouping the log hazard ratio is estimated only approximately. In some reviews it has been referred to as a log odds ratio (Early Breast Cancer Trialists' Collaborative Group 1990). When the time intervals are large, a more appropriate approach is one based on interval-censored survival (Collett 1994).

The third approach is to reconstruct approximate individual participant data from published Kaplan-Meier curves (Guyot et al 2012). This allows reanalysis of the data to estimate the hazard ratio, and also allows alternative approaches to analysis of the time-to-event data.

6.9 Conditional outcomes only available for subsets of participants

Some study outcomes may only be applicable to a proportion of participants. For example, in subfertility trials the proportion of clinical pregnancies that miscarry following treatment is often of interest to clinicians. By definition this outcome excludes participants who do not achieve an interim state (clinical pregnancy), so the comparison is not of all participants randomized. As a general rule it is better to re-define such outcomes so that the analysis includes all randomized participants. In this example, the outcome could be whether the woman has a 'successful pregnancy' (becoming pregnant and reaching, say, 24 weeks or term). If miscarriage is the outcome of interest, then appropriate analysis can be performed using individual participant data, but is rarely possible using summary data. Another example is provided by a morbidity outcome measured in the medium or long term (e.g. development of chronic lung disease), when there is a distinct possibility of a death preventing assessment of the morbidity. A convenient way to deal with such situations is to combine the outcomes, for example as 'death or chronic lung disease'.

Challenges arise when a continuous outcome (say a measure of functional ability or quality of life following stroke) is measured only on those who survive to the end of follow-up. Two unsatisfactory options are: (i) imputing zero functional ability scores for those who die (which may not appropriately represent the death state and will make the outcome severely skewed), and (ii) analysing the available data (which must be interpreted as a non-randomized comparison applicable only to survivors). The results of these analyses must be interpreted taking into account any disparity in the proportion of deaths between the two intervention groups. More sophisticated options are available, which may increasingly be applied by trial authors (Colantuoni et al 2018).

6.10 Chapter information

Editors: Julian PT Higgins, Tianjing Li, Jonathan J Deeks

Acknowledgements: This chapter builds on earlier versions of the *Handbook*. For details of previous authors and editors of the *Handbook*, see Preface. We are grateful to Judith Anzures, Mike Clarke, Miranda Cumpston, Peter Gøtzsche and Christopher Weir for helpful comments.

Funding: JPTH is a member of the National Institute for Health Research (NIHR) Biomedical Research Centre at University Hospitals Bristol NHS Foundation Trust and the University of Bristol. JJD received support from the NIHR Birmingham Biomedical Research Centre at the University Hospitals Birmingham NHS Foundation Trust and the University of Birmingham. JPTH received funding from National Institute for Health Research Senior Investigator award NF-SI-0617-10145. The views expressed are those of the author(s) and not necessarily those of the NHS, the NIHR or the Department of Health.

6.11 References

Abrams KR, Gillies CL, Lambert PC. Meta-analysis of heterogeneously reported trials assessing change from baseline. *Statistics in Medicine* 2005; **24**: 3823–3844.

Ades AE, Lu G, Dias S, Mayo-Wilson E, Kounali D. Simultaneous synthesis of treatment effects and mapping to a common scale: an alternative to standardisation. *Research Synthesis Methods* 2015; **6**: 96–107.

Agresti A. *An Introduction to Categorical Data Analysis*. New York (NY): John Wiley & Sons; 1996.

Anzures-Cabrera J, Sarpatwari A, Higgins JPT. Expressing findings from meta-analyses of continuous outcomes in terms of risks. *Statistics in Medicine* 2011; **30**: 2967–2985.

Bland M. Estimating mean and standard deviation from the sample size, three quartiles, minimum, and maximum. *International Journal of Statistics in Medical Research* 2015; **4**: 57–64.

Colantuoni E, Scharfstein DO, Wang C, Hashem MD, Leroux A, Needham DM, Girard TD. Statistical methods to compare functional outcomes in randomized controlled trials with high mortality. *BMJ* 2018; **360**: j5748.

Collett D. *Modelling Survival Data in Medical Research*. London (UK): Chapman & Hall; 1994.

Deeks J. Are you sure that's a standard deviation? (part 1). *Cochrane News* 1997a; **10**: 11–12.

Deeks J. Are you sure that's a standard deviation? (part 2). *Cochrane News* 1997b; **11**: 11–12.

Deeks JJ, Altman DG, Bradburn MJ. Statistical methods for examining heterogeneity and combining results from several studies in meta-analysis. In: Egger M, Davey Smith G, Altman DG, editors. *Systematic Reviews in Health Care: Meta-analysis in Context*. 2nd edition ed. London (UK): BMJ Publication Group; 2001. pp. 285–312.

Deeks JJ. Issues in the selection of a summary statistic for meta-analysis of clinical trials with binary outcomes. *Statistics in Medicine* 2002; **21**: 1575–1600.

Dubey SD, Lehnhoff RW, Radike AW. A statistical confidence interval for true per cent reduction in caries-incidence studies. *Journal of Dental Research* 1965; **44**: 921–923.

Early Breast Cancer Trialists' Collaborative Group. *Treatment of Early Breast Cancer. Volume 1: Worldwide Evidence 1985–1990*. Oxford (UK): Oxford University Press; 1990.

Follmann D, Elliott P, Suh I, Cutler J. Variance imputation for overviews of clinical trials with continuous response. *Journal of Clinical Epidemiology* 1992; **45**: 769–773.

Friedrich JO, Adhikari N, Herridge MS, Beyene J. Meta-analysis: low-dose dopamine increases urine output but does not prevent renal dysfunction or death. *Annals of Internal Medicine* 2005; **142**: 510–524.

Friedrich JO, Adhikari NK, Beyene J. The ratio of means method as an alternative to mean differences for analyzing continuous outcome variables in meta-analysis: a simulation study. *BMC Medical Research Methodology* 2008; **8**: 32.

Furukawa TA, Barbui C, Cipriani A, Brambilla P, Watanabe N. Imputing missing standard deviations in meta-analyses can provide accurate results. *Journal of Clinical Epidemiology* 2006; **59**: 7–10.

Guyot P, Ades AE, Ouwens MJ, Welton NJ. Enhanced secondary analysis of survival data: reconstructing the data from published Kaplan-Meier survival curves. *BMC Medical Research Methodology* 2012; **12**: 9.

Higgins JPT, White IR, Anzures-Cabrera J. Meta-analysis of skewed data: combining results reported on log-transformed or raw scales. *Statistics in Medicine* 2008; **27**: 6072–6092.

Hozo SP, Djulbegovic B, Hozo I. Estimating the mean and variance from the median, range, and the size of a sample. *BMC Medical Research Methodology* 2005; **5**: 13.

Johnston BC, Thorlund K, Schünemann HJ, Xie F, Murad MH, Montori VM, Guyatt GH. Improving the interpretation of quality of life evidence in meta-analyses: the application of minimal important difference units. *Health and Quality of Life Outcomes* 2010; **8**: 116.

Laupacis A, Sackett DL, Roberts RS. An assessment of clinically useful measures of the consequences of treatment. *New England Journal of Medicine* 1988; **318**: 1728–1733.

MacLennan JM, Shackley F, Heath PT, Deeks JJ, Flamank C, Herbert M, Griffiths H, Hatzmann E, Goilav C, Moxon ER. Safety, immunogenicity, and induction of immunologic memory by a serogroup C meningococcal conjugate vaccine in infants: a randomized controlled trial. *JAMA* 2000; **283**: 2795–2801.

Marinho VCC, Higgins JPT, Logan S, Sheiham A. Fluoride toothpaste for preventing dental caries in children and adolescents. *Cochrane Database of Systematic Reviews* 2003; **1**: CD002278.

Parmar MKB, Torri V, Stewart L. Extracting summary statistics to perform meta-analyses of the published literature for survival endpoints. *Statistics in Medicine* 1998; **17**: 2815–2834.

Sackett DL, Deeks JJ, Altman DG. Down with odds ratios! *Evidence Based Medicine* 1996; **1**: 164–166.

Sackett DL, Richardson WS, Rosenberg W, Haynes BR. *Evidence-Based Medicine: How to Practice and Teach EBM*. Edinburgh (UK): Churchill Livingstone; 1997.

Simmonds MC, Tierney J, Bowden J, Higgins JPT. Meta-analysis of time-to-event data: a comparison of two-stage methods. *Research Synthesis Methods* 2011; **2**: 139–149.

Sinclair JC, Bracken MB. Clinically useful measures of effect in binary analyses of randomized trials. *Journal of Clinical Epidemiology* 1994; **47**: 881–889.

Tierney JF, Stewart LA, Ghersi D, Burdett S, Sydes MR. Practical methods for incorporating summary time-to-event data into meta-analysis. *Trials* 2007; **8**.

Vickers AJ. The use of percentage change from baseline as an outcome in a controlled trial is statistically inefficient: a simulation study. *BMC Medical Research Methodology* 2001; **1**: 6.

Walter SD, Yao X. Effect sizes can be calculated for studies reporting ranges for outcome variables in systematic reviews. *Journal of Clinical Epidemiology* 2007; **60**: 849–852.

Wan X, Wang W, Liu J, Tong T. Estimating the sample mean and standard deviation from the sample size, median, range and/or interquartile range. *BMC Medical Research Methodology* 2014; **14**: 135.

Weir CJ, Butcher I, Assi V, Lewis SC, Murray GD, Langhorne P, Brady MC. Dealing with missing standard deviation and mean values in meta-analysis of continuous outcomes: a systematic review. *BMC Medical Research Methodology* 2018; **18**: 25.

Williamson PR, Smith CT, Hutton JL, Marson AG. Aggregate data meta-analysis with time-to-event outcomes. *Statistics in Medicine* 2002; **21**: 3337–3351.

7

Considering bias and conflicts of interest among the included studies

Isabelle Boutron, Matthew J Page, Julian PT Higgins, Douglas G Altman, Andreas Lundh, Asbjørn Hróbjartsson; on behalf of the Cochrane Bias Methods Group

KEY POINTS

- Review authors should seek to minimize bias. We draw a distinction between two places in which bias should be considered. The first is in the results of the individual studies included in a systematic review. The second is in the result of the meta-analysis (or other synthesis) of findings from the included studies.
- Problems with the design and execution of individual studies of healthcare interventions raise questions about the internal validity of their findings; empirical evidence provides support for this concern.
- An assessment of the internal validity of studies included in a Cochrane Review should emphasize the risk of bias in their results, that is, the risk that they will over-estimate or under-estimate the true intervention effect.
- Results of meta-analyses (or other syntheses) across studies may additionally be affected by bias due to the absence of results from studies that should have been included in the synthesis.
- Review authors should consider source of funding and conflicts of interest of authors of the study, which may inform the exploration of directness and heterogeneity of study results, assessment of risk of bias within studies, and assessment of risk of bias in syntheses owing to missing results.

7.1 Introduction

Cochrane Reviews seek to minimize bias. We define bias as a **systematic error**, or deviation from the truth, in results. Biases can lead to under-estimation or over-estimation of the true intervention effect and can vary in magnitude: some are small (and trivial compared with the observed effect) and some are substantial (so that an apparent

This chapter should be cited as: Boutron I, Page MJ, Higgins JPT, Altman DG, Lundh A, Hróbjartsson A. Chapter 7: Considering bias and conflicts of interest among the included studies. In: Higgins JPT, Thomas J, Chandler J, Cumpston M, Li T, Page MJ, Welch VA (editors). *Cochrane Handbook for Systematic Reviews of Interventions*. 2nd Edition. Chichester (UK): John Wiley & Sons, 2019: 177–204.

finding may be due entirely to bias). A source of bias may even vary in direction across studies. For example, bias due to a particular design flaw such as lack of allocation sequence concealment may lead to under-estimation of an effect in one study but over-estimation in another (Jüni et al 2001).

Bias can arise because of the actions of primary study investigators or because of the actions of review authors, or may be unavoidable due to constraints on how research can be undertaken in practice. Actions of authors can, in turn, be influenced by conflicts of interest. In this chapter we introduce issues of bias in the context of a Cochrane Review, covering both biases in the results of included studies and biases in the results of a synthesis. We introduce the general principles of assessing the risk that bias may be present, as well as the presentation of such assessments and their incorporation into analyses. Finally, we address how source of funding and conflicts of interest of study authors may impact on study design, conduct and reporting. Conflicts of interest held by review authors are also of concern; these should be addressed using editorial procedures and are not covered by this chapter (see Chapter 1, Section 1.3).

We draw a distinction between two places in which bias should be considered. The first is in the results of the *individual studies included in a systematic review*. Since the conclusions drawn in a review depend on the results of the included studies, if these results are biased, then a meta-analysis of the studies will produce a misleading conclusion. Therefore, review authors should systematically take into account **risk of bias in results of included studies** when interpreting the results of their review.

The second place in which bias should be considered is the result of the *meta-analysis (or other synthesis) of findings from the included studies*. This result will be affected by biases in the included studies, and may **additionally** be affected by bias due to the absence of results from studies that should have been included in the synthesis. Specifically, the conclusions of the review may be compromised when decisions about how, when and where to report results of eligible studies are influenced by the nature and direction of the results. This is the problem of 'non-reporting bias' (also described as 'publication bias' and 'selective reporting bias'). There is convincing evidence that results that are statistically non-significant and unfavourable to the experimental intervention are less likely to be published than statistically significant results, and hence are less easily identified by systematic reviews (see Section 7.2.3). This leads to results being missing systematically from syntheses, which can lead to syntheses over-estimating or under-estimating the effects of an intervention. For this reason, the assessment of **risk of bias due to missing results** is another essential component of a Cochrane Review.

Both the risk of bias in included studies and risk of bias due to missing results may be influenced by **conflicts of interest of study investigators or funders**. For example, investigators with a financial interest in showing that a particular drug works may exclude participants who did not respond favourably to the drug from the analysis, or fail to report unfavourable results of the drug in a manuscript.

Further discussion of assessing risk of bias in the results of an individual randomized trial is available in Chapter 8, and of a non-randomized study in Chapter 25. Further discussion of assessing risk of bias due to missing results is available in Chapter 13.

7.1.1 Why consider *risk* of bias?

There is good empirical evidence that particular features of the design, conduct and analysis of randomized trials lead to bias on average, and that some results of randomized trials are suppressed from dissemination because of their nature. However, it is usually impossible to know to what extent biases have affected the results of a particular study or analysis (Savović et al 2012). For these reasons, it is more appropriate to consider whether a result is at **risk of bias** rather than claiming with certainty that it is biased. Most recent tools for assessing the internal validity of findings from quantitative studies in health now focus on risk of bias, whereas previous tools targeted the broader notion of 'methodological quality' (see also Section 7.1.2).

Bias should not be confused with **imprecision**. Bias refers to *systematic error*, meaning that multiple replications of the same study would reach the wrong answer on average. Imprecision refers to *random error*, meaning that multiple replications of the same study will produce different effect estimates because of sampling variation, but would give the right answer on average. Precision depends on the number of participants and (for dichotomous outcomes) the number of events in a study, and is reflected in the confidence interval around the intervention effect estimate from each study. The results of smaller studies are subject to greater sampling variation and hence are less precise. A small trial may be at low risk of bias yet its result may be estimated very imprecisely, with a wide confidence interval. Conversely, the results of a large trial may be precise (narrow confidence interval) but also at a high risk of bias.

Bias should also not be confused with the **external validity** of a study, that is, the extent to which the results of a study can be generalized to other populations and settings. For example, a study may enrol participants who are not representative of the population who most commonly experience a particular clinical condition. The results of this study may have limited generalizability to the wider population, but will not necessarily give a biased estimate of the effect in the highly specific population on which it is based. Factors influencing the applicability of an included study to the review question are covered in Chapters 14 and 15.

7.1.2 From quality scales to domain-based tools

Critical assessment of included studies has long been an important component of a systematic review or meta-analysis, and methods have evolved greatly over time. Early appraisal tools were structured as quality 'scales', which combined information on several features into a single score. However, this approach was questioned after it was revealed that the type of quality scale used could significantly influence the interpretation of the meta-analysis results (Jüni et al 1999). That is, risk ratios of trials deemed 'high quality' by some scales suggested that the experimental intervention was superior, whereas when trials were deemed 'high quality' by other scales, the opposite was the case. The lack of a theoretical framework underlying the concept of 'quality' assessed by these scales resulted in tools mixing different concepts such as risk of bias, imprecision, relevance, applicability, ethics, and completeness of reporting. Furthermore, the summary score combining these components is difficult to interpret (Jüni et al 2001).

In 2008, Cochrane released the Cochrane risk-of-bias (RoB) tool, which was slightly revised in 2011 (Higgins et al 2011). The tool was built on the following key principles.

1) The tool focused on a single concept: risk of bias. It did not consider other concepts such as the quality of reporting, precision (the extent to which results are free of random errors), or external validity (directness, applicability or generalizability).
2) The tool was based on a domain-based (or component) approach, in which different types of bias are considered in turn. Users were asked to assess seven domains: random sequence generation, allocation sequence concealment, blinding of participants and personnel, blinding of outcome assessment, incomplete outcome data, selective outcome reporting, and other sources of bias. There was no scoring system in the tool.
3) The domains were selected to characterize mechanisms through which bias may be introduced into a trial, based on a combination of theoretical considerations and empirical evidence.
4) The assessment of risk of bias required judgement and should thus be completely transparent. Review authors provided a judgement for each domain, rated as 'low', 'high' or 'unclear' risk of bias, and provided reasons to support their judgement.

This tool has been implemented widely both in Cochrane Reviews and non-Cochrane reviews (Jørgensen et al 2016). However, user testing has raised some concerns related to the modest inter-rater reliability of some domains (Hartling et al 2013), the need to rethink the theoretical background of the 'selective outcome reporting' domain (Page and Higgins 2016), the misuse of the 'other sources of bias' domain (Jørgensen et al 2016), and the lack of appropriate consideration of the risk-of-bias assessment in the analyses and interpretation of results (Hopewell et al 2013).

To address these concerns, a new version of the Cochrane risk-of-bias tool, RoB 2, has been developed. The tool, described in Chapter 8, includes important innovations in the assessment of risk of bias in randomized trials. The structure of the tool is similar to that of the ROBINS-I tool for non-randomized studies of interventions (described in Chapter 25). Both tools include a fixed set of bias domains, which are intended to cover all issues that might lead to a risk of bias. To help reach risk-of-bias judgements, a series of 'signalling questions' are included within each domain. Also, the assessment is typically specific to a particular result. This is because the risk of bias may differ depending on how an outcome is measured and how the data for the outcome are analysed. For example, if two analyses for a single outcome are presented, one adjusted for baseline prognostic factors and the other not, then the risk of bias in the two results may be different. The risk of bias in at least one specific result for each included study should be assessed in all Cochrane Reviews (MECIR Box 7.1.a).

7.2 Empirical evidence of bias

Where possible, assessments of risk of bias in a systematic review should be informed by evidence. The following sections summarize some of the key evidence about bias that informs our guidance on risk-of-bias assessments in Cochrane Reviews.

MECIR Box 7.1.a Relevant expectations for conduct of intervention reviews	
C52: Assessing risk of bias (**Mandatory**)	
Assess the risk of bias in at least one specific result for each included study. For randomized trials, the RoB 2 tool should be used, involving judgements and support for those judgements across a series of domains of bias, as described in this Handbook.	The risk of bias in at least one specific result for every included study must be explicitly considered to determine the extent to which its findings can be believed, noting that risks of bias might vary by result. Recommendations for assessing bias in randomized studies included in Cochrane Reviews are now well established. The RoB 2 tool – as described in this *Handbook* – must be used for all randomized trials in new reviews. This does not prevent other tools being used.

7.2.1 Empirical evidence of bias in randomized trials: meta-epidemiologic studies

Many empirical studies have shown that methodological features of the design, conduct and reporting of studies are associated with biased intervention effect estimates. This evidence is mainly based on meta-epidemiologic studies using a large collection of meta-analyses to investigate the association between a reported methodological characteristic and intervention effect estimates in randomized trials. The first meta-epidemiologic study was published in 1995. It showed exaggerated intervention effect estimates when intervention allocation methods were inadequate or unclear and when trials were not described as double-blinded (Schulz et al 1995). These results were subsequently confirmed in several meta-epidemiologic studies, showing that lack of reporting of adequate random sequence generation, allocation sequence concealment, double blinding and more specifically blinding of outcome assessors tend to yield higher intervention effect estimates on average (Dechartres et al 2016a, Page et al 2016).

Evidence from meta-epidemiologic studies suggests that the influence of methodological characteristics such as lack of blinding and inadequate allocation sequence concealment varies by the type of outcome. For example, the extent of over-estimation is larger when the outcome is subjectively measured (e.g. pain) and therefore likely to be influenced by knowledge of the intervention received, and lower when the outcome is objectively measured (e.g. death) and therefore unlikely to be influenced by knowledge of the intervention received (Wood et al 2008, Savović et al 2012).

7.2.2 Trial characteristics explored in meta-epidemiologic studies that are not considered sources of bias

Researchers have also explored the influence of other trial characteristics that are not typically considered a threat to a direct causal inference for intervention effect estimates. Recent meta-epidemiologic studies have shown that effect estimates were lower in prospectively registered trials compared with trials not registered or registered retrospectively (Dechartres et al 2016b, Odutayo et al 2017). Others have shown an association between sample size and effect estimates, with larger effects observed in smaller trials (Dechartres et al 2013). Studies have also shown a consistent association between intervention effect and single or multiple centre status, with single-centre trials showing larger effect estimates, even after controlling for sample size (Dechartres et al 2011).

In some of these cases, plausible bias mechanisms can be hypothesized. For example, both the number of centres and sample size may be associated with intervention effect estimates because of non-reporting bias (e.g. single-centre studies and small studies may be more likely to be published when they have larger, statistically significant effects than when they have smaller, non-significant effects); or single-centre and small studies may be subject to less stringent controls and checks. However, alternative explanations are possible, such as differences in factors relating to external validity (e.g. participants in small, single-centre trials may be more homogenous than participants in other trials). Because of this, these factors are not directly captured by the risk-of-bias tools recommended by Cochrane. Review authors should record these characteristics systematically for each study included in the systematic review (e.g. in the 'Characteristics of included studies' table) where appropriate. For example, trial registration status should be recorded for all randomized trials identified.

7.2.3 Empirical evidence of non-reporting biases

A list of the key types of non-reporting biases is provided in Table 7.2.a. In the sections that follow, we provide some of the evidence that underlies this list.

Table 7.2.a Definitions of some types of non-reporting biases

Type of reporting bias	Definition
Publication bias	The *publication* or *non-publication* of research findings, depending on the nature and direction of the results.
Time-lag bias	The *rapid* or *delayed* publication of research findings, depending on the nature and direction of the results.
Language bias	The publication of research findings *in a particular language*, depending on the nature and direction of the results.
Citation bias	The *citation* or *non-citation* of research findings, depending on the nature and direction of the results.
Multiple (duplicate) publication bias	The *multiple* or *singular* publication of research findings, depending on the nature and direction of the results.
Location bias	The publication of research findings in journals with different *ease of access* or *levels of indexing* in standard databases, depending on the nature and direction of results.
Selective (non-) reporting bias	The *selective reporting* of some outcomes or analyses, but not others, depending on the nature and direction of the results.

7.2.3.1 Selective publication of study reports

There is convincing evidence that the publication of a study report is influenced by the nature and direction of its results (Chan et al 2014). Direct empirical evidence of such selective publication (or 'publication bias') is obtained from analysing a cohort of studies in which there is a full accounting of what is published and unpublished (Franco et al 2014). Schmucker and colleagues analysed the proportion of published studies in 39 cohorts (including 5112 studies identified from research ethics committees and 12,660 studies identified from trials registers) (Schmucker et al 2014). Only half of the studies were published, and studies with statistically significant results were more likely to be published than those with non-significant results (odds ratio (OR) 2.8; 95% confidence interval (CI) 2.2 to 3.5) (Schmucker et al 2014). Similar findings were observed by Scherer and colleagues, who conducted a systematic review of 425 studies that explored subsequent full publication of research initially presented at biomedical conferences (Scherer et al 2018). Only 37% of the 307,028 abstracts presented at conferences were published later in full (60% for randomized trials), and abstracts with statistically significant results in favour of the experimental intervention (versus results in favour of the comparator intervention) were more likely to be published in full (OR 1.17; 95% CI 1.07 to 1.28) (Scherer et al 2018). By examining a cohort of 164 trials submitted to the FDA for regulatory approval, Rising and colleagues found that trials with favourable results were more likely than those with unfavourable results to be published (OR 4.7; 95% CI 1.33 to 17.1) (Rising et al 2008).

In addition to being more likely than unpublished randomized trials to have statistically significant results, published trials also tend to report larger effect estimates in favour of the experimental intervention than trials disseminated elsewhere (e.g. in conference abstracts, theses, books or government reports) (ratio of odds ratios 0.90; 95% CI 0.82 to 0.98) (Dechartres et al 2018). This bias has been observed in studies in many scientific disciplines, including the medical, biological, physical and social sciences (Polanin et al 2016, Fanelli et al 2017).

7.2.3.2 Other types of selective dissemination of study reports

The length of time between completion of a study and publication of its results can be influenced by the nature and direction of the study results ('time-lag bias'). Several studies suggest that randomized trials with results that favour the experimental intervention are published in journals about one year earlier on average than trials with unfavourable results (Hopewell et al 2007, Urrutia et al 2016).

Investigators working in a non-English speaking country may publish some of their work in local, non-English language journals, which may not be indexed in the major biomedical databases ('language bias'). It has long been assumed that investigators are more likely to publish positive studies in English-language journals than in local, non-English language journals (Morrison et al 2012). Contrary to this belief, Dechartres and colleagues identified larger intervention effects in randomized trials published in a language other than English than in English (ratio of odds ratios 0.86; 95% CI 0.78 to 0.95), which the authors hypothesized may be related to the higher risk of bias observed in the non-English language trials (Dechartres et al 2018). Several studies have found that in most cases there were no major differences between summary estimates of meta-analyses restricted to English-language studies compared with meta-analyses including studies in languages other than English (Morrison et al 2012, Dechartres et al 2018).

The number of times a study report is cited appears to be influenced by the nature and direction of its results ('citation bias'). In a meta-analysis of 21 methodological studies, Duyx and colleagues observed that articles with statistically significant results were cited 1.57 times the rate of articles with non-significant results (rate ratio 1.57; 95% CI 1.34 to 1.83) (Duyx et al 2017). They also found that articles with results in a positive direction (regardless of their statistical significance) were cited at 2.14 times the rate of articles with results in a negative direction (rate ratio 2.14; 95% CI 1.29 to 3.56) (Duyx et al 2017). In an analysis of 33,355 studies across all areas of science, Fanelli and colleagues found that the number of citations received by a study was positively correlated with the magnitude of effects reported (Fanelli et al 2017). If positive studies are more likely to be cited, they may be more likely to be located, and thus more likely to be included in a systematic review.

Investigators may report the results of their study across multiple publications; for example, Blümle and colleagues found that of 807 studies approved by a research ethics committee in Germany from 2000 to 2002, 135 (17%) had more than one corresponding publication (Blümle et al 2014). Evidence suggests that studies with statistically significant results or larger treatment effects are more likely to lead to multiple publications ('multiple (duplicate) publication bias') (Easterbrook et al 1991, Tramèr et al 1997), which makes it more likely that they will be located and included in a meta-analysis.

Research suggests that the accessibility or level of indexing of journals is associated with effect estimates in trials ('location bias'). For example, a study of 61 meta-analyses found that trials published in journals indexed in Embase but not MEDLINE yielded smaller effect estimates than trials indexed in MEDLINE (ratio of odds ratios 0.71; 95% CI 0.56 to 0.90); however, the risk of bias due to not searching Embase may be minor, given the lower prevalence of Embase-unique trials (Sampson et al 2003). Also, Moher and colleagues estimate that 18,000 biomedical research studies are tucked away in 'predatory' journals, which actively solicit manuscripts and charge publications fees without providing robust editorial services (such as peer review and archiving or indexing of articles) (Moher et al 2017). The direction of bias associated with non-inclusion of studies published in predatory journals depends on whether they are publishing valid studies with null results or studies whose results are biased towards finding an effect.

7.2.3.3 Selective dissemination of study results

The need to compress a substantial amount of information into a few journal pages, along with a desire for the most noteworthy findings to be published, can lead to omission from publication of results for some outcomes because of the nature and direction of the findings. Particular results may not be reported at all ('**selective non-reporting of results**') or be reported incompletely ('**selective under-reporting of results**', e.g. stating only that "$P > 0.05$" rather than providing summary statistics or an effect estimate and measure of precision) (Kirkham et al 2010). In such instances, the data necessary to include the results in a meta-analysis are unavailable. Excluding such studies from the synthesis ignores the information that no significant difference was found, and biases the synthesis towards finding a difference (Schmid 2016).

Evidence of selective non-reporting and under-reporting of results in randomized trials has been obtained by comparing what was pre-specified in a trial protocol with what is available in the final trial report. In two landmark studies, Chan and colleagues found that results were not reported for at least one benefit outcome in 71% of randomized trials in one cohort (Chan et al 2004a) and 88% in another (Chan et al 2004b). Results were under-reported (e.g. stating only that "$P > 0.05$") for at least one benefit outcome in 92% of randomized trials in one cohort and 96% in another. Statistically significant results for benefit outcomes were twice as likely as non-significant results to be completely reported (range of odds ratios 2.4 to 2.7) (Chan et al 2004a, Chan et al 2004b). Reviews of studies investigating selective non-reporting and under-reporting of results suggest that it is more common for outcomes defined by trialists as secondary rather than primary (Jones et al 2015, Li et al 2018).

Selective non-reporting and under-reporting of results occurs for both benefit and harm outcomes. Examining the studies included in a sample of 283 Cochrane Reviews, Kirkham and colleagues suspected that 50% of 712 studies with results missing for the primary benefit outcome of the review were missing because of the nature of the results (Kirkham et al 2010). This estimate was slightly higher (63%) in 393 studies with results missing for the primary harm outcome of 322 systematic reviews (Saini et al 2014).

7.3 General procedures for risk-of-bias assessment

7.3.1 Collecting information for assessment of risk of bias

Information for assessing the risk of bias can be found in several sources, including published articles, trials registers, protocols, clinical study reports (i.e. documents prepared by pharmaceutical companies, which provide extensive detail on trial methods and results), and regulatory reviews (see also Chapter 5, Section 5.2).

Published articles are the most frequently used source of information for assessing risk of bias. This source is theoretically very valuable because it has been reviewed by editors and peer reviewers, who ideally will have prompted authors to report their methods transparently. However, the completeness of reporting of published articles is, in general, quite poor, and essential information for assessing risk of bias is frequently missing. For example, across 20,920 randomized trials included in 2001 Cochrane Reviews, the percentage of trials at unclear risk of bias was 49% for random sequence generation, 57% for allocation sequence concealment; 31% for blinding and 25% for incomplete outcome data (Dechartres et al 2017). Nevertheless, more recent trials were less likely to be judged at unclear risk of bias, suggesting that reporting is improving over time (Dechartres et al 2017).

Trials registers can be a useful source of information to obtain results of studies that have not yet been published (Riveros et al 2013). However, registers typically report only limited information about methods used in the trial to inform an assessment of risk of bias (Wieseler et al 2012). Protocols, which outline the objectives, design, methodology, statistical consideration and procedural aspects of a clinical study, may provide more detailed information on the methods used than that provided in the results report of a study. They are increasingly being published or made available by journals who publish the final report of a study. Protocols are also available in some trials registers, particularly ClinicalTrials.gov (Zarin et al 2016), on websites dedicated to data sharing such as ClinicalStudyDataRequest.com, or from drug regulatory authorities such as the European Medicines Agency. Clinical study reports are another highly useful source of information (Wieseler et al 2012, Jefferson et al 2014).

It may be necessary to contact study investigators to request access to the trial protocol, to clarify incompletely reported information or understand discrepant information available in different sources. To reduce the risk that study authors provide overly positive answers to questions about study design and conduct, we suggest review authors use open-ended questions. For example, to obtain information about the randomization process, review authors might consider asking: 'What process did you use to assign each participant to an intervention?' To obtain information about blinding of participants, it might be useful to request something like, 'Please describe any measures used to ensure that trial participants were unaware of the intervention to which they were assigned'. More focused questions can then be asked to clarify remaining uncertainties.

7.3.2 Performing assessments of risk of bias

Risk-of-bias assessments in Cochrane Reviews should be performed **independently by at least two people** (MECIR Box 7.3.a). Doing so can minimize errors in assessments and ensure that the judgement is not influenced by a single person's preconceptions. Review authors should also define in advance the process for resolving disagreements. For example, both assessors may attempt to resolve disagreements via discussion, and if that fails, call on another author to adjudicate the final judgement. Review authors assessing risk of bias should have either content or methodological expertise (or both), and an adequate understanding of the relevant methodological issues addressed by the risk-of-bias tool. There is some evidence that intensive, standardized training may significantly improve the reliability of risk-of-bias assessments (da Costa et al 2017). To improve reliability of assessments, a review team could consider piloting the risk-of-bias tool on a sample of articles. This may help ensure that criteria are applied consistently and that consensus can be reached. Three to six papers should provide a suitable sample for this. We do not recommend the use of statistical measures of agreement (such as kappa statistics) to describe the extent to which assessments by multiple authors were the same. It is more important that reasons for any disagreement are explored and resolved.

MECIR Box 7.3.a Relevant expectations for conduct of intervention reviews	
C53: Assessing risk of bias in duplicate (**Mandatory**)	
Use (at least) two people working independently to apply the risk-of-bias tool to each result in each included study, and define in advance the process for resolving disagreements.	Duplicating the risk-of-bias assessment reduces both the risk of making mistakes and the possibility that assessments are influenced by a single person's biases.

MECIR Box 7.3.b Relevant expectations for conduct of intervention reviews	
C54: Supporting judgements of risk of bias (**Mandatory**)	
Justify judgements of risk of bias (high, low and some concerns) and provide this information in the risk-of-bias tables (as 'Support for judgement').	Providing support for the judgement makes the process transparent.
C55: Providing sources of information for risk-of-bias assessments (**Mandatory**)	
Collect the source of information for each risk-of-bias judgement (e.g. quotation, summary of information from a trial report, correspondence with investigator, etc). Where judgements are based on assumptions made on the basis of information provided outside publicly available documents, this should be stated.	Readers, editors and referees should have the opportunity to see for themselves from where supports for judgements have been obtained.

The process for reaching risk-of-bias judgements should be transparent. In other words, readers should be able to discern why a particular result was rated at low risk of bias and why another was rated at high risk of bias. This can be achieved by review authors providing information in risk-of-bias tables to justify the judgement made. Such information may include direct quotes from study reports that articulate which methods were used, and an explanation for why such a method is flawed. Cochrane Review authors are expected to record the source of information (including the precise location within a document) that informed each risk-of-bias judgement (MECIR Box 7.3.b).

Many results are often available in trial reports, so review authors should think carefully about which results to assess for risk of bias. We suggest that review authors assess risk of bias in results for outcomes that are included in the 'Summary of findings' table (MECIR Box 7.3.c). Such tables typically include seven or fewer patient-important outcomes (for more details on constructing a 'Summary of findings' table, see Chapter 14).

Novel methods for assessing risk of bias are emerging, including machine learning systems designed to semi-automate risk-of-bias assessment (Marshall et al 2016, Millard et al 2016). These methods involve using a sample of previous risk-of-bias assessments to train machine learning models to predict risk of bias from PDFs of study reports, and extract supporting text for the judgements. Some of these approaches showed good performance for identifying relevant sentences to identify information pertinent to risk of bias from the full-text content of research articles describing clinical trials. A study showed that about one-third of articles could be assessed by just one reviewer if such a tool is used instead of the two required reviewers (Millard et al 2016). However, reliability in reaching judgements about risk of bias compared with human reviewers was slight to moderate depending on the domain assessed (Gates et al 2018).

MECIR Box 7.3.c Relevant expectations for conduct of intervention reviews	
C56: Ensuring results of outcomes included in 'Summary of findings' tables are assessed for risk of bias (**Highly desirable**)	
Ensure that assessments of risk of bias cover the outcomes included in the 'Summary of findings' table.	It may not be feasible to assess the risk of bias in every single result available across the included studies, particularly if a large number of studies and results are available. Review author should strive to assess risk of bias in the results of outcomes that are most important to patients. Such outcomes will typically be included in 'Summary of findings' tables, which present the findings of seven or fewer patient-important outcomes.

7.4 Presentation of assessment of risk of bias

Risk-of-bias assessments may be presented in a Cochrane Review in various ways. A full risk-of-bias table includes responses to each signalling question within each domain (see Chapter 8, Section 8.2) and risk-of-bias judgements, along with text to support each judgement. Such full tables are lengthy and are unlikely to be of great interest to readers, so should generally not be included in the main body of the review. It is nevertheless good practice to make these full tables available for reference.

We recommend the use of forest plots that present risk-of-bias judgements alongside the results of each study included in a meta-analysis (see Figure 7.4.a). This will give a visual impression of the relative contributions of the studies at different levels of risk of bias, especially when considered in combination with the weight given to each study. This may assist authors in reaching overall conclusions about the risk of bias of the synthesized result, as discussed in Section 7.6. Optionally, forest plots or other tables or graphs can be ordered (stratified) by judgements on each risk-of-bias domain or by the overall risk-of-bias judgement for each result.

Review authors may wish to generate bar graphs illustrating the relative contributions of studies with each of risk-of-bias judgement (low risk of bias, some concerns, and high risk of bias). When dividing up a bar into three regions for this purpose, it is preferable to determine the regions according to statistical information (e.g. precision, or weight in a meta-analysis) arising from studies in each category, rather than according to the number of studies in each category.

7.5 Summary assessments of risk of bias

Review authors should make explicit summary judgements about the risk of bias for important results both within studies and across studies (see MECIR Box 7.5.a). The tools currently recommended by Cochrane for assessing risk of bias within included

Study or Subgroup	MHFA training Mean	MHFA training SD	MHFA training Total	Control Mean	Control SD	Control Total	Weight	Std. Mean Difference IV, Random, 95% CI	Risk of Bias A	B	C	D	E	F
Burns 2017	13.62	2.287	59	12.72	2.015	81	12.5%	0.42 [0.08, 0.76]	+	+	−	+	+	−
Jensen 2016a	9.4	2.5	142	8.3	2.5	132	25.1%	0.44 [0.20, 0.68]	+	+	+	+	+	+
Jensen 2016b	9.5	2.5	145	8.1	2.7	143	26.1%	0.54 [0.30, 0.77]	+	+	+	+	+	+
Svensson 2014	8.7	2.1	199	7.3	2.4	207	36.3%	0.62 [0.42, 0.82]	+	+	+	+	+	+
Total (95% CI)			**545**			**563**	**100.0%**	**0.53 [0.41, 0.65]**						

Heterogeneity: $Tau^2 = 0.00$; $Chi^2 = 1.73$, $df = 3$ ($P = 0.63$); $I^2 = 0\%$

Test for overall effect: $Z = 8.61$ ($P < 0.00001$)

Test for subgroup differences: Not applicable

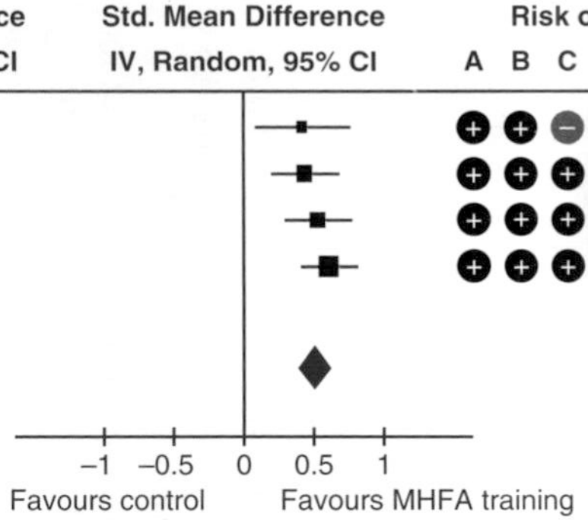

Risk of bias legend

(A) Bias arising from the randomization process

(B) Bias due to deviations from intended interventions

(C) Bias due to missing outcome data

(D) Bias in measurement of the outcome

(E) Bias in selection of the reported results

(F) Overall bias

Figure 7.4.a Forest plot displaying RoB 2 risk-of-bias judgements for each randomized trial included in a meta-analysis of mental health first aid (MHFA) knowledge scores. Adapted from Morgan et al (2018).

MECIR Box 7.5.a Relevant expectations for conduct of intervention reviews	
C57: Summarizing risk-of-bias assessments (**Highly desirable**)	
Summarize the risk of bias for each key outcome for each study.	This reinforces the link between the characteristics of the study design and their possible impact on the results of the study, and is an important prerequisite for the GRADE approach to assessing the certainty of the body of evidence.

studies (RoB 2 and ROBINS-I) produce an overall judgement of risk of bias for the result being assessed. These overall judgements are derived from assessments of individual bias domains as described, for example, in Chapter 8 (Section 8.2).

To summarize risk of bias across study results in a synthesis, review authors should follow guidance for assessing certainty in the body of evidence (e.g. using GRADE), as described in Chapter 14 (Section 14.2.2). When a meta-analysis is dominated by study results at high risk of bias, the certainty of the body of evidence may be rated as being lower than if such studies were excluded from the meta-analysis. Section 7.6 discusses some possible courses of action that may be preferable to retaining such studies in the synthesis.

7.6 Incorporating assessment of risk of bias into analyses

7.6.1 Introduction

When performing and presenting meta-analyses, review authors should address risk of bias in the results of included studies (MECIR Box 7.6.a). It is not appropriate to present

MECIR Box 7.6.a Relevant expectations for conduct of intervention reviews	
C58: Addressing risk of bias in the synthesis (**Highly desirable**)	
Address risk of bias in the synthesis (whether quantitative or non-quantitative). For example, present analyses stratified according to summary risk of bias, or restricted to studies at low risk of bias.	Review authors should consider how study biases affect results. This is useful in determining the strength of conclusions and how future research should be designed and conducted.
C59: Incorporating assessments of risk of bias (**Mandatory**)	
If randomized trials have been assessed using one or more tools in addition to the RoB 2 tool, *use the RoB 2 tool as the primary assessment of bias for interpreting results, choosing the primary analysis, and drawing conclusions.*	For consistency of approach across Cochrane Reviews of Interventions, the RoB 2 tool should take precedence when two or more tools are used for assessing risk of bias in randomized trials. The RoB 2 tool also feeds directly into the GRADE approach for assessing the certainty of the body of evidence.

analyses and interpretations while ignoring flaws identified during the assessment of risk of bias. In this section we present suitable strategies for addressing risk of bias in results from studies included in a meta-analysis, either in order to understand the impact of bias or to determine a suitable estimate of intervention effect (Section 7.6.2). For the latter, decisions often involve a trade-off between bias and precision. A meta-analysis that includes all eligible studies may produce a result with high precision (narrow confidence interval) but be seriously biased because of flaws in the conduct of some of the studies. However, including only the studies at low risk of bias in all domains assessed may produce a result that is unbiased but imprecise (if there are only a few studies at low risk of bias).

7.6.2 Including risk-of-bias assessments in analyses

Broadly speaking, studies at high risk of bias should be given reduced weight in meta-analyses compared with studies at low risk of bias. However, methodological approaches for weighting studies according to their risk of bias are not sufficiently well developed that they can currently be recommended for use in Cochrane Reviews.

When risks of bias vary across studies in a meta-analysis, four broad strategies are available to incorporate assessments into the analysis. The choice of strategy will influence which result to present as the main finding for a particular outcome (e.g. in the Abstract). The intended strategy should be described in the protocol for the review.

1) **Primary analysis restricted to studies at low risk of bias**

The first approach involves restricting the primary analysis to studies judged to be at low risk of bias overall. Review authors who restrict their primary analysis in this way are encouraged to perform **sensitivity analyses** to show how conclusions might be affected if studies at a high risk of bias were included.

2) **Present multiple (stratified) analyses**

Stratifying according to the overall risk of bias will produce multiple estimates of the intervention effect: for example, one based on all studies, one based on studies at low risk of bias, and one based on studies at high risk of bias. Two or more such estimates might be considered with equal prominence (e.g. the first and second of these). However, presenting the results in this way may be confusing for readers. In particular, people who need to make a decision usually require a single estimate of effect. Furthermore, 'Summary of findings' tables typically present only a single result for each outcome. On the other hand, a stratified forest plot presents all the information transparently. Though we would generally recommend stratification is done on the basis of overall risk of bias, review authors may choose to conduct subgroup analyses based on specific bias domains (e.g. risk of bias arising from the randomization process).

Formal comparisons of intervention effects according to risk of bias can be done with a test for differences across subgroups (e.g. comparing studies at high risk of bias with studies at low risk of bias), or by using meta-regression (for more details see Chapter 10, Section 10.11.4). However, review authors should be cautious in planning and carrying out such analyses, because an individual review may not have enough studies in each category of risk of bias to identify meaningful differences. Lack of a statistically significant difference between studies at high and low risk of bias should not be interpreted as absence of bias, because these analyses typically have low power.

The choice between strategies (1) and (2) should be based to large extent on the balance between the potential for bias and the loss of precision when studies at high or unclear risk of bias are excluded.

3) **Present all studies and provide a narrative discussion of risk of bias**

The simplest approach to incorporating risk-of-bias assessments in results is to present an estimated intervention effect based on all available studies, together with a description of the risk of bias in individual domains, or a description of the summary risk of bias, across studies. This is the only feasible option when all studies are at the same risk of bias. However, when studies have different risks of bias, we **discourage** such an approach for two reasons. First, detailed descriptions of risk of bias in the Results section, together with a cautious interpretation in the Discussion section, will often be lost in the Authors' conclusions, Abstract and 'Summary of findings' table, so that the final interpretation ignores the risk of bias and decisions continue to be based, at least in part, on compromised evidence. Second, such an analysis fails to down-weight studies at high risk of bias and so will lead to an overall intervention effect that is too precise, as well as being potentially biased.

When the primary analysis is based on all studies, summary assessments of risk of bias should be incorporated into explicit measures of the certainty of evidence for each important outcome, for example, by using the GRADE system (Guyatt et al 2008). This incorporation can help to ensure that judgements about the risk of bias, as well as other factors affecting the quality of evidence, such as imprecision, heterogeneity and publication bias, are considered appropriately when interpreting the results of the review (see Chapters 14 and 15).

4) **Adjust effect estimates for bias**

A final, more sophisticated, option is to adjust the result from each study in an attempt to remove the bias. Adjustments are usually undertaken within a Bayesian framework, with assumptions about the size of the bias and its uncertainty being expressed through prior distributions (see Chapter 10, Section 10.13). Prior distributions may be based on expert opinion or on meta-epidemiological findings (Turner et al 2009, Welton et al 2009). The approach is increasingly used in decision making, where adjustments can additionally be made for applicability of the evidence to the decision at hand. However, we do not encourage use of bias adjustments in the context of a Cochrane Review because the assumptions required are strong, limited methodological expertise is available, and it is not possible to account for issues of applicability due to the diverse intended audiences for Cochrane Reviews. The approach might be entertained as a sensitivity analysis in some situations.

7.7 Considering risk of bias due to missing results

The 2011 Cochrane risk-of-bias tool for randomized trials encouraged a study-level judgement about whether there has been selective reporting, in general, of the trial results. As noted in Section 7.2.3.3, selective reporting can arise in several ways: (1) selective non-reporting of results, where results for some of the analysed outcomes are selectively omitted from a published report; (2) selective under-reporting of data, where results for some outcomes are selectively reported with inadequate detail for the data to be included in a meta-analysis; and (3) bias in selection of the reported result, where a result has been selected for reporting by the study authors, on the basis of the results, from multiple measurements or analyses that have been generated for the outcome domain (Page and Higgins 2016).

The RoB 2 and ROBINS-I tools focus solely on risk of bias as it pertains to a specific trial result. With respect to selective reporting, RoB 2 and ROBINS-I examine whether a specific result from the trial is likely to have been selected from multiple possible results on the basis of the findings (scenario 3 above). Guidance on assessing the risk of bias in selection of the reported result is available in Chapter 8 (for randomized trials) and Chapter 25 (for non-randomized studies of interventions).

If there is no result (i.e. it has been omitted selectively from the report or under-reported), then a risk-of-bias assessment at the level of the study result is not applicable. Selective non-reporting of results and selective under-reporting of data are therefore not covered by the RoB 2 and ROBINS-I tools. Instead, selective non-reporting of results and under-reporting of data should be assessed at the level of the synthesis across studies. Both practices lead to a situation similar to that when an entire study report is unavailable because of the nature of the results (also known as publication bias). Regardless of whether an entire study report or only a particular result of a study is unavailable, the same consequence can arise: bias in a synthesis because available results differ systematically from missing results (Page et al 2018). Chapter 13 provides detailed guidance on assessing risk of bias due to missing results in a systematic review.

7.8 Considering source of funding and conflict of interest of authors of included studies

Readers of a trial report often need to reflect on whether conflicts of interest have influenced the design, conduct, analysis and reporting of a trial. It is therefore now common for scientific journals to require authors of trial reports to provide a declaration of conflicts of interest (sometimes called 'competing' or 'declarations of' interest), to report funding sources and to describe any funder's role in the trial.

In this section, we characterize conflicts of interest in randomized trials and discuss how conflicts of interest may impact on trial design and effect estimates. We also suggest how review authors can collect, process and use information on conflicts of interest in the assessment of:

- directness of studies to the review's research question;
- heterogeneity in results due to differences in the designs of eligible studies;
- risk of bias in results of included studies;
- risk of bias in a synthesis due to missing results.

At the time of writing, a formal Tool for Addressing Conflicts of Interest in Trials (TACIT) is being developed under the auspices of the Cochrane Bias Methods Group. The TACIT development process has informed the content of this section, and we encourage readers to check http://tacit.one for more detailed guidance that will become available.

7.8.1 Characteristics of conflicts of interest

The Institute of Medicine defined conflicts of interest as "a set of circumstances that creates a risk that professional judgment or actions regarding a primary interest will be unduly influenced by a secondary interest" (Lo et al 2009). In a clinical trial, the primary interest is to provide patients, clinicians and health policy makers with an unbiased and clinically relevant estimate of an intervention effect. Secondary interest may be both financial and non-financial.

Financial conflicts of interest involve both financial interests related to a specific trial (for example, a company funding a trial of a drug produced by the same company) and financial interests related to the authors of a trial report (for example, authors' ownership of stocks or employment by a drug company).

For drug and device companies and other manufacturers, the financial difference between a negative and positive pivotal trial can be considerable. For example, the mean stock price of the companies funding 23 positive pivotal oncology trials increased by 14% after disclosure of the results (Rothenstein et al 2011). Industry funding is common, especially in drug trials. In a study of 200 trial publications from 2015, 68 (38%) of 178 trials with funding declarations were industry funded (Hakoum et al 2017). Also, in a cohort of oncology drug trials, industry funded 44% of trials and authors declared conflicts of interest in 69% of trials (Riechelmann et al 2007).

The degree of funding, and the type of the involvement of industry funders, may differ across trials. In some situations, involvement includes only the provision of free study medication for a trial that has otherwise been planned and conducted independently, and funded largely, by public means. In other situations, a company fully funds and controls a trial. In rarer cases, head-to-head trials comparing two drugs may be funded by the two different companies producing the drugs.

A Cochrane Methodology Review analysed 75 studies of the association between industry funding and trial results (Lundh et al 2017). The authors concluded that trials funded by a drug or device company were more likely to have positive conclusions and statistically significant results, and that this association could not be explained by differences in risk of bias between industry and non-industry funded trials. However, industry and non-industry trials may differ in ways that may confound the association; for example due to choice of patient population, comparator interventions or outcomes. Only one of the included studies used a meta-epidemiological design and found no clear association between industry funding and the magnitude of intervention effects (Als-Nielsen et al 2003). Similar to the association with industry funding, other studies have reported that results of trials conducted by authors with a financial conflict of interest were more likely to be positive (Ahn et al 2017).

Conflicts of interest may also be non-financial (Viswanathan et al 2014). Characterizations of non-financial conflicts of interest differ somewhat, but typically distinguish between conflicts related mainly to an individual (e.g. adherence to a theory or ideology), relationships to other individuals (e.g. loyalty to friends, family members or close colleagues), or relationship to groups (e.g. work place or professional groups). In medicine, non-financial conflicts of interest have received less attention than financial conflicts of interest. In addition, financial and non-financial conflicts are often intertwined; for example, non-financial conflicts related to institutional association can be considered as indirect financial conflicts linked to employment. Definitions of what should be characterized as a 'non-financial' conflict of interest, and, in particular, whether personal beliefs, experiences or intellectual commitments should be considered conflicts of interest, have been debated (Bero and Grundy 2016).

It is useful to differentiate between non-financial conflicts of interest of a trial researcher and the basic interests and hopes involved in doing good trial research. Most researchers conducting a trial will have an interest in the scientific problem addressed, a well-articulated theoretical position, anticipation for a specific trial result, and hopes for publication in a respectable journal. This is not a conflict of interest but a basic condition for doing health research. However, individual researchers may lose sight of the primacy of the methodological neutrality at the heart of a scientific enquiry, and become unduly occupied with the secondary interest of how trial results may affect academic appearance or chances of future funding. Extreme examples are the publication of fabricated trial data or trials, some of which have had an impact on systematic reviews (Marret et al 2009).

Few empirical studies of non-financial conflicts of interest in randomized trials have been published, and to our knowledge there are none that assess the impact of non-financial conflicts of interest on trial results and conclusions. However, non-financial conflicts of interests have been investigated in other types of clinical research; for example, guideline authors' specialty appears to have influenced their voting behaviour while developing guidelines for mammography screening (Norris et al 2012).

7.8.2 Conflict of interest and trial design

Core decisions on designing a trial involve defining the type of participants to be included, the type of experimental intervention, the type of comparator, the outcomes (and timing of outcome assessments) and the choice of analysis. Such decisions will often reflect a compromise between what is clinically and scientifically ideal and what is practically possible. However, when investigators have important conflicts of interest, a trial may be designed in a way that increases its chances of detecting a positive trial result, at the expense of clinical applicability. For example, narrow eligibility criteria may exclude older and frail patients, thus reducing the possibility of detecting clinically relevant harms. Alternatively, trial designers may choose placebo as a comparator despite an effective intervention being in regular use, or they may focus on short-term surrogate outcomes rather than clinically relevant long-term outcomes (Estellat and Ravaud 2012, Wieland et al 2017).

Trial design choices may be more subtle. For example, a trial may be designed to favour an experimental drug by using an inferior comparator drug when better alternatives exist (Safer 2002) or by using a low dose of the comparator drug when the focus is efficacy and a high dose of the comparator drug when the focus is harms (Mann and Djulbegovic 2013). In a typical Cochrane Review with fairly broad eligibility criteria aiming to identify and summarize all relevant trials, it is pertinent to consider the degree to which a given trial result directly relates to the question posed by the review. If all or most identified trials have narrow eligibility criteria and short-term outcomes, a review question focusing on broad patient categories and long-term effects can only be answered indirectly by the included studies. This has implications for the assessment of the certainty of the evidence provided by the review, which is addressed through the concept of indirectness in the GRADE framework (see Chapter 14, Section 14.2).

If results in a meta-analysis display heterogeneity, then differences in design choices that are driven by conflicts of interest may be one reason for this. Thus, conflicts of interest may also affect reflections on the certainty of the evidence through the GRADE concept of inconsistency.

7.8.3 Conflicts of interest and risk of bias in a trial's effect estimate

Authors of Cochrane Reviews have sometimes included conflicts of interest as an 'other source of bias' while using the previous versions of the risk-of-bias tool (Jørgensen et al 2016). Consistent with previous versions of the *Handbook*, we discourage the inclusion of conflicts of interest *directly* in the risk-of-bias assessment. Adding conflicts of interest to the bias tool is inconsistent with the conceptual structure of the tool, which is built on mechanistically defined bias domains. Also, restricting consideration of the potential impact of conflicts of interest to a question of risk of bias in an individual trial result overlooks other important aspects, such as the design of the trial (see Section 7.8.2) and potential bias in a meta-analysis due to missing results (see Section 7.8.4).

Conflicts of interest may lead to bias in effect estimates from a trial through several mechanisms. For example, if those recruiting participants into a trial have important conflicts of interest and the allocation sequence is not concealed, then they may be more likely to subvert the allocation process to produce intervention groups that are systematically unbalanced in favour of their preferred intervention. Similarly, investigators with important conflicts of interests may decide to exclude from the analysis some patients who did not respond as anticipated to the experimental intervention, resulting in bias due to missing outcome data. Furthermore, selective reporting of a favourable result may be strongly associated with conflicts of interest (McGauran et al 2010), due to either selective reporting of particular outcome measurements or selective reporting of particular analyses (Eyding et al 2010, Vedula et al 2013). One study found that use of modified-intention-to-treat analysis and post-randomization exclusions occurred more often in trials with industry funding or author conflicts of interest (Montedori et al 2011). Accessing the trial protocol and statistical analysis plan to determine which outcomes and analyses were pre-specified is therefore especially important for a trial with relevant conflicts of interest.

Review authors should explain how consideration of conflicts of interest informed their risk-of-bias judgements. For example, when information on the analysis plans is lacking, review authors may judge the risk of bias in selection of the reported result to be high if the study investigators had important financial conflicts of interest. Conversely, if trial investigators have clearly used methods that are likely to minimize bias, review authors should not judge the risk of bias for each domain higher just because the investigators happen to have conflicts of interest. In addition, as an optional component in the revised risk-of-bias tool, review authors may reflect on the direction of bias (e.g. bias in favour of the experimental intervention). Information on conflicts of interest may inform the assessment of direction of bias.

7.8.4 Conflicts of interest and risk of bias in a synthesis of trial results

Conflicts of interest may also affect the decision not to report trial results. Conflicts of interest are probably one of several important reasons for decisions not to publish trials with negative findings, and not to publish unfavourable results (Sterne 2013). When relevant trial results are systematically missing from a meta-analysis because of the nature of the findings, the synthesis is at risk of bias due to missing results. Chapter 13 provides detailed guidance on assessing risk of bias due to missing results in a systematic review.

7.8.5 Practical approach to identifying and extracting information on conflicts of interest

When assessing conflicts of interest in a trial, review authors will, to a large degree, rely on declared conflicts. Source of funding may be reported in a trial publication, and conflicts of interest may be reported in an accompanying declaration, for example the International Committee of Medical Journal Editors (ICMJE) declaration. In a random sample of 1002 articles published in 2016, authors of 229 (23%) declared having a conflict of interest (Grundy et al 2018). Unfortunately, undeclared conflicts of interest and sources of funding are fairly common (Rasmussen et al 2015, Patel et al 2018).

It is always prudent to examine closely the conflicts of interest of lead and corresponding authors, based on information reported in the trial publication and the author declaration (for example, the ICMJE declaration form). Review authors should also consider examining conflicts of interest of trial co-authors and any commercial collaborators with conflicts of interest; for example, a commercial contract research organization hired by the funder to collect and analyse trial data or the involvement of a medical writing agency. Due to the high prevalence of undisclosed conflicts of interest, review authors should consider expanding their search for conflicts of interest data from other sources (e.g. disclosure in other publications by the authors, the trial protocol, the clinical study report, and public conflicts of interest registries (e.g. Open Payments database)).

We suggest that review authors balance the workload involved with the expected gain, and search additional sources of information on conflicts of interest when there is reason to suspect important conflicts of interest. As a rule of thumb, in trials with unclear funding source and no declaration of conflicts of interest from lead or corresponding authors, we suggest review authors search the Open Payments database, ClinicalTrials.gov, and conflicts of interest declarations in a few previous publications by the study authors. In trials with no commercial funding (including no company employee co-authors) and no declared conflicts of interest for lead or corresponding authors, we suggest review authors not bother to consult additional sources. Also, for trials where lead or corresponding authors have clear conflicts of interest, little additional information may be gained from checking conflicts of interest of co-authors.

Gaining access to relevant information on financial conflicts of interest is possible for a considerable number of trials, despite inherent problems of undeclared conflicts. We expect that the proportion of trials with relevant declarations will increase further.

Access to relevant information on non-financial conflicts of interest is more difficult to gain. Declaration of non-financial conflicts of interest is requested by approximately 50% of journals (Shawwa et al 2016). The term was deleted from ICMJE's declaration in 2010 in exchange for a broad category of "Other relationships or activities" (Drazen et al 2010).

Therefore, non-financial conflicts of interests are seldom self-declared, although if available, such information should be considered.

Non-financial conflicts of interest are difficult to address due to lack of relevant empirical studies on their impact on study results, lack of relevant thresholds for importance, and lack of declaration in many previous trials. However, as a rule of thumb, we suggest that review authors assume trial authors have no non-financial conflicts of interest unless there are clear suggestions of the opposite. Examples of such clues could be a considerable spin in trial publications (Boutron et al 2010), an institutional relationship pertinent to the intervention tested, or external evidence of a fixated ideological or theoretical position.

7.8.6 Judgement of notable concern about conflict of interest

Review authors should describe funding information and conflicts of interest of authors for all studies in the 'Characteristics of included studies' table (MECIR Box 7.8.a). Also, review authors may want to explore (e.g. in a subgroup analysis) whether trials with conflicts of interest have different intervention effect estimates, or more variable effect estimates, than trials without conflicts of interest. In both cases, review authors need to aim for a relevant threshold for when any conflict of interest is deemed important. If put too low, there is a risk that trivial conflicts of interest will cloud important ones; if set too high, there is the risk that important conflicts of interest are downplayed or ignored.

This judgement should take into account both the degree of conflicts of interest of study authors and also the extent of their involvement in the study. We pragmatically suggest review authors aim for a judgement about whether or not there is reason for 'notable concern' about conflicts of interest. This information could be displayed in a table with three columns:

1) trial identifier;
2) judgement (e.g. 'notable concern about conflict of interest' versus 'no notable concern about conflict of interest'); and
3) rationale for judgement, potentially subdivided according to who had conflicts of interest (e.g. lead or corresponding authors, other authors) and stage(s) of the trial to which they contributed (design, conduct, analysis, reporting).

A judgement of 'notable concern about conflict of interest' should be based on reflected assessment of identified conflicts of interest. A hypothetical possibility for undeclared conflicts of interest is, as a rule of thumb, not considered sufficient reason for 'notable concern'. By 'notable concern' we imply important conflicts of interest expected to have a potential impact on study design, risk of bias in study results or risk of bias in a synthesis due to missing results. For example, financial conflicts of interest are important in a trial initiated, designed, analysed and reported by drug or device company employees. Conversely, financial conflicts of interest are less important in a trial initiated, designed, analysed and reported by academics adhering to the arm's length principle when acquiring free trial medication from a drug company, and where lead authors have no conflicts of interest. Similarly, non-financial conflicts of interest may be important in a trial of a highly controversial and ideologically loaded question such as the adverse effect of male circumcision. Non-financial conflicts of interest are

MECIR Box 7.8.a Relevant expectations for conduct of intervention reviews	
C60: Addressing conflicts of interest in included trials (**Highly desirable**)	
Address conflict of interests in included trials, and reflect on possible impact on: (a) differences in study design; (b) risk of bias in trial result, and (c) risk of bias in synthesis result.	Review authors should consider assessing whether they judge a trial to be of 'notable concern about conflicts of interest'. This assessment is useful for exploration of possible heterogeneity between trials (e.g. in a subgroup analysis), and for reflection on relevant mechanisms for how conflict of interest may have biased trial results and synthesis results. Concerns about conflicts of interest can be reported in the 'Characteristics of included studies' table.

less concerning in a trial comparing two treatments in general use with no connotation to highly controversial scientific theories, ideology or professional groups. Mixing trivial conflicts of interest with important ones may mask the latter and will expand review author workload considerably.

7.9 Chapter information

Authors: Isabelle Boutron, Matthew J Page, Julian PT Higgins, Douglas G Altman, Andreas Lundh, Asbjørn Hróbjartsson

Acknowledgements: We thank Gerd Antes, Peter Gøtzsche, Peter Jüni, Steff Lewis, David Moher, Andrew Oxman, Ken Schulz, Jonathan Sterne and Simon Thompson for their contributions to previous versions of this chapter.

7.10 References

Ahn R, Woodbridge A, Abraham A, Saba S, Korenstein D, Madden E, Boscardin WJ, Keyhani S. Financial ties of principal investigators and randomized controlled trial outcomes: cross sectional study. *BMJ* 2017; **356**: i6770.

Als-Nielsen B, Chen W, Gluud C, Kjaergard LL. Association of funding and conclusions in randomized drug trials: a reflection of treatment effect or adverse events? *JAMA* 2003; **290**: 921–928.

Bero LA, Grundy Q. Why having a (nonfinancial) interest is not a conflict of interest. *PLoS Biology* 2016; **14**: e2001221.

Blümle A, Meerpohl JJ, Schumacher M, von Elm E. Fate of clinical research studies after ethical approval – follow-up of study protocols until publication. *PloS One* 2014; **9**: e87184.

Boutron I, Dutton S, Ravaud P, Altman DG. Reporting and interpretation of randomized controlled trials with statistically nonsignificant results for primary outcomes. *JAMA* 2010; **303**: 2058–2064.

Chan A-W, Song F, Vickers A, Jefferson T, Dickersin K, Gøtzsche PC, Krumholz HM, Ghersi D, van der Worp HB. Increasing value and reducing waste: addressing inaccessible research. *The Lancet* 2014; **383**: 257–266.

Chan AW, Hróbjartsson A, Haahr MT, Gøtzsche PC, Altman DG. Empirical evidence for selective reporting of outcomes in randomized trials: comparison of protocols to published articles. *JAMA* 2004a; **291**: 2457–2465.

Chan AW, Krleža-Jeric K, Schmid I, Altman DG. Outcome reporting bias in randomized trials funded by the Canadian Institutes of Health Research. *Canadian Medical Association Journal* 2004b; **171**: 735–740.

da Costa BR, Beckett B, Diaz A, Resta NM, Johnston BC, Egger M, Jüni P, Armijo-Olivo S. Effect of standardized training on the reliability of the Cochrane risk of bias assessment tool: a prospective study. *Systematic Reviews* 2017; **6**: 44.

Dechartres A, Boutron I, Trinquart L, Charles P, Ravaud P. Single-center trials show larger treatment effects than multicenter trials: evidence from a meta-epidemiologic study. *Annals of Internal Medicine* 2011; **155**: 39–51.

Dechartres A, Trinquart L, Boutron I, Ravaud P. Influence of trial sample size on treatment effect estimates: meta-epidemiological study. *BMJ* 2013; **346**: f2304.

Dechartres A, Trinquart L, Faber T, Ravaud P. Empirical evaluation of which trial characteristics are associated with treatment effect estimates. *Journal of Clinical Epidemiology* 2016a; **77**: 24–37.

Dechartres A, Ravaud P, Atal I, Riveros C, Boutron I. Association between trial registration and treatment effect estimates: a meta-epidemiological study. *BMC Medicine* 2016b; **14**: 100.

Dechartres A, Trinquart L, Atal I, Moher D, Dickersin K, Boutron I, Perrodeau E, Altman DG, Ravaud P. Evolution of poor reporting and inadequate methods over time in 20,920 randomised controlled trials included in Cochrane reviews: research on research study. *BMJ* 2017; **357**: j2490.

Dechartres A, Atal I, Riveros C, Meerpohl J, Ravaud P. Association between publication characteristics and treatment effect estimates: a meta-epidemiologic study. *Annals of Internal Medicine* 2018; **169**: 385–393.

Drazen JM, de Leeuw PW, Laine C, Mulrow C, DeAngelis CD, Frizelle FA, Godlee F, Haug C, Hébert PC, Horton R, Kotzin S, Marusic A, Reyes H, Rosenberg J, Sahni P, Van der Weyden MB, Zhaori G. Towards more uniform conflict disclosures: the updated ICMJE conflict of interest reporting form. *BMJ* 2010; **340**: c3239.

Duyx B, Urlings MJE, Swaen GMH, Bouter LM, Zeegers MP. Scientific citations favor positive results: a systematic review and meta-analysis. *Journal of Clinical Epidemiology* 2017; **88**: 92–101.

Easterbrook PJ, Berlin JA, Gopalan R, Matthews DR. Publication bias in clinical research. *The Lancet* 1991; **337**: 867–872.

Estellat C, Ravaud P. Lack of head-to-head trials and fair control arms: randomized controlled trials of biologic treatment for rheumatoid arthritis. *Archives of Internal Medicine* 2012; **172**: 237–244.

Eyding D, Lelgemann M, Grouven U, Harter M, Kromp M, Kaiser T, Kerekes MF, Gerken M, Wieseler B. Reboxetine for acute treatment of major depression: systematic review and meta-analysis of published and unpublished placebo and selective serotonin reuptake inhibitor controlled trials. *BMJ* 2010; **341**: c4737.

Fanelli D, Costas R, Ioannidis JPA. Meta-assessment of bias in science. *Proceedings of the National Academy of Sciences of the United States of America* 2017; **114**: 3714–3719.

Franco A, Malhotra N, Simonovits G. Social science. Publication bias in the social sciences: unlocking the file drawer. *Science* 2014; **345**: 1502–1505.

Gates A, Vandermeer B, Hartling L. Technology-assisted risk of bias assessment in systematic reviews: a prospective cross-sectional evaluation of the RobotReviewer machine learning tool. *Journal of Clinical Epidemiology* 2018; **96**: 54–62.

Grundy Q, Dunn AG, Bourgeois FT, Coiera E, Bero L. Prevalence of disclosed conflicts of interest in biomedical research and associations with journal impact factors and altmetric scores. *JAMA* 2018; **319**: 408–409.

Guyatt GH, Oxman AD, Vist GE, Kunz R, Falck-Ytter Y, Alonso-Coello P, Schünemann HJ. GRADE: an emerging consensus on rating quality of evidence and strength of recommendations. *BMJ* 2008; **336**: 924–926.

Hakoum MB, Jouni N, Abou-Jaoude EA, Hasbani DJ, Abou-Jaoude EA, Lopes LC, Khaldieh M, Hammoud MZ, Al-Gibbawi M, Anouti S, Guyatt G, Akl EA. Characteristics of funding of clinical trials: cross-sectional survey and proposed guidance. *BMJ Open* 2017; **7**: e015997.

Hartling L, Hamm MP, Milne A, Vandermeer B, Santaguida PL, Ansari M, Tsertsvadze A, Hempel S, Shekelle P, Dryden DM. Testing the risk of bias tool showed low reliability between individual reviewers and across consensus assessments of reviewer pairs. *Journal of Clinical Epidemiology* 2013; **66**: 973–981.

Higgins JPT, Altman DG, Gøtzsche PC, Jüni P, Moher D, Oxman AD, Savović J, Schulz KF, Weeks L, Sterne JAC. The Cochrane Collaboration's tool for assessing risk of bias in randomised trials. *BMJ* 2011; **343**: d5928.

Hopewell S, Clarke M, Stewart L, Tierney J. Time to publication for results of clinical trials. *Cochrane Database of Systematic Reviews* 2007; **2**: MR000011.

Hopewell S, Boutron I, Altman D, Ravaud P. Incorporation of assessments of risk of bias of primary studies in systematic reviews of randomised trials: a cross-sectional study. *BMJ Open* 2013; **3**: 8.

Jefferson T, Jones MA, Doshi P, Del Mar CB, Hama R, Thompson MJ, Onakpoya I, Heneghan CJ. Risk of bias in industry-funded oseltamivir trials: comparison of core reports versus full clinical study reports. *BMJ Open* 2014; **4**: e005253.

Jones CW, Keil LG, Holland WC, Caughey MC, Platts-Mills TF. Comparison of registered and published outcomes in randomized controlled trials: a systematic review. *BMC Medicine* 2015; **13**: 282.

Jørgensen L, Paludan-Muller AS, Laursen DR, Savović J, Boutron I, Sterne JAC, Higgins JPT, Hróbjartsson A. Evaluation of the Cochrane tool for assessing risk of bias in randomized clinical trials: overview of published comments and analysis of user practice in Cochrane and non-Cochrane reviews. *Systematic Reviews* 2016; **5**: 80.

Jüni P, Witschi A, Bloch R, Egger M. The hazards of scoring the quality of clinical trials for meta-analysis. *JAMA* 1999; **282**: 1054–1060.

Jüni P, Altman DG, Egger M. Systematic reviews in health care: assessing the quality of controlled clinical trials. *BMJ* 2001; **323**: 42–46.

Kirkham JJ, Dwan KM, Altman DG, Gamble C, Dodd S, Smyth R, Williamson PR. The impact of outcome reporting bias in randomised controlled trials on a cohort of systematic reviews. *BMJ* 2010; **340**: c365.

Li G, Abbade LPF, Nwosu I, Jin Y, Leenus A, Maaz M, Wang M, Bhatt M, Zielinski L, Sanger N, Bantoto B, Luo C, Shams I, Shahid H, Chang Y, Sun G, Mbuagbaw L, Samaan Z, Levine MAH, Adachi JD, Thabane L. A systematic review of comparisons between protocols or registrations and full reports in primary biomedical research. *BMC Medical Research Methodology* 2018; **18**: 9.

Lo B, Field MJ, Institute of Medicine (US) Committee on Conflict of Interest in Medical Research Education and Practice. *Conflict of Interest in Medical Research, Education, and Practice*. Washington, D.C.: National Academies Press (US); 2009.

Lundh A, Lexchin J, Mintzes B, Schroll JB, Bero L. Industry sponsorship and research outcome. *Cochrane Database of Systematic Reviews* 2017; **2**: MR000033.

Mann H, Djulbegovic B. Comparator bias: why comparisons must address genuine uncertainties. *Journal of the Royal Society of Medicine* 2013; **106**: 30–33.

Marret E, Elia N, Dahl JB, McQuay HJ, Møiniche S, Moore RA, Straube S, Tramèr MR. Susceptibility to fraud in systematic reviews: lessons from the Reuben case. *Anesthesiology* 2009; **111**: 1279–1289.

Marshall IJ, Kuiper J, Wallace BC. RobotReviewer: evaluation of a system for automatically assessing bias in clinical trials. *Journal of the American Medical Informatics Association* 2016; **23**: 193–201.

McGauran N, Wieseler B, Kreis J, Schuler YB, Kolsch H, Kaiser T. Reporting bias in medical research – a narrative review. *Trials* 2010; **11**: 37.

Millard LA, Flach PA, Higgins JPT. Machine learning to assist risk-of-bias assessments in systematic reviews. *International Journal of Epidemiology* 2016; **45**: 266–277.

Moher D, Shamseer L, Cobey KD, Lalu MM, Galipeau J, Avey MT, Ahmadzai N, Alabousi M, Barbeau P, Beck A, Daniel R, Frank R, Ghannad M, Hamel C, Hersi M, Hutton B, Isupov I, McGrath TA, McInnes MDF, Page MJ, Pratt M, Pussegoda K, Shea B, Srivastava A, Stevens A, Thavorn K, van Katwyk S, Ward R, Wolfe D, Yazdi F, Yu AM, Ziai H. Stop this waste of people, animals and money. *Nature* 2017; **549**: 23–25.

Montedori A, Bonacini MI, Casazza G, Luchetta ML, Duca P, Cozzolino F, Abraha I. Modified versus standard intention-to-treat reporting: are there differences in methodological quality, sponsorship, and findings in randomized trials? *A cross-sectional study. Trials* 2011; **12**: 58.

Morgan AJ, Ross A, Reavley NJ. Systematic review and meta-analysis of Mental Health First Aid training: effects on knowledge, stigma, and helping behaviour. *PloS One* 2018; **13**: e0197102.

Morrison A, Polisena J, Husereau D, Moulton K, Clark M, Fiander M, Mierzwinski-Urban M, Clifford T, Hutton B, Rabb D. The effect of English-language restriction on systematic review-based meta-analyses: a systematic review of empirical studies. *International Journal of Technology Assessment in Health Care* 2012; **28**: 138–144.

Norris SL, Burda BU, Holmer HK, Ogden LA, Fu R, Bero L, Schunemann H, Deyo R. Author's specialty and conflicts of interest contribute to conflicting guidelines for screening mammography. *Journal of Clinical Epidemiology* 2012; **65**: 725–733.

Odutayo A, Emdin CA, Hsiao AJ, Shakir M, Copsey B, Dutton S, Chiocchia V, Schlussel M, Dutton P, Roberts C, Altman DG, Hopewell S. Association between trial registration and positive study findings: cross-sectional study (Epidemiological Study of Randomized Trials-ESORT). *BMJ* 2017; **356**: j917.

Page MJ, Higgins JPT. Rethinking the assessment of risk of bias due to selective reporting: a cross-sectional study. *Systematic Reviews* 2016; **5**: 108.

Page MJ, Higgins JPT, Clayton G, Sterne JAC, Hróbjartsson A, Savović J. Empirical evidence of study design biases in randomized trials: systematic review of meta-epidemiological studies. *PloS One* 2016; **11**: 7.

Page MJ, McKenzie JE, Higgins JPT. Tools for assessing risk of reporting biases in studies and syntheses of studies: a systematic review. *BMJ Open* 2018; **8**: e019703.

Patel SV, Yu D, Elsolh B, Goldacre BM, Nash GM. Assessment of conflicts of interest in robotic surgical studies: validating author's declarations with the open payments database. *Annals of Surgery* 2018; **268**: 86–92.

Polanin JR, Tanner-Smith EE, Hennessy EA. Estimating the difference between published and unpublished effect sizes: a meta-review. *Review of Educational Research* 2016; **86**: 207–236.

Rasmussen K, Schroll J, Gøtzsche PC, Lundh A. Under-reporting of conflicts of interest among trialists: a cross-sectional study. *Journal of the Royal Society of Medicine* 2015; **108**: 101–107.

Riechelmann RP, Wang L, O'Carroll A, Krzyzanowska MK. Disclosure of conflicts of interest by authors of clinical trials and editorials in oncology. *Journal of Clinical Oncology* 2007; **25**: 4642–4647.

Rising K, Bacchetti P, Bero L. Reporting bias in drug trials submitted to the Food and Drug Administration: review of publication and presentation. *PLoS Medicine* 2008; **5**: e217.

Riveros C, Dechartres A, Perrodeau E, Haneef R, Boutron I, Ravaud P. Timing and completeness of trial results posted at ClinicalTrials.gov and published in journals. *PLoS Medicine* 2013; **10**: e1001566.

Rothenstein JM, Tomlinson G, Tannock IF, Detsky AS. Company stock prices before and after public announcements related to oncology drugs. *Journal of the National Cancer Institute* 2011; **103**: 1507–1512.

Safer DJ. Design and reporting modifications in industry-sponsored comparative psychopharmacology trials. *Journal of Nervous and Mental Disease* 2002; **190**: 583–592.

Saini P, Loke YK, Gamble C, Altman DG, Williamson PR, Kirkham JJ. Selective reporting bias of harm outcomes within studies: findings from a cohort of systematic reviews. *BMJ* 2014; **349**: g6501.

Sampson M, Barrowman NJ, Moher D, Klassen TP, Pham B, Platt R, St John PD, Viola R, Raina P. Should meta-analysts search Embase in addition to Medline? *Journal of Clinical Epidemiology* 2003; **56**: 943–955.

Savović J, Jones HE, Altman DG, Harris RJ, Jüni P, Pildal J, Als-Nielsen B, Balk EM, Gluud C, Gluud LL, Ioannidis JPA, Schulz KF, Beynon R, Welton NJ, Wood L, Moher D, Deeks JJ, Sterne JAC. Influence of reported study design characteristics on intervention effect estimates from randomized, controlled trials. *Annals of Internal Medicine* 2012; **157**: 429–438.

Scherer RW, Meerpohl JJ, Pfeifer N, Schmucker C, Schwarzer G, von Elm E. Full publication of results initially presented in abstracts. *Cochrane Database of Systematic Reviews* 2018; **11**: MR000005.

Schmid CH. Outcome reporting bias: a pervasive problem in published meta-analyses. *American Journal of Kidney Diseases* 2016; **69**: 172–174.

Schmucker C, Schell LK, Portalupi S, Oeller P, Cabrera L, Bassler D, Schwarzer G, Scherer RW, Antes G, von Elm E, Meerpohl JJ. Extent of non-publication in cohorts of studies approved by research ethics committees or included in trial registries. *PloS One* 2014; **9**: e114023.

Schulz KF, Chalmers I, Hayes RJ, Altman DG. Empirical evidence of bias. Dimensions of methodological quality associated with estimates of treatment effects in controlled trials. *JAMA* 1995; **273**: 408–412.

Shawwa K, Kallas R, Koujanian S, Agarwal A, Neumann I, Alexander P, Tikkinen KA, Guyatt G, Akl EA. Requirements of clinical journals for authors' disclosure of financial and non-financial conflicts of interest: a cross-sectional study. *PloS One* 2016; **11**: e0152301.

Sterne JAC. Why the Cochrane risk of bias tool should not include funding source as a standard item [editorial]. *Cochrane Database of Systematic Reviews* 2013; **12**: ED000076.

Tramèr MR, Reynolds DJ, Moore RA, McQuay HJ. Impact of covert duplicate publication on meta-analysis: a case study. *BMJ* 1997; **315**: 635–640.

Turner RM, Spiegelhalter DJ, Smith GC, Thompson SG. Bias modelling in evidence synthesis. *Journal of the Royal Statistical Society Series A (Statistics in Society)* 2009; **172**: 21–47.

Urrutia G, Ballesteros M, Djulbegovic B, Gich I, Roque M, Bonfill X. Cancer randomized trials showed that dissemination bias is still a problem to be solved. *Journal of Clinical Epidemiology* 2016; **77**: 84–90.

Vedula SS, Li T, Dickersin K. Differences in reporting of analyses in internal company documents versus published trial reports: comparisons in industry-sponsored trials in off-label uses of gabapentin. *PLoS Medicine* 2013; **10**: e1001378.

Viswanathan M, Carey TS, Belinson SE, Berliner E, Chang SM, Graham E, Guise JM, Ip S, Maglione MA, McCrory DC, McPheeters M, Newberry SJ, Sista P, White CM. A proposed approach may help systematic reviews retain needed expertise while minimizing bias from nonfinancial conflicts of interest. *Journal of Clinical Epidemiology* 2014; **67**: 1229–1238.

Welton NJ, Ades AE, Carlin JB, Altman DG, Sterne JAC. Models for potentially biased evidence in meta-analysis using empirically based priors. *Journal of the Royal Statistical Society: Series A (Statistics in Society)* 2009; **172**: 119–136.

Wieland LS, Berman BM, Altman DG, Barth J, Bouter LM, D'Adamo CR, Linde K, Moher D, Mullins CD, Treweek S, Tunis S, van der Windt DA, Zwarenstein M, Witt C. Rating of included trials on the efficacy-effectiveness spectrum: development of a new tool for systematic reviews. *Journal of Clinical Epidemiology* 2017; **84**.

Wieseler B, Kerekes MF, Vervoelgyi V, McGauran N, Kaiser T. Impact of document type on reporting quality of clinical drug trials: a comparison of registry reports, clinical study reports, and journal publications. *BMJ* 2012; **344**: d8141.

Wood L, Egger M, Gluud LL, Schulz K, Jüni P, Altman DG, Gluud C, Martin RM, Wood AJG, Sterne JAC. Empirical evidence of bias in treatment effect estimates in controlled trials with different interventions and outcomes: meta-epidemiological study. *BMJ* 2008; **336**: 601–605.

Zarin DA, Tse T, Williams RJ, Carr S. Trial reporting in ClinicalTrials.gov – The Final Rule. *New England Journal of Medicine* 2016; **375**: 1998–2004.

8

Assessing risk of bias in a randomized trial

Julian PT Higgins, Jelena Savović, Matthew J Page, Roy G Elbers, Jonathan AC Sterne

KEY POINTS

- This chapter details version 2 of the Cochrane risk-of-bias tool for randomized trials (RoB 2), the recommended tool for use in Cochrane Reviews.
- RoB 2 is structured into a fixed set of domains of bias, focusing on different aspects of trial design, conduct and reporting.
- Each assessment using the RoB 2 tool focuses on a specific result from a randomized trial.
- Within each domain, a series of questions ('signalling questions') aim to elicit information about features of the trial that are relevant to risk of bias.
- A judgement about the risk of bias arising from each domain is proposed by an algorithm, based on answers to the signalling questions. Judgements can be 'Low', or 'High' risk of bias, or can express 'Some concerns'.
- Answers to signalling questions and judgements about risk of bias should be supported by written justifications.
- The overall risk of bias for the result is the least favourable assessment across the domains of bias. Both the proposed domain-level and overall risk-of-bias judgements can be overridden by the review authors, with justification.

8.1 Introduction

Cochrane Reviews include an assessment of the risk of bias in each included study (see Chapter 7 for a general discussion of this topic). When randomized trials are included, the recommended tool is the revised version of the Cochrane tool, known as RoB 2, described in this chapter. The RoB 2 tool provides a framework for assessing the risk of bias in a single result (an estimate of the effect of an experimental intervention

This chapter should be cited as: Higgins JPT, Savović J, Page MJ, Elbers RG, Sterne JAC. Chapter 8: Assessing risk of bias in a randomized trial. In: Higgins JPT, Thomas J, Chandler J, Cumpston M, Li T, Page MJ, Welch VA (editors). *Cochrane Handbook for Systematic Reviews of Interventions*. 2nd Edition. Chichester (UK): John Wiley & Sons, 2019: 205–228.

compared with a comparator intervention on a particular outcome) from any type of randomized trial.

The RoB 2 tool is structured into domains through which bias might be introduced into the result. These domains were identified based on both empirical evidence and theoretical considerations. This chapter summarizes the main features of RoB 2 applied to individually randomized parallel-group trials. It describes the process of undertaking an assessment using the RoB 2 tool, summarizes the important issues for each domain of bias, and ends with a list of the key differences between RoB 2 and the earlier version of the tool. Variants of the RoB 2 tool specific to cluster-randomized trials and crossover trials are summarized in Chapter 23.

The full guidance document for the RoB 2 tool is available at www.riskofbias.info: it summarizes the empirical evidence underlying the tool and provides detailed explanations of the concepts covered and guidance on implementation.

8.2 Overview of RoB 2

8.2.1 Selecting which results to assess within the review

Before starting an assessment of risk of bias, authors will need to select which specific results from the included trials to assess. Because trials usually contribute multiple results to a systematic review, several risk-of-bias assessments may be needed for each trial, although it is unlikely to be feasible to assess every result for every trial in the review. It is important not to select results to assess based on the likely judgements arising from the assessment. An approach that focuses on the main outcomes of the review (the results contributing to the review's 'Summary of findings' table) may be the most appropriate approach (see also Chapter 7, Section 7.3.2).

8.2.2 Specifying the nature of the effect of interest: 'intention-to-treat' effects versus 'per-protocol' effects

Assessments for one of the RoB 2 domains, 'Bias due to deviations from intended interventions', differ according to whether review authors are interested in quantifying:

1) the effect of **assignment** to the interventions at baseline, regardless of whether the interventions are received as intended (the 'intention-to-treat effect'); or
2) the effect of **adhering to** the interventions as specified in the trial protocol (the 'per-protocol effect') (Hernán and Robins 2017).

If some patients do not receive their assigned intervention or deviate from the assigned intervention after baseline, these effects will differ, and will each be of interest. For example, the estimated effect of assignment to intervention would be the most appropriate to inform a health policy question about whether to recommend an intervention in a particular health system (e.g. whether to instigate a screening programme, or whether to prescribe a new cholesterol-lowering drug), whereas the estimated effect of adhering to the intervention as specified in the trial protocol would be the most appropriate to inform a care decision by an individual patient (e.g. whether to be screened, or whether to take the new drug). Review authors should define the intervention effect in which they are interested, and apply the risk-of-bias tool appropriately to this effect.

The effect of principal interest should be specified in the review protocol: most systematic reviews are likely to address the question of assignment rather than adherence to intervention. On occasion, review authors may be interested in both effects of interest.

The effect of **assignment** to intervention should be estimated by an **intention-to-treat (ITT) analysis** that includes all randomized participants (Fergusson et al 2002). The principles of ITT analyses are (Piantadosi 2005, Menerit 2012):

1) analyse participants in the intervention groups to which they were randomized, regardless of the intervention they actually received; and
2) include all randomized participants in the analysis, which requires measuring all participants' outcomes.

An ITT analysis maintains the benefit of randomization: that, on average, the intervention groups do not differ at baseline with respect to measured or unmeasured prognostic factors. Note that the term 'intention-to-treat' does not have a consistent definition and is used inconsistently in study reports (Hollis and Campbell 1999, Gravel et al 2007, Bell et al 2014).

Patients and other stakeholders are often interested in the effect of **adhering to** the intervention as described in the trial protocol (the 'per-protocol effect'), because it relates most closely to the implications of their choice between the interventions. However, two approaches to estimation of per-protocol effects that are commonly used in randomized trials may be seriously biased. These are:

- 'as-treated' analyses in which participants are analysed according to the intervention they actually received, even if their randomized allocation was to a different treatment group; and
- naïve 'per-protocol' analyses restricted to individuals who adhered to their assigned interventions.

Each of these analyses is problematic because prognostic factors may influence whether individuals adhere to their assigned intervention. If deviations are present, it is still possible to use data from a randomized trial to derive an unbiased estimate of the effect of adhering to intervention (Hernán and Robins 2017). However, appropriate methods require strong assumptions and published applications are relatively rare to date. When authors wish to assess the risk of bias in the estimated effect of adhering to intervention, use of results based on modern statistical methods may be at lower risk of bias than results based on 'as-treated' or naïve per-protocol analyses.

Trial authors often estimate the effect of intervention using more than one approach. They may not explain the reasons for their choice of analysis approach, or whether their aim is to estimate the effect of assignment or adherence to intervention. We recommend that when the effect of interest is that of assignment to intervention, the trial result included in meta-analyses, and assessed for risk of bias, should be chosen according to the following order of preference:

1) the result corresponding to a full ITT analysis, as defined above;

2) the result corresponding to an analysis (sometimes described as a 'modified intention-to-treat' (mITT) analysis) that adheres to ITT principles except that participants with missing outcome data are excluded (see Section 8.4.2; such an analysis does not prevent bias due to missing outcome data, which is addressed in the corresponding domain of the risk-of-bias assessment);
3) a result corresponding to an 'as-treated' or naïve 'per-protocol' analysis, or an analysis from which eligible trial participants were excluded.

8.2.3 Domains of bias and how they are addressed

The domains included in RoB 2 cover all types of bias that are currently understood to affect the results of randomized trials. These are:

1) bias arising from the randomization process;
2) bias due to deviations from intended interventions;
3) bias due to missing outcome data;
4) bias in measurement of the outcome; and
5) bias in selection of the reported result.

Each domain is required, and no additional domains should be added. Table 8.2.a summarizes the issues addressed within each bias domain.

For each domain, the tool comprises:

1) a series of 'signalling questions';
2) a judgement about risk of bias for the domain, which is facilitated by an algorithm that maps responses to the signalling questions to a proposed judgement;
3) free text boxes to justify responses to the signalling questions and risk-of-bias judgements; and
4) an option to predict (and explain) the likely direction of bias.

The **signalling questions** aim to provide a structured approach to eliciting information relevant to an assessment of risk of bias. They seek to be reasonably factual in nature, but some may require a degree of judgement. The response options are:

- Yes;
- Probably yes;
- Probably no;
- No;
- No information.

To maximize their simplicity and clarity, the signalling questions are phrased such that a response of 'Yes' may indicate either a low or high risk of bias, depending on the most natural way to ask the question. Responses of 'Yes' and 'Probably yes' have the same implications for risk of bias, as do responses of 'No' and 'Probably no'. The definitive responses ('Yes' and 'No') would typically imply that firm evidence is available in relation to the signalling question; the 'Probably' versions would typically imply that a judgement has been made. Although not required, if review authors wish to calculate measures of agreement (e.g. kappa statistics) for the answers to the signalling

Table 8.2.a Bias domains included in version 2 of the Cochrane risk-of-bias tool for randomized trials, with a summary of the issues addressed

Bias domain	Issues addressed*
Bias arising from the randomization process	Whether: • the allocation sequence was random; • the allocation sequence was adequately concealed; • baseline differences between intervention groups suggest a problem with the randomization process.
Bias due to deviations from intended interventions	Whether: • participants were aware of their assigned intervention during the trial; • carers and people delivering the interventions were aware of participants' assigned intervention during the trial. *When the review authors' interest is in the effect of assignment to intervention* (see Section 8.2.2): • (if applicable) deviations from the intended intervention arose because of the experimental context (i.e. do not reflect usual practice); and, if so, whether they were unbalanced between groups and likely to have affected the outcome; • an appropriate analysis was used to estimate the effect of assignment to intervention; and, if not, whether there was potential for a substantial impact on the result. *When the review authors' interest is in the effect of adhering to intervention* (see Section 8.2.2): • (if applicable) important non-protocol interventions were balanced across intervention groups; • (if applicable) failures in implementing the intervention could have affected the outcome; • (if applicable) study participants adhered to the assigned intervention regimen; • (if applicable) an appropriate analysis was used to estimate the effect of adhering to the intervention.
Bias due to missing outcome data	Whether: • data for this outcome were available for all, or nearly all, participants randomized; • (if applicable) there was evidence that the result was not biased by missing outcome data; • (if applicable) missingness in the outcome was likely to depend on its true value (e.g. the proportions of missing outcome data, or reasons for missing outcome data, differ between intervention groups).
Bias in measurement of the outcome	Whether: • the method of measuring the outcome was inappropriate; • measurement or ascertainment of the outcome could have differed between intervention groups; • outcome assessors were aware of the intervention received by study participants;

(*Continued*)

Table 8.2.a (Continued)

Bias domain	Issues addressed*
	• (if applicable) assessment of the outcome was likely to have been influenced by knowledge of intervention received.
Bias in selection of the reported result	Whether: • the trial was analysed in accordance with a pre-specified plan that was finalized before unblinded outcome data were available for analysis; • the numerical result being assessed is likely to have been selected, on the basis of the results, from multiple outcome measurements within the outcome domain; • the numerical result being assessed is likely to have been selected, on the basis of the results, from multiple analyses of the data.

* For the precise wording of signalling questions and guidance for answering each one, see the full risk-of-bias tool at www.riskofbias.info.

questions, we recommend treating 'Yes' and 'Probably yes' as the same response, and 'No' and 'Probably no' as the same response.

The 'No information' response should be used only when both (1) insufficient details are reported to permit a response of 'Yes', 'Probably yes', 'No' or 'Probably no', and (2) in the absence of these details it would be unreasonable to respond 'Probably yes' or 'Probably no' given the circumstances of the trial. For example, in the context of a large trial run by an experienced clinical trials unit for regulatory purposes, if specific information about the randomization methods is absent, it may still be reasonable to respond 'Probably yes' rather than 'No information' to the signalling question about allocation sequence concealment.

The implications of a 'No information' response to a signalling question differ according to the purpose of the question. If the question seeks to identify evidence of a problem, then 'No information' corresponds to no evidence of that problem. If the question relates to an item that is expected to be reported (such as whether any participants were lost to follow-up), then the absence of information leads to concerns about there being a problem.

A response option 'Not applicable' is available for signalling questions that are answered only if the response to a previous question implies that they are required.

Signalling questions should be answered independently: the answer to one question should not affect answers to other questions in the same or other domains other than through determining which subsequent questions are answered.

Once the signalling questions are answered, the next step is to reach a **risk-of-bias judgement**, and assign one of three levels to each domain:

- Low risk of bias;
- Some concerns; or
- High risk of bias.

The RoB 2 tool includes **algorithms that map responses to signalling questions to a proposed risk-of-bias judgement** for each domain (see the full documentation at www.riskofbias.info for details). The algorithms include specific mappings of each possible combination of responses to the signalling questions (including responses of 'No information') to judgements of low risk of bias, some concerns or high risk of bias.

Use of the word 'judgement' is important for the risk-of-bias assessment. The algorithms provide *proposed* judgements, but review authors should verify these and change them if they feel this is appropriate. In reaching final judgements, review authors should interpret 'risk of bias' as 'risk of material bias'. That is, concerns should be expressed only about issues that are likely to affect the ability to draw reliable conclusions from the study.

A **free text box** alongside the signalling questions and judgements provides space for review authors to present supporting information for each response. In some instances, when the same information is likely to be used to answer more than one question, one text box covers more than one signalling question. Brief, direct quotations from the text of the study report should be used whenever possible. It is important that reasons are provided for any judgements that do not follow the algorithms. The tool also provides space to indicate all the sources of information about the study obtained to inform the judgements (e.g. published papers, trial registry entries, additional information from the study authors).

RoB 2 includes optional judgements of the **direction of the bias** for each domain and overall. For some domains, the bias is most easily thought of as being towards or away from the null. For example, high levels of switching of participants from their assigned intervention to the other intervention may have the effect of reducing the observed difference between the groups, leading to the estimated effect of adhering to intervention (see Section 8.2.2) being biased towards the null. For other domains, the bias is likely to favour one of the interventions being compared, implying an increase or decrease in the effect estimate depending on which intervention is favoured. Examples include manipulation of the randomization process, awareness of interventions received influencing the outcome assessment and selective reporting of results. If review authors do not have a clear rationale for judging the likely direction of the bias, they should not guess it and can leave this response blank.

8.2.4 Reaching an overall risk-of-bias judgement for a result

The response options for an **overall risk-of-bias judgement** are the same as for individual domains. Table 8.2.b shows the approach to mapping risk-of-bias judgements within domains to an overall judgement for the outcome.

Judging a result to be at a particular level of risk of bias for an individual domain implies that the result has an overall risk of bias at least this severe. Therefore, a judgement of 'High' risk of bias within any domain should have similar implications for the result, irrespective of which domain is being assessed. In practice this means that if the answers to the signalling questions yield a proposed judgement of 'High' risk of bias, the assessors should consider whether any identified problems are of sufficient concern to warrant this judgement for that result overall. If this is not the case, the appropriate action would be to override the proposed default judgement and provide justification. 'Some concerns' in multiple domains may lead review authors to decide on an overall judgement of 'High' risk of bias for that result or group of results.

Table 8.2.b Reaching an overall risk-of-bias judgement for a specific outcome

Overall risk-of-bias judgement	Criteria
Low risk of bias	The trial is judged to be at **low risk of bias for all domains** for this result.
Some concerns	The trial is judged to raise **some concerns** in at least one domain for this result, but not to be at high risk of bias for any domain.
High risk of bias	The trial is judged to be at **high risk of bias** in at least one domain for this result. Or The trial is judged to have **some concerns** for **multiple domains** in a way that substantially lowers confidence in the result.

Once an overall judgement has been reached for an individual trial result, this information will need to be presented in the review and reflected in the analysis and conclusions. For discussion of the presentation of risk-of-bias assessments and how they can be incorporated into analyses, see Chapter 7. Risk-of-bias assessments also feed into one domain of the GRADE approach for assessing certainty of a body of evidence, as discussed in Chapter 14.

8.3 Bias arising from the randomization process

If successfully accomplished, randomization avoids the influence of either known or unknown prognostic factors (factors that predict the outcome, such as severity of illness or presence of comorbidities) on the assignment of individual participants to intervention groups. This means that, on average, each intervention group has the same prognosis before the start of intervention. If prognostic factors influence the intervention group to which participants are assigned then the estimated effect of intervention will be biased by 'confounding', which occurs when there are common causes of intervention group assignment and outcome. Confounding is an important potential cause of bias in intervention effect estimates from observational studies, because treatment decisions in routine care are often influenced by prognostic factors.

To randomize participants into a study, an allocation sequence that specifies how participants will be assigned to interventions is generated, based on a process that includes an element of chance. We call this **allocation sequence generation**. Subsequently, steps must be taken to prevent participants or trial personnel from knowing the forthcoming allocations until after recruitment has been confirmed. This process is often termed **allocation sequence concealment**.

Knowledge of the next assignment (e.g. if the sequence is openly posted on a bulletin board) can enable selective enrolment of participants on the basis of prognostic factors. Participants who would have been assigned to an intervention deemed to be 'inappropriate' may be rejected. Other participants may be directed to the 'appropriate' intervention, which can be accomplished by delaying their entry into the trial until the desired allocation appears. For this reason, successful allocation sequence concealment is a vital part of randomization.

Some review authors confuse allocation sequence concealment with blinding of assigned interventions during the trial. Allocation sequence concealment seeks to prevent bias in intervention assignment by preventing trial personnel and participants from knowing the allocation sequence before and until assignment. It can always be successfully implemented, regardless of the study design or clinical area (Schulz et al 1995, Jüni et al 2001). In contrast, blinding seeks to prevent bias after assignment (Jüni et al 2001, Schulz et al 2002) and cannot always be implemented. This is often the situation, for example, in trials comparing surgical with non-surgical interventions.

8.3.1 Approaches to sequence generation

Randomization with no constraints is called **simple randomization** or **unrestricted randomization**. Sometimes **blocked randomization (restricted randomization)** is used to ensure that the desired ratio of participants in the experimental and comparator intervention groups (e.g. 1 : 1) is achieved (Schulz and Grimes 2002, Schulz and Grimes 2006). This is done by ensuring that the numbers of participants assigned to each intervention group is balanced within blocks of specified size (e.g. for every 10 consecutively entered participants): the specified number of allocations to experimental and comparator intervention groups is assigned in random order within each block. If the block size is known to trial personnel and the intervention group is revealed after assignment, then the last allocation within each block can always be predicted. To avoid this problem multiple block sizes may be used, and randomly varied (random permuted blocks).

Stratified randomization, in which randomization is performed separately within subsets of participants defined by potentially important prognostic factors, such as disease severity and study centres, is also common. In practice, stratified randomization is usually performed together with blocked randomization. The purpose of combining these two procedures is to ensure that experimental and comparator groups are similar with respect to the specified prognostic factors other than intervention. If simple (rather than blocked) randomization is used in each stratum, then stratification offers no benefit, but the randomization is still valid.

Another approach that incorporates both general concepts of stratification and restricted randomization is **minimization**. Minimization algorithms assign the next intervention in a way that achieves the best balance between intervention groups in relation to a specified set of prognostic factors. Minimization generally includes a random element (at least for participants enrolled when the groups are balanced with respect to the prognostic factors included in the algorithm) and should be implemented along with clear strategies for allocation sequence concealment. Some methodologists are cautious about the acceptability of minimization, while others consider it to be an attractive approach (Brown et al 2005, Clark et al 2016).

8.3.2 Allocation sequence concealment and failures of randomization

If future assignments can be anticipated, leading to a failure of allocation sequence concealment, then bias can arise through selective enrolment of participants into a study, depending on their prognostic factors. Ways in which this can happen include:

1) knowledge of a deterministic assignment rule, such as by alternation, date of birth or day of admission;

2) knowledge of the sequence of assignments, whether randomized or not (e.g. if a sequence of random assignments is posted on the wall); and
3) ability to predict assignments successfully, based on previous assignments.

The last of these can occur when blocked randomization is used and assignments are known to the recruiter after each participant is enrolled into the trial. It may then be possible to predict future assignments for some participants, particularly when blocks are of a fixed size and are not divided across multiple recruitment centres (Berger 2005).

Attempts to achieve allocation sequence concealment may be undermined in practice. For example, unsealed allocation envelopes may be opened, while translucent envelopes may be held against a bright light to reveal the contents (Schulz 1995, Schulz et al 1995, Jüni et al 2001). Personal accounts suggest that many allocation schemes have been deduced by investigators because the methods of concealment were inadequate (Schulz 1995).

The success of randomization in producing comparable groups is often examined by comparing baseline values of important prognostic factors between intervention groups. Corbett and colleagues have argued that risk-of-bias assessments should consider whether participant characteristics are balanced between intervention groups (Corbett et al 2014). The RoB 2 tool includes consideration of situations in which baseline characteristics indicate that something may have gone wrong with the randomization process. **It is important that baseline imbalances that are consistent with chance are not interpreted as evidence of risk of bias.** Chance imbalances are not a source of systematic bias, and the RoB 2 tool does not aim to identify imbalances in baseline variables that have arisen due to chance.

8.4 Bias due to deviations from intended interventions

This domain relates to biases that arise when there are deviations from the intended interventions. Such differences could be the administration of additional interventions that are inconsistent with the trial protocol, failure to implement the protocol interventions as intended, or non-adherence by trial participants to their assigned intervention. Biases that arise due to deviations from intended interventions are sometimes referred to as performance biases.

The intended interventions are those specified in the trial protocol. It is often intended that interventions should change or evolve in response to the health of, or events experienced by, trial participants. For example, the investigators may intend that:

- in a trial of a new drug to control symptoms of rheumatoid arthritis, participants experiencing severe toxicities should receive additional care and/or switch to an alternative drug;
- in a trial of a specified cancer drug regimen, participants whose cancer progresses should switch to a second-line intervention; or
- in a trial comparing surgical intervention with conservative management of stable angina, participants who progress to unstable angina receive surgical intervention.

Unfortunately, trial protocols may not fully specify the circumstances in which deviations from the initial intervention should occur, or distinguish changes to intervention that are consistent with the intentions of the investigators from those that should be considered as deviations from the intended intervention. For example, a cancer trial protocol may not define progression, or specify the second-line drug that should be used in patients who progress (Hernán and Scharfstein 2018). It may therefore be necessary for review authors to document changes that are and are not considered to be deviations from intended intervention. Similarly, for trials in which the comparator intervention is 'usual care', the protocol may not specify interventions consistent with usual care or whether they are expected to be used alongside the experimental intervention. Review authors may therefore need to document what departures from usual care will be considered as deviations from intended intervention.

8.4.1 Non-protocol interventions

Non-protocol interventions that trial participants might receive during trial follow up and that are likely to affect the outcome of interest can lead to bias in estimated intervention effects. If possible, review authors should specify potential non-protocol interventions in advance (at review protocol writing stage). Non-protocol interventions may be identified through the expert knowledge of members of the review group, via reviews of the literature, and through discussions with health professionals.

8.4.2 The role of the effect of interest

As described in Section 8.2.2, assessments for this domain depend on the effect of interest. In RoB 2, the only deviations from the intended intervention that are addressed in relation to the effect of *assignment to the intervention* are those that:

1) are inconsistent with the trial protocol;
2) arise because of the experimental context; and
3) influence the outcome.

For example, in an unblinded study participants may feel unlucky to have been assigned to the comparator group and therefore seek the experimental intervention, or other interventions that improve their prognosis. Similarly, monitoring patients randomized to a novel intervention more frequently than those randomized to standard care would increase the risk of bias, unless such monitoring was an intended part of the novel intervention. **Deviations from intervention that do not arise because of the experimental context, such as a patient's choice to stop taking their assigned medication, do not lead to bias in the effect of assignment to intervention.**

To examine the effect of *adhering to the interventions* as specified in the trial protocol, it is important to specify what types of deviations from the intended intervention will be examined. These will be one or more of:

1) how well the intervention was implemented;
2) how well participants adhered to the intervention (without discontinuing or switching to another intervention);

3) whether non-protocol interventions were received alongside the intended intervention and (if so) whether they were balanced across intervention groups; and

If such deviations are present, review authors should consider whether appropriate statistical methods were used to adjust for their effects.

8.4.3 The role of blinding

Bias due to deviations from intended interventions can sometimes be reduced or avoided by implementing mechanisms that ensure the participants, carers and trial personnel (i.e. people delivering the interventions) are unaware of the interventions received. This is commonly referred to as 'blinding', although in some areas (including eye health) the term 'masking' is preferred. Blinding, if successful, should prevent knowledge of the intervention assignment from influencing contamination (application of one of the interventions in participants intended to receive the other), switches to non-protocol interventions or non-adherence by trial participants.

Trial reports often describe blinding in broad terms, such as 'double blind'. This term makes it difficult to know who was blinded (Schulz et al 2002). Such terms are also used inconsistently (Haahr and Hróbjartsson 2006). A review of methods used for blinding highlights the variety of methods used in practice (Boutron et al 2006).

Blinding during a trial can be difficult or impossible in some contexts, for example in a trial comparing a surgical with a non-surgical intervention. Non-blinded ('open') trials may take other measures to avoid deviations from intended intervention, such as treating patients according to strict criteria that prevent administration of non-protocol interventions.

Lack of blinding of participants, carers or people delivering the interventions may cause bias if it leads to deviations from intended interventions. For example, low expectations of improvement among participants in the comparator group may lead them to seek and receive the experimental intervention. Such deviations from intended intervention that arise due to the experimental context can lead to bias in the estimated effects of both assignment to intervention and of adhering to intervention.

An attempt to blind participants, carers and people delivering the interventions to intervention group does not ensure successful blinding in practice. For many blinded drug trials, the side effects of the drugs allow the possible detection of the intervention being received for some participants, unless the study compares similar interventions, for example drugs with similar side effects, or uses an active placebo (Boutron et al 2006, Bello et al 2017, Jensen et al 2017).

Deducing the intervention received, for example among participants experiencing side effects that are specific to the experimental intervention, does not in itself lead to a risk of bias. As discussed, cessation of a drug intervention because of toxicity will usually not be considered a deviation from intended intervention. See the elaborations that accompany the signalling questions in the full guidance at www.riskofbias.info for further discussion of this issue.

Risk of bias in this domain may differ between outcomes, even if the same people were aware of intervention assignments during the trial. For example, knowledge of the assigned intervention may affect behaviour (such as number of clinic visits), while not having an important impact on physiology (including risk of mortality).

Blinding of outcome assessors, to avoid bias in *measuring* the outcome, is considered separately, in the 'Bias in measurement of outcomes' domain. Bias due to differential rates of dropout (withdrawal from the study) is considered in the 'Bias due to missing outcome data' domain.

8.4.4 Appropriate analyses

For the effect of assignment to intervention, an appropriate analysis should follow the principles of ITT (see Section 8.2.2). Some authors may report a 'modified intention-to-treat' (mITT) analysis in which participants with missing outcome data are excluded. Such an analysis may be biased because of the missing outcome data: this is addressed in the domain 'Bias due to missing outcome data'. Note that the phrase 'modified intention-to-treat' is used in different ways, and may refer to inclusion of participants who received at least one dose of treatment (Abraha and Montedori 2010); our use of the term refers to missing data rather than to adherence to intervention.

Inappropriate analyses include 'as-treated' analyses, naïve 'per-protocol' analyses, and other analyses based on post-randomization exclusion of eligible trial participants on whom outcomes were measured (Hernán and Hernandez-Diaz 2012) (see also Section 8.2.2).

For the effect of adhering to intervention, appropriate analysis approaches are described by Hernán and Robins (Hernán and Robins 2017). Instrumental variable approaches can be used in some circumstances to estimate the effect of intervention among participants who received the assigned intervention.

8.5 Bias due to missing outcome data

Missing measurements of the outcome may lead to bias in the intervention effect estimate. Possible reasons for missing outcome data include (National Research Council 2010):

1) participants withdraw from the study or cannot be located ('loss to follow-up' or 'dropout');
2) participants do not attend a study visit at which outcomes should have been measured;
3) participants attend a study visit but do not provide relevant data;
4) data or records are lost or are unavailable for other reasons; and
5) participants can no longer experience the outcome, for example because they have died.

This domain addresses risk of bias due to missing outcome data, including biases introduced by procedures used to impute, or otherwise account for, the missing outcome data.

Some participants may be excluded from an analysis for reasons other than missing outcome data. In particular, a naïve 'per-protocol' analysis is restricted to participants who received the intended intervention. Potential bias introduced by such analyses, or by other exclusions of eligible participants for whom outcome data are available, is addressed in the domain 'Bias due to deviations from intended interventions' (see Section 8.4).

The ITT principle of measuring outcome data on all participants (see Section 8.2.2) is frequently difficult or impossible to achieve in practice. Therefore, it can often only be followed by making assumptions about the missing outcome values. Even when an analysis is described as ITT, it may exclude participants with missing outcome data and be at risk of bias (such analyses may be described as 'modified intention-to-treat' (mITT) analyses). Therefore, assessments of risk of bias due to missing outcome data should be based on the issues addressed in the signalling questions for this domain, and not on the way that trial authors described the analysis.

8.5.1 When do missing outcome data lead to bias?

Analyses excluding individuals with missing outcome data are examples of 'complete-case' analyses (analyses restricted to individuals in whom there were no missing values of included variables). To understand when missing outcome data lead to bias in such analyses, we need to consider:

1) the **true value of the outcome** in participants with missing outcome data: this is the value of the outcome that should have been measured but was not; and
2) the **missingness mechanism**, which is the process that led to outcome data being missing.

Whether missing outcome data lead to bias in complete case analyses depends on whether the missingness mechanism is related to the true value of the outcome. Equivalently, we can consider whether the measured (non-missing) outcomes differ systematically from the missing outcomes (the true values in participants with missing outcome data). For example, consider a trial of cognitive behavioural therapy compared with usual care for depression. If participants who are more depressed are less likely to return for follow-up, then whether a measurement of depression is missing depends on its true value, which implies that the measured depression outcomes will differ systematically from the true values of the missing depression outcomes.

The specific situations in which a complete case analysis suffers from bias (when there are missing data) are discussed in detail in the full guidance for the RoB 2 tool at www.riskofbias.info. In brief:

1) missing outcome data **will not lead to bias** if missingness in the outcome is unrelated to its true value, within each intervention group;
2) missing outcome data **will lead to bias** if missingness in the outcome depends on *both* the intervention group and the true value of the outcome; and
3) missing outcome data **will often lead to bias** if missingness is related to its true value and, additionally, the effect of the experimental intervention differs from that of the comparator intervention.

8.5.2 When is the amount of missing outcome data small enough to exclude bias?

It is tempting to classify risk of bias according to the proportion of participants with missing outcome data.

Unfortunately, there is no sensible threshold for 'small enough' in relation to the proportion of missing outcome data.

In situations where missing outcome data lead to bias, the extent of bias will increase as the amount of missing outcome data increases. There is a tradition of regarding a proportion of less than 5% missing outcome data as 'small' (with corresponding implications for risk of bias), and over 20% as 'large'. However, the potential impact of missing data on estimated intervention effects depends on the proportion of participants with missing data, the type of outcome and (for dichotomous outcome) the risk of the event. For example, consider a study of 1000 participants in the intervention group where the observed mortality is 2% for the 900 participants with outcome data (18 deaths). Even though the proportion of data missing is only 10%, if the mortality rate in the 100 missing participants is 20% (20 deaths), the overall true mortality of the intervention group would be nearly double (3.8% vs 2%) that estimated from the observed data.

8.5.3 Judging risk of bias due to missing outcome data

It is not possible to examine directly whether the chance that the outcome is missing depends on its true value: judgements of risk of bias will depend on the circumstances of the trial. Therefore, we can only be sure that there is no bias due to missing outcome data when: (1) the outcome is measured in all participants; (2) the proportion of missing outcome data is sufficiently low that any bias is too small to be of importance; or (3) sensitivity analyses (conducted by either the trial authors or the review authors) confirm that plausible values of the missing outcome data could make no important difference to the estimated intervention effect.

Indirect evidence that missing outcome data are likely to cause bias can come from examining: (1) differences between the proportion of missing outcome data in the experimental and comparator intervention groups; and (2) reasons that outcome data are missing.

If the effects of the experimental and comparator interventions on the outcome are different, and missingness in the outcome depends on its true value, then the proportion of participants with missing data is likely to differ between the intervention groups. Therefore, differing proportions of missing outcome data in the experimental and comparator intervention groups provide evidence of potential bias.

Trial reports may provide reasons why participants have missing data. For example, trials of haloperidol to treat dementia reported various reasons such as 'lack of efficacy', 'adverse experience', 'positive response', 'withdrawal of consent' and 'patient ran away', and 'patient sleeping' (Higgins et al 2008). It is likely that some of these (e.g. 'lack of efficacy' and 'positive response') are related to the true values of the missing outcome data. Therefore, these reasons increase the risk of bias if the effects of the experimental and comparator interventions differ, or if the reasons are related to intervention group (e.g. 'adverse experience').

In practice, our ability to assess risk of bias will be limited by the extent to which trial authors collected and reported reasons that outcome data were missing. The situation most likely to lead to bias is when reasons for missing outcome data differ between the intervention groups: for example if participants who became seriously unwell withdrew from the comparator group while participants who recovered withdrew from the experimental intervention group.

Trial authors may present statistical analyses (in addition to or instead of complete case analyses) that attempt to address the potential for bias caused by missing outcome data. Approaches include single imputation (e.g. assuming the participant had no event; last observation carried forward), multiple imputation and likelihood-based methods (see Chapter 10, Section 10.12.2). Imputation methods are unlikely to remove or reduce the bias that occurs when missingness in the outcome depends on its true value, unless they use information additional to intervention group assignment to predict the missing values. Review authors may attempt to address missing data using sensitivity analyses, as discussed in Chapter 10 (Section 10.12.3).

8.6 Bias in measurement of the outcome

Errors in measurement of outcomes can bias intervention effect estimates. These are often referred to as **measurement error** (for continuous outcomes), **misclassification** (for dichotomous or categorical outcomes) or **under-ascertainment/over-ascertainment** (for events). Measurement errors may be **differential** or **non-differential** in relation to intervention assignment:

- Differential measurement errors are related to intervention assignment. Such errors are systematically different between experimental and comparator intervention groups and are less likely when outcome assessors are blinded to intervention assignment.
- Non-differential measurement errors are unrelated to intervention assignment.

This domain relates primarily to differential errors. Non-differential measurement errors are not addressed in detail.

Risk of bias in this domain depends on the following five considerations.

1. Whether the method of measuring the outcome is appropriate. Outcomes in randomized trials should be assessed using appropriate outcome measures. For example, portable blood glucose machines used by trial participants may not reliably measure below 3.1 mmol, leading to an inability to detect differences in rates of severe hypoglycaemia between an insulin intervention and placebo, and under-representation of the true incidence of this adverse effect. Such a measurement would be inappropriate for this outcome.

2. Whether measurement or ascertainment of the outcome differs, or could differ, between intervention groups. The methods used to measure or ascertain outcomes should be the same across intervention groups. This is usually the case for pre-specified outcomes, but problems may arise with passive collection of outcome data, as is often the case for unexpected adverse effects. For example, in a placebo-controlled trial, severe headaches occur more frequently in participants assigned to a new drug than those assigned to placebo. These lead to more MRI scans being done in the experimental intervention group, and therefore to more diagnoses of symptomless brain tumours, even though the drug does not increase the incidence of brain tumours. Even for a pre-specified outcome measure, the nature of the intervention may lead to methods of measuring the outcome that are not comparable across intervention groups. For example, an intervention involving additional visits to a healthcare provider may lead to additional opportunities for outcome events to be identified, compared with the comparator intervention.

3. Who is the outcome assessor. The outcome assessor can be:

1) the participant, when the outcome is a participant-reported outcome such as pain, quality of life, or self-completed questionnaire;
2) the intervention provider, when the outcome is the result of a clinical examination, the occurrence of a clinical event or a therapeutic decision such as decision to offer a surgical intervention; or
3) an observer not directly involved in the intervention provided to the participant, such as an adjudication committee, or a health professional recording outcomes for inclusion in disease registries.

4. Whether the outcome assessor is blinded to intervention assignment. Blinding of outcome assessors is often possible even when blinding of participants and personnel during the trial is not feasible. However, it is particularly difficult for participant-reported outcomes: for example, in a trial comparing surgery with medical management when the outcome is pain at 3 months. The potential for bias cannot be ignored even if the outcome assessor cannot be blinded.

5. Whether the assessment of outcome is likely to be influenced by knowledge of intervention received. For trials in which outcome assessors were not blinded, the risk of bias will depend on whether the outcome assessment involves judgement, which depends on the type of outcome. We describe most situations in Table 8.6.a.

8.7 Bias in selection of the reported result

This domain addresses bias that arises because the reported result is selected (based on its direction, magnitude or statistical significance) from among multiple intervention effect estimates that were calculated by the trial authors. Consideration of risk of bias requires distinction between

- an **outcome domain**: this is a state or endpoint of interest, irrespective of how it is measured (e.g. presence or severity of depression);
- a specific **outcome measurement** (e.g. measurement of depression using the Hamilton rating scale 6 weeks after starting intervention); and
- an **outcome analysis**: this is a specific result obtained by analysing one or more outcome measurements (e.g. the difference in mean change in Hamilton rating scale scores from baseline to 6 weeks between experimental and comparator groups).

This domain does not address bias due to selective non-reporting (or incomplete reporting) of outcome domains that were measured and analysed by the trial authors (Kirkham et al 2010). For example, deaths of trial participants may be recorded by the trialists, but the reports of the trial might contain no data for deaths, or state only that

Table 8.6.a Considerations of risk of bias in measurement of the outcome for different types of outcomes

Outcome type	Description	Examples	Who is the outcome assessor?	Implications for risk of bias if the outcome assessor is aware of the intervention assignment
Participant-reported outcomes	Reports coming directly from participants about how they function or feel in relation to a health condition or intervention, without interpretation by anyone else. They include any evaluation obtained directly from participants through interviews, self-completed questionnaires or hand-held devices.	Pain, nausea and health-related quality of life.	The **participant**, even if a blinded interviewer is questioning the participant and completing a questionnaire on their behalf.	The outcome assessment is **potentially influenced** by knowledge of intervention received, leading to a judgement of at least 'Some concerns'. Review authors will need to judge whether it is **likely** that participants' reporting of the outcome was influenced by knowledge of intervention received, in which case risk of bias is considered high.
Observer-reported outcomes not involving judgement	Outcomes reported by an external observer (e.g. an intervention provider, independent researcher, or radiologist) that do *not* involve any judgement from the observer.	All-cause mortality or the result of an automated test.	The **observer**.	The assessment of outcome is usually **not likely to be influenced** by knowledge of intervention received.
Observer-reported outcomes involving some judgement	Outcomes reported by an external observer (e.g. an intervention provider, independent researcher, or radiologist) that involve some judgement.	Assessment of an X-ray or other image, clinical examination and clinical events other than death (e.g. myocardial infarction) that require judgements on clinical definitions or medical records.	The **observer**.	The assessment of outcome is **potentially influenced** by knowledge of intervention received, leading to a judgement of at least 'Some concerns'. Review authors will need to judge whether it is likely that assessment of the outcome was influenced by knowledge of intervention received, in which case risk of bias is considered high.

Outcomes that reflect decisions made by the intervention provider	Outcomes that reflect decisions made by the intervention provider, where recording of the decisions does not involve any judgement, but where the decision itself can be influenced by knowledge of intervention received.	Hospitalization, stopping treatment, referral to a different ward, performing a caesarean section, stopping ventilation and discharge of the participant.	The **care provider making the decision**.	Assessment of outcome is usually **likely to be influenced** by knowledge of intervention received, if the care provider is aware of this. This is particularly important when preferences or expectations regarding the effect of the experimental intervention are strong.
Composite outcomes	Combination of multiple end points into a single outcome. Typically, participants who have experienced any of a specified set of endpoints are considered to have experienced the composite outcome. Composite endpoints can also be constructed from continuous outcome measures.	Major adverse cardiac and cerebrovascular events.	Any of the above.	Assessment of risk of bias for composite outcomes should take into account the frequency or contribution of each component and the risk of bias due to the most influential components.

the effect estimate for mortality was not statistically significant. Such bias puts the result of a synthesis at risk because results are omitted based on their direction, magnitude or statistical significance. It should therefore be addressed at the review level, as part of an integrated assessment of the risk of reporting bias (Page and Higgins 2016). For further guidance, see Chapter 7 and Chapter 13.

Bias in selection of the reported result typically arises from a desire for findings to support vested interests or to be sufficiently noteworthy to merit publication. It can arise for both harms and benefits, although the motivations may differ. For example, in trials comparing an experimental intervention with placebo, trialists who have a preconception or vested interest in showing that the experimental intervention is beneficial and safe may be inclined to be selective in reporting efficacy estimates that are statistically significant and favourable to the experimental intervention, along with harm estimates that are not significantly different between groups. In contrast, other trialists may selectively report harm estimates that are statistically significant and unfavourable to the experimental intervention if they believe that publicizing the existence of a harm will increase their chances of publishing in a high impact journal.

This domain considers:

1. Whether the trial was analysed in accordance with a pre-specified plan that was finalized before unblinded outcome data were available for analysis. We strongly encourage review authors to attempt to retrieve the pre-specified analysis intentions for each trial (see Chapter 7, Section 7.3.1). Doing so allows for the identification of any outcome measures or analyses that have been omitted from, or added to, the results report, post hoc. Review authors should ideally ask the study authors to supply the study protocol and full statistical analysis plan if these are not publicly available. In addition, if outcome measures and analyses mentioned in an article, protocol or trial registration record are not reported, study authors could be asked to clarify whether those outcome measures were in fact analysed and, if so, to supply the data.

Trial protocols should describe how unexpected adverse outcomes (that potentially reflect unanticipated harms) will be collected and analysed. However, results based on spontaneously reported adverse outcomes may lead to concerns that these were selected based on the finding being noteworthy.

For some trials, the analysis intentions will not be readily available. It is still possible to assess the risk of bias in selection of the reported result. For example, outcome measures and analyses listed in the methods section of an article can be compared with those reported. Furthermore, outcome measures and analyses should be compared across different papers describing the trial.

2. Selective reporting of a particular outcome measurement (based on the results) from among estimates for multiple measurements assessed within an outcome domain. Examples include:

- reporting only one or a subset of time points at which the outcome was measured;
- use of multiple measurement instruments (e.g. pain scales) and only reporting data for the instrument with the most favourable result;
- having multiple assessors measure an outcome domain (e.g. clinician-rated and patient-rated depression scales) and only reporting data for the measure with the most favourable result; and

- reporting only the most favourable subscale (or a subset of subscales) for an instrument when measurements for other subscales were available.

3. Selective reporting of a particular analysis (based on the results) from multiple analyses estimating intervention effects for a specific outcome measurement. Examples include:

- carrying out analyses of both change scores and post-intervention scores adjusted for baseline and reporting only the more favourable analysis;
- multiple analyses of a particular outcome measurement with and without adjustment for prognostic factors (or with adjustment for different sets of prognostic factors);
- a continuously scaled outcome converted to categorical data on the basis of multiple cut-points; and
- effect estimates generated for multiple composite outcomes with full reporting of just one or a subset.

Either type of selective reporting will lead to bias if selection is based on the direction, magnitude or statistical significance of the effect estimate.

Insufficient detail in some documents may preclude full assessment of the risk of bias (e.g. trialists only state in the trial registry record that they will measure 'pain', without specifying the measurement scale, time point or metric that will be used). Review authors should indicate insufficient information alongside their responses to signalling questions.

8.8 Differences from the previous version of the tool

Version 2 of the tool replaces the first version, originally published in version 5 of the *Handbook* in 2008, and updated in 2011 (Higgins et al 2011). Research in the field has progressed, and RoB 2 reflects current understanding of how the causes of bias can influence study results, and the most appropriate ways to assess this risk.

Authors familiar with the previous version of the tool, which is used widely in Cochrane and other systematic reviews, will notice several changes:

1) assessment of bias is at the level of an individual result, rather than at a study or outcome level;
2) the names given to the bias domains describe more clearly the issues targeted and should reduce confusion arising from terms that are used in different ways or may be unfamiliar (such as 'selection bias' and 'performance bias') (Mansournia et al 2017);
3) signalling questions have been introduced, along with algorithms to assist authors in reaching a judgement about risk of bias for each domain;
4) a distinction is introduced between considering the effect of assignment to intervention and the effect of adhering to intervention, with implications for the assessment of bias due to deviations from intended interventions;
5) the assessment of bias arising from the exclusion of participants from the analysis (for example, as part of a naïve 'per-protocol' analysis) is under the domain of bias

due to deviations from the intended intervention, rather than bias due to missing outcome data;
6) the concept of selective reporting of a result is distinguished from that of selective *non-reporting* of a result, with the latter concept removed from the tool so that it can be addressed (more appropriately) at the level of the synthesis (see Chapter 13);
7) the option to add new domains has been removed;
8) an explicit process for reaching a judgement about the overall risk of bias in the result has been introduced.

Because most Cochrane Reviews published before 2019 used the first version of the tool, authors working on updating these reviews should refer to online Chapter IV for guidance on considering whether to change methodology when updating a review.

8.9 Chapter information

Authors: Julian PT Higgins, Jelena Savović, Matthew J Page, Roy G Elbers, Jonathan AC Sterne

Acknowledgements: Contributors to the development of bias domains were: Natalie Blencowe, Isabelle Boutron, Christopher Cates, Rachel Churchill, Mark Corbett, Nicky Cullum, Jonathan Emberson, Sally Hopewell, Asbjørn Hróbjartsson, Sharea Ijaz, Peter Jüni, Jamie Kirkham, Toby Lasserson, Tianjing Li, Barney Reeves, Sasha Shepperd, Ian Shrier, Lesley Stewart, Kate Tilling, Ian White, Penny Whiting. Other contributors were: Henning Keinke Andersen, Vincent Cheng, Mike Clarke, Jon Deeks, Miguel Hernán, Daniela Junqueira, Yoon Loke, Geraldine MacDonald, Alexandra McAleenan, Richard Morris, Mona Nasser, Nishith Patel, Jani Ruotsalainen, Holger Schünemann, Jayne Tierney, Sunita Vohra, Liliane Zorzela.

Funding: Development of RoB 2 was supported by the Medical Research Council (MRC) Network of Hubs for Trials Methodology Research (MR/L004933/2- N61) hosted by the MRC ConDuCT-II Hub (Collaboration and innovation for Difficult and Complex randomised controlled Trials In Invasive procedures – MR/K025643/1), by a Methods Innovation Fund grant from Cochrane and by MRC grant MR/M025209/1. JPTH and JACS are members of the National Institute for Health Research (NIHR) Biomedical Research Centre at University Hospitals Bristol NHS Foundation Trust and the University of Bristol, and the MRC Integrative Epidemiology Unit at the University of Bristol. JPTH, JS and JACS are members of the NIHR Collaboration for Leadership in Applied Health Research and Care West (CLAHRC West) at University Hospitals Bristol NHS Foundation Trust. JPTH and JACS received funding from NIHR Senior Investigator awards NF-SI-0617-10145 and NF-SI-0611-10168, respectively. MJP received funding from an Australian National Health and Medical Research Council (NHMRC) Early Career Fellowship (1088535). The views expressed are those of the authors and not necessarily those of the National Health Service, the NIHR, the UK Department of Health and Social Care, the MRC or the Australian NHMRC.

8.10 References

Abraha I, Montedori A. Modified intention to treat reporting in randomised controlled trials: systematic review. *BMJ* 2010; **340**: c2697.

Bell ML, Fiero M, Horton NJ, Hsu CH. Handling missing data in RCTs: a review of the top medical journals. *BMC Medical Research Methodology* 2014; **14**: 118.

Bello S, Moustgaard H, Hróbjartsson A. Unreported formal assessment of unblinding occurred in 4 of 10 randomized clinical trials, unreported loss of blinding in 1 of 10 trials. *Journal of Clinical Epidemiology* 2017; **81**: 42–50.

Berger VW. Quantifying the magnitude of baseline covariate imbalances resulting from selection bias in randomized clinical trials. *Biometrical Journal* 2005; **47**: 119–127.

Boutron I, Estellat C, Guittet L, Dechartres A, Sackett DL, Hróbjartsson A, Ravaud P. Methods of blinding in reports of randomized controlled trials assessing pharmacologic treatments: a systematic review. *PLoS Medicine* 2006; **3**: e425.

Brown S, Thorpe H, Hawkins K, Brown J. Minimization – reducing predictability for multi-centre trials whilst retaining balance within centre. *Statistics in Medicine* 2005; **24**: 3715–3727.

Clark L, Fairhurst C, Torgerson DJ. Allocation concealment in randomised controlled trials: are we getting better? *BMJ* 2016; **355**: i5663.

Corbett MS, Higgins JPT, Woolacott NF. Assessing baseline imbalance in randomised trials: implications for the Cochrane risk of bias tool. *Research Synthesis Methods* 2014; **5**: 79–85.

Fergusson D, Aaron SD, Guyatt G, Hebert P. Post-randomisation exclusions: the intention to treat principle and excluding patients from analysis. *BMJ* 2002; **325**: 652–654.

Gravel J, Opatrny L, Shapiro S. The intention-to-treat approach in randomized controlled trials: are authors saying what they do and doing what they say? *Clinical Trials (London, England)* 2007; **4**: 350–356.

Haahr MT, Hróbjartsson A. Who is blinded in randomized clinical trials? A study of 200 trials and a survey of authors. *Clinical Trials (London, England)* 2006; **3**: 360–365.

Hernán MA, Hernandez-Diaz S. Beyond the intention-to-treat in comparative effectiveness research. *Clinical Trials (London, England)* 2012; **9**: 48–55.

Hernán MA, Scharfstein D. Cautions as regulators move to end exclusive reliance on intention to treat. *Annals of Internal Medicine* 2018; **168**: 515–516.

Hernán MA, Robins JM. Per-protocol analyses of pragmatic trials. *New England Journal of Medicine* 2017; **377**: 1391–1398.

Higgins JPT, White IR, Wood AM. Imputation methods for missing outcome data in meta-analysis of clinical trials. *Clinical Trials* 2008; **5**: 225–239.

Higgins JPT, Altman DG, Gøtzsche PC, Jüni P, Moher D, Oxman AD, Savović J, Schulz KF, Weeks L, Sterne JAC. The Cochrane Collaboration's tool for assessing risk of bias in randomised trials. *BMJ* 2011; **343**: d5928.

Hollis S, Campbell F. What is meant by intention to treat analysis? Survey of published randomised controlled trials. *BMJ* 1999; **319**: 670–674.

Jensen JS, Bielefeldt AO, Hróbjartsson A. Active placebo control groups of pharmacological interventions were rarely used but merited serious consideration: a methodological overview. *Journal of Clinical Epidemiology* 2017; **87**: 35–46.

Jüni P, Altman DG, Egger M. Systematic reviews in health care: assessing the quality of controlled clinical trials. *BMJ* 2001; **323**: 42–46.

Kirkham JJ, Dwan KM, Altman DG, Gamble C, Dodd S, Smyth R, Williamson PR. The impact of outcome reporting bias in randomised controlled trials on a cohort of systematic reviews. *BMJ* 2010; **340**: c365.

Mansournia MA, Higgins JPT, Sterne JAC, Hernán MA. Biases in randomized trials: a conversation between trialists and epidemiologists. *Epidemiology* 2017; **28**: 54–59.

Menerit CL. *Clinical Trials – Design, Conduct, and Analysis*. 2nd ed. Oxford (UK): Oxford University Press; 2012.

National Research Council. *The Prevention and Treatment of Missing Data in Clinical Trials. Panel on Handling Missing Data in Clinical Trials. Committee on National Statistics, Division of Behavioral and Social Sciences and Education*. Washington, DC: The National Academies Press; 2010.

Page MJ, Higgins JPT. Rethinking the assessment of risk of bias due to selective reporting: a cross-sectional study. *Systematic Reviews* 2016; **5**: 108.

Piantadosi S. *Clinical Trials: A Methodologic Perspective*. 2nd ed. Hoboken (NJ): Wiley; 2005.

Schulz KF, Chalmers I, Hayes RJ, Altman DG. Empirical evidence of bias. Dimensions of methodological quality associated with estimates of treatment effects in controlled trials. *JAMA* 1995; **273**: 408–412.

Schulz KF. Subverting randomization in controlled trials. *JAMA* 1995; **274**: 1456–1458.

Schulz KF, Grimes DA. Generation of allocation sequences in randomised trials: chance, not choice. *Lancet* 2002; **359**: 515–519.

Schulz KF, Chalmers I, Altman DG. The landscape and lexicon of blinding in randomized trials. *Annals of Internal Medicine* 2002; **136**: 254–259.

Schulz KF, Grimes DA. *The Lancet Handbook of Essential Concepts in Clinical Research*. Edinburgh (UK): Elsevier; 2006.

9

Summarizing study characteristics and preparing for synthesis

Joanne E McKenzie, Sue E Brennan, Rebecca E Ryan, Hilary J Thomson, Renea V Johnston

KEY POINTS

- Synthesis is a process of bringing together data from a set of included studies with the aim of drawing conclusions about a body of evidence. This will include synthesis of study characteristics and, potentially, statistical synthesis of study findings.
- A general framework for synthesis can be used to guide the process of planning the comparisons, preparing for synthesis, undertaking the synthesis, and interpreting and describing the results.
- Tabulation of study characteristics aids the examination and comparison of PICO elements across studies, facilitates synthesis of these characteristics and grouping of studies for statistical synthesis.
- Tabulation of extracted data from studies allows assessment of the number of studies contributing to a particular meta-analysis, and helps determine what other statistical synthesis methods might be used if meta-analysis is not possible.

9.1 Introduction

Synthesis is a process of bringing together data from a set of included studies with the aim of drawing conclusions about a body of evidence. Most Cochrane Reviews on the effects of interventions will include some type of statistical synthesis. Most commonly this is the statistical combination of results from two or more separate studies (henceforth referred to as meta-analysis) of effect estimates.

An examination of the included studies always precedes statistical synthesis in Cochrane Reviews. For example, examination of the interventions studied is often needed to itemize their content so as to determine which studies can be grouped in a single synthesis. More broadly, synthesis of the PICO (Population, Intervention, Comparator and Outcome) elements of the included studies underpins interpretation

This chapter should be cited as: McKenzie JE, Brennan SE, Ryan RE, Thomson HJ, Johnston RV. Chapter 9: Summarizing study characteristics and preparing for synthesis. In: Higgins JPT, Thomas J, Chandler J, Cumpston M, Li T, Page MJ, Welch VA (editors). *Cochrane Handbook for Systematic Reviews of Interventions*. 2nd Edition. Chichester (UK): John Wiley & Sons, 2019: 229–240.

of review findings and is an important output of the review in its own right. This synthesis should encompass the characteristics of the interventions and comparators in included studies, the populations and settings in which the interventions were evaluated, the outcomes assessed, and the strengths and weaknesses of the body of evidence.

Chapter 2 defined three types of PICO criteria that may be helpful in understanding decisions that need to be made at different stages in the review.

- The **review PICO** (planned at the protocol stage) is the PICO on which eligibility of studies is based (what will be included and what excluded from the review).
- The **PICO for each synthesis** (also planned at the protocol stage) defines the question that the specific synthesis aims to answer, determining how the synthesis will be structured, specifying planned comparisons (including intervention and comparator groups, any grouping of outcome and population subgroups).
- The **PICO of the included studies** (determined at the review stage) is what was actually investigated in the included studies.

In this chapter, we focus on the **PICO for each synthesis** and the **PICO of the included studies**, as the basis for determining which studies can be grouped for statistical synthesis and for synthesizing study characteristics. We describe the preliminary steps undertaken before performing the statistical synthesis. Methods for the statistical synthesis are described in Chapters 10, 11 and 12.

9.2 A general framework for synthesis

Box 9.2.a provides a **general framework for synthesis** that can be applied irrespective of the methods used to synthesize results. Planning for the synthesis should start at protocol-writing stage, and Chapters 2 and 3 describe the steps involved in planning the review questions and comparisons between intervention groups. These steps included specifying which characteristics of the interventions, populations, outcomes and study design would be grouped together for synthesis (the PICO for each synthesis: stage 1 in Box 9.2.a).

This chapter primarily concerns stage 2 of the general framework in Box 9.2.a. After deciding which studies will be included in the review and extracting data, review authors can start implementing their plan, working through steps 2.1 to 2.5 of the framework. This process begins with a detailed examination of the characteristics of each study (step 2.1), and then comparison of characteristics across studies in order to determine which studies are similar enough to be grouped for synthesis (step 2.2). Examination of the type of data available for synthesis follows (step 2.3). These three steps inform decisions about whether any modification to the planned comparisons or outcomes is necessary, or new comparisons are needed (step 2.4). The last step of the framework covered in this chapter involves synthesis of the characteristics of studies contributing to each comparison (step 2.5). The chapter concludes with practical tips for checking data before synthesis (Section 9.4).

Steps 2.1, 2.2 and 2.5 involve analysis and synthesis of mainly qualitative information about study characteristics. The process used to undertake these steps is rarely

Box 9.2.a A general framework for synthesis that can be applied irrespective of the methods used to synthesize results

Stage 1. ***At protocol stage:***

Step 1.1. Set up the comparisons (Chapters 2 and 3).

Stage 2. ***Summarizing the included studies and preparing for synthesis:***

Step 2.1. Summarize the characteristics of each study in a 'Characteristics of included studies' table (see Chapter 5), including examining the interventions to itemize their content and other characteristics (Section 9.3.1).

Step 2.2. Determine which studies are similar enough to be grouped within each comparison by comparing the characteristics across studies (e.g. in a matrix) (Section 9.3.2).

Step 2.3. Determine what data are available for synthesis (Section 9.3.3; extraction of data and conversion to the desired format is discussed in Chapters 5 and 6).

Step 2.4. Determine if modification to the planned comparisons or outcomes is necessary, or new comparisons are needed, noting any deviations from the protocol plans (Section 9.3.4; and Chapters 2 and 3).

Step 2.5. Synthesize the characteristics of the studies contributing to each comparison (Section 9.3.5).

Stage 3. ***The synthesis itself:***

Step 3.1. Perform a statistical synthesis (if appropriate), or provide structured reporting of the effects (Section 9.5; and Chapters 10, 11 and 12).

Step 3.2. Interpret and describe the results, including consideration of the direction of effect, size of the effect, certainty of the evidence (Chapter 14), and the interventions tested and the populations in which they were tested.

described in reviews, yet can require many subjective decisions about the nature and similarity of the PICO elements of the included studies. The examples described in this section illustrate approaches for making this process more transparent.

9.3 Preliminary steps of a synthesis

9.3.1 Summarize the characteristics of each study (step 2.1)

A starting point for synthesis is to summarize the PICO characteristics of each study (i.e. the PICO of the included studies, see Chapter 3) and categorize these PICO elements in the groups (or domains) pre-specified in the protocol (i.e. the PICO for each synthesis). The resulting descriptions are reported in the 'Characteristics of included studies' table, and are used in step 2.2 to determine which studies can be grouped for synthesis.

In some reviews, the labels and terminology used in each study are retained when describing the PICO elements of the included studies. This may be sufficient in areas with consistent and widely understood terminology that matches the PICO for each synthesis. However, in most areas, terminology is variable, making it difficult to compare the PICO of each included study to the PICO for each synthesis, or to compare PICO elements across studies. Standardizing the description of PICO elements across studies facilitates these comparisons. This standardization includes applying the labels and terminology used to articulate the PICO for each synthesis (Chapter 3), and structuring the description of PICO elements. The description of interventions can be structured using the Template for Intervention Description and Replication (TIDIeR) checklist, for example (see Chapter 3 and Table 9.3.a).

Table 9.3.a illustrates the use of pre-specified groups to categorize and label interventions in a review of psychosocial interventions for smoking cessation in pregnancy (Chamberlain et al 2017). The main intervention strategy in each study was categorized into one of six groups: counselling, health education, feedback, incentive-based interventions, social support, and exercise. This categorization determined which studies were eligible for each comparison (e.g. counselling versus usual care; single or multi-component strategy). The extract from the 'Characteristics of included studies' table shows the diverse descriptions of interventions in three of the 54 studies for which the main intervention was categorized as 'counselling'. Other intervention characteristics, such as duration and frequency, were coded in pre-specified categories to standardize description of the intervention intensity and facilitate meta-regression (not shown here).

While this example focuses on categorizing and describing interventions according to groups pre-specified in the PICO for each synthesis, the same approach applies to other PICO elements.

9.3.2 Determine which studies are similar enough to be grouped within each comparison (step 2.2)

Once the PICO of included studies have been coded using labels and descriptions specified in the PICO for each synthesis, it will be possible to compare PICO elements across studies and determine which studies are similar enough to be grouped within each comparison.

Tabulating study characteristics can help to explore and compare PICO elements across studies, and is particularly important for reviews that are broad in scope, have diversity across one or more PICO elements, or include large numbers of studies. Data about study characteristics can be ordered in many different ways (e.g. by comparison or by specific PICO elements), and tables may include information about one or more PICO elements. Deciding on the best approach will depend on the purpose of the table and the stage of the review. A close examination of study characteristics will require detailed tables; for example, to identify differences in characteristics that were pre-specified as potentially important modifiers of the intervention effects. As the review progresses, this detail may be replaced by standardized description of PICO characteristics (e.g. the coding of counselling interventions presented in Table 9.3.a).

Table 9.3.b illustrates one approach to tabulating study characteristics to enable comparison and analysis across studies. This table presents a high-level summary of the characteristics that are most important for determining which comparisons can be made. The table was adapted from tables presented in a review of self-management education programmes for osteoarthritis (Kroon et al 2014). The authors presented a structured summary of intervention and comparator groups for each study, and then categorized intervention components thought to be important for enabling patients to manage their own condition. Table 9.3.b shows selected intervention components, the

Table 9.3.a Example of categorizing interventions into pre-defined groups

Definition of (selected) intervention groups from the PICO for each synthesis

- *Counselling*: "provide[s] motivation to quit, support to increase problem solving and coping skills, and may incorporate 'transtheoretical' models of change. … includes … motivational interviewing, cognitive behaviour therapy, psychotherapy, relaxation, problem solving facilitation, and other strategies."*
- *Incentives*: "women receive a financial incentive, contingent on their smoking cessation; these incentives may be gift vouchers. … Interventions that provided a 'chance' of incentive (e.g. lottery tickets) combined with counselling were coded as counselling."
- *Social support*: "interventions where the intervention explicitly included provision of support from a peer (including self-nominated peers, 'lay' peers trained by project staff, or support from healthcare professionals), or from partners" (Chamberlain et al 2017).

<table>
<tr><th>Study ID</th><th>Precis of intervention description from study</th><th>Main intervention strategy</th><th>Other intervention components</th></tr>
<tr><td>Study 1</td><td>• Assessment of smoking motivation and intention to quit.
• Bilingual health educators (Spanish and English) with bachelors degrees provided 15 minutes of individual counselling that included risk information and quit messages or reinforcement. Participants were asked to select a quit date and nominate a significant other as a 'quit buddy'.
• Self-help guide 'Time for a change' with an explanation of how to use it and behavioural counselling.
• Explanation of how to win prizes ($100) by completing activity sheets.
• Booster postcard one month after study entry.</td><td>Counselling</td><td>Incentive</td></tr>
<tr><td>Study 2</td><td>Routine prenatal advice on a range of health issues, from midwives and obstetricians plus:
• Structured one-to-one counselling by a trained facilitator (based on stages of change theory).
• Partners invited to be involved in the program.
• An information pack (developed in collaboration with a focus group of women), which included a self-help booklet.
• Invited to join a stop smoking support group.</td><td>Counselling</td><td>Social support</td></tr>
<tr><td>Study 3</td><td>Midwives received two and a half days of training on theory of transtheoretical model. Participants received a set of six stage-based self-help manuals 'Pro-Change programme for a healthy pregnancy'. The midwife assessed each participant's stage of change and pointed the woman to the appropriate manual. No more than 15 minutes was spent on the intervention.</td><td>Counselling</td><td>Nil</td></tr>
</table>

* The definition also specified eligible modes of delivery, intervention duration and personnel.

comparator, and outcomes measured in a subset of studies (some details are fictitious). Outcomes have been grouped by the outcome domains 'Pain' and 'Function' (column 'Outcome measure' Table 9.3.b). These pre-specified outcome domains are the chosen level for the synthesis as specified in the PICO for each synthesis. Authors will need to assess whether the measurement methods or tools used within each study provide an appropriate assessment of the domains (Chapter 3, Section 3.2.4). A next step is to group each measure into the pre-specified time points. In this example, outcomes are grouped into short-term (< 6 weeks) and long-term follow-up (≥ 6 weeks to 12 months) (column 'Time points (time frame)' Table 9.3.b).

Variations on the format shown in Table 9.3.b can be presented within a review to summarize the characteristics of studies contributing to each synthesis, which is important for interpreting findings (step 2.5).

9.3.3 Determine what data are available for synthesis (step 2.3)

Once the studies that are similar enough to be grouped together within each comparison have been determined, a next step is to examine what data are available for synthesis. Tabulating the measurement tools and time frames as shown in Table 9.3.b allows assessment of the potential for multiplicity (i.e. when multiple outcomes within a study and outcome domain are available for inclusion (Chapter 3, Section 3.2.4.3)). In this example, multiplicity arises in two ways. First, from multiple measurement instruments used to measure the same outcome domain within the same time frame (e.g. 'Short-term Pain' is measured using the 'Pain VAS' and 'Pain on walking VAS' scales in study 3). Second, from multiple time points measured within the same time frame (e.g. 'Short-term Pain' is measured using 'Pain VAS' at both 2 weeks and 1 month in study 6). Pre-specified methods to deal with the multiplicity can then be implemented (see Table 9.3.c for examples of approaches for dealing with multiplicity). In this review, the authors pre-specified a set of decision rules for selecting specific outcomes within the outcome domains. For example, for the outcome domain 'Pain', the selected outcome was the highest on the following list: global pain, pain on walking, WOMAC pain subscore, composite pain scores other than WOMAC, pain on activities other than walking, rest pain or pain during the night. The authors further specified that if there were multiple time points at which the outcome was measured within a time frame, they would select the longest time point. The selected outcomes from applying these rules to studies 3 and 6 are indicated by an asterisk in Table 9.3.b.

Table 9.3.b also illustrates an approach to tabulating the extracted data. The available statistics are tabulated in the column labelled 'Data', from which an assessment can be made as to whether the study contributes the required data for a meta-analysis (column 'Effect & SE') (Chapter 10). For example, of the seven studies comparing health-directed behaviour (BEH) with usual care, six measured 'Short-term Pain', four of which contribute required data for meta-analysis. Reordering the table by comparison, outcome and time frame, will more readily show the number of studies that will contribute to a particular meta-analysis, and help determine what other synthesis methods might be used if the data available for meta-analysis are limited.

Table 9.3.b Table of study characteristics illustrating similarity of PICO elements across studies

Study[1]	Comparator	Self-management intervention components							Outcome domain	Outcome measure	Time points (time frame)[2]	Data[3]	Effect & SE
1	Attention control	BEH			MON	CON	SKL	NAV	Pain	Pain VAS	1 mth (short), 8 mths (long)	Mean, N / group	Yes[4]
									Function	HAQ disability subscale	1 mth (short), 8 mths (long)	Median, IQR, N / group	Maybe[4]
2	Acupuncture	BEH		EMO		CON	SKL	NAV	Pain	Pain on walking VAS	1 mth (short), 12 mths (long)	MD from ANCOVA model, 95%CI	Yes
									Function	Dutch AIMS-SF	1 mth (short), 12 mths (long)	Median, range, N / group	Maybe[4]
4	Information	BEH	ENG	EMO	MON	CON	SKL	NAV	Pain	Pain VAS	1 mth (short)	MD, SE	Yes
									Function	Dutch AIMS-SF	1 mth (short)	Mean, SD, N / group	Yes
12	Information	BEH					SKL		Pain	WOMAC pain subscore	12 mths (long)	MD from ANCOVA model, 95%CI	Yes
3	Usual care	BEH		EMO	MON		SKL	NAV	Pain	Pain VAS* Pain on walking VAS	1 mth (short) 1 mth (short)	Mean, SD, N / group	Yes
5	Usual care	BEH	ENG	EMO	MON	CON	SKL		Pain	Pain on walking VAS	2 wks (short)	Mean, SD, N / group	Yes
6	Usual care	BEH			MON	CON	SKL	NAV	Pain	Pain VAS	2 wks (short), 1 mth (short)*	MD, t-value and P value for MD	Yes
									Function	WOMAC disability subscore	2 wks (short), 1 mth (short)*	Mean, N / group	Yes
7	Usual care	BEH			MON	CON	SKL	NAV	Pain	WOMAC pain subscore	1 mth (short)	Direction of effect	No
									Function	WOMAC disability subscore	1 mth (short)	Means, N / group; statistically significant difference	Yes[4]
8	Usual care				MON				Pain	Pain VAS	12 mths (long)	MD, 95%CI	Yes

(Continued)

Table 9.3.b (Continued)

Study[1]	Comparator	Self-management intervention components							Outcome domain	Outcome measure	Time points (time frame)[2]	Data[3]	Effect & SE
9	Usual care	BEH			MON		SKL		Function	Global disability	12 mths (long)	Direction of effect, NS	No
10	Usual care	BEH		EMO	MON	CON	SKL	NAV	Pain	Pain VAS	1 mth (short)	No information	No
									Function	Global disability	1 mth (short)	Direction of effect	No
11	Usual care	BEH			MON		SKL		Pain	WOMAC pain subscore	1 mth (short), 12 mths (long)	Mean, SD, N / group	Yes

BEH = health-directed behaviour; CON = constructive attitudes and approaches; EMO = emotional well-being; ENG = positive and active engagement in life; MON = self-monitoring and insight; NAV = health service navigation; SKL = skill and technique acquisition.

ANCOVA = Analysis of covariance; CI = confidence interval; IQR = interquartile range; MD = mean difference; SD = standard deviation; SE = standard error, NS = non-significant.

Pain and function measures: Dutch AIMS-SF = Dutch short form of the Arthritis Impact Measurement Scales; HAQ = Health Assessment Questionnaire; VAS = visual analogue scale; WOMAC = Western Ontario and McMaster Universities Osteoarthritis Index.

[1] Ordered by type of comparator; [2] Short-term (denoted 'immediate' in the review Kroon et al (2014)) follow-up is defined as < 6 weeks, long-term follow-up (denoted 'intermediate' in the review) is ≥ 6 weeks to 12 months; [3] For simplicity, in this example the available data are assumed to be the same for all outcomes within an outcome domain within a study. In practice, this is unlikely and the available data would likely vary by outcome; [4] Indicates that an effect estimate and its standard error may be computed through imputation of missing statistics, methods to convert between statistics (e.g. medians to means) or contact with study authors. * Indicates the selected outcome when there was multiplicity in the outcome domain and time frame.

Table 9.3.c Examples of approaches for selecting one outcome (effect estimate) for inclusion in a synthesis. Adapted from López-López et al (2018)

Approach	Description	Comment
Random selection	Randomly select an outcome (effect estimate) when multiple are available for an outcome domain	Assumes that the effect estimates are interchangeable measures of the domain and that random selection will yield a 'representative' effect for the meta-analysis.
Averaging of effect estimates	Calculate the average of the intervention effects when multiple are available for a particular outcome domain	Assumes that the effect estimates are interchangeable measures of the domain. The standard error of the average effect can be calculated using a simple method of averaging the variances of the effect estimates.
Median effect estimate	Rank the effect estimates of outcomes within an outcome domain and select the outcome with the middle value	An alternative to averaging effect estimates. Assumes that the effect estimates are interchangeable measures of the domain and that the median effect will yield a 'representative' effect for the meta-analysis. This approach is often adopted in Effective Practice and Organization of Care reviews that include broad outcome domains.
Decision rules	Select the most relevant outcome from multiple that are available for an outcome domain using a decision rule	Assumes that while the outcomes all provide a measure of the outcome domain, they are not completely interchangeable, with some being more relevant. The decision rules aim to select the most relevant. The rules may be based on clinical (e.g. content validity of measurement tools) or methodological (e.g. reliability of the measure) considerations. If multiple rules are specified, a hierarchy will need to be determined to specify the order in which they are applied.

9.3.4 Determine if modification to the planned comparisons or outcomes is necessary, or new comparisons are needed (step 2.4)

The previous steps may reveal the need to modify the planned comparisons. Important variations in the intervention may be identified leading to different or modified intervention groups. Few studies or sparse data, or both, may lead to different groupings of interventions, populations or outcomes. Planning contingencies for anticipated scenarios is likely to lead to less post-hoc decision making (Chapters 2 and 3); however, it is difficult to plan for all scenarios. In the latter circumstance, the rationale for any post-hoc changes should be reported. This approach was adopted in a review examining the effects of portion, package or tableware size for changing selection and consumption of food, alcohol and tobacco (Hollands et al 2015). After preliminary examination of the outcome data, the review authors changed their planned intervention groups. They judged that intervention groups based on 'size' and those based on 'shape' of the products were not conceptually comparable, and therefore should form separate comparisons. The authors provided a rationale for the change and noted that it was a post-hoc decision.

9.3.5 Synthesize the characteristics of the studies contributing to each comparison (step 2.5)

A final step, and one that is essential for interpreting combined effects, is to synthesize the characteristics of studies contributing to each comparison. This description should integrate information about key PICO characteristics across studies, and identify any potentially important differences in characteristics that were pre-specified as possible effect modifiers. The synthesis of study characteristics is also needed for GRADE assessments, informing judgements about whether the evidence applies directly to the review question (indirectness) and analyses conducted to examine possible explanations for heterogeneity (inconsistency) (see Chapter 14).

Tabulating study characteristics is generally preferable to lengthy description in the text, since the structure imposed by a table can make it easier and faster for readers to scan and identify patterns in the information presented. Table 9.3.b illustrates one such approach. Tabulating characteristics of studies that contribute to each comparison can also help to improve the transparency of decisions made around grouping of studies, while also ensuring that studies that do not contribute to the combined effect are accounted for.

9.4 Checking data before synthesis

Before embarking on a synthesis, it is important to be confident that the findings from the individual studies have been collated correctly. Therefore, review authors must compare the magnitude and direction of effects reported by studies with how they are to be presented in the review. This is a reasonably straightforward way for authors to check a number of potential problems, including typographical errors in studies' reports, accuracy of data collection and manipulation, and data entry into RevMan. For example, the direction of a standardized mean difference may accidentally be wrong in the review. A basic check is to ensure the same qualitative findings (e.g. direction of effect and statistical significance) between the data as presented in the review and the data as available from the original study.

Results in forest plots should agree with data in the original report (point estimate and confidence interval) if the same effect measure and statistical model is used. There are legitimate reasons for differences, however, including: using a different measure of intervention effect; making different choices between change-from-baseline measures, post-intervention measures alone or post-intervention measures adjusted for baseline values; grouping similar intervention groups; or making adjustments for unit-of-analysis errors in the reports of the primary studies.

9.5 Types of synthesis

The focus of this chapter has been describing the steps involved in implementing the planned comparisons between intervention groups (stage 2 of the general framework for synthesis (Box 9.2.a)). The next step (stage 3) is often performing a statistical synthesis. Meta-analysis of effect estimates, and its extensions have many advantages. There are circumstances under which a meta-analysis is not possible, however, and other statistical synthesis methods might be considered, so as to make best use of the available data. Available summary and synthesis methods, along with the questions they address and examples of associated plots, are described in Table 9.5.a.

Table 9.5.a Overview of available methods for summary and synthesis

	Summary	Statistical synthesis methods					
Methods	Text/Tabular	Vote counting	Combining P values	Summary of effect estimates	Pairwise meta-analysis	Network meta-analysis	Subgroup analysis/ meta-regression
Questions addressed	Narrative summary of evidence presented in either text or tabular form	Is there any evidence of an effect?	Is there evidence that there is an effect in at least one study?	What is the range and distribution of observed effects?	What is the common intervention effect? (fixed-effect model) What is the average intervention effect? (random effects model)	Which intervention of multiple is most effective?	What factors modify the magnitude of the intervention effects?
Example plots	Forest plot (plotting individual study effects without a combined effect estimate)	Harvest plot Effect direction plot	Albatross plot	Box and whisker plot Bubble plot	Forest plot	Forest plot Network diagram Rankogram plots	Forest plot Box and whisker plot Bubble plot

Chapters 10 and 11 discuss meta-analysis (of effect estimate) methods, while Chapter 12 focuses on the other statistical synthesis methods, along with approaches to tabulating, visually displaying and providing a structured presentation of the findings. An important part of planning the analysis strategy is building in contingencies to use alternative methods when the desired method cannot be used.

9.6 Chapter information

Authors: Joanne E McKenzie, Sue E Brennan, Rebecca E Ryan, Hilary J Thomson, Renea V Johnston

Acknowledgements: Sections of this chapter build on Chapter 9 of version 5.1 of the *Handbook*, with editors Jonathan Deeks, Julian Higgins and Douglas Altman. We are grateful to Julian Higgins, James Thomas and Tianjing Li for commenting helpfully on earlier drafts.

Funding: JM is supported by an NHMRC Career Development Fellowship (1143429). SB and RR's positions are supported by the NHMRC Cochrane Collaboration Funding Program. HT is funded by the UK Medical Research Council (MC_UU_12017-13 and MC_UU_12017-15) and Scottish Government Chief Scientist Office (SPHSU13 and SPHSU15). RJ's position is supported by the NHMRC Cochrane Collaboration Funding Program and Cabrini Institute.

9.7 References

Chamberlain C, O'Mara-Eves A, Porter J, Coleman T, Perlen SM, Thomas J, McKenzie JE. Psychosocial interventions for supporting women to stop smoking in pregnancy. *Cochrane Database of Systematic Reviews* 2017; **2**: CD001055.

Hollands GJ, Shemilt I, Marteau TM, Jebb SA, Lewis HB, Wei Y, Higgins JPT, Ogilvie D. Portion, package or tableware size for changing selection and consumption of food, alcohol and tobacco. *Cochrane Database of Systematic Reviews* 2015; **9**: CD011045.

Kroon FPB, van der Burg LRA, Buchbinder R, Osborne RH, Johnston RV, Pitt V. Self-management education programmes for osteoarthritis. *Cochrane Database of Systematic Reviews* 2014; **1**: CD008963.

López-López JA, Page MJ, Lipsey MW, Higgins JPT. Dealing with effect size multiplicity in systematic reviews and meta-analyses. *Research Synthesis Methods* 2018; **9**: 336–351.

10

Analysing data and undertaking meta-analyses

Jonathan J Deeks, Julian PT Higgins, Douglas G Altman; on behalf of the Cochrane Statistical Methods Group

KEY POINTS

- Meta-analysis is the statistical combination of results from two or more separate studies.
- Potential advantages of meta-analyses include an improvement in precision, the ability to answer questions not posed by individual studies, and the opportunity to settle controversies arising from conflicting claims. However, they also have the potential to mislead seriously, particularly if specific study designs, within-study biases, variation across studies, and reporting biases are not carefully considered.
- It is important to be familiar with the type of data (e.g. dichotomous, continuous) that result from measurement of an outcome in an individual study, and to choose suitable effect measures for comparing intervention groups.
- Most meta-analysis methods are variations on a weighted average of the effect estimates from the different studies.
- Studies with no events contribute no information about the risk ratio or odds ratio. For rare events, the Peto method has been observed to be less biased and more powerful than other methods.
- Variation across studies (heterogeneity) must be considered, although most Cochrane Reviews do not have enough studies to allow for the reliable investigation of its causes Random-effects meta-analyses allow for heterogeneity by assuming that underlying effects follow a normal distribution, but they must be interpreted carefully. Prediction intervals from random-effects meta-analyses are a useful device for presenting the extent of between-study variation.
- Many judgements are required in the process of preparing a meta-analysis. Sensitivity analyses should be used to examine whether overall findings are robust to potentially influential decisions.

This chapter should be cited as: Deeks JJ, Higgins JPT, Altman DG (editors). Chapter 10: Analysing data and undertaking meta-analyses. In: Higgins JPT, Thomas J, Chandler J, Cumpston M, Li T, Page MJ, Welch VA (editors). *Cochrane Handbook for Systematic Reviews of Interventions*. 2nd Edition. Chichester (UK): John Wiley & Sons, 2019: 241–284.

10.1 Do not start here!

It can be tempting to jump prematurely into a statistical analysis when undertaking a systematic review. The production of a diamond at the bottom of a plot is an exciting moment for many authors, but results of meta-analyses can be very misleading if suitable attention has not been given to formulating the review question; specifying eligibility criteria; identifying and selecting studies; collecting appropriate data; considering risk of bias; planning intervention comparisons; and deciding what data would be meaningful to analyse. Review authors should consult the chapters that precede this one before a meta-analysis is undertaken.

10.2 Introduction to meta-analysis

An important step in a systematic review is the thoughtful consideration of whether it is appropriate to combine the numerical results of all, or perhaps some, of the studies. Such a **meta-analysis** yields an overall statistic (together with its confidence interval) that summarizes the effectiveness of an experimental intervention compared with a comparator intervention. Potential advantages of meta-analyses include the following.

1) *To improve precision*. Many studies are too small to provide convincing evidence about intervention effects in isolation. Estimation is usually improved when it is based on more information.
2) *To answer questions not posed by the individual studies*. Primary studies often involve a specific type of participant and explicitly defined interventions. A selection of studies in which these characteristics differ can allow investigation of the consistency of effect across a wider range of populations and interventions. It may also, if relevant, allow reasons for differences in effect estimates to be investigated.
3) *To settle controversies arising from apparently conflicting studies or to generate new hypotheses*. Statistical synthesis of findings allows the degree of conflict to be formally assessed, and reasons for different results to be explored and quantified.

Of course, the use of statistical synthesis methods does not guarantee that the results of a review are valid, any more than it does for a primary study. Moreover, like any tool, statistical methods can be misused.

This chapter describes the principles and methods used to carry out a meta-analysis for a comparison of two interventions for the main types of data encountered. The use of network meta-analysis to compare more than two interventions is addressed in Chapter 11. Formulae for most of the methods described are provided in a supplementary document 'Statistical algorithms in Review Manager' (available via the *Handbook* web pages), and a longer discussion of many of the issues is available (Deeks et al 2001).

10.2.1 Principles of meta-analysis

The commonly used methods for meta-analysis follow the following basic principles.

1) Meta-analysis is typically a two-stage process. In the first stage, a summary statistic is calculated for each study, to describe the observed intervention effect in the same

way for every study. For example, the summary statistic may be a risk ratio if the data are dichotomous, or a difference between means if the data are continuous (see Chapter 6).

2) In the second stage, a summary (combined) intervention effect estimate is calculated as a weighted average of the intervention effects estimated in the individual studies. A weighted average is defined as

$$\text{weighted average} = \frac{\text{sum of}\left(\text{estimate} \times \text{weight}\right)}{\text{sum of weights}} = \frac{\sum Y_i W_i}{\sum W_i},$$

where Y_i is the intervention effect estimated in the ith study, W_i is the weight given to the ith study, and the summation is across all studies. Note that if all the weights are the same then the weighted average is equal to the mean intervention effect. The bigger the weight given to the ith study, the more it will contribute to the weighted average (see Section 10.3).

3) The combination of intervention effect estimates across studies may optionally incorporate an assumption that the studies are not all estimating the same intervention effect, but estimate intervention effects that follow a distribution across studies. This is the basis of a random-effects meta-analysis (see Section 10.10.4). Alternatively, if it is assumed that each study is estimating exactly the same quantity, then a fixed-effect meta-analysis is performed.
4) The standard error of the summary intervention effect can be used to derive a confidence interval, which communicates the precision (or uncertainty) of the summary estimate; and to derive a P value, which communicates the strength of the evidence against the null hypothesis of no intervention effect.
5) As well as yielding a summary quantification of the intervention effect, all methods of meta-analysis can incorporate an assessment of whether the variation among the results of the separate studies is compatible with random variation, or whether it is large enough to indicate inconsistency of intervention effects across studies (see Section 10.10).
6) The problem of missing data is one of the numerous practical considerations that must be thought through when undertaking a meta-analysis. In particular, review authors should consider the implications of missing outcome data from individual participants (due to losses to follow-up or exclusions from analysis) (see Section 10.12).

Meta-analyses are usually illustrated using a **forest plot**. An example appears in Figure 10.2.a. A forest plot displays effect estimates and confidence intervals for both individual studies and meta-analyses (Lewis and Clarke 2001). Each study is represented by a block at the point estimate of intervention effect with a horizontal line extending either side of the block. The area of the block indicates the weight assigned to that study in the meta-analysis while the horizontal line depicts the confidence interval (usually with a 95% level of confidence). The area of the block and the confidence interval convey similar information, but both make different contributions to the graphic. The confidence interval depicts the range of intervention effects compatible with the study's result. The size of the block draws the eye towards the studies with larger weight (usually those with narrower confidence intervals), which dominate the calculation of the summary result, presented as a diamond at the bottom.

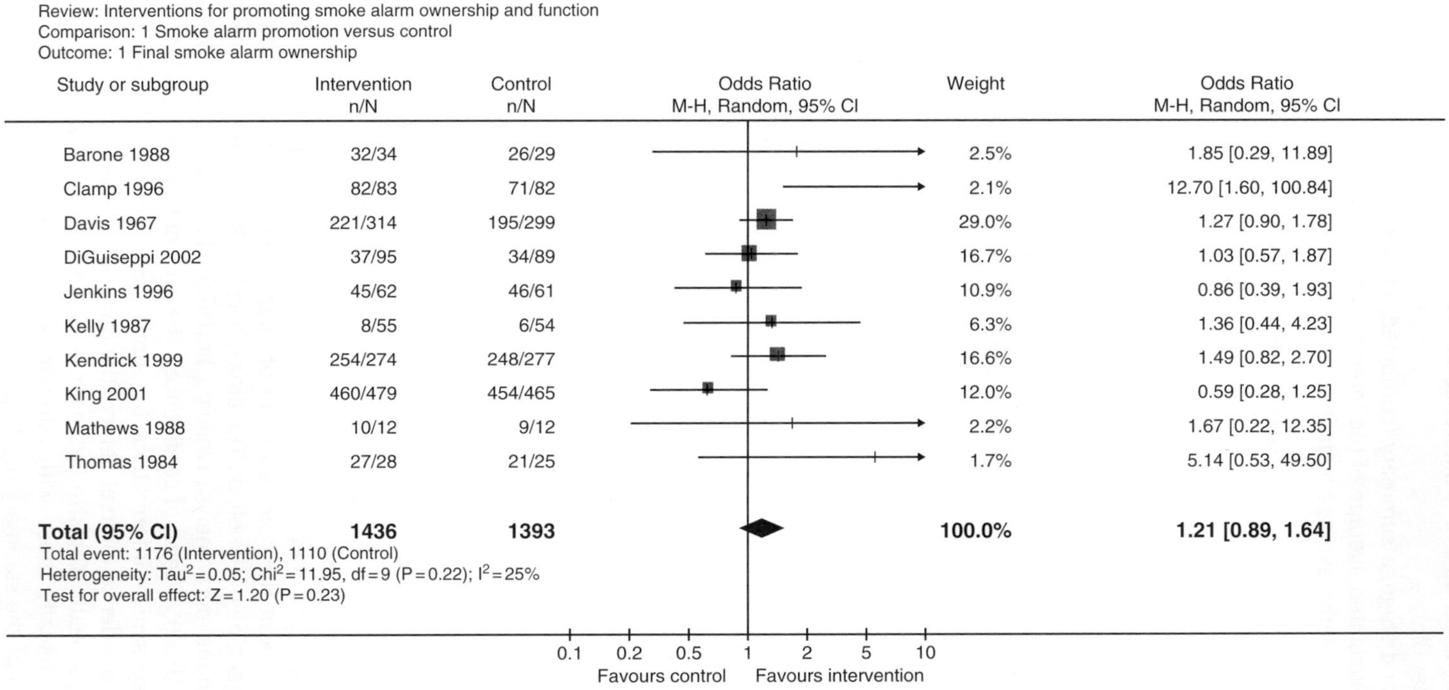

Review: Interventions for promoting smoke alarm ownership and function
Comparison: 1 Smoke alarm promotion versus control
Outcome: 1 Final smoke alarm ownership

Study or subgroup	Intervention n/N	Control n/N	Odds Ratio M-H, Random, 95% CI	Weight	Odds Ratio M-H, Random, 95% CI
Barone 1988	32/34	26/29		2.5%	1.85 [0.29, 11.89]
Clamp 1996	82/83	71/82		2.1%	12.70 [1.60, 100.84]
Davis 1967	221/314	195/299		29.0%	1.27 [0.90, 1.78]
DiGuiseppi 2002	37/95	34/89		16.7%	1.03 [0.57, 1.87]
Jenkins 1996	45/62	46/61		10.9%	0.86 [0.39, 1.93]
Kelly 1987	8/55	6/54		6.3%	1.36 [0.44, 4.23]
Kendrick 1999	254/274	248/277		16.6%	1.49 [0.82, 2.70]
King 2001	460/479	454/465		12.0%	0.59 [0.28, 1.25]
Mathews 1988	10/12	9/12		2.2%	1.67 [0.22, 12.35]
Thomas 1984	27/28	21/25		1.7%	5.14 [0.53, 49.50]
Total (95% CI)	**1436**	**1393**		**100.0%**	**1.21 [0.89, 1.64]**

Total event: 1176 (Intervention), 1110 (Control)
Heterogeneity: $Tau^2 = 0.05$; $Chi^2 = 11.95$, df = 9 (P = 0.22); $I^2 = 25\%$
Test for overall effect: Z = 1.20 (P = 0.23)

0.1 0.2 0.5 1 2 5 10
Favours control Favours intervention

Figure 10.2.a Example of a forest plot from a review of interventions to promote ownership of smoke alarms (DiGuiseppi and Higgins 2001). Reproduced with permission of John Wiley & Sons

10.3 A generic inverse-variance approach to meta-analysis

A very common and simple version of the meta-analysis procedure is commonly referred to as the **inverse-variance method**. This approach is implemented in its most basic form in RevMan, and is used behind the scenes in many meta-analyses of both dichotomous and continuous data.

The inverse-variance method is so named because the weight given to each study is chosen to be the inverse of the variance of the effect estimate (i.e. 1 over the square of its standard error). Thus, larger studies, which have smaller standard errors, are given more weight than smaller studies, which have larger standard errors. This choice of weights minimizes the imprecision (uncertainty) of the pooled effect estimate.

10.3.1 Fixed-effect method for meta-analysis

A fixed-effect meta-analysis using the inverse-variance method calculates a weighted average as:

$$\text{generic inverse-variance weighted average} = \frac{\sum Y_i\left(1/\text{SE}_i^2\right)}{\sum\left(1/\text{SE}_i^2\right)},$$

where Y_i is the intervention effect estimated in the ith study, SE_i is the standard error of that estimate, and the summation is across all studies. The basic data required for the analysis are therefore an estimate of the intervention effect and its standard error from each study. A fixed-effect meta-analysis is valid under an assumption that all effect estimates are estimating the same underlying intervention effect, which is referred to variously as a 'fixed-effect' assumption, a 'common-effect' assumption or an 'equal-effects' assumption. However, the result of the meta-analysis can be interpreted without making such an assumption (Rice et al 2018).

10.3.2 Random-effects methods for meta-analysis

A variation on the inverse-variance method is to incorporate an assumption that the different studies are estimating different, yet related, intervention effects (Higgins et al 2009). This produces a random-effects meta-analysis, and the simplest version is known as the DerSimonian and Laird method (DerSimonian and Laird 1986). Random-effects meta-analysis is discussed in detail in Section 10.10.4.

10.3.3 Performing inverse-variance meta-analyses

Most meta-analysis programs perform inverse-variance meta-analyses. Usually the user provides summary data from each intervention arm of each study, such as a 2 × 2 table when the outcome is dichotomous (see Chapter 6, Section 6.4), or means, standard deviations and sample sizes for each group when the outcome is continuous (see Chapter 6, Section 6.5). This avoids the need for the author to calculate effect estimates, and allows the use of methods targeted specifically at different types of data (see Sections 10.4 and 10.5).

When the data are conveniently available as summary statistics from each intervention group, the inverse-variance method can be implemented directly. For example, estimates and their standard errors may be entered directly into RevMan under the 'Generic inverse variance' outcome type. For ratio measures of intervention effect, the data must be entered into RevMan as natural logarithms (for example, as a log odds ratio and the standard error of the log odds ratio). However, it is straightforward to instruct the software to display results on the original (e.g. odds ratio) scale. It is possible to supplement or replace this with a column providing the sample sizes in the two groups. Note that the ability to enter estimates and standard errors creates a high degree of flexibility in meta-analysis. It facilitates the analysis of properly analysed crossover trials, cluster-randomized trials and non-randomized trials (see Chapter 23), as well as outcome data that are ordinal, time-to-event or rates (see Chapter 6).

10.4 Meta-analysis of dichotomous outcomes

There are four widely used methods of meta-analysis for dichotomous outcomes, three fixed-effect methods (Mantel-Haenszel, Peto and inverse variance) and one random-effects method (DerSimonian and Laird inverse variance). All of these methods are available as analysis options in RevMan. The Peto method can only combine odds ratios, whilst the other three methods can combine odds ratios, risk ratios or risk differences. Formulae for all of the meta-analysis methods are available elsewhere (Deeks et al 2001).

Note that having no events in one group (sometimes referred to as 'zero cells') causes problems with computation of estimates and standard errors with some methods: see Section 10.4.4.

10.4.1 Mantel-Haenszel methods

When data are sparse, either in terms of event risks being low or study size being small, the estimates of the standard errors of the effect estimates that are used in the inverse-variance methods may be poor. Mantel-Haenszel methods are fixed-effect meta-analysis methods using a different weighting scheme that depends on which effect measure (e.g. risk ratio, odds ratio, risk difference) is being used (Mantel and Haenszel 1959, Greenland and Robins 1985). They have been shown to have better statistical properties when there are few events. As this is a common situation in Cochrane Reviews, the Mantel-Haenszel method is generally preferable to the inverse variance method in fixed-effect meta-analyses. In other situations the two methods give similar estimates.

10.4.2 Peto odds ratio method

Peto's method can only be used to combine odds ratios (Yusuf et al 1985). It uses an inverse-variance approach, but uses an approximate method of estimating the log odds ratio, and uses different weights. An alternative way of viewing the Peto method is as a sum of 'O – E' statistics. Here, O is the observed number of events and E is an expected number of events in the experimental intervention group of each study under the null hypothesis of no intervention effect.

The approximation used in the computation of the log odds ratio works well when intervention effects are small (odds ratios are close to 1), events are not particularly common and the studies have similar numbers in experimental and comparator groups. In other situations it has been shown to give biased answers. As these criteria are not always fulfilled, Peto's method is not recommended as a default approach for meta-analysis.

Corrections for zero cell counts are not necessary when using Peto's method. Perhaps for this reason, this method performs well when events are very rare (Bradburn et al 2007); see Section 10.4.4.1. Also, Peto's method can be used to combine studies with dichotomous outcome data with studies using time-to-event analyses where log-rank tests have been used (see Section 10.9).

10.4.3 Which effect measure for dichotomous outcomes?

Effect measures for dichotomous data are described in Chapter 6, Section 6.4.1. The effect of an intervention can be expressed as either a relative or an absolute effect. The risk ratio (relative risk) and odds ratio are relative measures, while the risk difference and number needed to treat for an additional beneficial outcome are absolute measures. A further complication is that there are, in fact, two risk ratios. We can calculate the risk ratio of an event occurring or the risk ratio of no event occurring. These give different summary results in a meta-analysis, sometimes dramatically so.

The selection of a summary statistic for use in meta-analysis depends on balancing three criteria (Deeks 2002). First, we desire a summary statistic that gives values that are similar for all the studies in the meta-analysis and subdivisions of the population to which the interventions will be applied. The more consistent the summary statistic, the greater is the justification for expressing the intervention effect as a single summary number. Second, the summary statistic must have the mathematical properties required to perform a valid meta-analysis. Third, the summary statistic would ideally be easily understood and applied by those using the review. The summary intervention effect should be presented in a way that helps readers to interpret and apply the results appropriately. Among effect measures for dichotomous data, no single measure is uniformly best, so the choice inevitably involves a compromise.

Consistency Empirical evidence suggests that relative effect measures are, on average, more consistent than absolute measures (Engels et al 2000, Deeks 2002, Rucker et al 2009). For this reason, it is wise to avoid performing meta-analyses of risk differences, unless there is a clear reason to suspect that risk differences will be consistent in a particular clinical situation. On average there is little difference between the odds ratio and risk ratio in terms of consistency (Deeks 2002). When the study aims to reduce the incidence of an adverse event, there is empirical evidence that risk ratios of the adverse event are more consistent than risk ratios of the non-event (Deeks 2002). Selecting an effect measure based on what is the most consistent in a *particular* situation is not a generally recommended strategy, since it may lead to a selection that spuriously maximizes the precision of a meta-analysis estimate.

Mathematical properties The most important mathematical criterion is the availability of a reliable variance estimate. The number needed to treat for an additional beneficial outcome does not have a simple variance estimator and cannot easily be used directly in meta-analysis, although it can be computed from the meta-analysis result afterwards (see Chapter 15, Section 15.4.2). There is no consensus regarding the importance of two other often-cited mathematical properties: the fact that the behaviour of the odds ratio and the risk difference do not rely on which of the two outcome states is coded as the event, and the odds ratio being the only statistic which is unbounded (see Chapter 6, Section 6.3.1).

Ease of interpretation The odds ratio is the hardest summary statistic to understand and to apply in practice, and many practising clinicians report difficulties in using them. There are many published examples where authors have misinterpreted odds ratios from meta-analyses as risk ratios. Although odds ratios can be re-expressed for interpretation (as discussed here), there must be some concern that routine presentation of the results of systematic reviews as odds ratios will lead to frequent over-estimation of the benefits and harms of interventions when the results are applied in clinical practice. Absolute measures of effect are thought to be more easily interpreted by clinicians than relative effects (Sinclair and Bracken 1994), and allow trade-offs to be made between likely benefits and likely harms of interventions. However, they are less likely to be generalizable.

It is generally recommended that meta-analyses are undertaken using risk ratios (taking care to make a sensible choice over which category of outcome is classified as the event) or odds ratios. This is because it seems important to avoid using summary statistics for which there is empirical evidence that they are unlikely to give consistent estimates of intervention effects (the risk difference), and it is impossible to use statistics for which meta-analysis cannot be performed (the number needed to treat for an additional beneficial outcome). It may be wise to plan to undertake a sensitivity analysis to investigate whether choice of summary statistic (and selection of the event category) is critical to the conclusions of the meta-analysis (see Section 10.14).

It is often sensible to use one statistic for meta-analysis and to re-express the results using a second, more easily interpretable statistic. For example, often meta-analysis may be best performed using relative effect measures (risk ratios or odds ratios) and the results re-expressed using absolute effect measures (risk differences or numbers needed to treat for an additional beneficial outcome – see Chapter 15 (Section 15.4). This is one of the key motivations for 'Summary of findings' tables in Cochrane Reviews: see Chapter 14). If odds ratios are used for meta-analysis they can also be re-expressed as risk ratios (see Chapter 15, Section 15.4). In all cases the same formulae can be used to convert upper and lower confidence limits. However, all of these transformations require specification of a value of baseline risk that indicates the likely risk of the outcome in the 'control' population to which the experimental intervention will be applied. Where the chosen value for this assumed comparator group risk is close to the typical observed comparator group risks across the studies, similar estimates of absolute effect will be obtained regardless of whether odds ratios or risk ratios are used for meta-analysis. Where the assumed comparator risk differs from the typical observed comparator group risk, the predictions of absolute benefit will differ according to which summary statistic was used for meta-analysis.

10.4.4 Meta-analysis of rare events

For rare outcomes, meta-analysis may be the only way to obtain reliable evidence of the effects of healthcare interventions. Individual studies are usually under-powered to detect differences in rare outcomes, but a meta-analysis of many studies may have adequate power to investigate whether interventions do have an impact on the incidence of the rare event. However, many methods of meta-analysis are based on large sample approximations, and are unsuitable when events are rare. Thus authors must take care when selecting a method of meta-analysis (Efthimiou 2018).

There is no single risk at which events are classified as 'rare'. Certainly risks of 1 in 1000 constitute rare events, and many would classify risks of 1 in 100 the same way. However, the performance of methods when risks are as high as 1 in 10 may also be affected by the issues discussed in this section. What is typical is that a high proportion of the studies in the meta-analysis observe no events in one or more study arms.

10.4.4.1 Studies with no events in one or more arms

Computational problems can occur when no events are observed in one or both groups in an individual study. Inverse variance meta-analytical methods involve computing an intervention effect estimate and its standard error for each study. For studies where no events were observed in one or both arms, these computations often involve dividing by a zero count, which yields a computational error. Most meta-analytical software routines (including those in RevMan) automatically check for problematic zero counts, and add a fixed value (typically 0.5) to all cells of a 2 × 2 table where the problems occur. The Mantel-Haenszel methods require zero-cell corrections only if the same cell is zero in all the included studies, and hence need to use the correction less often. However, in many software applications the same correction rules are applied for Mantel-Haenszel methods as for the inverse-variance methods. Odds ratio and risk ratio methods require zero cell corrections more often than difference methods, except for the Peto odds ratio method, which encounters computation problems only in the extreme situation of no events occurring in all arms of all studies.

Whilst the fixed correction meets the objective of avoiding computational errors, it usually has the undesirable effect of biasing study estimates towards no difference and over-estimating variances of study estimates (consequently down-weighting inappropriately their contribution to the meta-analysis). Where the sizes of the study arms are unequal (which occurs more commonly in non-randomized studies than randomized trials), they will introduce a directional bias in the treatment effect. Alternative non-fixed zero-cell corrections have been explored by Sweeting and colleagues, including a correction proportional to the reciprocal of the size of the contrasting study arm, which they found preferable to the fixed 0.5 correction when arm sizes were not balanced (Sweeting et al 2004).

10.4.4.2 Studies with no events in either arm

The standard practice in meta-analysis of odds ratios and risk ratios is to exclude studies from the meta-analysis where there are no events in both arms. This is because such studies do not provide any indication of either the direction or magnitude of the relative treatment effect. Whilst it may be clear that events are very rare on both the experimental intervention and the comparator intervention, no information is provided as to which group is likely to have the higher risk, or on whether the risks are of the same or different orders of magnitude (when risks are very low, they are compatible with very large or very small ratios). Whilst one might be tempted to infer that the risk would be lowest in the group with the larger sample size (as the upper limit of the confidence interval would be lower), this is not justified as the sample size allocation was determined by the study investigators and is not a measure of the incidence of the event.

Risk difference methods superficially appear to have an advantage over odds ratio methods in that the risk difference is defined (as zero) when no events occur in either arm. Such studies are therefore included in the estimation process. Bradburn and colleagues undertook simulation studies which revealed that all risk difference methods yield confidence intervals that are too wide when events are rare, and have associated poor statistical power, which make them unsuitable for meta-analysis of rare events (Bradburn et al 2007). This is especially relevant when outcomes that focus on treatment safety are being studied, as the ability to identify correctly (or attempt to refute) serious adverse events is a key issue in drug development.

It is likely that outcomes for which no events occur in either arm may not be mentioned in reports of many randomized trials, precluding their inclusion in a meta-analysis. It is unclear, though, when working with published results, whether failure to mention a particular adverse event means there *were* no such events, or simply that such events were not included as a measured endpoint. Whilst the results of risk difference meta-analyses will be affected by non-reporting of outcomes with no events, odds and risk ratio based methods naturally exclude these data whether or not they are published, and are therefore unaffected.

10.4.4.3 Validity of methods of meta-analysis for rare events

Simulation studies have revealed that many meta-analytical methods can give misleading results for rare events, which is unsurprising given their reliance on asymptotic statistical theory. Their performance has been judged suboptimal either through results being biased, confidence intervals being inappropriately wide, or statistical power being too low to detect substantial differences.

In the following we consider the choice of statistical method for meta-analyses of odds ratios. Appropriate choices appear to depend on the comparator group risk, the likely size of the treatment effect and consideration of balance in the numbers of experimental and comparator participants in the constituent studies. We are not aware of research that has evaluated risk ratio measures directly, but their performance is likely to be very similar to corresponding odds ratio measurements. When events are rare, estimates of odds and risks are near identical, and results of both can be interpreted as ratios of probabilities.

Bradburn and colleagues found that many of the most commonly used meta-analytical methods were biased when events were rare (Bradburn et al 2007). The bias was greatest in inverse variance and DerSimonian and Laird odds ratio and risk difference methods, and the Mantel-Haenszel odds ratio method using a 0.5 zero-cell correction. As already noted, risk difference meta-analytical methods tended to show conservative confidence interval coverage and low statistical power when risks of events were low.

At event rates below 1% the Peto one-step odds ratio method was found to be the least biased and most powerful method, and provided the best confidence interval coverage, provided there was no substantial imbalance between treatment and comparator group sizes within studies, and treatment effects were not exceptionally large. This finding was consistently observed across three different meta-analytical scenarios, and was also observed by Sweeting and colleagues (Sweeting et al 2004).

This finding was noted despite the method producing only an approximation to the odds ratio. For very large effects (e.g. risk ratio = 0.2) when the approximation is known to be poor, treatment effects were under-estimated, but the Peto method still had the best performance of all the methods considered for event risks of 1 in 1000, and the bias was never more than 6% of the comparator group risk.

In other circumstances (i.e. event risks above 1%, very large effects at event risks around 1%, and meta-analyses where many studies were substantially imbalanced) the best performing methods were the Mantel-Haenszel odds ratio without zero-cell corrections, logistic regression and an exact method. None of these methods is available in RevMan.

Methods that should be avoided with rare events are the inverse-variance methods (including the DerSimonian and Laird random-effects method) (Efthimiou 2018). These directly incorporate the study's variance in the estimation of its contribution to the meta-analysis, but these are usually based on a large-sample variance approximation, which was not intended for use with rare events. We would suggest that incorporation of heterogeneity into an estimate of a treatment effect should be a secondary consideration when attempting to produce estimates of effects from sparse data – the primary concern is to discern whether there is any signal of an effect in the data.

10.5 Meta-analysis of continuous outcomes

An important assumption underlying standard methods for meta-analysis of continuous data is that the outcomes have a normal distribution in each intervention arm in each study. This assumption may not always be met, although it is unimportant in very large studies. It is useful to consider the possibility of skewed data (see Section 10.5.3).

10.5.1 Which effect measure for continuous outcomes?

The two summary statistics commonly used for meta-analysis of continuous data are the mean difference (MD) and the standardized mean difference (SMD). Other options are available, such as the ratio of means (see Chapter 6, Section 6.5.1). Selection of summary statistics for continuous data is principally determined by whether studies all report the outcome using the same scale (when the mean difference can be used) or using different scales (when the standardized mean difference is usually used). The ratio of means can be used in either situation, but is appropriate only when outcome measurements are strictly greater than zero. Further considerations in deciding on an effect measure that will facilitate interpretation of the findings appears in Chapter 15 (Section 15.5).

The different roles played in MD and SMD approaches by the standard deviations (SDs) of outcomes observed in the two groups should be understood.

For the mean difference approach, the SDs are used together with the sample sizes to compute the weight given to each study. Studies with small SDs are given relatively higher weight whilst studies with larger SDs are given relatively smaller weights. This is appropriate if variation in SDs between studies reflects differences in the reliability of outcome measurements, but is probably not appropriate if the differences in SD reflect real differences in the variability of outcomes in the study populations.

For the standardized mean difference approach, the SDs are used to standardize the mean differences to a single scale, as well as in the computation of study weights. Thus, studies with small SDs lead to relatively higher estimates of SMD, whilst studies with larger SDs lead to relatively smaller estimates of SMD. For this to be appropriate, it must be assumed that between-study variation in SDs reflects only differences in measurement scales and not differences in the reliability of outcome measures or variability among study populations, as discussed in Chapter 6 (Section 6.5.1.2).

These assumptions of the methods should be borne in mind when unexpected variation of SDs is observed across studies.

10.5.2 Meta-analysis of change scores

In some circumstances an analysis based on changes from baseline will be more efficient and powerful than comparison of post-intervention values, as it removes a component of between-person variability from the analysis. However, calculation of a change score requires measurement of the outcome twice and in practice may be less efficient for outcomes that are unstable or difficult to measure precisely, where the measurement error may be larger than true between-person baseline variability. Change-from-baseline outcomes may also be preferred if they have a less skewed distribution than post-intervention measurement outcomes. Although sometimes used as a device to 'correct' for unlucky randomization, this practice is not recommended.

The preferred statistical approach to accounting for baseline measurements of the outcome variable is to include the baseline outcome measurements as a covariate in a regression model or analysis of covariance (ANCOVA). These analyses produce an 'adjusted' estimate of the intervention effect together with its standard error. These analyses are the least frequently encountered, but as they give the most precise and least biased estimates of intervention effects they should be included in the analysis when they are available. However, they can only be included in a meta-analysis using the generic inverse-variance method, since means and SDs are not available for each intervention group separately.

In practice an author is likely to discover that the studies included in a review include a mixture of change-from-baseline and post-intervention value scores. However, mixing of outcomes is not a problem when it comes to meta-analysis of MDs. There is no statistical reason why studies with change-from-baseline outcomes should not be combined in a meta-analysis with studies with post-intervention measurement outcomes when using the (unstandardized) MD method. In a randomized study, MD based on changes from baseline can usually be assumed to be addressing exactly the same underlying intervention effects as analyses based on post-intervention measurements. That is to say, the difference in mean post-intervention values will on average be the same as the difference in mean change scores. If the use of change scores does increase precision, appropriately, the studies presenting change scores will be given higher weights in the analysis than they would have received if post-intervention values had been used, as they will have smaller SDs.

When combining the data on the MD scale, authors must be careful to use the appropriate means and SDs (either of post-intervention measurements or of changes from baseline) for each study. Since the mean values and SDs for the two types of outcome may differ substantially, it may be advisable to place them in separate subgroups to avoid confusion for the reader, but the results of the subgroups can legitimately be pooled together.

In contrast, post-intervention value and change scores should not in principle be combined using standard meta-analysis approaches when the effect measure is an SMD. This is because the SDs used in the standardization reflect different things. The SD when standardizing post-intervention values reflects between-person variability at a single point in time. The SD when standardizing change scores reflects variation in between-person changes over time, so will depend on both within-person and between-person variability; within-person variability in turn is likely to depend on the length of time between measurements. Nevertheless, an empirical study of 21 meta-analyses in osteoarthritis did not find a difference between combined SMDs based on post-intervention values and combined SMDs based on change scores (da Costa et al 2013). One option is to standardize SMDs using post-intervention SDs rather than change score SDs. This would lead to valid synthesis of the two approaches, but we are not aware that an appropriate standard error for this has been derived.

A common practical problem associated with including change-from-baseline measures is that the SD of changes is not reported. Imputation of SDs is discussed in Chapter 6 (Section 6.4.2.8).

10.5.3 Meta-analysis of skewed data

Analyses based on means are appropriate for data that are at least approximately normally distributed, and for data from very large trials. If the true distribution of outcomes is asymmetrical, then the data are said to be skewed. Review authors should consider the possibility and implications of skewed data when analysing continuous outcomes (see MECIR Box 10.5.a). Skew can sometimes be diagnosed from the means and SDs of the outcomes. A rough check is available, but it is only valid if a lowest or highest possible value for an outcome is known to exist. Thus, the check may be used

MECIR Box 10.5.a Relevant expectations for conduct of intervention reviews	
C65: Addressing skewed data (**Highly desirable**)	
Consider the possibility and implications of skewed data when analysing continuous outcomes.	Skewed data are sometimes not summarized usefully by means and standard deviations. While statistical methods are approximately valid for large sample sizes, skewed outcome data can lead to misleading results when studies are small.

for outcomes such as weight, volume and blood concentrations, which have lowest possible values of 0, or for scale outcomes with minimum or maximum scores, but it may not be appropriate for change-from-baseline measures. The check involves calculating the observed mean minus the lowest possible value (or the highest possible value minus the observed mean), and dividing this by the SD. A ratio less than 2 suggests skew (Altman and Bland 1996). If the ratio is less than 1, there is strong evidence of a skewed distribution.

Transformation of the original outcome data may reduce skew substantially. Reports of trials may present results on a transformed scale, usually a log scale. Collection of appropriate data summaries from the trialists, or acquisition of individual patient data, is currently the approach of choice. Appropriate data summaries and analysis strategies for the individual patient data will depend on the situation. Consultation with a knowledgeable statistician is advised.

Where data have been analysed on a log scale, results are commonly presented as geometric means and ratios of geometric means. A meta-analysis may be then performed on the scale of the log-transformed data; an example of the calculation of the required means and SD is given in Chapter 6 (Section 6.5.2.4). This approach depends on being able to obtain transformed data for all studies; methods for transforming from one scale to the other are available (Higgins et al 2008b). Log-transformed and untransformed data should not be mixed in a meta-analysis.

10.6 Combining dichotomous and continuous outcomes

Occasionally authors encounter a situation where data for the same outcome are presented in some studies as dichotomous data and in other studies as continuous data. For example, scores on depression scales can be reported as means, or as the percentage of patients who were depressed at some point after an intervention (i.e. with a score above a specified cut-point). This type of information is often easier to understand, and more helpful, when it is dichotomized. However, deciding on a cut-point may be arbitrary, and information is lost when continuous data are transformed to dichotomous data.

There are several options for handling combinations of dichotomous and continuous data. Generally, it is useful to summarize results from all the relevant, valid studies in a similar way, but this is not always possible. It may be possible to collect missing data from investigators so that this can be done. If not, it may be useful to summarize the data in three ways: by entering the means and SDs as continuous outcomes, by entering the counts as dichotomous outcomes and by entering all of the data in text form as 'Other data' outcomes.

There are statistical approaches available that will re-express odds ratios as SMDs (and vice versa), allowing dichotomous and continuous data to be combined (Anzures-Cabrera et al 2011). A simple approach is as follows. Based on an assumption that the underlying continuous measurements in each intervention group follow a logistic distribution (which is a symmetrical distribution similar in shape to the normal distribution, but with more data in the distributional tails), and that the variability of the outcomes is the same in both experimental and comparator participants, the odds ratios can be re-expressed as a SMD according to the following simple formula (Chinn 2000):

$$\text{SMD} = \frac{\sqrt{3}}{\pi}\ln\text{OR}.$$

The standard error of the log odds ratio can be converted to the standard error of a SMD by multiplying by the same constant ($\sqrt{3}/\pi = 0.5513$). Alternatively SMDs can be re-expressed as log odds ratios by multiplying by $\pi/\sqrt{3} = 1.814$. Once SMDs (or log odds ratios) and their standard errors have been computed for all studies in the meta-analysis, they can be combined using the generic inverse-variance method. Standard errors can be computed for all studies by entering the data as dichotomous and continuous outcome type data, as appropriate, and converting the confidence intervals for the resulting log odds ratios and SMDs into standard errors (see Chapter 6, Section 6.3).

10.7 Meta-analysis of ordinal outcomes and measurement scales

Ordinal and measurement scale outcomes are most commonly meta-analysed as dichotomous data (if so, see Section 10.4) or continuous data (if so, see Section 10.5) depending on the way that the study authors performed the original analyses.

Occasionally it is possible to analyse the data using proportional odds models. This is the case when ordinal scales have a small number of categories, the numbers falling into each category for each intervention group can be obtained, and the same ordinal scale has been used in all studies. This approach may make more efficient use of all available data than dichotomization, but requires access to statistical software and results in a summary statistic for which it is challenging to find a clinical meaning.

The proportional odds model uses the proportional odds ratio as the measure of intervention effect (Agresti 1996) (see Chapter 6, Section 6.6), and can be used for conducting a meta-analysis in advanced statistical software packages (Whitehead and Jones 1994). Estimates of log odds ratios and their standard errors from a proportional odds model may be meta-analysed using the generic inverse-variance method (see Section 10.3.3). If the same ordinal scale has been used in all studies, but in some reports has been presented as a dichotomous outcome, it may still be possible to include all studies in the meta-analysis. In the context of the three-category model, this might mean that for some studies category 1 constitutes a success, while for others both categories 1 and 2 constitute a success. Methods are available for dealing with this, and for combining data from scales that are related but have different definitions for their categories (Whitehead and Jones 1994).

10.8 Meta-analysis of counts and rates

Results may be expressed as **count data** when each participant may experience an event, and may experience it more than once (see Chapter 6, Section 6.7). For example, 'number of strokes', or 'number of hospital visits' are counts. These events may not happen at all, but if they do happen there is no theoretical maximum number of occurrences for an individual. Count data may be analysed using methods for dichotomous data if the counts are dichotomized for each individual (see Section 10.4), continuous data (see Section 10.5) and time-to-event data (see Section 10.9), as well as being analysed as rate data.

Rate data occur if counts are measured for each participant along with the time over which they are observed. This is particularly appropriate when the events being counted are rare. For example, a woman may experience two strokes during a follow-up period of two years. Her rate of strokes is one per year of follow-up (or, equivalently 0.083 per month of follow-up). Rates are conventionally summarized at the group level. For example, participants in the comparator group of a clinical trial may experience 85 strokes during a total of 2836 person-years of follow-up. An underlying assumption associated with the use of rates is that the risk of an event is constant across participants and over time. This assumption should be carefully considered for each situation. For example, in contraception studies, rates have been used (known as Pearl indices) to describe the number of pregnancies per 100 women-years of follow-up. This is now considered inappropriate since couples have different risks of conception, and the risk for each woman changes over time. Pregnancies are now analysed more often using life tables or time-to-event methods that investigate the time elapsing before the first pregnancy.

Analysing count data as rates is not always the most appropriate approach and is uncommon in practice. This is because:

1) the assumption of a constant underlying risk may not be suitable; and
2) the statistical methods are not as well developed as they are for other types of data.

The results of a study may be expressed as a **rate ratio**, that is the ratio of the rate in the experimental intervention group to the rate in the comparator group. The (natural) logarithms of the rate ratios may be combined across studies using the generic inverse-variance method (see Section 10.3.3). Alternatively, Poisson regression approaches can be used (Spittal et al 2015).

In a randomized trial, rate ratios may often be very similar to risk ratios obtained after dichotomizing the participants, since the average period of follow-up should be similar in all intervention groups. Rate ratios and risk ratios will differ, however, if an intervention affects the likelihood of some participants experiencing multiple events.

It is possible also to focus attention on the rate difference (see Chapter 6, Section 6.7.1). The analysis again can be performed using the generic inverse-variance method (Hasselblad and McCrory 1995, Guevara et al 2004).

10.9 Meta-analysis of time-to-event outcomes

Two approaches to meta-analysis of time-to-event outcomes are readily available to Cochrane Review authors. The choice of which to use will depend on the type of data that have been extracted from the primary studies, or obtained from re-analysis of individual participant data.

If 'O – E' and 'V' statistics have been obtained (see Chapter 6, Section 6.8.2), either through re-analysis of individual participant data or from aggregate statistics presented in the study reports, then these statistics may be entered directly into RevMan using the 'O – E and Variance' outcome type. There are several ways to calculate these 'O – E' and 'V' statistics. Peto's method applied to dichotomous data (Section 10.4.2) gives rise to an odds ratio; a log-rank approach gives rise to a hazard ratio; and a variation of the Peto method for analysing time-to-event data gives rise to something in between (Simmonds et al 2011). The appropriate effect measure should be specified. Only fixed-effect meta-analysis methods are available in RevMan for 'O – E and Variance' outcomes.

Alternatively, if estimates of log hazard ratios and standard errors have been obtained from results of Cox proportional hazards regression models, study results can be combined using generic inverse-variance methods (see Section 10.3.3).

If a mixture of log-rank and Cox model estimates are obtained from the studies, all results can be combined using the generic inverse-variance method, as the log-rank estimates can be converted into log hazard ratios and standard errors using the approaches discussed in Chapter 6 (Section 6.8).

10.10 Heterogeneity

10.10.1 What is heterogeneity?

Inevitably, studies brought together in a systematic review will differ. Any kind of variability among studies in a systematic review may be termed heterogeneity. It can be helpful to distinguish between different types of heterogeneity. Variability in the participants, interventions and outcomes studied may be described as **clinical diversity** (sometimes called clinical heterogeneity), and variability in study design, outcome measurement tools and risk of bias may be described as **methodological diversity** (sometimes called methodological heterogeneity). Variability in the intervention effects being evaluated in the different studies is known as **statistical heterogeneity**, and is a consequence of clinical or methodological diversity, or both, among the studies. Statistical heterogeneity manifests itself in the observed intervention effects being more different from each other than one would expect due to random error (chance) alone. We will follow convention and refer to **statistical heterogeneity** simply as **heterogeneity**.

Clinical variation will lead to heterogeneity if the intervention effect is affected by the factors that vary across studies; most obviously, the specific interventions or patient characteristics. In other words, the true intervention effect will be different in different studies.

Differences between studies in terms of methodological factors, such as use of blinding and concealment of allocation sequence, or if there are differences between studies in the way the outcomes are defined and measured, may be expected to lead to differences in the observed intervention effects. Significant statistical heterogeneity arising from methodological diversity or differences in outcome assessments suggests that the studies are not all estimating the same quantity, but does not necessarily suggest that the true intervention effect varies. In particular, heterogeneity associated solely with methodological diversity would indicate that the studies suffer from different degrees of bias. Empirical evidence suggests that some aspects of design can affect the result of clinical trials, although this is not always the case. Further discussion appears in Chapters 7 and 8.

The scope of a review will largely determine the extent to which studies included in a review are diverse. Sometimes a review will include studies addressing a variety of questions, for example when several different interventions for the same condition are of interest (see also Chapter 11) or when the differential effects of an intervention in different populations are of interest. Meta-analysis should only be considered when a group of studies is sufficiently homogeneous in terms of participants, interventions and outcomes to provide a meaningful summary. It is often appropriate to take a broader perspective in a meta-analysis than in a single clinical trial. A common analogy is that systematic reviews bring together apples and oranges, and that combining these can yield a meaningless result. This is true if apples and oranges are of intrinsic interest on their own, but may not be if they are used to contribute to a wider question about fruit. For example, a meta-analysis may reasonably evaluate the average effect of a class of drugs by combining results from trials where each evaluates the effect of a different drug from the class.

There may be specific interest in a review in investigating how clinical and methodological aspects of studies relate to their results. Where possible these investigations should be specified a priori (i.e. in the protocol for the systematic review). It is legitimate for a systematic review to focus on examining the relationship between some clinical characteristic(s) of the studies and the size of intervention effect, rather than on obtaining a summary effect estimate across a series of studies (see Section 10.11). Meta-regression may best be used for this purpose, although it is not implemented in RevMan (see Section 10.11.4).

10.10.2 Identifying and measuring heterogeneity

It is essential to consider the extent to which the results of studies are consistent with each other (see MECIR Box 10.10.a). If confidence intervals for the results of individual studies (generally depicted graphically using horizontal lines) have poor overlap, this generally indicates the presence of statistical heterogeneity. More formally, a statistical

MECIR Box 10.10.a Relevant expectations for conduct of intervention reviews	
C63: Assessing statistical heterogeneity (**Mandatory**)	
Assess the presence and extent of between-study variation when undertaking a meta-analysis.	The presence of heterogeneity affects the extent to which generalizable conclusions can be formed. It is important to identify heterogeneity in case there is sufficient information to explain it and offer new insights. Authors should recognize that there is much uncertainty in measures such as I^2 and Tau^2 when there are few studies. Thus, use of simple thresholds to diagnose heterogeneity should be avoided.

test for heterogeneity is available. This Chi^2 (χ^2, or chi-squared) test is included in the forest plots in Cochrane Reviews. It assesses whether observed differences in results are compatible with chance alone. A low P value (or a large Chi^2 statistic relative to its degree of freedom) provides evidence of heterogeneity of intervention effects (variation in effect estimates beyond chance).

Care must be taken in the interpretation of the Chi^2 test, since it has low power in the (common) situation of a meta-analysis when studies have small sample size or are few in number. This means that while a statistically significant result may indicate a problem with heterogeneity, a non-significant result must not be taken as evidence of no heterogeneity. This is also why a P value of 0.10, rather than the conventional level of 0.05, is sometimes used to determine statistical significance. A further problem with the test, which seldom occurs in Cochrane Reviews, is that when there are many studies in a meta-analysis, the test has high power to detect a small amount of heterogeneity that may be clinically unimportant.

Some argue that, since clinical and methodological diversity always occur in a meta-analysis, statistical heterogeneity is inevitable (Higgins et al 2003). Thus, the test for heterogeneity is irrelevant to the choice of analysis; heterogeneity will always exist whether or not we happen to be able to detect it using a statistical test. Methods have been developed for quantifying inconsistency across studies that move the focus away from testing whether heterogeneity is present to assessing its impact on the meta-analysis. A useful statistic for quantifying inconsistency is:

$$I^2 = \left(\frac{Q - \mathrm{df}}{Q}\right) \times 100\%.$$

In this equation, Q is the Chi^2 statistic and df is its degrees of freedom (Higgins and Thompson 2002, Higgins et al 2003). I^2 describes the percentage of the variability in effect estimates that is due to heterogeneity rather than sampling error (chance).

Thresholds for the interpretation of the I^2 statistic can be misleading, since the importance of inconsistency depends on several factors. A rough guide to interpretation in the context of meta-analyses of randomized trials is as follows:

- 0% to 40%: might not be important;
- 30% to 60%: may represent moderate heterogeneity*;
- 50% to 90%: may represent substantial heterogeneity*;
- 75% to 100%: considerable heterogeneity*.

*The importance of the observed value of I^2 depends on (1) magnitude and direction of effects, and (2) strength of evidence for heterogeneity (e.g. P value from the Chi^2 test, or a confidence interval for I^2: uncertainty in the value of I^2 is substantial when the number of studies is small).

10.10.3 Strategies for addressing heterogeneity

Review authors must take into account any statistical heterogeneity when interpreting results, particularly when there is variation in the direction of effect (see MECIR Box 10.10.b). A number of options are available if heterogeneity is identified among a group of studies that would otherwise be considered suitable for a meta-analysis.

MECIR Box 10.10.b Relevant expectations for conduct of intervention reviews	
C69: Considering statistical heterogeneity when interpreting the results (**Mandatory**)	
Take into account any statistical heterogeneity when interpreting the results, particularly when there is variation in the direction of effect.	The presence of heterogeneity affects the extent to which generalizable conclusions can be formed. If a fixed-effect analysis is used, the confidence intervals ignore the extent of heterogeneity. If a random-effects analysis is used, the result pertains to the mean effect across studies. In both cases, the implications of notable heterogeneity should be addressed. It may be possible to understand the reasons for the heterogeneity if there are sufficient studies.

1) *Check again that the data are correct.* Severe apparent heterogeneity can indicate that data have been incorrectly extracted or entered into meta-analysis software. For example, if standard errors have mistakenly been entered as SDs for continuous outcomes, this could manifest itself in overly narrow confidence intervals with poor overlap and hence substantial heterogeneity. Unit-of-analysis errors may also be causes of heterogeneity (see Chapter 6, Section 6.2).
2) *Do not do a meta-analysis.* A systematic review need not contain any meta-analyses. If there is considerable variation in results, and particularly if there is inconsistency in the direction of effect, it may be misleading to quote an average value for the intervention effect.
3) *Explore heterogeneity.* It is clearly of interest to determine the causes of heterogeneity among results of studies. This process is problematic since there are often many characteristics that vary across studies from which one may choose. Heterogeneity may be explored by conducting subgroup analyses (see Section 10.11.3) or meta-regression (see Section 10.11.4). Reliable conclusions can only be drawn from analyses that are truly pre-specified before inspecting the studies' results, and even these conclusions should be interpreted with caution. Explorations of heterogeneity that are devised after heterogeneity is identified can at best lead to the generation of hypotheses. They should be interpreted with even more caution and should generally not be listed among the conclusions of a review. Also, investigations of heterogeneity when there are very few studies are of questionable value.
4) *Ignore heterogeneity.* Fixed-effect meta-analyses ignore heterogeneity. The summary effect estimate from a fixed-effect meta-analysis is normally interpreted as being the best estimate of the intervention effect. However, the existence of heterogeneity suggests that there may not be a single intervention effect but a variety of intervention effects. Thus, the summary fixed-effect estimate may be an intervention effect that does not actually exist in any population, and therefore have a confidence interval that is meaningless as well as being too narrow (see Section 10.10.4).

5) *Perform a random-effects meta-analysis.* A random-effects meta-analysis may be used to incorporate heterogeneity among studies. This is not a substitute for a thorough investigation of heterogeneity. It is intended primarily for heterogeneity that cannot be explained. An extended discussion of this option appears in Section 10.10.4.
6) *Reconsider the effect measure.* Heterogeneity may be an artificial consequence of an inappropriate choice of effect measure. For example, when studies collect continuous outcome data using different scales or different units, extreme heterogeneity may be apparent when using the mean difference but not when the more appropriate standardized mean difference is used. Furthermore, choice of effect measure for dichotomous outcomes (odds ratio, risk ratio, or risk difference) may affect the degree of heterogeneity among results. In particular, when comparator group risks vary, homogeneous odds ratios or risk ratios will necessarily lead to heterogeneous risk differences, and vice versa. However, it remains unclear whether homogeneity of intervention effect in a particular meta-analysis is a suitable criterion for choosing between these measures (see also Section 10.4.3).
7) *Exclude studies.* Heterogeneity may be due to the presence of one or two outlying studies with results that conflict with the rest of the studies. In general it is unwise to exclude studies from a meta-analysis on the basis of their results as this may introduce bias. However, if an obvious reason for the outlying result is apparent, the study might be removed with more confidence. Since usually at least one characteristic can be found for any study in any meta-analysis which makes it different from the others, this criterion is unreliable because it is all too easy to fulfil. It is advisable to perform analyses both with and without outlying studies as part of a sensitivity analysis (see Section 10.14). Whenever possible, potential sources of clinical diversity that might lead to such situations should be specified in the protocol.

10.10.4 Incorporating heterogeneity into random-effects models

The random-effects meta-analysis approach incorporates an assumption that the different studies are estimating different, yet related, intervention effects (DerSimonian and Laird 1986, Borenstein et al 2010). The approach allows us to address heterogeneity that cannot readily be explained by other factors. A random-effects meta-analysis model involves an assumption that the effects being estimated in the different studies follow some distribution. The model represents our lack of knowledge about why real, or apparent, intervention effects differ, by considering the differences as if they were random. The centre of the assumed distribution describes the average of the effects, while its width describes the degree of heterogeneity. The conventional choice of distribution is a normal distribution. It is difficult to establish the validity of any particular distributional assumption, and this is a common criticism of random-effects meta-analyses. The importance of the assumed shape for this distribution has not been widely studied.

To undertake a random-effects meta-analysis, the standard errors of the study-specific estimates (SE_i in Section 10.3.1) are adjusted to incorporate a measure of the extent of variation, or heterogeneity, among the intervention effects observed in different studies (this variation is often referred to as Tau-squared, τ^2, or Tau^2). The amount of variation, and hence the adjustment, can be estimated from the intervention effects and standard errors of the studies included in the meta-analysis.

In a heterogeneous set of studies, a random-effects meta-analysis will award relatively more weight to smaller studies than such studies would receive in a fixed-effect meta-analysis. This is because small studies are more informative for learning about the distribution of effects across studies than for learning about an assumed common intervention effect.

Note that a random-effects model does not 'take account' of the heterogeneity, in the sense that it is no longer an issue. It is always preferable to explore possible causes of heterogeneity, although there may be too few studies to do this adequately (see Section 10.11).

10.10.4.1 Fixed or random effects?

A fixed-effect meta-analysis provides a result that may be viewed as a 'typical intervention effect' from the studies included in the analysis. In order to calculate a confidence interval for a fixed-effect meta-analysis the assumption is usually made that the true effect of intervention (in both magnitude and direction) is the same value in every study (i.e. fixed across studies). This assumption implies that the observed differences among study results are due solely to the play of chance (i.e. that there is no statistical heterogeneity).

A random-effects model provides a result that may be viewed as an 'average intervention effect', where this average is explicitly defined according to an assumed distribution of effects across studies. Instead of assuming that the intervention effects are the same, we assume that they follow (usually) a normal distribution. The assumption implies that the observed differences among study results are due to a combination of the play of chance and some genuine variation in the intervention effects.

The random-effects method and the fixed-effect method will give identical results when there is no heterogeneity among the studies.

When heterogeneity is present, a confidence interval around the random-effects summary estimate is wider than a confidence interval around a fixed-effect summary estimate. This will happen whenever the I^2 statistic is greater than zero, even if the heterogeneity is not detected by the Chi^2 test for heterogeneity (see Section 10.10.2).

Sometimes the central estimate of the intervention effect is different between fixed-effect and random-effects analyses. In particular, if results of smaller studies are systematically different from results of larger ones, which can happen as a result of publication bias or within-study bias in smaller studies (Egger et al 1997, Poole and Greenland 1999, Kjaergard et al 2001), then a random-effects meta-analysis will exacerbate the effects of the bias (see also Chapter 13, Section 13.3.5.5). A fixed-effect analysis will be affected less, although strictly it will also be inappropriate.

The decision between fixed- and random-effects meta-analyses has been the subject of much debate, and we do not provide a universal recommendation. Some considerations in making this choice are as follows.

1) Many have argued that the decision should be based on an expectation of whether the intervention effects are truly identical, preferring the fixed-effect model if this is likely and a random-effects model if this is unlikely (Borenstein et al 2010). Since it is generally considered to be implausible that intervention effects across studies are identical (unless the intervention has no effect at all), this leads many to advocate use of the random-effects model.

2) Others have argued that a fixed-effect analysis can be interpreted in the presence of heterogeneity, and that it makes fewer assumptions than a random-effects meta-analysis. They then refer to it as a 'fixed-effects' meta-analysis (Peto et al 1995, Rice et al 2018).
3) Under any interpretation, a fixed-effect meta-analysis ignores heterogeneity. If the method is used, it is therefore important to supplement it with a statistical investigation of the extent of heterogeneity (see Section 10.10.2).
4) In the presence of heterogeneity, a random-effects analysis gives relatively more weight to smaller studies and relatively less weight to larger studies. If there is additionally some funnel plot asymmetry (i.e. a relationship between intervention effect magnitude and study size), then this will push the results of the random-effects analysis towards the findings in the smaller studies. In the context of randomized trials, this is generally regarded as an unfortunate consequence of the model.
5) A pragmatic approach is to plan to undertake both a fixed-effect and a random-effects meta-analysis, with an intention to present the random-effects result if there is no indication of funnel plot asymmetry. If there is an indication of funnel plot asymmetry, then both methods are problematic. It may be reasonable to present both analyses or neither, or to perform a sensitivity analysis in which small studies are excluded or addressed directly using meta-regression (see Chapter 13, Section 13.3.5.6).
6) The choice between a fixed-effect and a random-effects meta-analysis should never be made on the basis of a statistical test for heterogeneity.

10.10.4.2 Interpretation of random-effects meta-analyses

The summary estimate and confidence interval from a random-effects meta-analysis refer to the centre of the distribution of intervention effects, but do not describe the width of the distribution. Often the summary estimate and its confidence interval are quoted in isolation and portrayed as a sufficient summary of the meta-analysis. This is inappropriate. The confidence interval from a random-effects meta-analysis describes uncertainty in the location of the mean of systematically different effects in the different studies. It does not describe the degree of heterogeneity among studies, as may be commonly believed. For example, when there are many studies in a meta-analysis, we may obtain a very tight confidence interval around the random-effects estimate of the mean effect even when there is a large amount of heterogeneity. A solution to this problem is to consider a **prediction interval** (see Section 10.10.4.3).

Methodological diversity creates heterogeneity through biases variably affecting the results of different studies. The random-effects summary estimate will only correctly estimate the average intervention effect if the biases are symmetrically distributed, leading to a mixture of over-estimates and under-estimates of effect, which is unlikely to be the case. In practice it can be very difficult to distinguish whether heterogeneity results from clinical or methodological diversity, and in most cases it is likely to be due to both, so these distinctions are hard to draw in the interpretation.

When there is little information, either because there are few studies or if the studies are small with few events, a random-effects analysis will provide poor estimates of the amount of heterogeneity (i.e. of the width of the distribution of intervention effects). Fixed-effect methods such as the Mantel-Haenszel method will provide more robust estimates of the average intervention effect, but at the cost of ignoring any heterogeneity.

10.10.4.3 Prediction intervals from a random-effects meta-analysis

An estimate of the between-study variance in a random-effects meta-analysis is typically presented as part of its results. The square root of this number (i.e. Tau) is the estimated standard deviation of underlying effects across studies. Prediction intervals are a way of expressing this value in an interpretable way.

To motivate the idea of a prediction interval, note that for absolute measures of effect (e.g. risk difference, mean difference, standardized mean difference), an approximate 95% range of normally distributed underlying effects can be obtained by creating an interval from 1.96 × Tau below the random-effects mean, to 1.96 × Tau above it. (For relative measures such as the odds ratio and risk ratio, an equivalent interval needs to be based on the natural logarithm of the summary estimate.) In reality, both the summary estimate and the value of Tau are associated with uncertainty. A prediction interval seeks to present the range of effects in a way that acknowledges this uncertainty (Higgins et al 2009). A simple 95% prediction interval can be calculated as:

$$M \pm t_{k-2} \times \sqrt{\mathrm{Tau}^2 + \mathrm{SE}(M)^2},$$

where M is the summary mean from the random-effects meta-analysis, t_{k-2} is the 95% percentile of a t-distribution with $k-2$ degrees of freedom, k is the number of studies, Tau^2 is the estimated amount of heterogeneity and SE(M) is the standard error of the summary mean.

The term 'prediction interval' relates to the use of this interval to predict the possible underlying effect in a new study that is similar to the studies in the meta-analysis. A more useful interpretation of the interval is as a summary of the spread of underlying effects in the studies included in the random-effects meta-analysis.

Prediction intervals have proved a popular way of expressing the amount of heterogeneity in a meta-analysis (Riley et al 2011). They are, however, strongly based on the assumption of a normal distribution for the effects across studies, and can be very problematic when the number of studies is small, in which case they can appear spuriously wide or spuriously narrow. Nevertheless, we encourage their use when the number of studies is reasonable (e.g. more than ten) and there is no clear funnel plot asymmetry.

10.10.4.4 Implementing random-effects meta-analyses

As introduced in Section 10.3.2, the random-effects model can be implemented using an inverse-variance approach, incorporating a measure of the extent of heterogeneity into the study weights. RevMan implements a version of random-effects meta-analysis that is described by DerSimonian and Laird, making use of a 'moment-based' estimate of the between-study variance (DerSimonian and Laird 1986). The attraction of this method is that the calculations are straightforward, but it has a theoretical disadvantage in that the confidence intervals are slightly too narrow to encompass full uncertainty resulting from having estimated the degree of heterogeneity.

For many years, RevMan has implemented two random-effects methods for dichotomous data: a Mantel-Haenszel method and an inverse-variance method. Both use the moment-based approach to estimating the amount of between-studies variation. The difference between the two is subtle: the former estimates the between-study variation by comparing each study's result with a Mantel-Haenszel fixed-effect meta-analysis result, whereas the latter estimates it by comparing each study's result with an inverse-variance fixed-effect meta-analysis result. In practice, the difference is likely to be trivial.

There are alternative methods for performing random-effects meta-analyses that have better technical properties than the DerSimonian and Laird approach with a moment-based estimate (Veroniki et al 2016). Most notable among these is an adjustment to the confidence interval proposed by Hartung and Knapp and by Sidik and Jonkman (Hartung and Knapp 2001, Sidik and Jonkman 2002). This adjustment widens the confidence interval to reflect uncertainty in the estimation of between-study heterogeneity, and it should be used if available to review authors. An alternative option to encompass full uncertainty in the degree of heterogeneity is to take a Bayesian approach (see Section 10.13).

An empirical comparison of different ways to estimate between-study variation in Cochrane meta-analyses has shown that they can lead to substantial differences in estimates of heterogeneity, but seldom have major implications for estimating summary effects (Langan et al 2015). Several simulation studies have concluded that an approach proposed by Paule and Mandel should be recommended (Langan et al 2017); whereas a comprehensive recent simulation study recommended a restricted maximum likelihood approach, although noted that no single approach is universally preferable (Langan et al 2019). Review authors are encouraged to select one of these options if it is available to them.

10.11 Investigating heterogeneity

10.11.1 Interaction and effect modification

Does the intervention effect vary with different populations or intervention characteristics (such as dose or duration)? Such variation is known as interaction by statisticians and as effect modification by epidemiologists. Methods to search for such interactions include subgroup analyses and meta-regression. All methods have considerable pitfalls.

10.11.2 What are subgroup analyses?

Subgroup analyses involve splitting all the participant data into subgroups, often in order to make comparisons between them. Subgroup analyses may be done for subsets of participants (such as males and females), or for subsets of studies (such as different geographical locations). Subgroup analyses may be done as a means of investigating heterogeneous results, or to answer specific questions about particular patient groups, types of intervention or types of study.

Subgroup analyses of subsets of participants within studies are uncommon in systematic reviews based on published literature because sufficient details to extract data about separate participant types are seldom published in reports. By contrast, such subsets of participants are easily analysed when individual participant data have been collected (see Chapter 26). The methods we describe in the remainder of this chapter are for subgroups of studies.

Findings from multiple subgroup analyses may be misleading. Subgroup analyses are observational by nature and are not based on randomized comparisons. False negative and false positive significance tests increase in likelihood rapidly as more subgroup analyses are performed. If their findings are presented as definitive conclusions there is clearly a risk of people being denied an effective intervention or treated with an ineffective (or even harmful) intervention. Subgroup analyses can also generate misleading recommendations about directions for future research that, if followed, would waste scarce resources.

It is useful to distinguish between the notions of 'qualitative interaction' and 'quantitative interaction' (Yusuf et al 1991). Qualitative interaction exists if the direction of effect is reversed, that is if an intervention is beneficial in one subgroup but is harmful in another. Qualitative interaction is rare. This may be used as an argument that the most appropriate result of a meta-analysis is the overall effect across all subgroups. Quantitative interaction exists when the size of the effect varies but not the direction, that is if an intervention is beneficial to different degrees in different subgroups.

10.11.3 Undertaking subgroup analyses

Meta-analyses can be undertaken in RevMan both within subgroups of studies as well as across all studies irrespective of their subgroup membership. It is tempting to compare effect estimates in different subgroups by considering the meta-analysis results from each subgroup separately. This should only be done informally by comparing the magnitudes of effect. Noting that either the effect or the test for heterogeneity in one subgroup is statistically significant whilst that in the other subgroup is not statistically significant does not indicate that the subgroup factor explains heterogeneity. Since different subgroups are likely to contain different amounts of information and thus have different abilities to detect effects, it is extremely misleading simply to compare the statistical significance of the results.

10.11.3.1 Is the effect different in different subgroups?

Valid investigations of whether an intervention works differently in different subgroups involve comparing the subgroups with each other. It is a mistake to compare within-subgroup inferences such as P values. If one subgroup analysis is statistically significant and another is not, then the latter may simply reflect a lack of information rather than a smaller (or absent) effect. When there are only two subgroups, non-overlap of the confidence intervals indicates statistical significance, but note that the confidence intervals can overlap to a small degree and the difference still be statistically significant.

A formal statistical approach should be used to examine differences among subgroups (see MECIR Box 10.11.a). A simple significance test to investigate differences between two or more subgroups can be performed (Borenstein and Higgins 2013). This procedure consists of undertaking a standard test for heterogeneity across subgroup results rather than across individual study results. When the meta-analysis uses a fixed-effect inverse-variance weighted average approach, the method is exactly equivalent to the test described by Deeks and colleagues (Deeks et al 2001). An I^2 statistic is also computed for subgroup differences. This describes the percentage of the variability in effect estimates from the different subgroups that is due to genuine subgroup differences rather than sampling error (chance). Note that these methods for examining subgroup

MECIR Box 10.11.a Relevant expectations for conduct of intervention reviews	
C67: Comparing subgroups (**Mandatory**)	
If subgroup analyses are to be compared, and there are judged to be sufficient studies to do this meaningfully, use a formal statistical test to compare them.	Concluding that there is a difference in effect in different subgroups on the basis of differences in the level of statistical significance within subgroups can be very misleading.

differences should be used only when the data in the subgroups are independent (i.e. they should not be used if the same study participants contribute to more than one of the subgroups in the forest plot).

If fixed-effect models are used for the analysis within each subgroup, then these statistics relate to differences in typical effects across different subgroups. If random-effects models are used for the analysis within each subgroup, then the statistics relate to variation in the mean effects in the different subgroups.

An alternative method for testing for differences between subgroups is to use meta-regression techniques, in which case a random-effects model is generally preferred (see Section 10.11.4). Tests for subgroup differences based on random-effects models may be regarded as preferable to those based on fixed-effect models, due to the high risk of false-positive results when a fixed-effect model is used to compare subgroups (Higgins and Thompson 2004).

10.11.4 Meta-regression

If studies are divided into subgroups (see Section 10.11.2), this may be viewed as an investigation of how a categorical study characteristic is associated with the intervention effects in the meta-analysis. For example, studies in which allocation sequence concealment was adequate may yield different results from those in which it was inadequate. Here, allocation sequence concealment, being either adequate or inadequate, is a categorical characteristic at the study level. Meta-regression is an extension to subgroup analyses that allows the effect of continuous, as well as categorical, characteristics to be investigated, and in principle allows the effects of multiple factors to be investigated simultaneously (although this is rarely possible due to inadequate numbers of studies) (Thompson and Higgins 2002). Meta-regression should generally not be considered when there are fewer than ten studies in a meta-analysis.

Meta-regressions are similar in essence to simple regressions, in which an **outcome variable** is predicted according to the values of one or more **explanatory variables**. In meta-regression, the outcome variable is the effect estimate (for example, a mean difference, a risk difference, a log odds ratio or a log risk ratio). The explanatory variables are characteristics of studies that might influence the size of intervention effect. These are often called ‘potential effect modifiers’ or covariates. Meta-regressions usually differ from simple regressions in two ways. First, larger studies have more influence on the relationship than smaller studies, since studies are weighted by the precision of their respective effect estimate. Second, it is wise to allow for the residual heterogeneity among intervention effects not modelled by the explanatory variables. This gives rise to the term 'random-effects meta-regression', since the extra variability is incorporated in the same way as in a random-effects meta-analysis (Thompson and Sharp 1999).

The regression coefficient obtained from a meta-regression analysis will describe how the outcome variable (the intervention effect) changes with a unit increase in the explanatory variable (the potential effect modifier). The statistical significance of the regression coefficient is a test of whether there is a linear relationship between intervention effect and the explanatory variable. If the intervention effect is a ratio measure, the log-transformed value of the intervention effect should always be used in the regression model (see Chapter 6, Section 6.1.2.1), and the exponential of the regression coefficient will give an estimate of the relative change in intervention effect with a unit increase in the explanatory variable.

Meta-regression can also be used to investigate differences for categorical explanatory variables as done in subgroup analyses. If there are J subgroups, membership of particular subgroups is indicated by using J minus 1 dummy variables (which can only take values of zero or one) in the meta-regression model (as in standard linear regression modelling). The regression coefficients will estimate how the intervention effect in each subgroup differs from a nominated reference subgroup. The P value of each regression coefficient will indicate the strength of evidence against the null hypothesis that the characteristic is not associated with the intervention effect.

Meta-regression may be performed using the 'metareg' macro available for the Stata statistical package, or using the 'metafor' package for R, as well as other packages.

10.11.5 Selection of study characteristics for subgroup analyses and meta-regression

Authors need to be cautious about undertaking subgroup analyses, and interpreting any that they do. Some considerations are outlined here for selecting characteristics (also called explanatory variables, potential effect modifiers or covariates) that will be investigated for their possible influence on the size of the intervention effect. These considerations apply similarly to subgroup analyses and to meta-regressions. Further details may be obtained elsewhere (Oxman and Guyatt 1992, Berlin and Antman 1994).

10.11.5.1 Ensure that there are adequate studies to justify subgroup analyses and meta-regressions

It is very unlikely that an investigation of heterogeneity will produce useful findings unless there is a substantial number of studies. Typical advice for undertaking simple regression analyses: that at least ten observations (i.e. ten studies in a meta-analysis) should be available for each characteristic modelled. However, even this will be too few when the covariates are unevenly distributed across studies.

10.11.5.2 Specify characteristics in advance

Authors should, whenever possible, pre-specify characteristics in the protocol that later will be subject to subgroup analyses or meta-regression. The plan specified in the protocol should then be followed (data permitting), without undue emphasis on any particular findings (see MECIR Box 10.11.b). Pre-specifying characteristics reduces the likelihood of spurious findings, first by limiting the number of subgroups investigated,

MECIR Box 10.11.b Relevant expectations for conduct of intervention reviews

C68: Interpreting subgroup analyses (**Mandatory**)

If subgroup analyses are conducted, *follow the subgroup analysis plan specified in the protocol without undue emphasis on particular findings.*	Selective reporting, or over-interpretation, of particular subgroups or particular subgroup analyses should be avoided. This is a problem especially when multiple subgroup analyses are performed. This does not preclude the use of sensible and honest post hoc subgroup analyses.

and second by preventing knowledge of the studies' results influencing which subgroups are analysed. True pre-specification is difficult in systematic reviews, because the results of some of the relevant studies are often known when the protocol is drafted. If a characteristic was overlooked in the protocol, but is clearly of major importance and justified by external evidence, then authors should not be reluctant to explore it. However, such post-hoc analyses should be identified as such.

10.11.5.3 Select a small number of characteristics

The likelihood of a false-positive result among subgroup analyses and meta-regression increases with the number of characteristics investigated. It is difficult to suggest a maximum number of characteristics to look at, especially since the number of available studies is unknown in advance. If more than one or two characteristics are investigated it may be sensible to adjust the level of significance to account for making multiple comparisons.

10.11.5.4 Ensure there is scientific rationale for investigating each characteristic

Selection of characteristics should be motivated by biological and clinical hypotheses, ideally supported by evidence from sources other than the included studies. Subgroup analyses using characteristics that are implausible or clinically irrelevant are not likely to be useful and should be avoided. For example, a relationship between intervention effect and year of publication is seldom in itself clinically informative, and if identified runs the risk of initiating a post-hoc data dredge of factors that may have changed over time.

Prognostic factors are those that predict the outcome of a disease or condition, whereas effect modifiers are factors that influence how well an intervention works in affecting the outcome. Confusion between prognostic factors and effect modifiers is common in planning subgroup analyses, especially at the protocol stage. Prognostic factors are not good candidates for subgroup analyses unless they are also believed to modify the effect of intervention. For example, being a smoker may be a strong predictor of mortality within the next ten years, but there may not be reason for it to influence the effect of a drug therapy on mortality (Deeks 1998). Potential effect modifiers may include participant characteristics (age, setting), the precise interventions (dose of active intervention, choice of comparison intervention), how the study was done (length of follow-up) or methodology (design and quality).

10.11.5.5 Be aware that the effect of a characteristic may not always be identified

Many characteristics that might have important effects on how well an intervention works cannot be investigated using subgroup analysis or meta-regression. These are characteristics of participants that might vary substantially within studies, but that can only be summarized at the level of the study. An example is age. Consider a collection of clinical trials involving adults ranging from 18 to 60 years old. There may be a strong relationship between age and intervention effect that is apparent within each study. However, if the mean ages for the trials are similar, then no relationship will be apparent by looking at trial mean ages and trial-level effect estimates. The problem is one of aggregating individuals' results and is variously known as aggregation bias, ecological bias or the ecological fallacy (Morgenstern 1982, Greenland 1987, Berlin et al 2002). It is even possible for the direction of the relationship across studies be the opposite of the direction of the relationship observed within each study.

10.11.5.6 Think about whether the characteristic is closely related to another characteristic (confounded)

The problem of 'confounding' complicates interpretation of subgroup analyses and meta-regressions and can lead to incorrect conclusions. Two characteristics are confounded if their influences on the intervention effect cannot be disentangled. For example, if those studies implementing an intensive version of a therapy happened to be the studies that involved patients with more severe disease, then one cannot tell which aspect is the cause of any difference in effect estimates between these studies and others. In meta-regression, co-linearity between potential effect modifiers leads to similar difficulties (Berlin and Antman 1994). Computing correlations between study characteristics will give some information about which study characteristics may be confounded with each other.

10.11.6 Interpretation of subgroup analyses and meta-regressions

Appropriate interpretation of subgroup analyses and meta-regressions requires caution (Oxman and Guyatt 1992).

1) *Subgroup comparisons are observational.* It must be remembered that subgroup analyses and meta-regressions are entirely observational in their nature. These analyses investigate differences between studies. Even if individuals are randomized to one group or other within a clinical trial, they are not randomized to go in one trial or another. Hence, subgroup analyses suffer the limitations of any observational investigation, including possible bias through confounding by other study-level characteristics. Furthermore, even a genuine difference between subgroups is not necessarily due to the classification of the subgroups. As an example, a subgroup analysis of bone marrow transplantation for treating leukaemia might show a strong association between the age of a sibling donor and the success of the transplant. However, this probably does not mean that the age of donor is important.

In fact, the age of the recipient is probably a key factor and the subgroup finding would simply be due to the strong association between the age of the recipient and the age of their sibling.

2) *Was the analysis pre-specified or post hoc?* Authors should state whether subgroup analyses were pre-specified or undertaken after the results of the studies had been compiled (post hoc). More reliance may be placed on a subgroup analysis if it was one of a small number of pre-specified analyses. Performing numerous post-hoc subgroup analyses to explain heterogeneity is a form of data dredging. Data dredging is condemned because it is usually possible to find an apparent, but false, explanation for heterogeneity by considering lots of different characteristics.
3) *Is there indirect evidence in support of the findings?* Differences between subgroups should be clinically plausible and supported by other external or indirect evidence, if they are to be convincing.
4) *Is the magnitude of the difference practically important?* If the magnitude of a difference between subgroups will not result in different recommendations for different subgroups, then it may be better to present only the overall analysis results.
5) *Is there a statistically significant difference between subgroups?* To establish whether there is a different effect of an intervention in different situations, the magnitudes of effects in different subgroups should be compared directly with each other. In particular, statistical significance of the results within separate subgroup analyses should not be compared (see Section 10.11.3.1).
6) *Are analyses looking at within-study or between-study relationships?* For patient and intervention characteristics, differences in subgroups that are observed within studies are more reliable than analyses of subsets of studies. If such within-study relationships are replicated across studies then this adds confidence to the findings.

10.11.7 Investigating the effect of underlying risk

One potentially important source of heterogeneity among a series of studies is when the underlying average risk of the outcome event varies between the studies. The underlying risk of a particular event may be viewed as an aggregate measure of case-mix factors such as age or disease severity. It is generally measured as the observed risk of the event in the comparator group of each study (the comparator group risk, or CGR). The notion is controversial in its relevance to clinical practice since underlying risk represents a summary of both known and unknown risk factors. Problems also arise because comparator group risk will depend on the length of follow-up, which often varies across studies. However, underlying risk has received particular attention in meta-analysis because the information is readily available once dichotomous data have been prepared for use in meta-analyses. Sharp provides a full discussion of the topic (Sharp 2001).

Intuition would suggest that participants are more or less likely to benefit from an effective intervention according to their risk status. However, the relationship between underlying risk and intervention effect is a complicated issue. For example, suppose an intervention is equally beneficial in the sense that for all patients it reduces the risk of an event, say a stroke, to 80% of the underlying risk. Then it is not equally beneficial in terms of absolute differences in risk in the sense that it reduces a 50% stroke rate by 10 percentage points to 40% (number needed to treat = 10), but a 20% stroke rate by 4 percentage points to 16% (number needed to treat = 25).

Use of different summary statistics (risk ratio, odds ratio and risk difference) will demonstrate different relationships with underlying risk. Summary statistics that show close to no relationship with underlying risk are generally preferred for use in meta-analysis (see Section 10.4.3).

Investigating any relationship between effect estimates and the comparator group risk is also complicated by a technical phenomenon known as regression to the mean. This arises because the comparator group risk forms an integral part of the effect estimate. A high risk in a comparator group, observed entirely by chance, will on average give rise to a higher than expected effect estimate, and vice versa. This phenomenon results in a false correlation between effect estimates and comparator group risks. There are methods, which require sophisticated software, that correct for regression to the mean (McIntosh 1996, Thompson et al 1997). These should be used for such analyses, and statistical expertise is recommended.

10.11.8 Dose-response analyses

The principles of meta-regression can be applied to the relationships between intervention effect and dose (commonly termed dose-response), treatment intensity or treatment duration (Greenland and Longnecker 1992, Berlin et al 1993). Conclusions about differences in effect due to differences in dose (or similar factors) are on stronger ground if participants are randomized to one dose or another within a study and a consistent relationship is found across similar studies. While authors should consider these effects, particularly as a possible explanation for heterogeneity, they should be cautious about drawing conclusions based on between-study differences. Authors should be particularly cautious about claiming that a dose-response relationship does not exist, given the low power of many meta-regression analyses to detect genuine relationships.

10.12 Missing data

10.12.1 Types of missing data

There are many potential sources of missing data in a systematic review or meta-analysis (see Table 10.12.a). For example, a whole study may be missing from the review, an outcome may be missing from a study, summary data may be missing for an outcome, and individual participants may be missing from the summary data. Here we discuss a variety of potential sources of missing data, highlighting where more detailed discussions are available elsewhere in the *Handbook*.

Whole **studies** may be missing from a review because they are never published, are published in obscure places, are rarely cited, or are inappropriately indexed in databases. Thus, review authors should always be aware of the possibility that they have failed to identify relevant studies. There is a strong possibility that such studies are missing because of their 'uninteresting' or 'unwelcome' findings (that is, in the presence

Table 10.12.a Types of missing data in a meta-analysis

Type of missing data	Some possible reasons for missing data
Missing studies	Publication bias Search not sufficiently comprehensive
Missing outcomes	Outcome not measured Selective reporting bias
Missing summary data	Selective reporting bias Incomplete reporting
Missing individuals	Lack of intention-to-treat analysis Attrition from the study Selective reporting bias
Missing study-level characteristics (for subgroup analysis or meta-regression)	Characteristic not measured Incomplete reporting

of publication bias). This problem is discussed at length in Chapter 13. Details of comprehensive search methods are provided in Chapter 4.

Some studies might not report any information on **outcomes** of interest to the review. For example, there may be no information on quality of life, or on serious adverse effects. It is often difficult to determine whether this is because the outcome was not measured or because the outcome was not reported. Furthermore, failure to report that outcomes were measured may be dependent on the unreported results (selective outcome reporting bias; see Chapter 7, Section 7.2.3.3). Similarly, **summary data** for an outcome, in a form that can be included in a meta-analysis, may be missing. A common example is missing standard deviations (SDs) for continuous outcomes. This is often a problem when change-from-baseline outcomes are sought. We discuss imputation of missing SDs in Chapter 6 (Section 6.5.2.8). Other examples of missing summary data are missing sample sizes (particularly those for each intervention group separately), numbers of events, standard errors, follow-up times for calculating rates, and sufficient details of time-to-event outcomes. Inappropriate analyses of studies, for example of cluster-randomized and crossover trials, can lead to missing summary data. It is sometimes possible to approximate the correct analyses of such studies, for example by imputing correlation coefficients or SDs, as discussed in Chapter 23 (Section 23.1) for cluster-randomized studies and Chapter 23 (Section 23.2) for cross-over trials. As a general rule, most methodologists believe that missing summary data (e.g. 'no usable data') should not be used as a reason to exclude a study from a systematic review. It is more appropriate to include the study in the review, and to discuss the potential implications of its absence from a meta-analysis.

It is likely that in some, if not all, included studies, there will be **individuals** missing from the reported results. Review authors are encouraged to consider this problem

MECIR Box 10.12.a Relevant expectations for conduct of intervention reviews	
C64: Addressing missing outcome data (**Highly desirable**)	
Consider the implications of missing outcome data from individual participants (due to losses to follow-up or exclusions from analysis).	Incomplete outcome data can introduce bias. In most circumstances, authors should follow the principles of intention-to-treat analyses as far as possible (this may not be appropriate for adverse effects or if trying to demonstrate equivalence). Risk of bias due to incomplete outcome data is addressed in the Cochrane risk-of-bias tool. However, statistical analyses and careful interpretation of results are additional ways in which the issue can be addressed by review authors. Imputation methods can be considered (accompanied by, or in the form of, sensitivity analyses).

carefully (see MECIR Box 10.12.a). We provide further discussion of this problem in Section 10.12.3; see also Chapter 8 (Section 8.5).

Missing data can also affect subgroup analyses. If subgroup analyses or meta-regressions are planned (see Section 10.11), they require details of the **study-level characteristics** that distinguish studies from one another. If these are not available for all studies, review authors should consider asking the study authors for more information.

10.12.2 General principles for dealing with missing data

There is a large literature of statistical methods for dealing with missing data. Here we briefly review some key concepts and make some general recommendations for Cochrane Review authors. It is important to think *why* data may be missing. Statisticians often use the terms 'missing at random' and 'not missing at random' to represent different scenarios.

Data are said to be 'missing at random' if the fact that they are missing is unrelated to actual values of the missing data. For instance, if some quality-of-life questionnaires were lost in the postal system, this would be unlikely to be related to the quality of life of the trial participants who completed the forms. In some circumstances, statisticians distinguish between data 'missing at random' and data 'missing completely at random', although in the context of a systematic review the distinction is unlikely to be important. Data that are missing at random may not be important. Analyses based on the available data will often be unbiased, although based on a smaller sample size than the original data set.

Data are said to be 'not missing at random' if the fact that they are missing is related to the actual missing data. For instance, in a depression trial, participants who had a relapse of depression might be less likely to attend the final follow-up interview, and more likely to have missing outcome data. Such data are 'non-ignorable' in the sense that an analysis of the available data alone will typically be biased. Publication bias and selective reporting bias lead by definition to data that are 'not missing at random', and attrition and exclusions of individuals within studies often do as well.

The principal options for dealing with missing data are:

1) analysing only the available data (i.e. ignoring the missing data);
2) imputing the missing data with replacement values, and treating these as if they were observed (e.g. last observation carried forward, imputing an assumed outcome such as assuming all were poor outcomes, imputing the mean, imputing based on predicted values from a regression analysis);
3) imputing the missing data and accounting for the fact that these were imputed with uncertainty (e.g. multiple imputation, simple imputation methods (as point 2) with adjustment to the standard error); and
4) using statistical models to allow for missing data, making assumptions about their relationships with the available data.

Option 2 is practical in most circumstances and very commonly used in systematic reviews. However, it fails to acknowledge uncertainty in the imputed values and results, typically, in confidence intervals that are too narrow. Options 3 and 4 would require involvement of a knowledgeable statistician.

Five general recommendations for dealing with missing data in Cochrane Reviews are as follows.

- Whenever possible, contact the original investigators to request missing data.
- Make explicit the assumptions of any methods used to address missing data: for example, that the data are assumed missing at random, or that missing values were assumed to have a particular value such as a poor outcome.
- Follow the guidance in Chapter 8 to assess risk of bias due to missing outcome data in randomized trials.
- Perform sensitivity analyses to assess how sensitive results are to reasonable changes in the assumptions that are made (see Section 10.14).
- Address the potential impact of missing data on the findings of the review in the Discussion section.

10.12.3 Dealing with missing outcome data from individual participants

Review authors may undertake sensitivity analyses to assess the potential impact of missing outcome data, based on assumptions about the relationship between missingness in the outcome and its true value. Several methods are available (Akl et al 2015). For dichotomous outcomes, Higgins and colleagues propose a strategy involving different assumptions about how the risk of the event among the missing participants differs from the risk of the event among the observed participants, taking account of uncertainty introduced by the assumptions (Higgins et al 2008a). Akl and colleagues propose a suite of simple imputation methods, including a similar approach to that of Higgins and colleagues based on relative risks of the event in missing versus observed participants. Similar ideas can be applied to continuous outcome data (Ebrahim et al 2013, Ebrahim et al 2014). Particular care is required to avoid double counting events, since it can be unclear whether reported numbers of events in trial reports apply to the full randomized sample or only to those who did not drop out (Akl et al 2016).

Although there is a tradition of implementing 'worst case' and 'best case' analyses clarifying the extreme boundaries of what is theoretically possible, such analyses may not be informative for the most plausible scenarios (Higgins et al 2008a).

10.13 Bayesian approaches to meta-analysis

Bayesian statistics is an approach to statistics based on a different philosophy from that which underlies significance tests and confidence intervals. It is essentially about updating of evidence. In a Bayesian analysis, initial uncertainty is expressed through a **prior distribution** about the quantities of interest. Current data and assumptions concerning how they were generated are summarized in the **likelihood**. The **posterior distribution** for the quantities of interest can then be obtained by combining the prior distribution and the likelihood. The likelihood summarizes both the data from studies included in the meta-analysis (for example, 2 × 2 tables from randomized trials) and the meta-analysis model (for example, assuming a fixed effect or random effects). The result of the analysis is usually presented as a point estimate and 95% credible interval from the posterior distribution for each quantity of interest, which look much like classical estimates and confidence intervals. Potential advantages of Bayesian analyses are summarized in Box 10.13.a. Bayesian analysis may be performed using WinBUGS software (Smith et al 1995, Lunn et al 2000), within R (Röver 2017), or – for some applications – using standard meta-regression software with a simple trick (Rhodes et al 2016).

A difference between Bayesian analysis and classical meta-analysis is that the interpretation is directly in terms of belief: a 95% credible interval for an odds ratio is that region in which we believe the odds ratio to lie with probability 95%. This is how many

Box 10.13.a Some potential advantages of Bayesian meta-analysis

Some potential advantages of Bayesian approaches over classical methods for meta-analyses are that they:

- incorporate external evidence, such as on the effects of interventions or the likely extent of among-study variation;
- extend a meta-analysis to decision-making contexts, by incorporating the notion of the *utility* of various clinical outcome states;
- allow naturally for the imprecision in the estimated between-study variance estimate (see Section 10.10.4);
- investigate the relationship between underlying risk and treatment benefit (see Section 10.11.7);
- perform complex analyses (e.g. network meta-analysis: see Chapter 11); and
- examine the extent to which data would change people's beliefs (Higgins and Thompson 2002).

practitioners actually interpret a classical confidence interval, but strictly in the classical framework the 95% refers to the long-term frequency with which 95% intervals contain the true value. The Bayesian framework also allows a review author to calculate the probability that the odds ratio has a particular range of values, which cannot be done in the classical framework. For example, we can determine the probability that the odds ratio is less than 1 (which might indicate a beneficial effect of an experimental intervention), or that it is no larger than 0.8 (which might indicate a clinically important effect). It should be noted that these probabilities are specific to the choice of the prior distribution. Different meta-analysts may analyse the same data using different prior distributions and obtain different results. It is therefore important to carry out sensitivity analyses to investigate how the results depend on any assumptions made.

In the context of a meta-analysis, prior distributions are needed for the particular intervention effect being analysed (such as the odds ratio or the mean difference) and – in the context of a random-effects meta-analysis – on the amount of heterogeneity among intervention effects across studies. Prior distributions may represent subjective belief about the size of the effect, or may be derived from sources of evidence not included in the meta-analysis, such as information from non-randomized studies of the same intervention or from randomized trials of other interventions. The width of the prior distribution reflects the degree of uncertainty about the quantity. When there is little or no information, a 'non-informative' prior can be used, in which all values across the possible range are equally likely.

Most Bayesian meta-analyses use non-informative (or very weakly informative) prior distributions to represent beliefs about intervention effects, since many regard it as controversial to combine objective trial data with subjective opinion. However, prior distributions are increasingly used for the extent of among-study variation in a random-effects analysis. This is particularly advantageous when the number of studies in the meta-analysis is small, say fewer than five or ten. Libraries of data-based prior distributions are available that have been derived from re-analyses of many thousands of meta-analyses in the *Cochrane Database of Systematic Reviews* (Turner et al 2012).

Statistical expertise is strongly recommended for review authors who wish to carry out Bayesian analyses. There are several good texts (Sutton et al 2000, Sutton and Abrams 2001, Spiegelhalter et al 2004).

10.14 Sensitivity analyses

The process of undertaking a systematic review involves a sequence of decisions. Whilst many of these decisions are clearly objective and non-contentious, some will be somewhat arbitrary or unclear. For instance, if eligibility criteria involve a numerical value, the choice of value is usually arbitrary: for example, defining groups of older people may reasonably have lower limits of 60, 65, 70 or 75 years, or any value in between. Other decisions may be unclear because a study report fails to include the required information. Some decisions are unclear because the included studies themselves never obtained the information required: for example, the outcomes of those who were lost to follow-up. Further decisions are unclear because there is no consensus on the best statistical method to use for a particular problem.

MECIR Box 10.14.a Relevant expectations for conduct of intervention reviews	
C71: Sensitivity analysis (**Highly desirable**)	
Use sensitivity analyses to assess the robustness of results, such as the impact of notable assumptions, imputed data, borderline decisions and studies at high risk of bias.	It is important to be aware when results are robust, since the strength of the conclusion may be strengthened or weakened.

It is highly desirable to prove that the findings from a systematic review are not dependent on such arbitrary or unclear decisions by using sensitivity analysis (see MECIR Box 10.14.a). A sensitivity analysis is a repeat of the primary analysis or meta-analysis in which alternative decisions or ranges of values are substituted for decisions that were arbitrary or unclear. For example, if the eligibility of some studies in the meta-analysis is dubious because they do not contain full details, sensitivity analysis may involve undertaking the meta-analysis twice: the first time including all studies and, second, including only those that are definitely known to be eligible. A sensitivity analysis asks the question, 'Are the findings robust to the decisions made in the process of obtaining them?'

There are many decision nodes within the systematic review process that can generate a need for a sensitivity analysis. Examples include:

Searching for studies:

1) Should abstracts whose results cannot be confirmed in subsequent publications be included in the review?

Eligibility criteria:

1) Characteristics of participants: where a majority but not all people in a study meet an age range, should the study be included?
2) Characteristics of the intervention: what range of doses should be included in the meta-analysis?
3) Characteristics of the comparator: what criteria are required to define usual care to be used as a comparator group?
4) Characteristics of the outcome: what time point or range of time points are eligible for inclusion?
5) Study design: should blinded and unblinded outcome assessment be included, or should study inclusion be restricted by other aspects of methodological criteria?

What data should be analysed?

1) Time-to-event data: what assumptions of the distribution of censored data should be made?
2) Continuous data: where standard deviations are missing, when and how should they be imputed? Should analyses be based on change scores or on post-intervention values?

3) Ordinal scales: what cut-point should be used to dichotomize short ordinal scales into two groups?
4) Cluster-randomized trials: what values of the intraclass correlation coefficient should be used when trial analyses have not been adjusted for clustering?
5) Crossover trials: what values of the within-subject correlation coefficient should be used when this is not available in primary reports?
6) All analyses: what assumptions should be made about missing outcomes? Should adjusted or unadjusted estimates of intervention effects be used?

Analysis methods:

1) Should fixed-effect or random-effects methods be used for the analysis?
2) For dichotomous outcomes, should odds ratios, risk ratios or risk differences be used?
3) For continuous outcomes, where several scales have assessed the same dimension, should results be analysed as a standardized mean difference across all scales or as mean differences individually for each scale?

Some sensitivity analyses can be pre-specified in the study protocol, but many issues suitable for sensitivity analysis are only identified during the review process where the individual peculiarities of the studies under investigation are identified. When sensitivity analyses show that the overall result and conclusions are not affected by the different decisions that could be made during the review process, the results of the review can be regarded with a higher degree of certainty. Where sensitivity analyses identify particular decisions or missing information that greatly influence the findings of the review, greater resources can be deployed to try and resolve uncertainties and obtain extra information, possibly through contacting trial authors and obtaining individual participant data. If this cannot be achieved, the results must be interpreted with an appropriate degree of caution. Such findings may generate proposals for further investigations and future research.

Reporting of sensitivity analyses in a systematic review may best be done by producing a summary table. Rarely is it informative to produce individual forest plots for each sensitivity analysis undertaken.

Sensitivity analyses are sometimes confused with subgroup analysis. Although some sensitivity analyses involve restricting the analysis to a subset of the totality of studies, the two methods differ in two ways. First, sensitivity analyses do not attempt to estimate the effect of the intervention in the group of studies removed from the analysis, whereas in subgroup analyses, estimates are produced for each subgroup. Second, in sensitivity analyses, informal comparisons are made between different ways of estimating the same thing, whereas in subgroup analyses, formal statistical comparisons are made across the subgroups.

10.15 Chapter information

Editors: Jonathan J Deeks, Julian PT Higgins, Douglas G Altman; on behalf of the Cochrane Statistical Methods Group

Contributing authors: Douglas Altman, Deborah Ashby, Jacqueline Birks, Michael Borenstein, Marion Campbell, Jonathan Deeks, Matthias Egger, Julian Higgins,

Joseph Lau, Keith O'Rourke, Gerta Rücker, Rob Scholten, Jonathan Sterne, Simon Thompson, Anne Whitehead

Acknowledgements: We are grateful to the following for commenting helpfully on earlier drafts: Bodil Als-Nielsen, Deborah Ashby, Jesse Berlin, Joseph Beyene, Jacqueline Birks, Michael Bracken, Marion Campbell, Chris Cates, Wendong Chen, Mike Clarke, Albert Cobos, Esther Coren, Francois Curtin, Roberto D'Amico, Keith Dear, Heather Dickinson, Diana Elbourne, Simon Gates, Paul Glasziou, Christian Gluud, Peter Herbison, Sally Hollis, David Jones, Steff Lewis, Tianjing Li, Joanne McKenzie, Philippa Middleton, Nathan Pace, Craig Ramsey, Keith O'Rourke, Rob Scholten, Guido Schwarzer, Jack Sinclair, Jonathan Sterne, Simon Thompson, Andy Vail, Clarine van Oel, Paula Williamson and Fred Wolf.

Funding: JJD received support from the National Institute for Health Research (NIHR) Birmingham Biomedical Research Centre at the University Hospitals Birmingham NHS Foundation Trust and the University of Birmingham. JPTH is a member of the NIHR Biomedical Research Centre at University Hospitals Bristol NHS Foundation Trust and the University of Bristol. JPTH received funding from National Institute for Health Research Senior Investigator award NF-SI-0617-10145. The views expressed are those of the author(s) and not necessarily those of the NHS, the NIHR or the Department of Health.

10.16 References

Agresti A. *An Introduction to Categorical Data Analysis*. New York (NY): John Wiley & Sons; 1996.

Akl EA, Kahale LA, Agoritsas T, Brignardello-Petersen R, Busse JW, Carrasco-Labra A, Ebrahim S, Johnston BC, Neumann I, Sola I, Sun X, Vandvik P, Zhang Y, Alonso-Coello P, Guyatt G. Handling trial participants with missing outcome data when conducting a meta-analysis: a systematic survey of proposed approaches. *Systematic Reviews* 2015; **4**: 98.

Akl EA, Kahale LA, Ebrahim S, Alonso-Coello P, Schünemann HJ, Guyatt GH. Three challenges described for identifying participants with missing data in trials reports, and potential solutions suggested to systematic reviewers. *Journal of Clinical Epidemiology* 2016; **76**: 147–154.

Altman DG, Bland JM. Detecting skewness from summary information. *BMJ* 1996; **313**: 1200.

Anzures-Cabrera J, Sarpatwari A, Higgins JPT. Expressing findings from meta-analyses of continuous outcomes in terms of risks. *Statistics in Medicine* 2011; **30**: 2967–2985.

Berlin JA, Longnecker MP, Greenland S. Meta-analysis of epidemiologic dose-response data. *Epidemiology* 1993; **4**: 218–228.

Berlin JA, Antman EM. Advantages and limitations of metaanalytic regressions of clinical trials data. *Online Journal of Current Clinical Trials* 1994; **Doc No 134**.

Berlin JA, Santanna J, Schmid CH, Szczech LA, Feldman KA, Group A-LAITS. Individual patient-versus group-level data meta-regressions for the investigation of treatment effect modifiers: ecological bias rears its ugly head. *Statistics in Medicine* 2002; **21**: 371–387.

Borenstein M, Hedges LV, Higgins JPT, Rothstein HR. A basic introduction to fixed-effect and random-effects models for meta-analysis. *Research Synthesis Methods* 2010; **1**: 97–111.

Borenstein M, Higgins JPT. Meta-analysis and subgroups. *Prevention Science* 2013; **14**: 134–143.

Bradburn MJ, Deeks JJ, Berlin JA, Russell Localio A. Much ado about nothing: a comparison of the performance of meta-analytical methods with rare events. *Statistics in Medicine* 2007; **26**: 53–77.

Chinn S. A simple method for converting an odds ratio to effect size for use in meta-analysis. *Statistics in Medicine* 2000; **19**: 3127–3131.

da Costa BR, Nuesch E, Rutjes AW, Johnston BC, Reichenbach S, Trelle S, Guyatt GH, Jüni P. Combining follow-up and change data is valid in meta-analyses of continuous outcomes: a meta-epidemiological study. *Journal of Clinical Epidemiology* 2013; **66**: 847–855.

Deeks JJ. Systematic reviews of published evidence: miracles or minefields? *Annals of Oncology* 1998; **9**: 703–709.

Deeks JJ, Altman DG, Bradburn MJ. Statistical methods for examining heterogeneity and combining results from several studies in meta-analysis. In: Egger M, Davey Smith G, Altman DG, editors. *Systematic Reviews in Health Care: Meta-analysis in Context*. 2nd ed. London (UK): BMJ Publication Group; 2001. p. 285–312.

Deeks JJ. Issues in the selection of a summary statistic for meta-analysis of clinical trials with binary outcomes. *Statistics in Medicine* 2002; **21**: 1575–1600.

DerSimonian R, Laird N. Meta-analysis in clinical trials. *Controlled Clinical Trials* 1986; **7**: 177–188.

DiGuiseppi C, Higgins JPT. Interventions for promoting smoke alarm ownership and function. *Cochrane Database of Systematic Reviews* 2001; **2**: CD002246.

Ebrahim S, Akl EA, Mustafa RA, Sun X, Walter SD, Heels-Ansdell D, Alonso-Coello P, Johnston BC, Guyatt GH. Addressing continuous data for participants excluded from trial analysis: a guide for systematic reviewers. *Journal of Clinical Epidemiology* 2013; **66**: 1014–1021 e1011.

Ebrahim S, Johnston BC, Akl EA, Mustafa RA, Sun X, Walter SD, Heels-Ansdell D, Alonso-Coello P, Guyatt GH. Addressing continuous data measured with different instruments for participants excluded from trial analysis: a guide for systematic reviewers. *Journal of Clinical Epidemiology* 2014; **67**: 560–570.

Efthimiou O. Practical guide to the meta-analysis of rare events. *Evidence-Based Mental Health* 2018; **21**: 72–76.

Egger M, Davey Smith G, Schneider M, Minder C. Bias in meta-analysis detected by a simple, graphical test. *BMJ* 1997; **315**: 629–634.

Engels EA, Schmid CH, Terrin N, Olkin I, Lau J. Heterogeneity and statistical significance in meta-analysis: an empirical study of 125 meta-analyses. *Statistics in Medicine* 2000; **19**: 1707–1728.

Greenland S, Robins JM. Estimation of a common effect parameter from sparse follow-up data. *Biometrics* 1985; **41**: 55–68.

Greenland S. Quantitative methods in the review of epidemiologic literature. *Epidemiologic Reviews* 1987; **9**: 1–30.

Greenland S, Longnecker MP. Methods for trend estimation from summarized dose-response data, with applications to meta-analysis. *American Journal of Epidemiology* 1992; **135**: 1301–1309.

Guevara JP, Berlin JA, Wolf FM. Meta-analytic methods for pooling rates when follow-up duration varies: a case study. *BMC Medical Research Methodology* 2004; **4**: 17.

Hartung J, Knapp G. A refined method for the meta-analysis of controlled clinical trials with binary outcome. *Statistics in Medicine* 2001; **20**: 3875–3889.

Hasselblad V, McCrory DC. Meta-analytic tools for medical decision making: a practical guide. *Medical Decision Making* 1995; **15**: 81–96.

Higgins JPT, Thompson SG. Quantifying heterogeneity in a meta-analysis. *Statistics in Medicine* 2002; **21**: 1539–1558.

Higgins JPT, Thompson SG, Deeks JJ, Altman DG. Measuring inconsistency in meta-analyses. *BMJ* 2003; **327**: 557–560.

Higgins JPT, Thompson SG. Controlling the risk of spurious findings from meta-regression. *Statistics in Medicine* 2004;**23**: 1663–1682.

Higgins JPT, White IR, Wood AM. Imputation methods for missing outcome data in meta-analysis of clinical trials. *Clinical Trials* 2008a; **5**: 225–239.

Higgins JPT, White IR, Anzures-Cabrera J. Meta-analysis of skewed data: combining results reported on log-transformed or raw scales. *Statistics in Medicine* 2008b; **27**: 6072–6092.

Higgins JPT, Thompson SG, Spiegelhalter DJ. A re-evaluation of random-effects meta-analysis. *Journal of the Royal Statistical Society: Series A (Statistics in Society)* 2009; **172**: 137–159.

Kjaergard LL, Villumsen J, Gluud C. Reported methodologic quality and discrepancies between large and small randomized trials in meta-analyses. *Annals of Internal Medicine* 2001; **135**: 982–989.

Langan D, Higgins JPT, Simmonds M. An empirical comparison of heterogeneity variance estimators in 12 894 meta-analyses. *Research Synthesis Methods* 2015; **6**: 195–205.

Langan D, Higgins JPT, Simmonds M. Comparative performance of heterogeneity variance estimators in meta-analysis: a review of simulation studies. *Research Synthesis Methods* 2017; **8**: 181–198.

Langan D, Higgins JPT, Jackson D, Bowden J, Veroniki AA, Kontopantelis E, Viechtbauer W, Simmonds M. A comparison of heterogeneity variance estimators in simulated random-effects meta-analyses. *Research Synthesis Methods* 2019; **10**: 83–98.

Lewis S, Clarke M. Forest plots: trying to see the wood and the trees. *BMJ* 2001; **322**: 1479–1480.

Lunn DJ, Thomas A, Best N, Spiegelhalter D. WinBUGS – A Bayesian modelling framework: concepts, structure, and extensibility. *Statistics and Computing* 2000; **10**: 325–337.

Mantel N, Haenszel W. Statistical aspects of the analysis of data from retrospective studies of disease. *Journal of the National Cancer Institute* 1959; **22**: 719–748.

McIntosh MW. The population risk as an explanatory variable in research synthesis of clinical trials. *Statistics in Medicine* 1996; **15**: 1713–1728.

Morgenstern H. Uses of ecologic analysis in epidemiologic research. *American Journal of Public Health* 1982; **72**: 1336–1344.

Oxman AD, Guyatt GH. A consumers guide to subgroup analyses. *Annals of Internal Medicine* 1992; **116**: 78–84.

Peto R, Collins R, Gray R. Large-scale randomized evidence: large, simple trials and overviews of trials. *Journal of Clinical Epidemiology* 1995; **48**: 23–40.

Poole C, Greenland S. Random-effects meta-analyses are not always conservative. *American Journal of Epidemiology* 1999; **150**: 469–475.

Rhodes KM, Turner RM, White IR, Jackson D, Spiegelhalter DJ, Higgins JPT. Implementing informative priors for heterogeneity in meta-analysis using meta-regression and pseudo data. *Statistics in Medicine* 2016; **35**: 5495–5511.

Rice K, Higgins JPT, Lumley T. A re-evaluation of fixed effect(s) meta-analysis. *Journal of the Royal Statistical Society Series A (Statistics in Society)* 2018; **181**: 205–227.

Riley RD, Higgins JPT, Deeks JJ. Interpretation of random effects meta-analyses. *BMJ* 2011; **342**: d549.

Röver C. Bayesian random-effects meta-analysis using the bayesmeta R package 2017. https://arxiv.org/abs/1711.08683.

Rücker G, Schwarzer G, Carpenter J, Olkin I. Why add anything to nothing? The arcsine difference as a measure of treatment effect in meta-analysis with zero cells. *Statistics in Medicine* 2009; **28**: 721–738.

Sharp SJ. Analysing the relationship between treatment benefit and underlying risk: precautions and practical recommendations. In: Egger M, Davey Smith G, Altman DG, editors. *Systematic Reviews in Health Care: Meta-analysis in Context*. 2nd ed. London (UK): BMJ Publication Group; 2001: 176–188.

Sidik K, Jonkman JN. A simple confidence interval for meta-analysis. *Statistics in Medicine* 2002; **21**: 3153–3159.

Simmonds MC, Tierney J, Bowden J, Higgins JPT. Meta-analysis of time-to-event data: a comparison of two-stage methods. *Research Synthesis Methods* 2011; **2**: 139–149.

Sinclair JC, Bracken MB. Clinically useful measures of effect in binary analyses of randomized trials. *Journal of Clinical Epidemiology* 1994; **47**: 881–889.

Smith TC, Spiegelhalter DJ, Thomas A. Bayesian approaches to random-effects meta-analysis: a comparative study. *Statistics in Medicine* 1995; **14**: 2685–2699.

Spiegelhalter DJ, Abrams KR, Myles JP. *Bayesian Approaches to Clinical Trials and Health-Care Evaluation*. Chichester (UK): John Wiley & Sons; 2004.

Spittal MJ, Pirkis J, Gurrin LC. Meta-analysis of incidence rate data in the presence of zero events. *BMC Medical Research Methodology* 2015; **15**: 42.

Sutton AJ, Abrams KR, Jones DR, Sheldon TA, Song F. *Methods for Meta-analysis in Medical Research*. Chichester (UK): John Wiley & Sons; 2000.

Sutton AJ, Abrams KR. Bayesian methods in meta-analysis and evidence synthesis. *Statistical Methods in Medical Research* 2001; **10**: 277–303.

Sweeting MJ, Sutton AJ, Lambert PC. What to add to nothing? Use and avoidance of continuity corrections in meta-analysis of sparse data. *Statistics in Medicine* 2004; **23**: 1351–1375.

Thompson SG, Smith TC, Sharp SJ. Investigating underlying risk as a source of heterogeneity in meta-analysis. *Statistics in Medicine* 1997; **16**: 2741–2758.

Thompson SG, Sharp SJ. Explaining heterogeneity in meta-analysis: a comparison of methods. *Statistics in Medicine* 1999; **18**: 2693–2708.

Thompson SG, Higgins JPT. How should meta-regression analyses be undertaken and interpreted? *Statistics in Medicine* 2002; **21**: 1559–1574.

Turner RM, Davey J, Clarke MJ, Thompson SG, Higgins JPT. Predicting the extent of heterogeneity in meta-analysis, using empirical data from the Cochrane Database of Systematic Reviews. *International Journal of Epidemiology* 2012; **41**: 818–827.

Veroniki AA, Jackson D, Viechtbauer W, Bender R, Bowden J, Knapp G, Kuss O, Higgins JPT, Langan D, Salanti G. Methods to estimate the between-study variance and its uncertainty in meta-analysis. *Research Synthesis Methods* 2016; **7**: 55–79.

Whitehead A, Jones NMB. A meta-analysis of clinical trials involving different classifications of response into ordered categories. *Statistics in Medicine* 1994; **13**: 2503–2515.

Yusuf S, Peto R, Lewis J, Collins R, Sleight P. Beta blockade during and after myocardial infarction: an overview of the randomized trials. *Progress in Cardiovascular Diseases* 1985; **27**: 335–371.

Yusuf S, Wittes J, Probstfield J, Tyroler HA. Analysis and interpretation of treatment effects in subgroups of patients in randomized clinical trials. *JAMA* 1991; **266**: 93–98.

11

Undertaking network meta-analyses

Anna Chaimani, Deborah M Caldwell, Tianjing Li, Julian PT Higgins, Georgia Salanti

KEY POINTS

- Network meta-analysis is a technique for comparing three or more interventions simultaneously in a single analysis by combining both direct and indirect evidence across a network of studies.
- Network meta-analysis produces estimates of the relative effects between any pair of interventions in the network, and usually yields more precise estimates than a single direct or indirect estimate. It also allows estimation of the ranking and hierarchy of interventions.
- A valid network meta-analysis relies on the assumption that the different sets of studies included in the analysis are similar, on average, in all important factors that may affect the relative effects.
- Incoherence (also called inconsistency) occurs when different sources of information (e.g. direct and indirect) about a particular intervention comparison disagree.
- Grading confidence in evidence from a network meta-analysis begins by evaluating confidence in each direct comparison. Domain-specific assessments are combined to determine the overall confidence in the evidence.

11.1 What is network meta-analysis?

Most Cochrane Reviews present comparisons between pairs of interventions (an experimental intervention and a comparator intervention) for a specific condition and in a specific population or setting. However, it is usually the case that several, perhaps even numerous, competing interventions are available for any given condition. People who need to decide between alternative interventions would benefit

This chapter should be cited as: Chaimani A, Caldwell DM, Li T, Higgins JPT, Salanti G. Chapter 11: Undertaking network meta-analyses. In: Higgins JPT, Thomas J, Chandler J, Cumpston M, Li T, Page MJ, Welch VA (editors). *Cochrane Handbook for Systematic Reviews of Interventions*. 2nd Edition. Chichester (UK): John Wiley & Sons, 2019: 285–320.

from a single review that includes all relevant interventions, and presents their comparative effectiveness and potential for harm. Network meta-analysis provides an analysis option for such a review.

Any set of studies that links three or more interventions via direct comparisons forms a **network of interventions**. In a network of interventions there can be multiple ways to make **indirect comparisons** between the interventions. These are comparisons that have not been made directly within studies, and they can be estimated using mathematical combinations of the direct intervention effect estimates available. **Network meta-analysis** combines direct and indirect estimates across a network of interventions in a single analysis. Synonymous terms, less often used, are mixed treatment comparisons and multiple treatments meta-analysis.

11.1.1 Network diagrams

A **network diagram** is a graphical depiction of the structure of a network of interventions (Chaimani et al 2013). It consists of nodes representing the interventions in the network and lines showing the available direct comparisons between pairs of interventions. An example of a network diagram with four interventions is given in Figure 11.1.a. In this example, distinct lines forming a closed triangular loop have been added to illustrate the presence of a three-arm study. Note that for large and complex networks, such presentation of multi-arm studies may give complicated and unhelpful network diagrams; in this case it might be preferable to show multi-arm studies in a tabular format. Further discussion of displaying networks is available in Section 11.6.1.

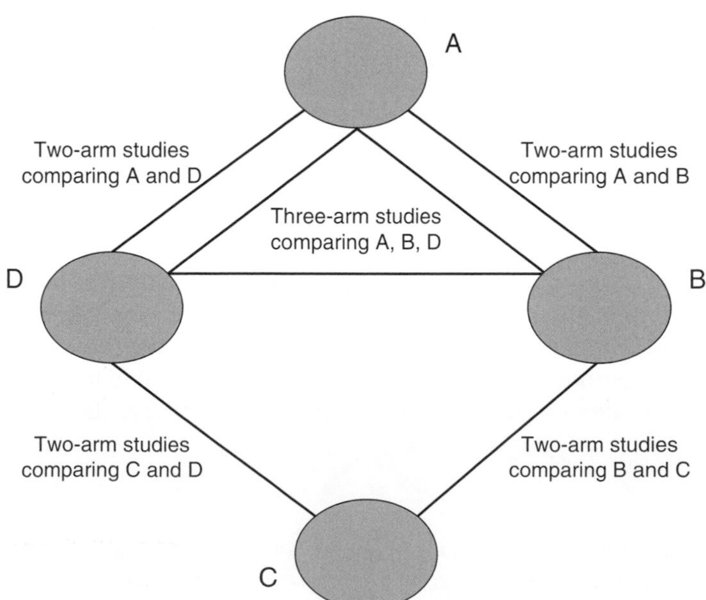

Figure 11.1.a Example of network diagram with four competing interventions and information on the presence of multi-arm randomized trials

11.1.2 Advantages of network meta-analysis

A network meta-analysis exploits all available direct and indirect evidence. Empirical studies have suggested it yields more precise estimates of the intervention effects in comparison with a single direct or indirect estimate (Cooper et al 2011, Caldwell et al 2015). In addition, network meta-analysis can provide information for comparisons between pairs of interventions that have never been evaluated within individual randomized trials. The simultaneous comparison of all interventions of interest in the same analysis enables the estimation of their relative ranking for a given outcome (see Section 11.4.3.3 for more discussion of ranking).

11.1.3 Outline of this chapter

This chapter provides an overview of the concepts, assumptions and methods that relate to network meta-analyses and to the indirect intervention comparisons on which they are built. Section 11.2 first describes what an indirect comparison is and how it can be made in a simple trio of interventions. It then introduces the notion of transitivity (and its statistical analogue, coherence) as the core assumption underlying the validity of an indirect comparison. Examples are provided where this assumption is likely to hold or be violated.

Section 11.3 provides guidance on the design of a Cochrane Review with multiple interventions and the appropriate definition of the research question with respect to selecting studies, outcomes and interventions. Section 11.4 briefly describes the available statistical methods for synthesizing the data, estimating the relative ranking and assessing coherence in a network of interventions. Finally, Sections 11.5 and 11.6 provide approaches for evaluating confidence in the evidence and presenting the evidence base and the results from a network meta-analysis. Note that the chapter only introduces the statistical aspects of network meta-analysis; authors will need a knowledgeable statistician to plan and execute these methods.

11.2 Important concepts

At the heart of network meta-analysis methodology is the concept of an **indirect comparison**. Indirect comparisons are necessary to estimate the relative effect of two interventions when no studies have compared them directly.

11.2.1 Indirect comparisons

Indirect comparisons allow us to estimate the relative effects of two interventions that have not been compared directly within a trial. For example, suppose there are randomized trials directly comparing provision of dietary advice by a dietitian (which we refer to as intervention A) with advice given by a doctor (intervention B). Suppose there are also randomized trials comparing dietary advice given by a dietitian (intervention A) with advice given by a nurse (intervention C). Suppose further that these randomized trials have been combined in standard, pair-wise meta-analyses separately to derive **direct estimates** of intervention effects for *A versus B* (sometimes depicted 'AB')

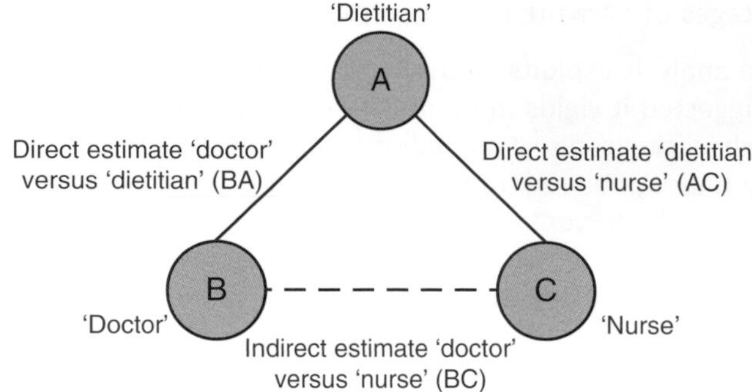

Figure 11.2.a Illustration of an indirect estimate that compares the effectiveness of 'doctor' (B) and 'nurse' (C) in providing dietary advice through a common comparator 'dietitian' (A)

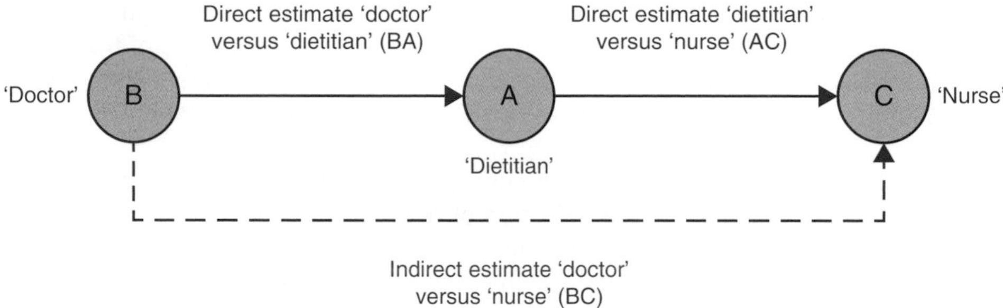

Figure 11.2.b Graphical representation of the indirect comparison 'doctor' (B) versus 'nurse' (C) via 'dietitian' (A)

and *A versus C* ('AC'), measured as mean difference (MD) in weight reduction (see Chapter 6, Section 6.5.1.1). The situation is illustrated in Figure 11.2.a, where the solid straight lines depict available evidence. We wish to learn about the relative effect of advice by a doctor versus a nurse (*B versus C*); the dashed line depicts this comparison, for which there is no direct evidence.

One way to understand an indirect comparison is to think of the BC comparison (of *B versus C*) as representing the benefit of B over C. All else being equal, the benefit of B over C is equivalent to the benefit of B over A plus the benefit of A over C. Thus, for example, the indirect comparison describing benefit of 'doctor' over 'nurse' may be thought of as the benefit of 'doctor' over 'dietitian' plus the benefit of 'dietitian' over 'nurse' (these 'benefits' may be positive or negative; we do not intend to imply any particular superiority among these three types of people offering dietary advice). This is represented graphically in Figure 11.2.b.

Mathematically, the sum can be written:

$$\text{indirect MD}(\text{BvsC}) = \text{direct MD}(\text{BvsA}) + \text{direct MD}(\text{AvsC}).$$

We usually write this in the form of subtraction:

$$\text{indirect MD}(\text{BvsC}) = \text{direct MD}(\text{AvsC}) - \text{direct MD}(\text{AvsB}),$$

such that the difference between the summary statistics of the intervention effect in the direct *A versus C* and *A versus B* meta-analyses provides an indirect estimate of the *B versus C* intervention effect.

For this simple case where we have two direct comparisons (three interventions) the analysis can be conducted by performing subgroup analyses using standard meta-analysis routines (including RevMan): studies addressing the two direct comparisons (i.e. *A versus B* and *A versus C*) can be treated as two subgroups in the meta-analysis. The difference between the summary effects from the two subgroups gives an estimate for the indirect comparison.

Most software will provide a P value for the statistical significance of the difference between the subgroups based on the estimated variance of the indirect effect estimate (Bucher et al 1997):

$$\text{Variance}[\text{indirect MD}(\text{BvsC})] = \text{Variance}[\text{direct MD}(\text{AvsC})] + \text{Variance}[\text{direct MD}(\text{AvsB})],$$

where variance[direct MD(AvsC)] and variance[direct MD(AvsB)] are the variances of the respective direct estimates (from the two subgroup analyses).

A 95% confidence interval for the indirect summary effect is constructed by the formula:

$$\left[\text{indirect MD}(\text{BvsC}) \pm 1.96 \times \sqrt{\text{Variance}[\text{indirect MD}(\text{BvsC})]}\right].$$

This method uses the intervention effects from each group of randomized trials and therefore preserves within-trial randomization. If we had instead pooled single arms across the studies (e.g. all B arms and all C arms, ignoring the A arms) and then performed a direct comparison between the pooled B and C arms (i.e. treating the data as if they came from a single large randomized trial), then our analysis would discard the benefits of within-trial randomization (Li and Dickersin 2013). This approach should not be used.

When four or more competing interventions are available, indirect estimates can be derived via multiple routes. The only requirement is that two interventions are 'connected' and not necessarily via a single common comparator. An example of this situation is provided in Figure 11.2.c. Here 'doctor' (B) and 'pharmacist' (D) do not have a common comparator, but we can compare them indirectly via the route 'doctor' (B) – 'dietitian' (A) – 'nurse' (C) – 'pharmacist (D) by an extension of the arguments set out earlier.

11.2.2 Transitivity

11.2.2.1 Validity of an indirect comparison

The underlying assumption of indirect comparisons is that we can learn about the true relative effect of B versus C via treatment A by combining the true relative effects *A versus B* and *A versus C*. This relationship can be written mathematically as

$$\text{effect of B versus C} = (\text{effect of A versus C}) - (\text{effect of A versus B}).$$

In words, this means that we can compare interventions B and C via intervention A (Figure 11.2.a).

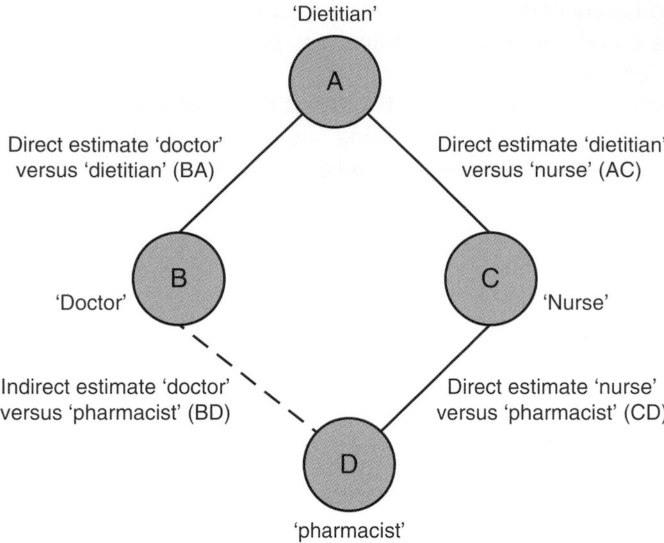

Figure 11.2.c Example of deriving indirect estimate that compares the effectiveness of 'doctor' (B) and 'pharmacist' (D) in providing dietary advice through a connected loop

Indirect comparisons provide observational evidence across randomized trials and may suffer the biases of observational studies, such as confounding (see Chapter 10, Sections 10.11.5 and 10.11.6). The validity of an indirect comparison requires that the different sets of randomized trials are similar, on average, in all important factors other than the intervention comparison being made (Song et al 2003, Glenny et al 2005, Donegan et al 2010, Salanti 2012). We use the term **transitivity** to refer to this requirement. It is closely related to the statistical notion of coherence (see Section 11.2.3.2); the distinction is a little like that between diversity and (statistical) heterogeneity in pair-wise meta-analysis (see Chapter 10, Section 10.10.1).

Studies that compare different interventions may differ in a wide range of characteristics. Sometimes these characteristics are associated with the effect of an intervention. We refer to such characteristics as effect modifiers; they are the aspects of diversity that induce heterogeneity in pairwise meta-analyses. If the *A versus B* and *A versus C* randomized trials differ with respect to their effect modifiers, then it would not be appropriate to make an indirect comparison.

Transitivity requires that intervention A is similar when it appears in *A versus B* studies and *A versus C* studies with respect to characteristics (effect modifiers) that may affect the two relative effects (Salanti et al 2009). For example, in the dietary advice network the common comparator 'dietitian' might differ with respect to the frequency of advice sessions between trials that compare dietitian with doctor (*A versus B*) and trials that compare dietitian with nurse (*A versus C*). If the participants visit the dietitian once a week in AB studies and once a month in AC studies, transitivity may be violated. Similarly, any other effect modifiers should not differ between AB and AC studies.

Transitivity requires all competing interventions of a systematic review to be **jointly randomizable**. That is, we can imagine all interventions being compared simultaneously in a single multi-arm randomized trial. Another way of viewing this is that, in any particular trial, the 'missing' interventions (those not included in trial) may be considered to be missing for reasons unrelated to their effects (Caldwell et al 2005, Salanti 2012).

11.2.2.2 Assessing transitivity

Clinical and methodological differences are inevitable between studies in a systematic review. Researchers undertaking indirect comparisons should assess whether such differences are sufficiently large to induce **intransitivity**. In principle, transitivity can be evaluated by comparing the distribution of effect modifiers across the different comparisons (Salanti 2012, Cipriani et al 2013, Jansen and Naci 2013). Imbalanced distributions would threaten the plausibility of the transitivity assumption and thus the validity of indirect comparison. In practice, however, this requires that the effect modifiers are known and have been measured. There are also some statistical options for assessing whether the transitive relationship holds in some circumstances, which we discuss in Section 11.4.4.

Extended guidance on considerations of potential effect modifiers is provided in discussions of heterogeneity in Chapter 10 (Section 10.11). For example, we may believe that age is a potential effect modifier so that the effect of an intervention differs between younger and older populations. If the average age in *A versus B* randomized trials is substantially older or younger than in *A versus C* randomized trials, transitivity may be implausible, and an indirect comparison *B versus C* may be invalid.

Figure 11.2.d shows hypothetical examples of valid and invalid indirect comparisons for the dietary advice example. Suppose a single effect modifier is severity of disease (e.g. obesity measured by the BMI score). The top row depicts a situation in which all patients in all trials have moderate severity. There are AB studies and AC studies in this population. Estimation of BC is valid here because there is no difference in the effect modifier. The second row depicts a similar situation in a second population of patients who all have severe disease. A valid indirect estimate of *B versus C* for this population can also be made. In the third row we depict a situation in which all AB trials are conducted only in moderately obese populations and all AC trials are conducted only in severely obese populations. In this situation, the distribution of effect modifiers is different in the two direct comparisons, so the indirect effect based on this row is invalid (due to intransitivity).

In practice, differences in effect modifiers are usually less extreme than this hypothetical scenario; for example, AB randomized trials may have 80% moderately obese population and 20% severely obese, and AC randomized trials may have 20% moderately obese and 80% severely obese population. Intransitivity would probably still invalidate the indirect estimate *B versus C* if severity is an important effect modifier.

11.2.3 Indirect comparisons and the validity of network meta-analysis

11.2.3.1 Combining direct and indirect evidence

Often there is direct evidence for a specific comparison of interventions as well as a possibility of making an indirect comparison of the interventions via one or more common comparators. If the key assumption of transitivity is considered reasonable, direct and indirect estimates should be considered jointly. When both direct and indirect intervention effects are available for a particular comparison, these can be synthesized into a single effect estimate. This summary effect is sometimes called a **combined** or

Population with *moderate* disease

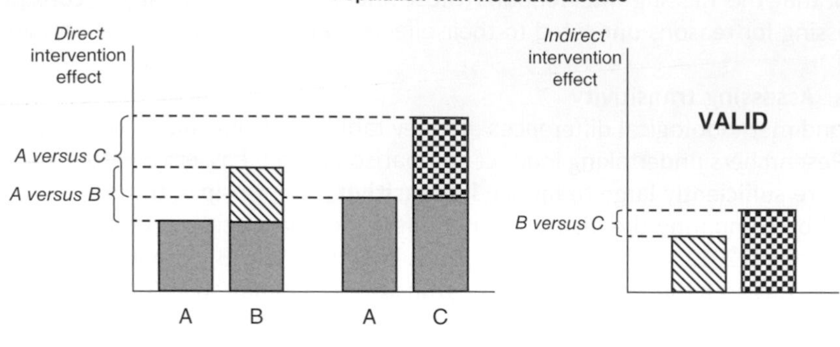

Population with *severe* disease

Direct intervention effect

A versus C

A versus B

A B A C

Indirect intervention effect

VALID

B versus C

Population with *moderate* obesity for *A versus B*
Population with *severe* obesity for *A versus C*

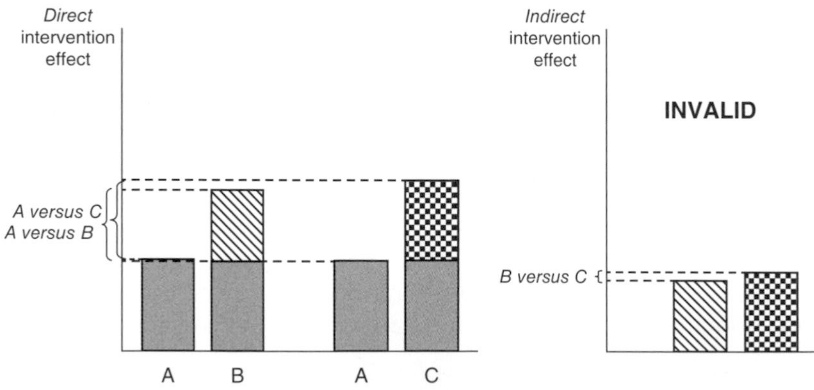

Figure 11.2.d Example of valid and invalid indirect comparisons when the severity of disease acts as effect modifier and its distribution differs between the two direct comparisons. The shaded boxes represent the treatment effect estimates from each source of evidence (striped box for *A versus B* and checked box for *A versus C*). In the first row, randomized trials of *A versus B* and of *A versus C* are all conducted in moderately obese populations; in the second row randomized trials are all conducted in severely obese populations. In both of these the indirect comparisons of the treatment effect estimates would be valid. In the last row, the *A versus B* and *A versus C* randomized trials are conducted in different populations. As severity is an effect modifier, the indirect comparison based on these would not be valid (Jansen et al 2014). Reproduced with permission of Elsevier

mixed estimate of the intervention effect. We will use the former term in this chapter. A combined estimate can be computed as an inverse variance weighted average (see Chapter 10, Section 10.3) of the direct and indirect summary estimates.

Since combined estimates incorporate indirect comparisons, they rely on the transitivity assumption. Violation of transitivity threatens the validity of both indirect and combined estimates. Of course, biased direct intervention effects for any of the comparisons also challenge the validity of a combined effect (Madan et al 2011).

11.2.3.2 Coherence (or consistency)

The key assumption of transitivity relates to potential clinical and methodological variation across the different comparisons. These differences may be reflected in the data in the form of disagreement in estimates between different sources of evidence. The statistical manifestation of transitivity and is typically called either **coherence** or **consistency**. We will use the former to distinguish the notion from inconsistency (or heterogeneity) within standard meta-analyses (e.g. as is measured using the I^2 statistic; see Chapter 10, Section 10.10.2). Coherence implies that the different sources of evidence (direct and indirect) agree with each other.

The coherence assumption is expressed mathematically by the **coherence equations**, which state that the true direct and indirect intervention effects for a specific comparison are identical:

$$\text{'true'MD}(\text{BvsC}) = \text{'true'MD}(\text{AvsC}) - \text{'true'MD}(\text{AvsB}).$$

Some methods for testing this assumption are presented in Section 11.4.4.

11.2.3.3 Validity of network meta-analysis

The validity of network meta-analysis relies on the fulfilment of underlying assumptions. Transitivity should hold for every possible indirect comparison, and coherence should hold in every loop of evidence within the network (see Section 11.4.4). Considerations about heterogeneity within each direct comparison in the network should follow the existing recommendations for standard pair-wise meta-analysis (see Chapter 10, Section 10.10).

11.3 Planning a Cochrane Review to compare multiple interventions

11.3.1 Expertise required in the review team

Because of the complexity of network meta-analysis, it is important to establish a multidisciplinary review team that includes a statistician skilled in network meta-analysis methodology early and throughout. Close collaboration between the statistician and the content area expert is essential to ensure that the studies selected for a network meta-analysis are similar except for the interventions being compared (see Section 11.2.2). Because basic meta-analysis software such as RevMan does not support network meta-analysis, the statistician will have to rely on statistical software packages such as Stata, R, WinBUGS or OpenBUGS for analysis.

11.3.2 The importance of a well-defined research question

Defining the research question of a systematic review that intends to compare multiple interventions should follow the general guidelines described in Chapter 2 and should be stated in the objectives of the review. In this section, we summarize and highlight key issues that are pertinent to systematic review with a network meta-analysis.

Because network meta-analysis could be used to estimate the relative ranking of the included interventions (Salanti et al 2011, Chaimani et al 2013), reviews that aim to rank the competing interventions should specify this in their objectives (Chaimani et al 2017). Review authors should consider obtaining an estimate of relative ranking as a secondary objective to supplement the relative effects. An extended discussion on the relative ranking of interventions is provided in Section 11.4.3.3.

11.3.2.1 Defining the population and choosing the interventions

Populations and interventions often need to be considered together given the potential for intransitivity (see Section 11.2.2). A driving principle is that any eligible participant should be eligible for randomization to any included intervention (Salanti 2012, Jansen and Naci 2013). Review authors should select their target population with this consideration in mind. Particular care is needed in the definition of the eligible interventions, as discussed in Chaimani and colleagues (Chaimani et al 2017). For example, suppose a systematic review aims to compare four chemotherapy regimens for a specific cancer. Regimen (D) is appropriate for stage II patients exclusively and regimen (A) is appropriate for both stage I and stage II patients. The remaining two regimens (B) and (C) are appropriate for stage I patients exclusively. Now suppose A and D were compared in stage II patients, and A, B and C were compared in stage I patients (see Figure 11.3.a). The four interventions forming the network are unlikely to satisfy the transitivity assumption because regimen D is not given to the same patient population as regimens B and C. Thus, a four-arm randomized trial comparing all interventions (A, B, C and D) simultaneously is not a reasonable study to conduct.

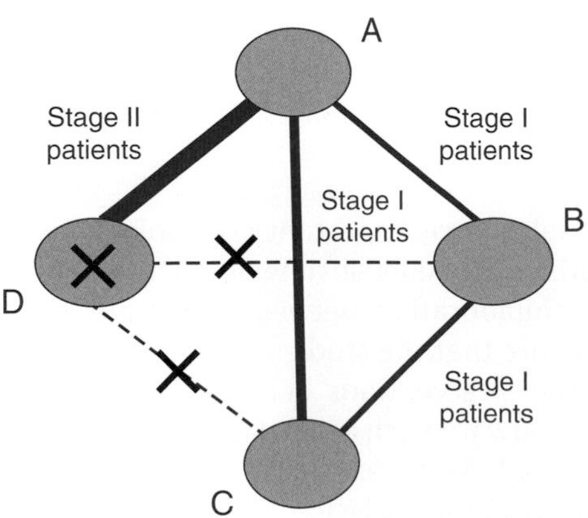

Figure 11.3.a Example of a network comparing four chemotherapy regimens, where transitivity is violated due to incomparability between the interventions

11.3.2.2 Decision sets and supplementary sets of interventions

Usually there is a specific set of interventions of direct interest when planning a network meta-analysis, and these are sometimes referred to as the **decision set**. These are the options among which patients and health professionals would be choosing in practice with respect to the outcomes under investigation. In selecting which competing interventions to include in the decision set, review authors should ensure that the transitivity assumption is likely to hold (see also Section 11.2.2) (Salanti 2012).

The ability of network meta-analysis to incorporate indirect evidence means that inclusion of interventions that are not of direct interest to the review authors might provide additional information in the network. For example, placebo is often included in network meta-analysis even though it is not a reasonable treatment option, because many studies have compared active interventions against placebo. In such cases, excluding placebo would result in ignoring a considerable amount of indirect evidence. Similar considerations apply to historical or legacy interventions.

We use the term **supplementary set** to refer to interventions, such as placebo, that are included in the network meta-analysis for the purpose of improving inference among interventions in the decision set. The full set of interventions, the decision set plus the supplementary set, has been called in the literature the **synthesis comparator set** (Ades et al 2013, Caldwell et al 2015).

When review authors decide to include a supplementary set of interventions in a network, they need to be cautious regarding the plausibility of the transitivity assumption. In general, broadening the network challenges the transitivity assumption. Thus, supplementary interventions should be added when their value outweighs the risk of violating the transitivity assumption. The addition of supplementary interventions in the analysis might be considered more valuable for sparse networks that include only a few trials per comparison. In these networks the benefit of improving the precision of estimates by incorporating supplementary indirect evidence may be quite important. There is limited empirical evidence to inform the decision of how far one should go in constructing the network evidence base (König et al 2013, Caldwell et al 2015). Inevitably it will require some judgement, and the robustness of decisions can be evaluated in sensitivity analyses and discussed in the review.

11.3.2.3 Grouping variants of an intervention (defining nodes in the network diagram)

The definition of nodes needs careful consideration in situations where variants of one or more interventions are expected to appear in the eligible trials (James et al 2018). The appropriateness of merging, for example, different doses of the same drug or different drugs within a class depends to a large extent on the research question. Lumping and splitting the variants of the competing interventions might be interesting to both review authors and evidence users; in such a case this should be stated clearly in the objectives of the review and the potential for intransitivity should be evaluated in every network. A decision on how the nodes of an expanded network could be merged is not always straightforward and researchers should act based on predefined criteria where possible. These criteria should be formed in such a way that maximizes similarity of the interventions within a node and minimizes similarity across nodes.

The following example refers to a network that used two criteria to classify electronic interventions for smoking cessation into five categories: "To be able to draw generalizable conclusions on the different types of electronic interventions, we developed a categorization system that brought similar interventions together in a limited number of categories. We sought advice from experts in smoking cessation on the key dimensions that would influence the effectiveness of smoking cessation programmes. Through this process, two dimensions for evaluating interventions were identified. The first dimension was related to whether the intervention offered generic advice or tailored its feedback to information provided by the user in some way. The second dimension related to whether the intervention used a single channel or multiple channels. From these dimensions, we developed a system with five categories..., ranging from interventions that provide generic information through a single channel, e.g. a static Web site or mass e-mail (category e1) to complex interventions with multiple channels delivering tailored information, e.g. an interactive Web site plus an interactive forum (category e5)" (Madan et al 2014).

Empirical evidence is currently lacking on whether more or less expanded networks are more prone to important intransitivity or incoherence. Extended discussions of how different dosages can be modelled in network meta-analysis are available (Giovane et al 2013, Owen et al 2015, Mawdsley et al 2016).

11.3.2.4 Defining eligible comparisons of interventions (defining lines in the network diagram)

Once the nodes of the network have been specified, every study that meets the eligibility criteria and compares any pair of the eligible interventions should be included in the review. The exclusion of specific direct comparisons without a rationale may introduce bias in the analysis and should be avoided.

11.3.3 Selecting outcomes to examine

In the context of a network meta-analysis, outcomes should be specified a priori regardless of the number of interventions the review intends to compare or the number of studies the review is able to include. Review authors should be aware that some characteristics may be effect modifiers for some outcomes but not for other outcomes. This implies that sometimes the potential for intransitivity should be examined separately for each outcome before undertaking the analyses.

11.3.4 Study designs to include

Randomized designs are generally preferable to non-randomized designs to ensure an increased level of validity of the summary estimates (see Chapter 3, Section 3.3). Sometimes observational data from non-randomized studies may form a useful source of evidence (see Chapter 24). In general, combining randomized with observational studies in a network meta-analysis is not recommended. In the case of sparse networks (i.e. networks with a few studies but many interventions), observational data might be used to supplement the analysis; for example, to form prior knowledge or provide information on baseline characteristics (Schmitz et al 2013, Soares et al 2014).

11.4 Synthesis of results

11.4.1 What does a network meta-analysis estimate?

In a connected network, the coherence equations provide mathematical links between the intervention effects, so that some effects can be computed from others using transitivity assumptions. This means that not all pair-wise comparisons are independently estimated. In fact, the number of comparisons that need to be estimated in a network meta-analysis equals the number of interventions minus one. In practice, we select a particular set of comparisons of this size, and we often label these the **basic comparisons** for the analysis (Lu and Ades 2006). For example, in the network of four interventions for heavy menstrual bleeding illustrated in Figure 11.4.a we might choose the following three basic comparisons: 'Hysterectomy versus first generation hysteroscopic techniques', 'Mirena versus first generation hysteroscopic techniques' and 'second generation non-hysteroscopic techniques versus first generation hysteroscopic techniques'. All other comparisons in the network (e.g. 'Mirena versus hysterectomy', 'Mirena versus second generation non-hysteroscopic techniques', etc.) can be computed from the three basic comparisons.

The main result of a network meta-analysis is a set of **network estimates** of the intervention effects for all basic comparisons. We obtain estimates for the other comparisons after the analysis using the coherence equations (see Section 11.2.3.2). It does not matter which set of comparisons we select as the basic comparisons. Often we would identify one intervention as a reference, and define the basic comparisons as the effect of each of the other interventions against this reference.

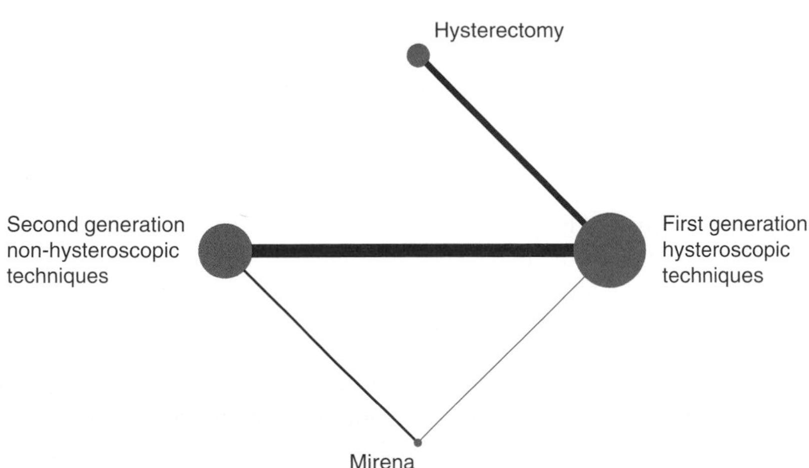

Figure 11.4.a Network graph of four interventions for heavy menstrual bleeding (Middleton et al 2010). The size of the nodes is proportional to the number of participants assigned to the intervention and the thickness of the lines is proportional to the number of randomized trials that studied the respective direct comparison. Reproduced with permission of BMJ Publishing Group

11.4.2 Synthesizing direct and indirect evidence using meta-regression

Network meta-analysis can be performed using several approaches (Salanti et al 2008). The main technical requirement for all approaches is that all interventions included in the analysis form a 'connected' network. A straightforward approach that be used for many networks is to use meta-regression (see Chapter 10, Section 10.11.4). This approach works as long as there are no multi-arm trials in the network (otherwise, other methods are more appropriate).

We introduced indirect comparisons in Section 11.2.1 in the context of subgroup analysis, where the subgroups are defined by the comparisons. Differences between subgroups of studies can also be investigated via meta-regression. When standard meta-regression is used to conduct a single indirect comparison, a single dummy variable is used to specify whether the result of each study relates to one direct comparison or the other (a dummy variable is coded as 1 or 0 to indicate which comparison is made in the study). For example, in the dietary advice network containing only three intervention nodes (see Section 11.2.1, Figure 11.2.a) the dummy variable might be used to indicate the comparison 'dietitian versus nurse'. This variable takes the value 1 for a study that involves that corresponding comparison and 0 if it involves the comparison 'dietitian versus doctor', and is included as a single covariate in the meta-regression. In this way, the meta-regression model would have an intercept and a regression coefficient (slope). The estimated intercept gives the meta-analytic direct summary estimate for the comparison 'dietitian versus doctor' while the sum of the estimated regression coefficient and intercept gives the direct summary estimate for 'dietitian versus nurse'. Consequently, the estimated coefficient is the indirect summary estimate for the comparison 'doctor versus nurse'.

An alternative way to perform the same analysis of an indirect comparison is to re-parameterize the meta-regression model by using two dummy variables and no intercept, instead of one dummy variable and an intercept. The first dummy variable would indicate the comparison 'dietitian versus doctor', and the second the comparison 'dietitian versus nurse'. The estimated regression coefficients then give the summary estimates for these two comparisons, and it is convenient to consider these as the two basic comparisons for this analysis. The difference between the two regression coefficients is the summary estimate for the indirect comparison 'doctor versus nurse'.

The coding of each basic comparison using a dummy variable, and the omission of the intercept, proves to be a useful approach for implementing network meta-analysis using meta-regression, and helps explain the role of the coherence equations. Specifically, suppose now that in the dietary advice example, studies that directly compare 'doctor versus nurse' are also available. Because we are already estimating all of the basic comparisons required for three interventions, we do not require a third dummy variable (under coherence, the comparison 'doctor versus nurse' can be expressed as the difference between the other two comparisons: see Section 11.2.3.2). This means that studies comparing 'doctor versus nurse' inform us about the difference between the two comparisons already in the analysis. Consequently, we need to assign values −1 and 1 to the dummies 'dietitian versus doctor' and 'dietitian versus nurse', respectively. The meta-regression is again fitted including both dummy variables without an intercept. The interpretations of the estimated regression coefficients are the same as for the indirect comparison.

11.4.3 Performing network meta-analysis

We now consider approaches designed specifically for network meta-analysis that can be used when we have multi-arm trials. An overview of methodological developments can be found in Efthimiou and colleagues (Efthimiou et al 2016).

A popular approach to conducting network meta-analysis is using hierarchical models, commonly implemented within a Bayesian framework (Sobieraj et al 2013, Petropoulou et al 2016). Detailed descriptions of hierarchical models for network meta-analysis can be found elsewhere (Lu and Ades 2004, Salanti et al 2008, Dias et al 2018). Software options for a Bayesian approach include WinBUGS and OpenBUGS.

Multivariate meta-analysis methods, initially developed to synthesize multiple outcomes jointly (Jackson et al 2011, Mavridis and Salanti 2013), offer an alternative approach to conducting network meta-analysis. A multivariate meta-analysis approach focuses the analysis on the set of basic comparisons (e.g. each intervention against a common reference intervention) and treats these as analogous to different outcomes. A study can report on one or more of the basic comparisons; for example, there are two comparisons in a three-arm randomized trial. For studies that do not target any of the basic comparisons (e.g. a study that does not include the common reference intervention), a technique known as data augmentation can be used to allow the appropriate parameterization (White et al 2012). The method is implemented in the **network** macro available for Stata (White 2015). A detailed description of the concepts and the implementation of this approach is available (White et al 2012).

Methodology from electrical networks and graphic theory also can be used to fit network meta-analysis and is outlined in by Rücker (Rücker 2012). This approach has been implemented in the R package **netmeta** (Rücker and Schwarzer 2013).

11.4.3.1 Illustrating example

To illustrate the advantages of network meta-analysis, Figure 11.4.a presents a network of four interventions for heavy menstrual bleeding (Middleton et al 2010). Data are available for four out of six possible direct comparisons. Table 11.4.a presents the results from direct (pair-wise) meta-analyses and a network meta-analysis using the meta-regression approach. Network meta-analysis provides evidence about the comparisons 'Hysterectomy versus second generation non-hysteroscopic techniques' and 'Hysterectomy versus Mirena', which no individual randomized trial has assessed. Also, the network meta-analysis results are more precise (narrower confidence intervals) than the pair-wise meta-analysis results for two comparisons ('Mirena versus first generation hysteroscopic techniques' and 'Second generation non-hysteroscopic techniques versus Mirena'). Note that precision is not gained for all comparisons; this is because for some comparisons (e.g. 'Hysterectomy versus first generation hysteroscopic techniques'), the heterogeneity among studies in the network as a whole is larger than the heterogeneity within the direct comparison, and therefore some uncertainty is added in the network estimates (see Section 11.4.3.2).

11.4.3.2 Assumptions about heterogeneity

Heterogeneity reflects the underlying differences between the randomized trials that directly compare the same pair of interventions (see Chapter 10, Section 10.10). In a pair-wise meta-analysis, the presence of important heterogeneity can make the

Table 11.4.a Intervention effects, measured as odds ratios of patient dissatisfaction at 12 months of four interventions for heavy menstrual bleeding with 95% confidence intervals. Odds ratios lower than 1 favour the column-defining intervention for the network meta-analysis results (lower triangle) and the row-defining intervention for the pair-wise meta-analysis results (upper triangle)

Pair-wise meta-analysis			
Hysterectomy	–	–	0.38 (0.22 to 0.65)
0.45 (0.24 to 0.82)	**Second generation non-hysteroscopic techniques**	1.35 (0.45 to 4.08)	0.82 (0.60 to 1.12)
0.43 (0.18 to 1.06)	0.96 (0.48 to 1.91)	**Mirena**	2.84 (0.51 to 15.87)
0.38 (0.23 to 0.65)	0.85 (0.63 to 1.15)	0.88 (0.43 to 1.84)	**First generation hysteroscopic techniques**
Network meta-analysis			

interpretation of the summary effect challenging. Network meta-analysis estimates are a combination of the available direct estimates via both direct and indirect comparisons, so heterogeneity among studies for one comparison can impact on findings for many other comparisons.

It is important to specify assumptions about heterogeneity in the network meta-analysis model. Heterogeneity can be specific to each comparison, or assumed to the same for every pair-wise comparison. The idea is similar to a subgroup analysis: the different subgroups could have a common heterogeneity or different heterogeneities. The latter can be estimated accurately only if enough studies are available in each subgroup.

It is common to assume that the amount of heterogeneity is the same for every comparison in the network (Higgins and Whitehead 1996). This has three advantages compared with assuming comparison-specific heterogeneities. First, it shares information across comparisons, so that comparisons with only one or two trials can borrow information about heterogeneity from comparisons with several trials. Second, heterogeneity is estimated more precisely because more data contribute to the estimate, resulting usually in more precise estimates of intervention effects. Third, assuming common heterogeneity makes model estimation computationally easier than assuming comparison-specific heterogeneity (Lu and Ades 2009).

The choice of heterogeneity assumption should be based on clinical and methodological understanding of the data, and assessment of the plausibility of the assumption, in addition to statistical properties.

11.4.3.3 Ranking interventions

One hallmark feature of network meta-analysis is that it can estimate relative rankings of the competing interventions for a particular outcome. **Ranking probability**, the probability that an intervention is at a specific rank (first, second, etc.) when compared with the other interventions in the network, is frequently used. Ranking probabilities may vary for different outcomes. As for any estimated quantity, ranking probabilities are estimated with some variability. Therefore, inference based solely on the probability of being ranked as the best, without accounting for the variability, is misleading and should be avoided.

Ranking measures such as the **mean ranks**, **median ranks** and the **cumulative ranking probabilities** summarize the estimated probabilities for all possible ranks and account for uncertainty in relative ranking. Further discussion of ranking measures is available elsewhere (Salanti et al 2011, Chaimani et al 2013, Tan et al 2014, Rücker and Schwarzer 2015).

The estimated ranking probabilities for the heavy menstrual bleeding network (see Section 11.4.3.2) are presented in Table 11.4.b. 'Hysterectomy' is the most effective intervention according to mean rank.

11.4.4 Disagreement between evidence sources (incoherence)

11.4.4.1 What is incoherence?

Incoherence refers to the violation of the coherence assumption in a network of interventions (see Section 11.2.3.2). Incoherence occurs when different sources of information for a particular relative effect are in disagreement (Song et al 2003, Lu and Ades 2006, Salanti 2012). In much of the literature on network meta-analysis, the term **inconsistency** has been used, rather than incoherence.

The amount of incoherence in a closed loop of evidence in a network graph can be measured as the absolute difference between the direct and indirect summary estimates for any of the pair-wise comparisons in the loop (Bucher et al 1997, Song et al 2011, Veroniki et al 2013). We refer to this method of detecting incoherence as the 'loop-specific approach'. The obtained statistic is usually called an **incoherence factor** or **inconsistency factor** (IF). For example, in the dietary advice network the incoherence factor would be estimated as:

$$\text{IF} = |\text{direct MD}(\text{BvsC}) - \text{indirect MD}(\text{BvsC})|$$

Table 11.4.b Ranking probabilities and mean ranks for intervention effectiveness in heavy menstrual bleeding. Lower mean rank values indicate that the interventions are associated with less mortality

	Rank	Hysterectomy	Second generation non-hysteroscopic techniques	Mirena	First generation hysteroscopic techniques
Probabilities	**1**	96%	1%	4%	0%
	2	4%	46%	40%	9%
	3	0%	46%	19%	35%
	4	0%	7%	37%	56%
Mean rank		1	3	3	4

IF measures the level of disagreement between the direct and indirect effect estimates.

The standard error of the incoherence factor is obtained from

$$\text{Variance}[\text{IF}] = \text{Variance}[\text{direct MD}(\text{BvsC})] + \text{Variance}[\text{indirect MD}(\text{BvsC})]$$

and can be used to construct a 95% confidence interval for the IF:

$$\text{IF} \pm 1.96 \times \text{SE}(\text{IF}).$$

Several approaches have been suggested for evaluating incoherence in a network of interventions with many loops (Donegan et al 2013, Veroniki et al 2013), broadly categorized as **local** and **global** approaches. Local approaches evaluate regions of network separately to detect possible 'incoherence spots', whereas global approaches evaluate coherence in the entire network.

11.4.4.2 Approaches to evaluating local incoherence

A recommended local approach for investigating incoherence is SIDE (Separating Indirect from Direct Evidence). This evaluates the IF for every pair-wise comparison in a network by contrasting a direct estimate (when available) with an indirect estimate; the latter being estimated from the entire network once the direct evidence has been removed. The method was first introduced by Dias and colleagues (Dias et al 2010) under the name 'node-splitting'. The SIDE approach has been implemented in the **network** macro for Stata (White 2015) and the **netmeta** command in R (Schwarzer et al 2015). For example, Table 11.4.c presents the incoherence results of a network that compares the effectiveness of four active interventions and placebo in preventing serious vascular events after transient ischaemic attack or stroke (Thijs et al 2008). Data are available for seven out of ten possible direct comparisons and none of them was found to be statistically significant in terms of incoherence.

In the special case where direct and several independent indirect estimates are available, the 'composite Chi^2 statistic' can be used instead (Caldwell et al 2010).

Table 11.4.c Results based on the SIDE approach to evaluating local incoherence. P values less than 0.05 suggest statistically significant incoherence

	Direct		Indirect		Incoherence factor		
Comparison	**Estimate**	**Standard error**	**Estimate**	**Standard error**	**Estimate**	**Standard error**	***P value***
A versus C	−0.15	0.05	−0.21	0.10	0.07	0.12	*0.56*
A versus D	−0.45	0.07	−0.32	0.11	−0.14	0.13	*0.28*
A versus E	−0.26	0.14	−0.23	0.07	−0.03	0.16	*0.85*
B versus C	0.18	0.11	0.13	0.08	0.05	0.14	*0.70*
B versus E	0.07	0.07	0.12	0.12	−0.05	0.14	*0.70*
C versus D	−0.23	0.06	−0.35	0.12	0.12	0.13	*0.38*
C versus E	−0.06	0.05	−0.11	0.10	0.05	0.11	*0.66*

The loop-specific approach described in Section 11.4.4.1 can be extended to networks with many interventions by evaluating incoherence separately in each closed loop of evidence. The approach can be performed using the *ifplot* macro available for Stata (Chaimani and Salanti 2015). However, unlike the SIDE approach, this method does not incorporate the information from the entire network when estimating the indirect evidence.

Tests for incoherence have low power and therefore may fail to detect incoherence as statistically significant even when it is present (Song et al 2012, Veroniki et al 2014). This means that the absence of statistically significant incoherence is not evidence for the absence of incoherence. Review authors should consider the confidence intervals for incoherence factors and decide whether they include values that are sufficiently large to suggest clinically important discrepancies between direct and indirect evidence.

11.4.4.3 Approaches to evaluating global incoherence

Global incoherence in a network can be evaluated and detected via **incoherence models**. These models differ from the **coherence** models described in Section 11.4.3.1 by relaxing the coherence equations (see Section 11.2.3.2) and allowing intervention effects to vary when estimated directly and indirectly (Lu and Ades 2006). The models add additional terms, equivalent to the incoherence factors (IFs) defined in Section 11.4.4.1, to the coherence equations. For example, in the dietary advice network the coherence equation given in Section 11.2.3.2 would be modified to:

$$\text{'true'indirect MD}(\text{BvsC}) = \text{'true'direct MD}(\text{AvsC}) - \text{'true'direct MD}(\text{AvsB}) + \text{IF}_{ABC}.$$

The quantity IF_{ABC} measures incoherence in the evidence loop 'dietitian-doctor-nurse'. Obviously, complex networks will have several IFs. For a network to be coherent, all IF need to be close to zero. This can be formally tested via a Chi^2 statistic test which is available in Stata in the **network** macro (White 2015). An extension of this model has been suggested where incoherence measures the disagreement when an effect size is measured in studies that involve different sets of interventions (termed 'design incoherence') (Higgins et al 2012).

Measures like the Q-test and the I^2 statistic, which are commonly used for the evaluation of heterogeneity in a pair-wise meta-analysis (see Chapter 10, Section 10.10.2), have been developed for the assessment of heterogeneity and incoherence in network meta-analysis (Krahn et al 2013, Rücker and Schwarzer 2013, Jackson et al 2014). These have been implemented in the package **netmeta** in R (Schwarzer et al 2015).

11.4.4.4 Forming conclusions about incoherence

We suggest review authors use both local and global approaches and consider their results jointly to make inferences about incoherence. The approaches presented in Sections 11.4.4.2 and 11.4.4.3 for evaluating incoherence have limitations. As for tests for statistical heterogeneity in a standard pair-wise meta-analysis, tests for detecting incoherence often lack power to detect incoherence when it is present, as shown in simulations and empirical studies (Song et al 2012, Veroniki et al 2014). Also, different assumptions and different methods in the estimation of heterogeneity may have an impact on the findings about incoherence (Veroniki et al 2013, Veroniki et al 2014). Empirical evidence suggests that review authors sometimes assess the presence of incoherence, if at all, using inappropriate methods (Veroniki et al 2013, Nikolakopoulou et al 2014, Petropoulou et al 2016).

Conclusions should be drawn not just from consideration of statistical significance but by interpreting the range of values included in confidence intervals of the incoherence factors. Researchers should remember that the absence of statistically significant incoherence does not ensure transitivity in the network, which should always be assessed by examining effect modifiers before undertaking the analysis (see Section 11.2.2.2).

Once incoherence is detected, possible explanations should be sought. Errors in data collection, broad eligibility criteria and imbalanced distributions of effect modifiers may have introduced incoherence. Possible analytical strategies in the presence of incoherence are available (Salanti 2012, Jansen and Naci 2013).

11.5 Evaluating confidence in the results of a network meta-analysis

The GRADE approach is recommended for use in Cochrane Reviews to assess the confidence of the evidence for each pair-wise comparison of interventions (see Chapter 14). The approach starts by assuming high confidence in the evidence for randomized trials of a specific pair-wise comparison and then rates down the evidence for considerations of five issues: study limitations, indirectness, inconsistency, imprecision and publication bias.

Rating the confidence in the evidence from a network of interventions is more challenging than pair-wise meta-analysis (Dumville et al 2012). To date, two frameworks have been suggested in the literature to extend the GRADE system to indirect comparisons and network meta-analyses: Salanti and colleagues (Salanti et al 2014) and Puhan and colleagues (Puhan et al 2014). Section 11.5.1 describes the principles of each approach, noting similarities and differences.

11.5.1 Available approaches for evaluating confidence in the evidence

The two available approaches to evaluating confidence in evidence from a network meta-analysis acknowledge that the confidence in each combined comparison depends on the confidence in the direct and indirect comparisons that contribute to it, and that the confidence in each indirect comparison in turn depends on the confidence in the pieces of direct evidence that contribute to it. Therefore, all GRADE assessments are built to some extent on applying GRADE ideas for direct evidence. The two approaches diverge in the way they combine the considerations when thinking about an indirect or combined comparison, as illustrated in Table 11.5.a using the dietary advice example.

The framework by Salanti and colleagues is driven by the ability to express each estimated intervention effect from a network meta-analysis as a weighted sum of all the available direct comparisons (see Section 11.4) (Lu et al 2011, König et al 2013, Krahn et al 2013). The weight is determined, under some assumptions, by the **contribution matrix,** which has been implemented in the *netweight* macro (Chaimani and Salanti 2015) available for the Stata statistical package and programmed in an online tool – CINeMA – which assesses 'Confidence in Network Meta-Analysis' (http://cinema.ispm.ch/). The matrix contains the percentage of information attributable to each direct

Table 11.5.a Steps to obtain the overall confidence ratings (across all GRADE domains) for every combined comparison of the dietary advice example. A ✓ or x indicates whether a particular step is needed in order to proceed to the next step

		Step 1		Step 2				Step 3	
		Domain-specific ratings for direct comparisons		*Overall rating across domains for direct comparisons*		*Domain-specific ratings for combined comparisons*		*Overall rating across domains for combined comparisons*	
Direct comparisons	GRADE domains	Salanti et al	Puhan et al	Salanti et al	Puhan et al	Salanti et al	Puhan et al	Salanti et al	Puhan et al
Dietitian versus nurse	Study limitations	✓	✓	x	✓	✓	x	✓	✓
	Indirectness	✓	✓			✓	x		
	Inconsistency	✓	✓			✓	x		
	Imprecision	-	-			✓	x		
	Publication bias	✓	✓			✓	x		
Dietitian versus doctor	Study limitations	✓	✓	x	✓	✓	x	✓	✓
	Indirectness	✓	✓			✓	x		
	Inconsistency	✓	✓			✓	x		
	Imprecision	-	-			✓	x		
	Publication bias	✓	✓			✓	x		
Nurse versus doctor	Study limitations	✓	✓	x	✓	✓	x	✓	✓
	Indirectness	✓	✓			✓	x		
	Inconsistency	✓	✓			✓	x		
	Imprecision	-	-			✓	x		
	Publication bias	✓	✓			✓	x		

comparison estimate and can be interpreted as the **contributions** of the direct comparison estimates. Then, the confidence in an indirect or combined comparison is estimated by combining the confidence assessment for the available direct comparison estimates with their contribution to the combined (or network) comparison. This approach is similar to the process of evaluating the likely impact of a high risk-of-bias study by looking at its weight in a pair-wise meta-analysis to decide whether to downgrade or not in a standard GRADE assessment.

As an example, in the dietary advice network (Figure 11.2.a) suppose that most of the evidence involved in the indirect comparison (i.e. the trials including dietitians) is at low risk of bias, and that there are studies of 'doctor versus nurse' that are mostly at high risk of bias. If the direct evidence on 'doctor versus nurse' has a very large contribution to the network meta-analysis estimate of the same comparison, then we would judge this result to be at high risk of bias. If the direct evidence has a very low contribution, we might judge the result to be at moderate, or possibly low, risk of bias. This approach might be preferable when there are indirect or mixed comparisons informed by many loops within a network, and for a specific comparison these loops lead to different risk-of-bias assessments. The contributions of the direct comparisons and the risk-of-bias assessments may be presented jointly in a bar graph, with bars proportional to the contributions of direct comparisons and different colours representing the different judgements. The bar graph for the heavy menstrual bleeding example is available in Figure 11.5.a,

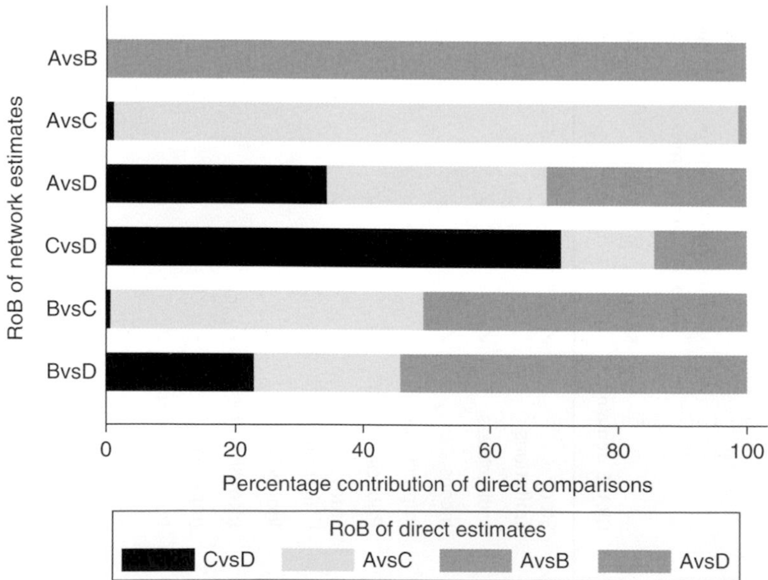

Figure 11.5.a Bar graph illustrating the percentage of information for every comparison that comes from low (dark grey), moderate (light grey) or high (blue) risk-of-bias (RoB) studies with respect to both randomization and compliance to treatment for the heavy menstrual bleeding network (Middleton et al 2010). The risk of bias of the direct comparisons was defined based on Appendix 3 of the original paper. The intervention labels are: A, first generation hysteroscopic techniques; B, hysterectomy; C, second generation non-hysteroscopic techniques; D, Mirena. Reproduced with permission of BMJ Publishing Group

which suggests that there are two comparisons ('First generation hysteroscopic techniques versus Mirena' and 'Second generation non-hysteroscopic techniques versus Mirena') for which a substantial amount of information comes from studies at high risk of bias.

Regardless of whether a review contains a network meta-analysis or a simple indirect comparison, Puhan and colleagues propose to focus on so-called 'most influential' loops only. These are the connections between a pair of interventions of interest that involve exactly one common comparator. This implies that the assessment for the indirect comparison is dependent only on confidence in the two other direct comparisons in this loop. To illustrate, consider the dietary advice network described in Section 11.2 (Figure 11.2.a), where we are interested in confidence in the evidence for the indirect comparison 'doctor versus nurse'. According to Puhan and colleagues, the lower confidence rating between the two direct comparisons 'dietitian versus doctor' and 'dietitian versus nurse' would be chosen to inform the confidence rating for the indirect comparison. If there are also studies directly comparing doctor versus nurse, the confidence in the combined comparison would be the higher rated source between the direct evidence and the indirect evidence. The main rationale for this is that, in general, the higher rated comparison is expected to be the more precise (and thus the dominating) body of evidence. Also, in the absence of important incoherence, the lower rated evidence is only supportive of the higher rated evidence; thus it is not very likely to reduce the confidence in the estimated intervention effects. One disadvantage of this approach is that investigators need to identify the most influential loop; this loop might be relatively uninfluential when there are many loops in a network, which is often the case when there are many interventions. In large networks, many loops with comparable influence may exist and it is not clear how many of those equally influential loops should be considered under this approach.

At the time of writing, no formal comparison has been performed to evaluate the degree of agreement between these two methods. Thus, at this point we do not prescribe using one approach or the other. However, when indirect comparisons are built on existing pair-wise meta-analyses, which have already been rated with respect to their confidence, it may be reasonable to follow the approach of Puhan and colleagues. On the other hand, when the body of evidence is built from scratch, or when a large number of interventions are involved, it may be preferable to consider the approach of Salanti and colleagues whose application is facilitated via the online tool CINeMA.

Since network meta-analysis produces estimates for several intervention effects, the confidence in the evidence should be assessed for each intervention effect that is reported in the results. In addition, network meta-analysis may also provide information on the relative ranking of interventions, and review authors should consider also assessing confidence in results for relative ranking when these are reported. Salanti and colleagues address confidence in the ranking based on the contributions of the direct comparisons to the *entire* network as well as on the use of measures and graphs that aim to assess the different GRADE domains in the network as a whole (e.g. measures of global incoherence) (see Section 11.4.4).

The two approaches modify the standard GRADE domains to fit network meta-analysis to varying degrees. These modifications are briefly described in Box 11.5.a; more details and examples are available in the original articles (Puhan et al 2014, Salanti et al 2014).

Box 11.5.a Modifications to the five domains of the standard GRADE system to fit network meta-analysis.

Study limitations (i.e. classical risk-of-bias items) Salanti and colleagues suggest a bar graph with bars proportional to the contributions of direct comparisons and different colours representing the different confidence ratings (e.g. green, yellow, red for low, moderate or high risk of bias) with respect to study limitations (Figure 11.5.a). The decision about downgrading or not is then formed by interpreting this graph. Such a graph can be used to rate the confidence of evidence for each combined *comparison* and for the relative ranking.

Indirectness The assessment of indirectness in the context of network meta-analysis should consider two components: the similarity of the studies in the analysis to the target question (PICO); and the similarity of the studies in the analysis to each other. The first addresses the extent to which the evidence at hand relates to the population, intervention(s), comparators and outcomes of interest, and the second relates to the evaluation of the transitivity assumption. A common view of the two approaches is that they do not support the idea of downgrading indirect evidence by default. They suggest that indirectness should be considered in conjunction with the risk of intransitivity.

Inconsistency Salanti and colleagues propose to create a common domain to consider jointly both types of inconsistency that may occur: heterogeneity within direct comparisons and incoherence. More specifically, they evaluate separately the presence of the two types of variation and then consider them jointly to infer whether downgrading for inconsistency is appropriate or not. It is usual in network meta-analysis to assume a common heterogeneity variance. They propose the use of prediction intervals to facilitate the assessment of heterogeneity for each combined comparison. Prediction intervals are the intervals expected to include the true intervention effects in future studies (Higgins et al 2009, Riley et al 2011) and they incorporate the extent of between-study variation; in the presence of important heterogeneity they are wide enough to include intervention effects with different implications for practice. The potential for incoherence for a particular comparison can be assessed using existing approaches for evaluating local and global incoherence (see Section 11.5). We may downgrade for one or two levels due to the presence of heterogeneity or incoherence, or both. The judgement for the relative ranking is based on the magnitude of the common heterogeneity as well as the use of global incoherence tests (see Section 11.4).

Imprecision Both approaches suggest that imprecision of the combined comparisons can be judged based on their 95% confidence intervals. Imprecision for relative treatment ranking is the variability in the relative order of the interventions. This is reflected by the overlap in the distributions of the ranking probabilities; i.e. when all or some of the interventions have similar probabilities of being at a particular rank.

Publication bias The potential for publication bias in a network meta-analysis can be difficult to judge. If a natural common comparator exists, a 'comparison-adjusted funnel plot' can be employed to identify possible small-study effects in a network meta-analysis (Chaimani and Salanti 2012, Chaimani et al 2013). This is a modified funnel plot that allows putting together all the studies of the network irrespective of the interventions they compare. However, the primary considerations for both the combined comparisons and relative ranking should be non-statistical. Review authors should consider whether there might be unpublished studies for every possible pair-wise comparison in the network.

11.6 Presenting network meta-analyses

The PRISMA Extension Statement for Reporting of Systematic Reviews Incorporating Network Meta-analyses of Health Care Interventions should be considered when reporting the results from network meta-analysis (Hutton et al 2015). Key graphical and numerical summaries include the network plot (e.g. Figure 11.4.a), a league table of the relative effects between all treatments with associated uncertainty (e.g. Table 11.4.a) and measures of heterogeneity and incoherence.

11.6.1 Presenting the evidence base of a network meta-analysis

Network diagrams provide a convenient way to describe the structure of the network (see Section 11.1.1). They may be modified to incorporate information on study-level or comparison-level characteristics. For instance, the thickness of the lines might reflect the number of studies or patients included in each direct comparison (e.g. Figure 11.4.a), or the comparison-specific average of a potential effect modifier. Using the latter device, network diagrams can be considered as a first step for the evaluation of transitivity in a network. In the example of Figure 11.6.a the age of the participants has been considered as a potential effect modifier. The thickness of the line implies that the average age within comparisons *A versus D* and *C versus D* seems quite different to the other three direct comparisons.

The inclusion of studies with design limitations in a network (e.g. lack of blinding, inadequate allocation sequence concealment) often threatens the validity of findings. The use of coloured lines in a network of interventions can reveal the presence of such studies in specific direct comparisons. Further discussion on issues related to confidence in the evidence is available in Section 11.5.

11.6.2 Tabular presentation of the network structure

For networks including many competing interventions and multiple different study designs, network diagrams might not be the most appropriate tool for presenting the data. An alternative way to present the structure of the network is to use a table, in which the columns represent the competing interventions and the rows represent the different study designs in terms of interventions being compared (Table 11.6.a)

Figure 11.6.a Example of network diagram with lines weighted according to the average age within each pair-wise comparison. Thicker lines correspond to greater average age within the respective comparison

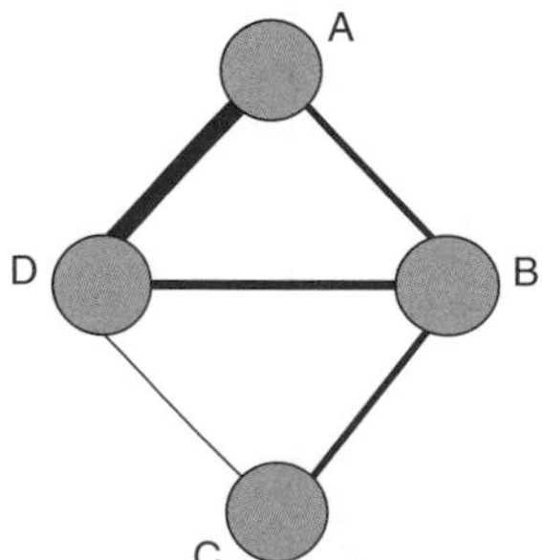

Table 11.6.a Example of table presenting a network that compares seven interventions and placebo for controlling exacerbation of episodes in chronic obstructive pulmonary disease (Baker et al 2009). Reproduced with permission of John Wiley & Sons

Number of studies	Placebo	Fluticasone	Budesonide	Salmeterol	Formoterol	Tiotropium	Fluticasone + salmeterol	Budesonide + formoterol
4	x	x		x			x	
4	x	x						
2	x		x		x			x
2	x			x		x		
2	x			x			x	
8	x			x				
2	x				x			
10	x					x		
1	x						x	
1				x		x		
1				x			x	
1					x	x		
1						x	x	

(Lu and Ades 2006). Additional information, such as the number of participants in each arm, may be presented in the non-empty cells.

11.6.3 Presenting the flow of evidence in a network

Another way to map the evidence in a network of interventions is to consider how much each of the included direct comparisons contributes to the final combined effect estimates. The percentage information that direct evidence contributes to each relative effect estimated in a network meta-analysis can be presented in the contribution matrix (see Section 11.4), and could help investigators understand the flow of information in the network (Chaimani et al 2013, Chaimani and Salanti 2015).

Figure 11.6.b presents the contribution matrix for the example of the network of interventions for heavy menstrual bleeding (obtained from the *netweight* macro in Stata). The indirect treatment effect for second generation non-hysteroscopic techniques versus hysterectomy (*B versus C*) can be estimated using information from the four direct relative treatment effects; these contribute information in different proportions depending on the precision of the direct treatment effects and the structure of the network. Evidence from the direct comparison of first generation hysteroscopic

Network meta-analysis estimates		Direct comparisons in the network (% contribution): A–B	A–C	A–D	C–D
Mixed estimates					
	A–B	100.0			
	A–C	·	97.8	1.1	1.1
	A–D	·	34.5	31.1	34.5
	C–D	·	14.4	14.4	71.2
Indirect estimates					
	B–C	49.6	48.9	0.7	0.7
	B–D	38.5	23.0	15.5	23.0
Entire network		31.4	36.4	10.5	21.7
Included studies		5	11	1	3

Figure 11.6.b Contribution matrix for the network on interventions for heavy menstrual bleeding presented in Figure 11.4.a. Four direct comparisons in the network are presented in the columns, and their contributions to the combined treatment effect are presented in the rows. The entries of the matrix are the percentage weights attributed to each direct comparison. The intervention labels are: A, first generation hysteroscopic techniques; B, hysterectomy; C, second generation non-hysteroscopic techniques; D, Mirena

techniques versus hysterectomy (*A versus B*) has the largest contribution to the indirect comparisons hysterectomy versus second generation non-hysteroscopic techniques (*B versus C*) (49.6%) and hysterectomy versus Mirena (*B versus D*) (38.5%), for both of which no direct evidence exists.

11.6.4 Presentation of results

Unlike pair-wise meta-analysis, the results from network meta-analysis cannot be easily summarized in a single figure such as a standard forest plot. Especially for networks with many competing interventions that involve many comparisons, presentation of findings in a concise and comprehensible way is challenging.

Summary statistics of the intervention effects for all pairs of interventions are the most important output from network meta-analysis. Results from a subset of comparisons are sometimes presented due to space limitations and the choice of the findings to be reported is based on the research question and the target audience (Tan et al 2013). In such cases, the use of additional figures and tables to present all results in detail is necessary. Additionally, review authors might wish to report the relative ranking of interventions (see Section 11.4.3.3) as a supplementary output, which provides a concise summary of the findings and might facilitate decision making. For this purpose, joint presentation of both relative effects and relative ranking is recommended (see Figure 11.6.c or Table 11.4.a of Section 11.4.3.1).

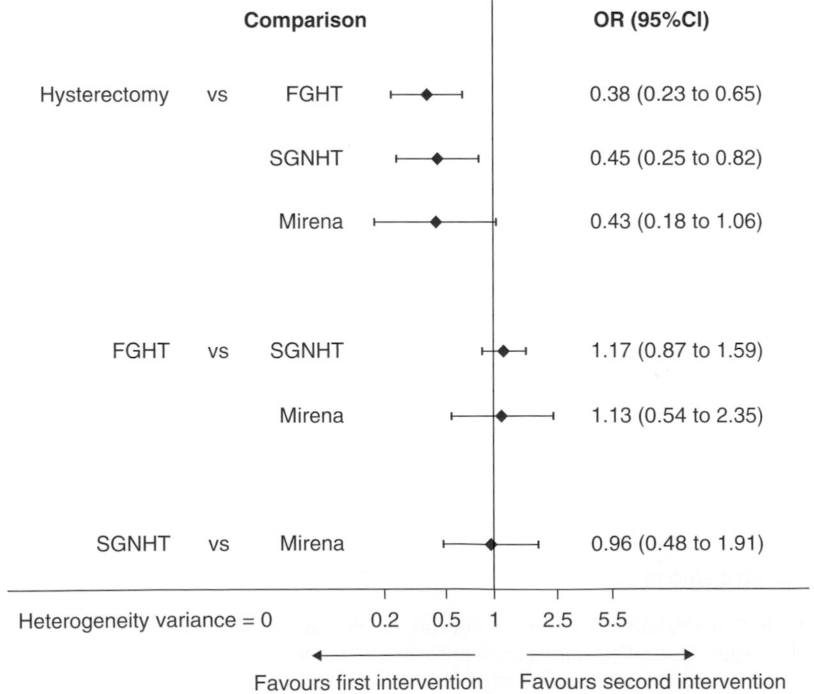

Figure 11.6.c Forest plot for effectiveness in heavy menstrual bleeding between four interventions. FGHT, first generation hysteroscopic techniques; SGNHT, second generation non-hysteroscopic techniques

In the presence of many competing interventions, the results across different outcomes (e.g. efficacy and acceptability) might conflict with respect to which interventions work best. To avoid drawing misleading conclusions, review authors may consider the simultaneous presentation of results for outcomes in these two categories.

Interpretation of the findings from network meta-analysis should always be considered with the evidence characteristics: risk of bias in included studies, heterogeneity, incoherence and selection bias. Reporting results with respect to the evaluation of incoherence and heterogeneity (such as I^2 statistic for incoherence) is important for drawing meaningful conclusions.

11.6.4.1 Presentation of intervention effects and ranking

A table presenting direct, indirect and network summary relative effects along with their confidence ratings is a helpful format (Puhan et al 2014). In addition, various graphical tools have been suggested for the presentation of results from network meta-analyses (Salanti et al 2011, Chaimani et al 2013, Tan et al 2014). Summary relative effects for pair-wise comparisons with their confidence intervals can be presented in a forest plot. For example, Figure 11.6.c shows the summary relative effects for each intervention versus a common reference intervention for the 'heavy menstrual bleeding' network.

Ranking probabilities for all possible ranks may be presented by drawing probability lines, which are known as **rankograms**, and show the distribution of ranking probabilities for each intervention (Salanti et al 2011). The rankograms for the heavy menstrual bleeding network example are shown in Figure 11.6.d. The graph suggests that 'Hysterectomy' has the highest probability of being the best intervention, 'First generation hysteroscopic techniques' have the highest probability of being worst followed by 'Mirena' and 'Second generation non-hysteroscopic techniques' have equal chances of being second or third.

The relative ranking for two (competing) outcomes can be presented jointly in a two-dimensional scatterplot (Chaimani et al 2013). An extended discussion on different ways to present jointly relative effects and relative ranking from network meta-analysis is available in Tan and colleagues (Tan et al 2013).

11.6.4.2 Presentation of heterogeneity and incoherence

The level of heterogeneity in a network of interventions can be expressed via the magnitude of the between-study variance Tau^2, typically assumed to be common in all comparisons in the network. A judgement on whether the estimated Tau^2 suggests the presence of important heterogeneity depends on the clinical outcome and the type of interventions being compared. More extended discussion on the expected values of Tau^2 specific to a certain clinical setting is available (Turner et al 2012, Nikolakopoulou et al 2014).

Forest plots that present all the estimated incoherence factors in the network and their uncertainty may be employed for the presentation of local incoherence (Salanti et al 2009, Chaimani et al 2013). The results from evaluating global incoherence can be summarized in the P value of the Chi^2 statistic incoherence test and the I^2 statistic for incoherence (see Chapter 10, Section 10.10.2).

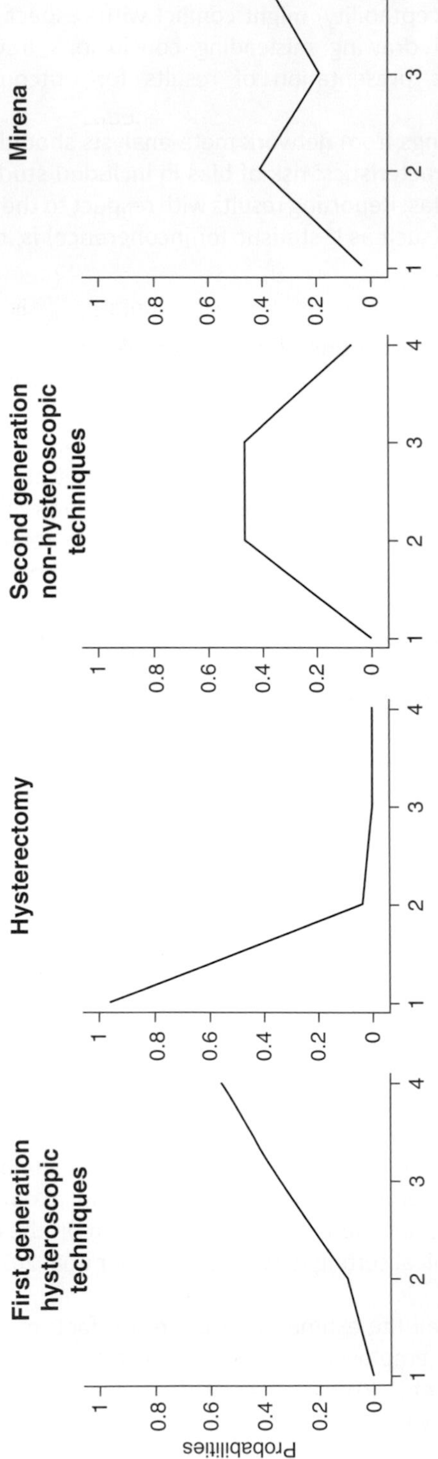

Figure 11.6.d Ranking probabilities (rankograms) for the effectiveness of interventions in heavy menstrual bleeding. The horizontal axis shows the possible ranks and the vertical axis the ranking probabilities. Each line connects the estimated probabilities of being at a particular rank for every intervention

11.6.4.3 'Summary of findings' tables

The purpose of 'Summary of findings' tables in Cochrane Reviews is to provide concisely the key information in terms of available data, confidence in the evidence and intervention effects (see Chapter 14). Providing such a table is more challenging in reviews that compare multiple interventions simultaneously, which very often involve a large number of comparisons between pairs of interventions. A general principle is that the comparison of multiple interventions is the main feature of a network meta-analysis, so is likely to drive the structure of the 'Summary of findings' table. This is in contrast to the 'Summary of findings' table for a pair-wise comparison, whose main strength is to facilitate comparison of effects on different outcomes. Nevertheless, it remains important to be able to compare network meta-analysis results across different outcomes. This provides presentational challenges that are almost impossible to resolve in two dimensions. One potential solution is an interactive electronic display such that the user can choose whether to emphasize the comparisons across interventions or the comparisons across outcomes.

For small networks of interventions (perhaps including up to five competing interventions) a separate 'Summary of findings' table might be produced for each main outcome. However, in the presence of many (more than five) competing interventions, researchers would typically need to select and report a reduced number of pair-wise comparisons. Review authors should provide a clear rationale for the choice of the comparisons they report in the 'Summary of findings' tables. For example, they may consider including only pair-wise comparisons that correspond to the decision set of interventions; that is, the group of interventions of direct interest for drawing conclusions (see Section 11.3.2.1). The distinction between the decision set and the wider synthesis comparator set (all interventions included in the analysis) should be made in the protocol of the review. If the decision set is still too large, researchers may be able to select the comparisons for the 'Summary of findings' table based on the most important information for clinical practice. For example, reporting the comparisons between the three or four most effective interventions with the most commonly used intervention as a comparator.

11.7 Concluding remarks

Network meta-analysis is a method that can inform comparative effectiveness of multiple interventions, but care needs to be taken using this method because it is more statistically complex than a standard meta-analysis. In addition, as network meta-analyses generally ask broader research questions, they usually involve more studies at each step of systematic review, from screening to analysis, than standard meta-analysis. It is therefore important to anticipate the expertise, time and resource required before embarking on one.

A valid indirect comparison and network meta-analysis requires a coherent evidence base. When formulating the research question and deciding the eligibility criteria, populations and interventions in relation to the assumption of transitivity need to be considered. Network meta-analysis is only valid when studies comparing different sets of interventions are similar enough to be combined. When conducted properly, it provides more precise estimates of relative effect than a single direct or indirect estimate. Network meta-analysis can yield estimates between any pairs of interventions, including those that have never been compared directly against each other. Network meta-analysis also allows the estimation of the ranking and hierarchy of interventions. Much care should be taken when interpreting the results and drawing conclusions from network meta-analysis, especially in the presence of incoherence or other potential biases.

11.8 Chapter information

Authors: Anna Chaimani, Deborah M Caldwell, Tianjing Li, Julian PT Higgins, Georgia Salanti

Acknowledgements: Lorne Becker contributed important insights in the discussion of separating Overview from Intervention Reviews with network meta-analysis. Gordon Guyatt provided helpful comments on earlier version of the chapter and Jeroen Jansen provided helpful contributions on Section 11.2.

Funding: This work was supported by the Methods Innovation Fund Program of the Cochrane Collaboration (MIF1) under the project 'Methods for comparing multiple interventions in Intervention reviews and Overviews of reviews'.

11.9 References

Ades AE, Caldwell DM, Reken S, Welton NJ, Sutton AJ, Dias S. Evidence synthesis for decision making 7: a reviewer's checklist. *Medical Decision Making* 2013; **33**: 679–691.

Baker WL, Baker EL, Coleman CI. Pharmacologic treatments for chronic obstructive pulmonary disease: a mixed-treatment comparison meta-analysis. *Pharmacotherapy* 2009; **29**: 891–905.

Bucher HC, Guyatt GH, Griffith LE, Walter SD. The results of direct and indirect treatment comparisons in meta-analysis of randomized controlled trials. *Journal of Clinical Epidemiology* 1997; **50**: 683–691.

Caldwell DM, Ades AE, Higgins JPT. Simultaneous comparison of multiple treatments: combining direct and indirect evidence. *BMJ* 2005; **331**: 897–900.

Caldwell DM, Welton NJ, Ades AE. Mixed treatment comparison analysis provides internally coherent treatment effect estimates based on overviews of reviews and can reveal inconsistency. *Journal of Clinical Epidemiology* 2010; **63**: 875–882.

Caldwell DM, Dias S, Welton NJ. Extending treatment networks in health technology assessment: how far should we go? *Value in Health* 2015; **18**: 673–681.

Chaimani A, Salanti G. Using network meta-analysis to evaluate the existence of small-study effects in a network of interventions. *Research Synthesis Methods* 2012; **3**: 161–176.

Chaimani A, Higgins JPT, Mavridis D, Spyridonos P, Salanti G. Graphical tools for network meta-analysis in STATA. *PloS One* 2013; **8**: e76654.

Chaimani A, Salanti G. Visualizing assumptions and results in network meta-analysis: the network graphs package. *Stata Journal* 2015; **15**: 905–950.

Chaimani A, Caldwell DM, Li T, Higgins JPT, Salanti G. Additional considerations are required when preparing a protocol for a systematic review with multiple interventions. *Journal of Clinical Epidemiology* 2017; **83**: 65–74.

Cipriani A, Higgins JPT, Geddes JR, Salanti G. Conceptual and technical challenges in network meta-analysis. *Annals of Internal Medicine* 2013; **159**: 130–137.

Cooper NJ, Peters J, Lai MC, Jüni P, Wandel S, Palmer S, Paulden M, Conti S, Welton NJ, Abrams KR, Bujkiewicz S, Spiegelhalter D, Sutton AJ. How valuable are multiple treatment comparison methods in evidence-based health-care evaluation? *Value in Health* 2011; **14**: 371–380.

Dias S, Welton NJ, Caldwell DM, Ades AE. Checking consistency in mixed treatment comparison meta-analysis. *Statistics in Medicine* 2010; **29**: 932–944.

Dias S, Ades AE, Welton NJ, Jansen JP, Sutton AJ. *Network meta-analysis for decision-making*. Chichester (UK): Wiley; 2018.

Donegan S, Williamson P, Gamble C, Tudur-Smith C. Indirect comparisons: a review of reporting and methodological quality. *PloS One* 2010; **5**: e11054.

Donegan S, Williamson P, D'Alessandro U, Tudur Smith C. Assessing key assumptions of network meta-analysis: a review of methods. *Research Synthesis Methods* 2013; **4**: 291–323.

Dumville JC, Soares MO, O'Meara S, Cullum N. Systematic review and mixed treatment comparison: dressings to heal diabetic foot ulcers. *Diabetologia* 2012; **55**: 1902–1910.

Efthimiou O, Debray TPA, Valkenhoef G, Trelle S, Panayidou K, Moons KGM, Reitsma JB, Shang A, Salanti G, GetReal Methods Review Group. GetReal in network meta-analysis: a review of the methodology. *Research Synthesis Methods* 2016; **7**: 236–263.

Giovane CD, Vacchi L, Mavridis D, Filippini G, Salanti G. Network meta-analysis models to account for variability in treatment definitions: application to dose effects. *Statistics in Medicine* 2013; **32**: 25–39.

Glenny AM, Altman DG, Song F, Sakarovitch C, Deeks JJ, D'Amico R, Bradburn M, Eastwood AJ. Indirect comparisons of competing interventions. *Health Technology Assessment* 2005; **9**: 1–iv.

Higgins JPT, Whitehead A. Borrowing strength from external trials in a meta-analysis. *Statistics in Medicine* 1996; **15**: 2733–2749.

Higgins JPT, Thompson SG, Spiegelhalter DJ. A re-evaluation of random-effects meta-analysis. *Journal of the Royal Statistical Society Series A (Statistics in Society)* 2009; **172**: 137–159.

Higgins JPT, Jackson D, Barrett JK, Lu G, Ades AE, White IR. Consistency and insconsistency in network meta-analysis: concepts and models for multi-arm studies. *Research Synthesis Methods* 2012; **3**: 98–110.

Hutton B, Salanti G, Caldwell DM, Chaimani A, Schmid CH, Cameron C, Ioannidis JPA, Straus S, Thorlund K, Jansen JP, Mulrow C, Catalá-López F, Gøtzsche PC, Dickersin K, Boutron I, Altman DG, Moher D. The PRISMA extension statement for reporting of systematic reviews incorporating network meta-analyses of health care interventions: checklist and explanations. *Annals of Internal Medicine* 2015; **162**: 777–784.

Jackson D, Riley R, White IR. Multivariate meta-analysis: potential and promise. *Statistics in Medicine* 2011; **30**: 2481–2498.

Jackson D, Barrett JK, Rice S, White IR, Higgins JPT. A design-by-treatment interaction model for network meta-analysis with random inconsistency effects. *Statistics in Medicine* 2014; **33**: 3639–3654.

James A, Yavchitz A, Ravaud P, Boutron I. Node-making process in network meta-analysis of nonpharmacological treatment are poorly reported. *Journal of Clinical Epidemiology* 2018; **97**: 95–102.

Jansen JP, Naci H. Is network meta-analysis as valid as standard pairwise meta-analysis? It all depends on the distribution of effect modifiers. *BMC Medicine* 2013; **11**: 159.

Jansen JP, Trikalinos T, Cappelleri JC, Daw J, Andes S, Eldessouki R, Salanti G. Indirect treatment comparison/network meta-analysis study questionnaire to assess relevance and credibility to inform health care decision making: an ISPOR-AMCP-NPC good practice task force report. *Value in Health* 2014; **17**: 157–173.

König J, Krahn U, Binder H. Visualizing the flow of evidence in network meta-analysis and characterizing mixed treatment comparisons. *Statistics in Medicine* 2013; **32**: 5414–5429.

Krahn U, Binder H, Konig J. A graphical tool for locating inconsistency in network meta-analyses. *BMC Medical Research Methodology* 2013; **13**: 35.

Li T, Dickersin K. Citation of previous meta-analyses on the same topic: a clue to perpetuation of incorrect methods? *Ophthalmology* 2013; **120**: 1113–1119.

Lu G, Ades AE. Combination of direct and indirect evidence in mixed treatment comparisons. *Statistics in Medicine* 2004; **23**: 3105–3124.

Lu G, Ades AE. Assessing evidence inconsistency in mixed treatment comparisons. *Journal of the American Statistical Association* 2006; **101**: 447–459.

Lu G, Ades A. Modeling between-trial variance structure in mixed treatment comparisons. *Biostatistics* 2009; **10**: 792–805.

Lu G, Welton NJ, Higgins JPT, White IR, Ades AE. Linear inference for mixed treatment comparison meta-analysis: a two-stage approach. *Research Synthesis Methods* 2011; **2**: 43–60.

Madan J, Stevenson MD, Cooper KL, Ades AE, Whyte S, Akehurst R. Consistency between direct and indirect trial evidence: is direct evidence always more reliable? *Value in Health* 2011; **14**: 953–960.

Madan J, Chen Y-F, Aveyard P, Wang D, Yahaya I, Munafo M, Bauld L, Welton N. Synthesis of evidence on heterogeneous interventions with multiple outcomes recorded over multiple follow-up times reported inconsistently: a smoking cessation case-study. *Journal of the Royal Statistical Society: Series A (Statistics in Society)* 2014; **177**: 295–314.

Mavridis D, Salanti G. A practical introduction to multivariate meta-analysis. *Statistical Methods in Medical Research* 2013; **22**: 133–158.

Mawdsley D, Bennetts M, Dias S, Boucher M, Welton N. Model-based network meta-analysis: a framework for evidence synthesis of clinical trial data. *CPT: Pharmacometrics & Systems Pharmacology* 2016; **5**: 393–401.

Middleton LJ, Champaneria R, Daniels JP, Bhattacharya S, Cooper KG, Hilken NH, O'Donovan P, Gannon M, Gray R, Khan KS, International Heavy Menstrual Bleeding Individual Patient Data Meta-analysis Collaborative G, Abbott J, Barrington J, Bhattacharya S, Bongers MY, Brun JL, Busfield R, Sowter M, Clark TJ, Cooper J, Cooper KG, Corson SL, Dickersin K, Dwyer N, Gannon M, Hawe J, Hurskainen R, Meyer WR, O'Connor H, Pinion S, Sambrook AM, Tam WH, Zon-Rabelink IAA, Zupi E. Hysterectomy, endometrial destruction, and levonorgestrel releasing intrauterine system (Mirena) for heavy menstrual bleeding: systematic review and meta-analysis of data from individual patients. *BMJ* 2010; **341**: c3929.

Nikolakopoulou A, Chaimani A, Veroniki AA, Vasiliadis HS, Schmid CH, Salanti G. Characteristics of networks of interventions: a description of a database of 186 published networks. *PloS One* 2014; **9**: e86754.

Owen RK, Tincello DG, Keith RA. Network meta-analysis: development of a three-level hierarchical modeling approach incorporating dose-related constraints. *Value in Health* 2015; **18**: 116–126.

Petropoulou M, Nikolakopoulou A, Veroniki AA, Rios P, Vafaei A, Zarin W, Giannatsi M, Sullivan S, Tricco AC, Chaimani A, Egger M, Salanti G. Bibliographic study showed improving statistical methodology of network meta-analyses published between 1999 and 2015. *Journal of Clinical Epidemiology* 2016; **82**: 20–28.

Puhan MA, Schünemann HJ, Murad MH, Li T, Brignardello-Petersen R, Singh JA, Kessels AG, Guyatt GH; GRADE Working Group. A GRADE Working Group approach for rating the quality of treatment effect estimates from network meta-analysis. *BMJ* 2014; **349**: g5630.

Riley RD, Higgins JPT, Deeks JJ. Interpretation of random effects meta-analyses. *BMJ* 2011; **342**: d549.

Rücker G. Network meta-analysis, electrical networks and graph theory. *Research Synthesis Methods* 2012; **3**: 312–324.

Rücker G, Schwarzer G. netmeta: an R package for network meta-analysis 2013. http://www.r-project.org.

Rücker G, Schwarzer G. Ranking treatments in frequentist network meta-analysis works without resampling methods. *BMC Medical Research Methodology* 2015; **15**: 58.

Salanti G, Higgins JPT, Ades AE, Ioannidis JPA. Evaluation of networks of randomized trials. *Statistical Methods in Medical Research* 2008; **17**: 279–301.

Salanti G, Marinho V, Higgins JPT. A case study of multiple-treatments meta-analysis demonstrates that covariates should be considered. *Journal of Clinical Epidemiology* 2009; **62**: 857–864.

Salanti G, Ades AE, Ioannidis JPA. Graphical methods and numerical summaries for presenting results from multiple-treatment meta-analysis: an overview and tutorial. *Journal of Clinical Epidemiology* 2011; **64**: 163–171.

Salanti G. Indirect and mixed-treatment comparison, network, or multiple-treatments meta-analysis: many names, many benefits, many concerns for the next generation evidence synthesis tool. *Research Synthesis Methods* 2012; **3**: 80–97.

Salanti G, Del Giovane C, Chaimani A, Caldwell DM, Higgins JPT. Evaluating the quality of evidence from a network meta-analysis. *PloS One* 2014; **9**: e99682.

Schmitz S, Adams R, Walsh C. Incorporating data from various trial designs into a mixed treatment comparison model. *Statistics in Medicine* 2013; **32**: 2935–2949.

Schwarzer G, Carpenter JR, Rücker G. *Meta-analysis with R*. Cham: Springer; 2015.

Soares MO, Dumville JC, Ades AE, Welton NJ. Treatment comparisons for decision making: facing the problems of sparse and few data. *Journal of the Royal Statistical Society Series A (Statistics in Society)* 2014; **177**: 259–279.

Sobieraj DM, Cappelleri JC, Baker WL, Phung OJ, White CM, Coleman CI. Methods used to conduct and report Bayesian mixed treatment comparisons published in the medical literature: a systematic review. *BMJ Open* 2013; **3**: pii.

Song F, Altman DG, Glenny AM, Deeks JJ. Validity of indirect comparison for estimating efficacy of competing interventions: empirical evidence from published meta-analyses. *BMJ* 2003; **326**: 472.

Song F, Xiong T, Parekh-Bhurke S, Loke YK, Sutton AJ, Eastwood AJ, Holland R, Chen YF, Glenny AM, Deeks JJ, Altman DG. Inconsistency between direct and indirect comparisons of competing interventions: meta-epidemiological study. *BMJ* 2011; **343**: d4909.

Song F, Clark A, Bachmann MO, Maas J. Simulation evaluation of statistical properties of methods for indirect and mixed treatment comparisons. *BMC Medical Research Methodology* 2012; **12**: 138.

Tan SH, Bujkiewicz S, Sutton A, Dequen P, Cooper N. Presentational approaches used in the UK for reporting evidence synthesis using indirect and mixed treatment comparisons. *Journal of Health Services Research and Policy* 2013; **18**: 224–232.

Tan SH, Cooper NJ, Bujkiewicz S, Welton NJ, Caldwell DM, Sutton AJ. Novel presentational approaches were developed for reporting network meta-analysis. *Journal of Clinical Epidemiology* 2014; **67**: 672–680.

Thijs V, Lemmens R, Fieuws S. Network meta-analysis: simultaneous meta-analysis of common antiplatelet regimens after transient ischaemic attack or stroke. *European Heart Journal* 2008; **29**: 1086–1092.

Turner RM, Davey J, Clarke MJ, Thompson SG, Higgins JPT. Predicting the extent of heterogeneity in meta-analysis, using empirical data from the Cochrane Database of Systematic Reviews. *International Journal of Epidemiology* 2012; **41**: 818–827.

Veroniki AA, Vasiliadis HS, Higgins JPT, Salanti G. Evaluation of inconsistency in networks of interventions. *International Journal of Epidemiology* 2013; **42**: 332–345.

Veroniki AA, Mavridis D, Higgins JPT, Salanti G. Characteristics of a loop of evidence that affect detection and estimation of inconsistency: a simulation study. *BMC Medical Research Methodology* 2014; **14**: 106.

White IR, Barrett JK, Jackson D, Higgins JPT. Consistency and inconsistency in network meta-analysis: model estimation using multivariate meta-regression. *Research Synthesis Methods* 2012; **3**: 111–125.

White IR. Network meta-analysis. *Stata Journal* 2015; **15**: 951–985.

12

Synthesizing and presenting findings using other methods

Joanne E McKenzie, Sue E Brennan

KEY POINTS

- Meta-analysis of effect estimates has many advantages, but other synthesis methods may need to be considered in the circumstance where there is incompletely reported data in the primary studies.
- Alternative synthesis methods differ in the completeness of the data they require, the hypotheses they address, and the conclusions and recommendations that can be drawn from their findings.
- These methods provide more limited information for healthcare decision making than meta-analysis, but may be superior to a narrative description where some results are privileged above others without appropriate justification.
- Tabulation and visual display of the results should always be presented alongside any synthesis, and are especially important for transparent reporting in reviews without meta-analysis.
- Alternative synthesis and visual display methods should be planned and specified in the protocol. When writing the review, details of the synthesis methods should be described.
- Synthesis methods that involve vote counting based on statistical significance have serious limitations and are unacceptable.

12.1 Why a meta-analysis of effect estimates may not be possible

Meta-analysis of effect estimates has many potential advantages (see Chapters 10 and 11). However, there are circumstances where it may not be possible to undertake a meta-analysis and other statistical synthesis methods may be considered (McKenzie and Brennan 2014).

Some common reasons why it may not be possible to undertake a meta-analysis are outlined in Table 12.1.a. Legitimate reasons include limited evidence; incompletely

This chapter should be cited as: McKenzie JE, Brennan SE. Chapter 12: Synthesizing and presenting findings using other methods. In: Higgins JPT, Thomas J, Chandler J, Cumpston M, Li T, Page MJ, Welch VA (editors). *Cochrane Handbook for Systematic Reviews of Interventions*. 2nd Edition. Chichester (UK): John Wiley & Sons, 2019: 321–348.

Table 12.1.a Scenarios that may preclude meta-analysis, with possible solutions

Scenario	Description	Examples of possible solutions*
Limited evidence for a pre-specified comparison	Meta-analysis is not possible with no studies, or only one study. This circumstance may reflect the infancy of research in a particular area, or that the specified **PICO for the synthesis** aims to address a narrow question.	Build contingencies into the analysis plan to group one or more of the PICO elements at a broader level (Chapter 2, Section 2.5.3).
Incompletely reported outcome or effect estimate	Within a study, the intervention effects may be incompletely reported (e.g. effect estimate with no measure of precision; direction of effect with P value or statement of statistical significance; only the direction of effect).	Calculate the effect estimate and measure of precision from the available statistics if possible (Chapter 6). Impute missing statistics (e.g. standard deviations) where possible (Chapter 6, Section 6.4.2). *Use other synthesis method(s) (Section 12.2), along with methods to display and present available effects visually (Section 12.3).*
Different effect measures	Across studies, the same outcome could be treated differently (e.g. a time-to-event outcome has been dichotomized in some studies) or analysed using different methods. Both scenarios could lead to different effect measures (e.g. hazard ratios and odds ratios).	Calculate the effect estimate and measure of precision for the same effect measure from the available statistics if possible (Chapter 6). Transform effect measures (e.g. convert standardized mean difference to an odds ratio) where possible (Chapter 10, Section 10.6). *Use other synthesis method(s) (Section 12.2), along with methods to display and present available effects visually (Section 12.3).*
Bias in the evidence	Concerns about missing studies, missing outcomes within the studies (Chapter 13), or bias in the studies (Chapters 8 and 25), are legitimate reasons for not undertaking a meta-analysis. These concerns similarly apply to other synthesis methods (Section 12.2).	*When there are major concerns about bias in the evidence, use structured reporting of the available effects using tables and visual displays (Section 12.3).*
	Incompletely reported outcomes/effects may bias meta-analyses, but not necessarily other synthesis methods.	*For incompletely reported outcomes/effects, also consider other synthesis methods in addition to meta-analysis (Section 12.2).*

Clinical and methodological diversity	Concerns about diversity in the populations, interventions, outcomes, study designs, are often cited reasons for not using meta-analysis (Ioannidis et al 2008). Arguments against using meta-analysis because of too much diversity equally apply to the other synthesis methods (Valentine et al 2010).	Modify planned comparisons, providing rationale for post-hoc changes (Chapter 9).
Statistical heterogeneity	Statistical heterogeneity is an often cited reason for not reporting the meta-analysis result (Ioannidis et al 2008). Presentation of an average combined effect in this circumstance can be misleading, particularly if the estimated effects across the studies are both harmful and beneficial.	Attempt to reduce heterogeneity (e.g. checking the data, correcting an inappropriate choice of effect measure) (Chapter 10, Section 10.10). Attempt to explain heterogeneity (e.g. using subgroup analysis) (Chapter 10, Section 10.11). Consider (if possible) presenting a prediction interval, which provides a predicted range for the true intervention effect in an individual study (Riley et al 2011), thus clearly demonstrating the uncertainty in the intervention effects.

* Italicized text indicates possible solutions discussed in this chapter.

reported outcome/effect estimates, or different effect measures used across studies; and bias in the evidence. Other commonly cited reasons for not using meta-analysis are because of too much clinical or methodological diversity, or statistical heterogeneity (Achana et al 2014). However, meta-analysis methods should be considered in these circumstances, as they may provide important insights if undertaken and interpreted appropriately.

12.2 Statistical synthesis when meta-analysis of effect estimates is not possible

A range of statistical synthesis methods are available, and these may be divided into three categories based on their preferability (Table 12.2.a). Preferable methods are the meta-analysis methods outlined in Chapters 10 and 11, and are not discussed in detail here. This chapter focuses on methods that might be considered when a meta-analysis of effect estimates is not possible due to incompletely reported data in the primary studies. These methods divide into those that are 'acceptable' and 'unacceptable'. The 'acceptable' methods differ in the data they require, the hypotheses they address, limitations around their use, and the conclusions and recommendations that can be drawn (see Section 12.2.1). The 'unacceptable' methods in common use are described (see Section 12.2.2), along with the reasons for why they are problematic.

Compared with meta-analysis methods, the 'acceptable' synthesis methods provide more limited information for healthcare decision making. However, these 'acceptable' methods may be superior to a narrative that describes results study by study, which comes with the risk that some studies or findings are privileged above others without appropriate justification. Further, in reviews with little or no synthesis, readers are left to make sense of the research themselves, which may result in the use of seemingly simple yet problematic synthesis methods such as vote counting based on statistical significance (see Section 12.2.2.1).

All methods first involve calculation of a 'standardized metric', followed by application of a synthesis method. In applying any of the following synthesis methods, it is important that only one outcome per study (or other independent unit, for example one comparison from a trial with multiple intervention groups) contributes to the synthesis. Chapter 9 outlines approaches for selecting an outcome when multiple have been measured. Similar to meta-analysis, sensitivity analyses can be undertaken to examine if the findings of the synthesis are robust to potentially influential decisions (see Chapter 10, Section 10.14 and Section 12.4 for examples).

Authors should report the specific methods used in lieu of meta-analysis (including approaches used for presentation and visual display), rather than stating that they have conducted a 'narrative synthesis' or 'narrative summary' without elaboration. The limitations of the chosen methods must be described, and conclusions worded with appropriate caution. The aim of reporting this detail is to make the synthesis process more transparent and reproducible, and help ensure use of appropriate methods and interpretation.

Table 12.2.a Summary of preferable and acceptable synthesis methods

Synthesis method	Question answered	Minimum data required				Purpose	Limitations
		Estimate of effect	Variance	Direction of effect	Precise P value		
Preferable							
Meta-analysis of effect estimates and extensions (Chapters 10 and 11)	What is the common intervention effect? What is the average intervention effect? Which intervention, of multiple, is most effective? What factors modify the magnitude of the intervention effects?	✓	✓			Can be used to synthesize results when effect estimates and their variances are reported (or can be calculated). Provides a combined estimate of average intervention effect (random effects), and precision of this estimate (95% CI). Can be used to synthesize evidence from multiple interventions, with the ability to rank them (network meta-analysis). Can be used to detect, quantify and investigate heterogeneity (meta-regression/ subgroup analysis). **Associated plots:** forest plot, funnel plot, network diagram, rankogram plot	Requires effect estimates and their variances. Extensions (network meta-analysis, meta-regression/subgroup analysis) require a reasonably large number of studies. Meta-regression/subgroup analysis involves observational comparisons and requires careful interpretation. High risk of false positive conclusions for sources of heterogeneity. Network meta-analysis is more complicated to undertake and requires careful assessment of the assumptions.
Acceptable							
Summarizing effect estimates	What is the range and distribution of observed effects?	✓				Can be used to synthesize results when it is difficult to undertake a meta-analysis (e.g. missing variances of effects, unit of analysis errors).	Does not account for differences in the relative sizes of the studies. Performance of these statistics applied in the context of summarizing effect estimates has not been evaluated.

(*Continued*)

Table 12.2.a (Continued)

Synthesis method	Question answered	Minimum data required: Estimate of effect	Variance	Direction of effect	Precise P value	Purpose	Limitations
						Provides information on the magnitude and range of effects (median, interquartile range, range). **Associated plots:** box-and-whisker plot, bubble plot	
Combining P values	Is there evidence that there is an effect in at least one study?			✓	✓	Can be used to synthesize results when studies report: • no, or minimal, information beyond P values and direction of effect; • results of non-parametric analyses; • results of different types of outcomes and statistical tests; • outcomes are different across studies (e.g. different serious side effects). **Associated plot:** albatross plot	Provides no information on the magnitude of effects. Does not distinguish between evidence from large studies with small effects and small studies with large effects. Difficult to interpret the test results when statistically significant, since the null hypothesis can be rejected on the basis of an effect in only one study (Jones 1995). When combining P values from few, small studies, failure to reject the null hypotheses should not be interpreted as evidence of no effect in all studies.
Vote counting based on direction of effect	Is there any evidence of an effect?			✓		Can be used to synthesize results when only direction of effect is reported, or there is inconsistency in the effect measures or data reported across studies. **Associated plots:** harvest plot, effect direction plot	Provides no information on the magnitude of effects (Borenstein et al 2009). Does not account for differences in the relative sizes of the studies (Borenstein et al 2009). Less powerful than methods used to combine P values.

12.2.1 Acceptable synthesis methods

12.2.1.1 Summarizing effect estimates

Description of method Summarizing effect estimates might be considered in the circumstance where estimates of intervention effect are available (or can be calculated), but the variances of the effects are not reported or are incorrect (and cannot be calculated from other statistics, or reasonably imputed) (Grimshaw et al 2003). Incorrect calculation of variances arises more commonly in non-standard study designs that involve clustering or matching (Chapter 23). While missing variances may limit the possibility of meta-analysis, the (standardized) effects can be summarized using descriptive statistics such as the median, interquartile range, and the range. Calculating these statistics addresses the question 'What is the range and distribution of observed effects?'

Reporting of methods and results The statistics that will be used to summarize the effects (e.g. median, interquartile range) should be reported. Box-and-whisker or bubble plots will complement reporting of the summary statistics by providing a visual display of the distribution of observed effects (Section 12.3.3). Tabulation of the available effect estimates will provide transparency for readers by linking the effects to the studies (Section 12.3.1). Limitations of the method should be acknowledged (Table 12.2.a).

12.2.1.2 Combining P values

Description of method Combining P values can be considered in the circumstance where there is no, or minimal, information reported beyond P values and the direction of effect; the types of outcomes and statistical tests differ across the studies; or results from non-parametric tests are reported (Borenstein et al 2009). Combining P values addresses the question 'Is there evidence that there is an effect in at least one study?' There are several methods available (Loughin 2004), with the method proposed by Fisher outlined here (Becker 1994).

Fisher's method combines the P values from statistical tests across *k* studies using the formula:

$$\text{Chi}^2 = -2\sum_{i=1}^{k}\ln(P_i).$$

One-sided P values are used, since these contain information about the direction of effect. However, these P values must reflect the same directional hypothesis (e.g. all testing if intervention A is more effective than intervention B). This is analogous to standardizing the direction of effects before undertaking a meta-analysis. Two-sided P values, which do not contain information about the direction, must first be converted to one-sided P values. If the effect is consistent with the directional hypothesis (e.g. intervention A is beneficial compared with B), then the one-sided P value is calculated as

$$P_{1\text{-}sided} = \frac{P_{2\text{-}sided}}{2};$$

otherwise,

$$P_{1\text{-}sided} = 1 - \left(\frac{P_{2\text{-}sided}}{2}\right).$$

In studies that do not report an exact P value but report a conventional level of significance (e.g. $P < 0.05$), a conservative option is to use the threshold (e.g. 0.05). The P values must have been computed from statistical tests that appropriately account for the features of the design, such as clustering or matching, otherwise they will likely be incorrect.

The Chi^2 statistic will follow a chi-squared distribution with $2k$ degrees of freedom if there is no effect in every study. A large Chi^2 statistic compared to the degrees of freedom (with a corresponding low P value) provides evidence of an effect in at least one study (see Section 12.4.2.2 for guidance on implementing Fisher's method for combining P values).

Reporting of methods and results There are several methods for combining P values (Loughin 2004), so the chosen method should be reported, along with details of sensitivity analyses that examine if the results are sensitive to the choice of method. The results from the test should be reported alongside any available effect estimates (either individual results or meta-analysis results of a subset of studies) using text, tabulation and appropriate visual displays (Section 12.3). The albatross plot is likely to complement the analysis (Section 12.3.4). Limitations of the method should be acknowledged (Table 12.2.a).

12.2.1.3 Vote counting based on the direction of effect

Description of method Vote counting based on the direction of effect might be considered in the circumstance where the direction of effect is reported (with no further information), or there is no consistent effect measure or data reported across studies. The essence of vote counting is to compare the number of effects showing benefit to the number of effects showing harm for a particular outcome. However, there is wide variation in the implementation of the method due to differences in how 'benefit' and 'harm' are defined. Rules based on subjective decisions or statistical significance are problematic and should be avoided (see Section 12.2.2).

To undertake vote counting properly, each effect estimate is first categorized as showing benefit or harm based on the observed direction of effect alone, thereby creating a standardized binary metric. A count of the number of effects showing benefit is then compared with the number showing harm. Neither statistical significance nor the size of the effect are considered in the categorization. A sign test can be used to answer the question 'is there any evidence of an effect?' If there is no effect, the study effects will be distributed evenly around the null hypothesis of no difference. This is equivalent to testing if the true proportion of effects favouring the intervention (or comparator) is equal to 0.5 (Bushman and Wang 2009) (see Section 12.4.2.3 for guidance on implementing the sign test). An estimate of the proportion of effects favouring the intervention can be calculated ($p = u/n$, where u = number of effects favouring the intervention, and n = number of studies) along with a confidence interval (e.g. using the Wilson or Jeffreys interval methods (Brown et al 2001)). Unless there are many studies contributing effects to the analysis, there will be large uncertainty in this estimated proportion.

Reporting of methods and results The vote counting method should be reported in the 'Data synthesis' section of the review. Failure to recognize vote counting as a synthesis method has led to it being applied informally (and perhaps unintentionally) to summarize results (e.g. through the use of wording such as '3 of 10 studies showed improvement in the outcome with intervention compared to control'; 'most studies found'; 'the majority of studies'; 'few studies' etc). In such instances, the method is rarely reported, and it may not be possible to determine whether an unacceptable (invalid) rule has been used to define benefit and harm (Section 12.2.2). The results from vote counting should be reported alongside any available effect estimates (either individual results or meta-analysis results of a subset of studies) using text, tabulation and appropriate visual displays (Section 12.3). The number of studies contributing to a synthesis based on vote counting may be larger than a meta-analysis, because only minimal statistical information (i.e. direction of effect) is required from each study to vote count. Vote counting results are used to derive the harvest and effect direction plots, although often using unacceptable methods of vote counting (see Section 12.3.5). Limitations of the method should be acknowledged (Table 12.2.a).

12.2.2 Unacceptable synthesis methods

12.2.2.1 Vote counting based on statistical significance

Conventional forms of vote counting use rules based on statistical significance and direction to categorize effects. For example, effects may be categorized into three groups: those that favour the intervention and are statistically significant (based on some predefined P value), those that favour the comparator and are statistically significant, and those that are statistically non-significant (Hedges and Vevea 1998). In a simpler formulation, effects may be categorized into two groups: those that favour the intervention and are statistically significant, and all others (Friedman 2001). Regardless of the specific formulation, when based on statistical significance, all have serious limitations and can lead to the wrong conclusion.

The conventional vote counting method fails because underpowered studies that do not rule out clinically important effects are counted as not showing benefit. Suppose, for example, the effect sizes estimated in two studies were identical. However, only one of the studies was adequately powered, and the effect in this study was statistically significant. Only this one effect (of the two identical effects) would be counted as showing 'benefit'. Paradoxically, Hedges and Vevea showed that as the number of studies increases, the power of conventional vote counting tends to zero, except with large studies and at least moderate intervention effects (Hedges and Vevea 1998). Further, conventional vote counting suffers the same disadvantages as vote counting based on direction of effect, namely, that it does not provide information on the magnitude of effects and does not account for differences in the relative sizes of the studies.

12.2.2.2 Vote counting based on subjective rules

Subjective rules, involving a combination of direction, statistical significance and magnitude of effect, are sometimes used to categorize effects. For example, in a review examining the effectiveness of interventions for teaching quality improvement to clinicians, the authors categorized results as 'beneficial effects', 'no effects' or 'detrimental effects' (Boonyasai et al 2007). Categorization was based on direction of effect and statistical significance (using a predefined P value of 0.05) when available. If statistical significance was not reported, effects greater than 10% were categorized as 'beneficial' or 'detrimental', depending on their direction. These subjective rules often vary in the elements, cut-offs and algorithms used to categorize effects, and while detailed descriptions of the rules may provide a veneer of legitimacy, such rules have poor performance validity (Ioannidis et al 2008).

A further problem occurs when the rules are not described in sufficient detail for the results to be reproduced (e.g. ter Wee et al 2012, Thornicroft et al 2016). This lack of transparency does not allow determination of whether an acceptable or unacceptable vote counting method has been used (Valentine et al 2010).

12.3 Visual display and presentation of the data

Visual display and presentation of data is especially important for transparent reporting in reviews without meta-analysis, and should be considered irrespective of whether synthesis is undertaken (see Table 12.2.a for a summary of plots associated with each synthesis method). Tables and plots structure information to show patterns in the data and convey detailed information more efficiently than text. This aids interpretation and helps readers assess the veracity of the review findings.

12.3.1 Structured tabulation of results across studies

Ordering studies alphabetically by study ID is the simplest approach to tabulation; however, more information can be conveyed when studies are grouped in subpanels or ordered by a characteristic important for interpreting findings. The grouping of studies in tables should generally follow the structure of the synthesis presented in the text, which should closely reflect the review questions. This grouping should help readers identify the data on which findings are based and verify the review authors' interpretation.

If the purpose of the table is comparative, grouping studies by any of following characteristics might be informative:

- comparisons considered in the review, or outcome domains (according to the structure of the synthesis);
- study characteristics that may reveal patterns in the data, for example potential effect modifiers including population subgroups, settings or intervention components.

If the purpose of the table is complete and transparent reporting of data, then ordering the studies to increase the prominence of the most relevant and trustworthy evidence should be considered. Possibilities include:

- certainty of the evidence (synthesized result or individual studies if no synthesis);
- risk of bias, study size or study design characteristics; and
- characteristics that determine how directly a study addresses the review question, for example relevance and validity of the outcome measures.

One disadvantage of grouping by study characteristics is that it can be harder to locate specific studies than when tables are ordered by study ID alone, for example when cross-referencing between the text and tables. Ordering by study ID within categories may partly address this.

The value of standardizing intervention and outcome labels is discussed in Chapter 3 (Sections 3.2.2 and 3.4), while the importance and methods for standardizing effect estimates is described in Chapter 6. These practices can aid readers' interpretation of tabulated data, especially when the purpose of a table is comparative.

12.3.2 Forest plots

Forest plots and methods for preparing them are described elsewhere (Chapter 10, Section 10.2). Some mention is warranted here of their importance for displaying study results when meta-analysis is not undertaken (i.e. without the summary diamond). Forest plots can aid interpretation of individual study results and convey overall patterns in the data, especially when studies are ordered by a characteristic important for interpreting results (e.g. dose and effect size, sample size). Similarly, grouping studies in subpanels based on characteristics thought to modify effects, such as population subgroups, variants of an intervention, or risk of bias, may help explore and explain differences across studies (Schriger et al 2010). These approaches to ordering provide important techniques for informally exploring heterogeneity in reviews without meta-analysis, and should be considered in preference to alphabetical ordering by study ID alone (Schriger et al 2010).

12.3.3 Box-and-whisker plots and bubble plots

Box-and-whisker plots (see Figure 12.4.a, Panel A) provide a visual display of the distribution of effect estimates (Section 12.2.1.1). The plot conventionally depicts five values. The upper and lower limits (or 'hinges') of the box, represent the 75th and 25th percentiles, respectively. The line within the box represents the 50th percentile (median), and the whiskers represent the extreme values (McGill et al 1978). Multiple box plots can be juxtaposed, providing a visual comparison of the distributions of effect estimates (Schriger et al 2006). For example, in a review examining the effects of audit and feedback on professional practice, the format of the feedback (verbal, written, both verbal and written) was hypothesized to be an effect modifier (Ivers et al 2012). Box-and-whisker plots of the risk differences were presented separately by the format of feedback, to allow visual comparison of the impact of format on the distribution of effects. When presenting multiple box-and-whisker plots, the width of the box can be varied to indicate the number of studies contributing to each. The plot's common usage facilitates rapid and correct interpretation by readers (Schriger et al 2010). The individual studies contributing to the plot are not identified (as in a forest plot), however, and the plot is not appropriate when there are few studies (Schriger et al 2006).

A bubble plot (see Figure 12.4.a, Panel B) can also be used to provide a visual display of the distribution of effects, and is more suited than the box-and-whisker plot when there are few studies (Schriger et al 2006). The plot is a scatter plot that can display multiple dimensions through the location, size and colour of the bubbles. In a review examining the effects of educational outreach visits on professional practice, a bubble plot was used to examine visually whether the distribution of effects was modified by the targeted behaviour (O'Brien et al 2007). Each bubble represented the effect size (y-axis) and whether the study targeted a prescribing or other behaviour (x-axis).

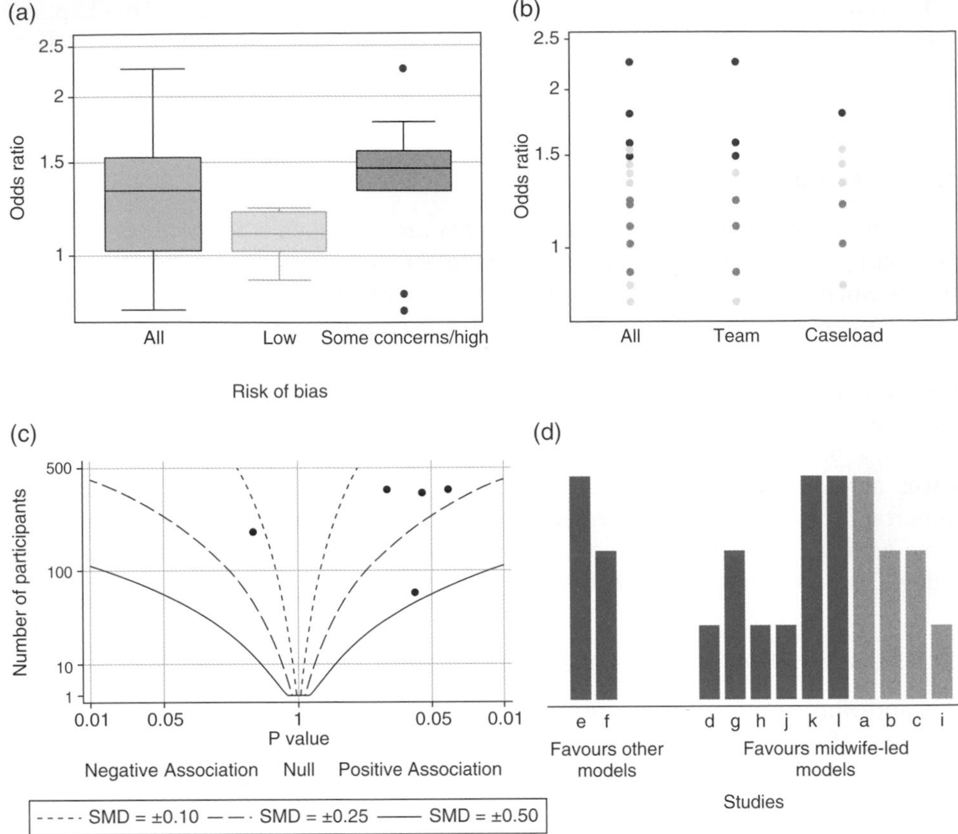

Figure 12.4.a Possible graphical displays of different types of data. (A) Box-and-whisker plots of odds ratios for all outcomes and separately by overall risk of bias. (B) Bubble plot of odds ratios for all outcomes and separately by the model of care. The colours of the bubbles represent the overall risk of bias judgement (dark grey = low risk of bias; light grey = some concerns; blue = high risk of bias). (C) Albatross plot of the study sample size against P values (for the five continuous outcomes in Table 12.4.c, column 6). The effect contours represent standardized mean differences. (D) Harvest plot (height depicts overall risk of bias judgement (tall = low risk of bias; medium = some concerns; short = high risk of bias), shading depicts model of care (light grey = caseload; dark grey = team), alphabet characters represent the studies)

The size of the bubbles reflected the number of study participants. However, different formulations of the bubble plot can display other characteristics of the data (e.g. precision, risk-of-bias assessments).

12.3.4 Albatross plot

The albatross plot (see Figure 12.4.a, Panel C) allows approximate examination of the underlying intervention effect sizes where there is minimal reporting of results within studies (Harrison et al 2017). The plot only requires a two-sided P value, sample size and direction of effect (or equivalently, a one-sided P value and a sample size) for each result. The plot is a scatter plot of the study sample sizes against two-sided P values, where the results are separated by the direction of effect. Superimposed on the plot are 'effect size contours' (inspiring the plot's name). These contours are specific to the type of data (e.g. continuous, binary) and statistical methods used to calculate the P values. The contours allow interpretation of the approximate effect sizes of the studies, which would otherwise not be possible due to the limited reporting of the results. Characteristics of studies (e.g. type of study design) can be identified using different colours or symbols, allowing informal comparison of subgroups.

The plot is likely to be more inclusive of the available studies than meta-analysis, because of its minimal data requirements. However, the plot should complement the results from a statistical synthesis, ideally a meta-analysis of available effects.

12.3.5 Harvest and effect direction plots

Harvest plots (see Figure 12.4.a, Panel D) provide a visual extension of vote counting results (Ogilvie et al 2008). In the plot, studies based on the categorization of their effects (e.g. 'beneficial effects', 'no effects' or 'detrimental effects') are grouped together. Each study is represented by a bar positioned according to its categorization. The bars can be 'visually weighted' (by height or width) and annotated to highlight study and outcome characteristics (e.g. risk-of-bias domains, proximal or distal outcomes, study design, sample size) (Ogilvie et al 2008, Crowther et al 2011). Annotation can also be used to identify the studies. A series of plots may be combined in a matrix that displays, for example, the vote counting results from different interventions or outcome domains.

The methods papers describing harvest plots have employed vote counting based on statistical significance (Ogilvie et al 2008, Crowther et al 2011). For the reasons outlined in Section 12.2.2.1, this can be misleading. However, an acceptable approach would be to display the results based on direction of effect.

The effect direction plot is similar in concept to the harvest plot in the sense that both display information on the direction of effects (Thomson and Thomas 2013). In the first version of the effect direction plot, the direction of effects for *each outcome within a single study* are displayed, while the second version displays the direction of the effects for *outcome domains across studies*. In this second version, an algorithm is first applied to 'synthesize' the directions of effect for all outcomes within a domain (e.g. outcomes 'sleep disturbed by wheeze', 'wheeze limits speech', 'wheeze during exercise' in the outcome domain 'respiratory'). This algorithm is based on the proportion of effects that are in a consistent direction and statistical significance. Arrows are used to indicate the reported direction of effect (for either outcomes or outcome domains). Features such as statistical significance, study design and sample size are denoted using size and colour. While this version of the plot conveys a large amount of information, it requires further development before its use can be recommended since the algorithm underlying the plot is likely to have poor performance validity.

12.4 Worked example

The example that follows uses four scenarios to illustrate methods for presentation and synthesis when meta-analysis is not possible. The first scenario contrasts a common approach to tabulation with alternative presentations that may enhance the transparency of reporting and interpretation of findings. Subsequent scenarios show the application of the synthesis approaches outlined in preceding sections of the chapter. Box 12.4.a summarizes the review comparisons and outcomes, and decisions taken by the review authors

Box 12.4.a The review

The review used in this example examines the effects of midwife-led continuity models versus other models of care for childbearing women. One of the outcomes considered in the review, and of interest to many women choosing a care option, is maternal satisfaction with care. The review included 15 randomized trials, all of which reported a measure of satisfaction. Overall, 32 satisfaction outcomes were reported, with between one and 11 outcomes reported per study. There were differences in the concepts measured (e.g. global satisfaction; specific domains such as of satisfaction with information), the measurement period (i.e. antenatal, intrapartum, postpartum care), and the measurement tools (different scales; variable evidence of validity and reliability).

Before conducting their synthesis, the review authors did the following.

1) **Specified outcome groups in their protocol** (see Chapter 3). Five types of satisfaction outcomes were defined (global measures, satisfaction with information, satisfaction with decisions, satisfaction with care, sense of control), any of which would be grouped for synthesis since they all broadly reflect satisfaction with care. The review authors hypothesized that the period of care (antenatal, intrapartum, postpartum) might influence satisfaction with a model of care, so planned to analyse outcomes for each period separately. The review authors specified that outcomes would be synthesized across periods if data were sparse.
2) **Specified decision rules in their protocol for dealing with multiplicity of outcomes** (Chapter 3). For studies that reported multiple satisfaction outcomes per period, one outcome would be chosen by (i) selecting the most relevant outcome (a global measure > satisfaction with care > sense of control > satisfaction with decisions > satisfaction with information), and if there were two or more equally relevant outcomes, then (ii) selecting the measurement tool with best evidence of validity and reliability.
3) **Examined study characteristics to determine which studies were similar enough for synthesis** (Chapter 9). All studies had similar models of care as a comparator. Satisfaction outcomes from each study were categorized into one of the five prespecified categories, and then the decision rules were applied to select the most relevant outcome for synthesis.
4) **Determined what data were available for synthesis** (Chapter 9). All measures of satisfaction were ordinal; however, outcomes were treated differently across studies (see Tables 12.4.a, 12.4.b and 12.4.c). In some studies, the outcome was dichotomized, while in others it was treated as ordinal or continuous. Based on their pre-specified synthesis methods, the review authors selected the preferred method for the available data. In this example, four scenarios, with progressively fewer data, are used to illustrate the application of alternative synthesis methods.
5) **Determined if modification to the planned comparison or outcomes was needed**. No changes were required to comparisons or outcome groupings.

in planning their synthesis. While the example is loosely based on an actual review, the review description, scenarios and data are fabricated for illustration.

12.4.1 Scenario 1: structured reporting of effects

We first address a scenario in which review authors have decided that the tools used to measure satisfaction measured concepts that were too dissimilar across studies for synthesis to be appropriate. Setting aside three of the 15 studies that reported on the birth partner's satisfaction with care, a structured summary of effects is sought of the remaining 12 studies. To keep the example table short, only one outcome is shown per study for each of the measurement periods (antenatal, intrapartum or postpartum).

Table 12.4.a depicts a common yet suboptimal approach to presenting results. Note two features.

- Studies are ordered by study ID, rather than grouped by characteristics that might enhance interpretation (e.g. risk of bias, study size, validity of the measures, certainty of the evidence (GRADE)).
- Data reported are as extracted from each study; effect estimates were not calculated by the review authors and, where reported, were not standardized across studies (although data were available to do both).

Table 12.4.b shows an improved presentation of the same results. In line with best practice, here effect estimates have been calculated by the review authors for all outcomes, and a common metric computed to aid interpretation (in this case an odds ratio; see Chapter 6 for guidance on conversion of statistics to the desired format). Redundant information has been removed ('statistical test' and 'P value' columns). The studies have been re-ordered, first to group outcomes by period of care (intrapartum outcomes are shown here), and then by risk of bias. This re-ordering serves two purposes. Grouping by period of care aligns with the plan to consider outcomes for each period separately and ensures the table structure matches the order in which results are described in the text. Re-ordering by risk of bias increases the prominence of studies at lowest risk of bias, focusing attention on the results that should most influence conclusions. Had the review authors determined that a synthesis would be informative, then ordering to facilitate comparison across studies would be appropriate; for example, ordering by the type of satisfaction outcome (as pre-defined in the protocol, starting with global measures of satisfaction), or the comparisons made in the studies.

The results may also be presented in a forest plot, as shown in Figure 12.4.b. In both the table and figure, studies are grouped by risk of bias to focus attention on the most trustworthy evidence. The pattern of effects across studies is immediately apparent in Figure 12.4.b and can be described efficiently without having to interpret each estimate (e.g. difference between studies at low and high risk of bias emerge), although these results should be interpreted with caution in the absence of a formal test for subgroup differences (see Chapter 10, Section 10.11). Only outcomes measured during the intrapartum period are displayed, although outcomes from other periods could be added, maximizing the information conveyed.

An example description of the results from Scenario 1 is provided in Box 12.4.b. It shows that describing results study by study becomes unwieldy with more than a

Table 12.4.a Scenario 1: table ordered by study ID, data as reported by study authors

Outcome (scale details*)	Intervention	Control	Effect estimate (metric)	95% CI	Statistical test	P value
Barry 2005	% (N)	% (N)				
Experience of labour	37% (246)	32% (223)	5% (RD)			P > 0.05
Biro 2000	n/N	n/N				
Perception of care: labour/birth	260/344	192/287	1.13 (RR)	1.02 to 1.25	z = 2.36	0.018
Crowe 2010	Mean (SD) N	Mean (SD) N				
Experience of antenatal care (0 to 24 points)	21.0 (5.6) 182	19.7 (7.3) 186	1.3 (MD)	–0.1 to 2.7	t = 1.88	0.061
Experience of labour/birth (0 to 18 points)	9.8 (3.1) 182	9.3 (3.3) 186	0.5 (MD)	–0.2 to 1.2	t = 1.50	0.135
Experience of postpartum care (0 to 18 points)	11.7 (2.9) 182	10.9 (4.2) 186	0.8 (MD)	0.1 to 1.5	t = 2.12	0.035
Flint 1989	n/N	n/N				
Care from staff during labour	240/275	208/256	1.07 (RR)	1.00 to 1.16	z = 1.89	0.059
Frances 2000						
Communication: labour/birth			0.90 (OR)	0.61 to 1.33	z = –0.52	0.606
Harvey 1996	Mean (SD) N	Mean (SD) N				
Labour & Delivery Satisfaction Index (37 to 222 points)	182 (14.2) 101	185 (30) 93			t = –0.90 for MD	0.369 for MD

Johns 2004	n/N	n/N				
Satisfaction with intrapartum care	605/1163	363/826	8.1% (RD)	3.6 to 12.5		<0.001
Mac Vicar 1993	n/N	n/N				
Birth satisfaction	849/1163	496/826	13.0% (RD)	8.8 to 17.2	z = 6.04	0.000
Parr 2002						
Experience of childbirth			0.85 (OR)	0.39 to 1.86	z = -0.41	0.685
Rowley 1995						
Encouraged to ask questions			1.02 (OR)	0.66 to 1.58	z = 0.09	0.930
Turnbull 1996	Mean (SD) N	Mean (SD) N				
Intrapartum care rating (−2 to 2 points)	1.2 (0.57) 35	0.93 (0.62) 30				P > 0.05
Zhang 2011	N	N				
Perception of antenatal care	359	322	1.23 (POR)	0.68 to 2.21	z = 0.69	0.490
Perception of care: labour/birth	355	320	1.10 (POR)	0.91 to 1.34	z = 0.95	0.341

* All scales operate in the same direction; higher scores indicate greater satisfaction.

CI = confidence interval; MD = mean difference; OR = odds ratio; POR = proportional odds ratio; RD = risk difference; RR = risk ratio.

Table 12.4.b Scenario 1: intrapartum outcome table ordered by risk of bias, standardized effect estimates calculated for all studies

Outcome* (scale details)	Intervention	Control	Mean difference (95% CI)**	Odds ratio (95% CI)†
Low risk of bias				
Barry 2005	n/N	n/N		
Experience of labour	90/246	72/223		1.21 (0.82 to 1.79)
Frances 2000	n/N	n/N		
Communication: labour/birth				0.90 (0.61 to 1.34)
Rowley 1995	n/N	n/N		
Encouraged to ask questions [during labour/birth]				1.02 (0.66 to 1.58)
Some concerns				
Biro 2000	n/N	n/N		
Perception of care: labour/birth	260/344	192/287		1.54 (1.08 to 2.19)
Crowe 2010	Mean (SD) N	Mean (SD) N		
Experience of labour/birth (0 to 18 points)	9.8 (3.1) 182	9.3 (3.3) 186	0.5 (–0.15 to 1.15)	1.32 (0.91 to 1.92)
Harvey 1996	Mean (SD) N	Mean (SD) N		
Labour & Delivery Satisfaction Index (37 to 222 points)	182 (14.2) 101	185 (30) 93	–3 (–10 to 4)	0.79 (0.48 to 1.32)
Johns 2004	n/N	n/N		
Satisfaction with intrapartum care	605/1163	363/826		1.38 (1.15 to 1.64)
Parr 2002	n/N	n/N		
Experience of childbirth				0.85 (0.39 to 1.87)

Zhang 2011	n/N	n/N		
Perception of care: labour and birth	N = 355	N = 320		POR 1.11 (0.91 to 1.34)
High risk of bias				
Flint 1989	n/N	n/N		
Care from staff during labour	240/275	208/256		1.58 (0.99 to 2.54)
Mac Vicar 1993	n/N	n/N		
Birth satisfaction	849/1163	496/826		1.80 (1.48 to 2.19)
Turnbull 1996	Mean (SD) N	Mean (SD) N		
Intrapartum care rating (–2 to 2 points)	1.2 (0.57) 35	0.93 (0.62) 30	0.27 (–0.03 to 0.57)	2.27 (0.92 to 5.59)

* Outcomes operate in the same direction. A higher score, or an event, indicates greater satisfaction.

** Mean difference calculated for studies reporting continuous outcomes.

† For binary outcomes, odds ratios were calculated from the reported summary statistics or were directly extracted from the study. For continuous outcomes, standardized mean differences were calculated and converted to odds ratios (see Chapter 6).

CI = confidence interval; POR = proportional odds ratio.

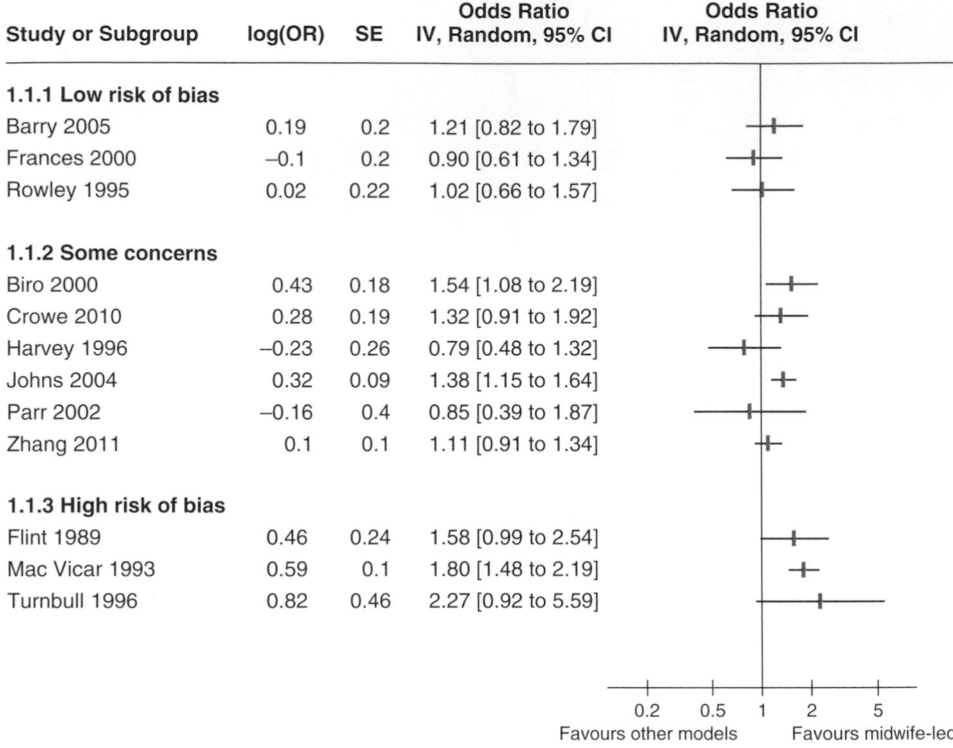

Study or Subgroup	log(OR)	SE	Odds Ratio IV, Random, 95% CI
1.1.1 Low risk of bias			
Barry 2005	0.19	0.2	1.21 [0.82 to 1.79]
Frances 2000	–0.1	0.2	0.90 [0.61 to 1.34]
Rowley 1995	0.02	0.22	1.02 [0.66 to 1.57]
1.1.2 Some concerns			
Biro 2000	0.43	0.18	1.54 [1.08 to 2.19]
Crowe 2010	0.28	0.19	1.32 [0.91 to 1.92]
Harvey 1996	–0.23	0.26	0.79 [0.48 to 1.32]
Johns 2004	0.32	0.09	1.38 [1.15 to 1.64]
Parr 2002	–0.16	0.4	0.85 [0.39 to 1.87]
Zhang 2011	0.1	0.1	1.11 [0.91 to 1.34]
1.1.3 High risk of bias			
Flint 1989	0.46	0.24	1.58 [0.99 to 2.54]
Mac Vicar 1993	0.59	0.1	1.80 [1.48 to 2.19]
Turnbull 1996	0.82	0.46	2.27 [0.92 to 5.59]

Figure 12.4.b Forest plot depicting standardized effect estimates (odds ratios) for satisfaction

few studies, highlighting the importance of tables and plots. It also brings into focus the risk of presenting results without any synthesis, since it seems likely that the reader will try to make sense of the results by drawing inferences across studies. Since a synthesis was considered inappropriate, GRADE was applied to individual studies and then used to prioritize the reporting of results, focusing attention on the most relevant and trustworthy evidence. An alternative might be to report results at low risk of bias, an approach analogous to limiting a meta-analysis to studies at low risk of bias. Where possible, these and other approaches to prioritizing (or ordering) results from individual studies in text and tables should be pre-specified at the protocol stage.

12.4.2 Overview of scenarios 2–4: synthesis approaches

We now address three scenarios in which review authors have decided that the outcomes reported in the 15 studies all broadly reflect satisfaction with care. While the measures were quite diverse, a synthesis is sought to help decision makers understand whether women and their birth partners were generally more satisfied with the care received in midwife-led continuity models compared with other models. The three scenarios differ according to the data available (see Table 12.4.c), with each reflecting progressively less complete reporting of the effect estimates. The data available determine the synthesis method that can be applied.

Box 12.4.b How to describe the results from this structured summary

Scenario 1. Structured reporting of effects (no synthesis)

Table 12.4.b and Figure 12.4.b present results for the 12 included studies that reported a measure of maternal satisfaction with care during labour and birth (hereafter 'satisfaction'). Results from these studies were not synthesized for the reasons reported in the data synthesis methods. Here, we summarize results from studies providing high or moderate certainty evidence (based on GRADE) for which results from a valid measure of global satisfaction were available. Barry 2015 found a small increase in satisfaction with midwife-led care compared to obstetrician-led care (4 more women per 100 were satisfied with care; 95% CI 4 fewer to 15 more per 100 women; 469 participants, 1 study; moderate certainty evidence). Harvey 1996 found a small possibly unimportant decrease in satisfaction with midwife-led care compared with obstetrician-led care (3-point reduction on a 185-point LADSI scale, higher scores are more satisfied; 95% CI 10 points lower to 4 higher; 367 participants, 1 study; moderate certainty evidence). The remaining 10 studies reported specific aspects of satisfaction (Frances 2000, Rowley 1995, ...), used tools with little or no evidence of validity and reliability (Parr 2002, ...) or provided low or very low certainty evidence (Turnbull 1996, ...).

Note: While it is tempting to make statements about consistency of effects across studies (...the majority of studies showed improvement in ..., X of Y studies found ...), be aware that this may contradict claims that a synthesis is inappropriate and constitute unintentional vote counting.

- Scenario 2: effect estimates available without measures of precision (illustrating synthesis of summary statistics).
- Scenario 3: P values available (illustrating synthesis of P values).
- Scenario 4: directions of effect available (illustrating synthesis using vote-counting based on direction of effect).

For studies that reported multiple satisfaction outcomes, one result is selected for synthesis using the decision rules in Box 12.4.a (point 2).

12.4.2.1 Scenario 2: summarizing effect estimates

In Scenario 2, effect estimates are available for all outcomes. However, for most studies, a measure of variance is not reported, or cannot be calculated from the available data. We illustrate how the effect estimates may be summarized using descriptive statistics. In this scenario, it is possible to calculate odds ratios for all studies. For the continuous outcomes, this involves first calculating a standardized mean difference, and then converting this to an odds ratio (Chapter 10, Section 10.6). The median odds ratio is 1.32 with an interquartile range of 1.02 to 1.53 (15 studies). Box-and-whisker plots may be used to display these results and examine informally whether the distribution of effects differs by the overall risk-of-bias assessment (Figure 12.4.a, Panel A). However, because there are relatively few effects, a reasonable alternative would be to present bubble plots (Figure 12.4.a, Panel B).

An example description of the results from the synthesis is provided in Box 12.4.c.

Table 12.4.c Scenarios 2, 3 and 4: available data for the selected outcome from each study

			Scenario 2. Summary statistics		Scenario 3. Combining P values		Scenario 4. Vote counting	
Study ID	Outcome (scale details*)	Overall RoB judgement	Available data**	Stand. metric OR (SMD)	Available data** (2-sided P value)	Stand. metric (1-sided P value)	Available data**	Stand. metric
Continuous			Mean (SD)					
Crowe 2010	Expectation of labour/birth (0 to 18 points)	Some concerns	Intervention 9.8 (3.1); Control 9.3 (3.3)	1.3 (0.16)	Favours intervention, P = 0.135, N = 368	0.068	NS	—
Finn 1997	Experience of labour/birth (0 to 24 points)	Some concerns	Intervention 21 (5.6); Control 19.7 (7.3)	1.4 (0.20)	Favours intervention, P = 0.061, N = 351	0.030	MD 1.3, NS	1
Harvey 1996	Labour & Delivery Satisfaction Index (37 to 222 points)	Some concerns	Intervention 182 (14.2); Control 185 (30)	0.8 (−0.13)	MD −3, P = 0.368, N = 194	0.816	MD −3, NS	0
Kidman 2007	Control during labour/birth (0 to 18 points)	High	Intervention 11.7 (2.9); Control 10.9 (4.2)	1.5 (0.22)	MD 0.8, P = 0.035, N = 368	0.017	MD 0.8 (95% CI 0.1 to 1.5)	1
Turnbull 1996	Intrapartum care rating (−2 to 2 points)	High	Intervention 1.2 (0.57); Control 0.93 (0.62)	2.3 (0.45)	MD 0.27, P = 0.072, N = 65	0.036	MD 0.27 (95% CI0.03 to 0.57)	1
Binary								
Barry 2005	Experience of labour	Low	Intervention 90/246; Control 72/223	1.21	NS	—	RR 1.13, NS	1
Biro 2000	Perception of care: labour/birth	Some concerns	Intervention 260/344; Control 192/287	1.53	RR 1.13, P = 0.018	0.009	RR 1.13, P < 0.05	1

Flint 1989	Care from staff during labour	High	Intervention 240/275; Control 208/256	1.58	Favours intervention, P = 0.059	0.029	RR 1.07 (95% CI 1.00 to 1.16)	1
Frances 2000	Communication: labour/birth	Low	OR 0.90	0.90	Favours control, P = 0.606	0.697	Favours control, NS	0
Johns 2004	Satisfaction with intrapartum care	Some concerns	Intervention 605/ 1163; Control 363/ 826	1.38	Favours intervention, P < 0.001	0.0005	RD 8.1% (95% CI 3.6% to 12.5%)	1
Mac Vicar 1993	Birth satisfaction	High	OR 1.80, P < 0.001	1.80	Favours intervention, P < 0.001	0.0005	RD 13.0% (95% CI 8.8% to 17.2%)	1
Parr 2002	Experience of childbirth	Some concerns	OR 0.85	0.85	OR 0.85, P = 0.685	0.658	NS	—
Rowley 1995	Encouraged to ask questions	Low	OR 1.02, NS	1.02	P = 0.685	—	NS	—
Ordinal								
Waldenstrom 2001	Perception of intrapartum care	Low	POR 1.23, P = 0.490	1.23	POR 1.23, P = 0.490	0.245	POR 1.23, NS	1
Zhang 2011	Perception of care: labour/birth	Low	POR 1.10, P > 0.05	1.10	POR 1.1, P = 0.341	0.170	Favours intervention	1

* All scales operate in the same direction. Higher scores indicate greater satisfaction.

** For a particular scenario, the 'available data' column indicates the data that were directly reported, or were calculated from the reported statistics, in terms of: effect estimate, direction of effect, confidence interval, precise P value, or statement regarding statistical significance (either statistically significant, or not).

CI = confidence interval; direction = direction of effect reported or can be calculated; MD = mean difference; NS = not statistically significant; OR = odds ratio; RD = risk difference; RoB = risk of bias; RR = risk ratio; sig. = statistically significant; SMD = standardized mean difference; Stand. = standardized.

Box 12.4.c How to describe the results from this synthesis

Scenario 2. Synthesis of summary statistics

'The median odds ratio of satisfaction was 1.32 for midwife-led models of care compared with other models (interquartile range 1.02 to 1.53; 15 studies). Only five of the 15 effects were judged to be at a low risk of bias, and informal visual examination suggested the size of the odds ratios may be smaller in this group.'

12.4.2.2 Scenario 3: combining P values

In Scenario 3, there is minimal reporting of the data, and the type of data and statistical methods and tests vary. However, 11 of the 15 studies provide a precise P value and direction of effect, and a further two report a P value less than a threshold (< 0.001) and direction. We use this scenario to illustrate a synthesis of P values. Since the reported P values are two-sided (Table 12.4.c, column 6), they must first be converted to one-sided P values, which incorporate the direction of effect (Table 12.4.c, column 7).

Fisher's method for combining P values involved calculating the following statistic:

$$X^2 = -2\sum_{i=1}^{k}\ln(P_i) = -2 \times (\ln(0.068) + \ldots + \ln(0.170)) = -2 \times -41.2 = 82.3$$

where P_i is the one-sided P value from study i, and k is the total number of P values. This formula can be implemented using a standard spreadsheet package. The statistic is then compared against the chi-squared distribution with 26 (= 2 × 13) degrees of freedom to obtain the P value. Using a Microsoft Excel spreadsheet, this can be obtained by typing =CHIDIST(82.3, 26) into any cell. In Stata or R, the packages (both named) **metap** could be used. These packages include a range of methods for combining P values.

The combination of P values suggests there is strong evidence of benefit of midwife-led models of care in at least one study (P < 0.001 from a Chi^2 test, 13 studies). Restricting this analysis to those studies judged to be at an overall low risk of bias (sensitivity analysis), there is no longer evidence to reject the null hypothesis of no benefit of midwife-led model of care in any studies (P = 0.314, 3 studies). For the five studies reporting continuous satisfaction outcomes, sufficient data (precise P value, direction, total sample size) are reported to construct an albatross plot (Figure 12.4.a, Panel C). The location of the points relative to the standardized mean difference contours indicate that the likely effects of the intervention in these studies are small.

An example description of the results from the synthesis is provided in Box 12.4.d.

Box 12.4.d How to describe the results from this synthesis

Scenario 3. Synthesis of P values

'There was strong evidence of benefit of midwife-led models of care in at least one study (P < 0.001, 13 studies). However, a sensitivity analysis restricted to studies with an overall low risk of bias suggested there was no effect of midwife-led models of care in any of the trials (P = 0.314, 3 studies). Estimated standardized mean differences for five of the outcomes were small (ranging from –0.13 to 0.45) (Figure 12.4.a, Panel C).'

12.4.2.3 Scenario 4: vote counting based on direction of effect

In Scenario 4, there is minimal reporting of the data, and the type of effect measure (when used) varies across the studies (e.g. mean difference, proportional odds ratio). Of the 15 results, only five report data suitable for meta-analysis (effect estimate and measure of precision; Table 12.4.c, column 8), and no studies reported precise P values. We use this scenario to illustrate vote counting based on direction of effect. For each study, the effect is categorized as beneficial or harmful based on the direction of effect (indicated as a binary metric; Table 12.4.c, column 9).

Of the 15 studies, we exclude three because they do not provide information on the direction of effect, leaving 12 studies to contribute to the synthesis. Of these 12, 10 effects favour midwife-led models of care (83%). The probability of observing this result if midwife-led models of care are truly ineffective is 0.039 (from a binomial probability test, or equivalently, the sign test). The 95% confidence interval for the percentage of effects favouring midwife-led care is wide (55% to 95%).

The binomial test can be implemented using standard computer spreadsheet or statistical packages. For example, the two-sided P value from the binomial probability test presented can be obtained from Microsoft Excel by typing =2*BINOM.DIST(2, 12, 0.5, TRUE) into any cell in the spreadsheet. The syntax requires the smaller of the 'number of effects favouring the intervention' or 'the number of effects favouring the control' (here, the smaller of these counts is 2), the number of effects (here 12), and the null value (true proportion of effects favouring the intervention = 0.5). In Stata, the **bitest** command could be used (e.g. **bitesti 12 10 0.5**).

A harvest plot can be used to display the results (Figure 12.4.a, Panel D), with characteristics of the studies represented using different heights and shading. A sensitivity analysis might be considered, restricting the analysis to those studies judged to be at an overall low risk of bias. However, only four studies were judged to be at a low risk of bias (of which, three favoured midwife-led models of care), precluding reasonable interpretation of the count.

An example description of the results from the synthesis is provided in Box 12.4.e.

12.5 Chapter information

Authors: Joanne E McKenzie, Sue E Brennan

Acknowledgements: Sections of this chapter build on chapter 9 of version 5.1 of the *Handbook*, with editors Jonathan J Deeks, Julian PT Higgins and Douglas G Altman.

Box 12.4.e How to describe the results from this synthesis
Scenario 4. Synthesis using vote counting based on direction of effects
'There was evidence that midwife-led models of care had an effect on satisfaction, with 10 of 12 studies favouring the intervention (83% (95% CI 55% to 95%), P = 0.039) (Figure 12.4.a, Panel D). Four of the 12 studies were judged to be at a low risk of bias, and three of these favoured the intervention. The available effect estimates are presented in [review] Table X.'

We are grateful to the following for commenting helpfully on earlier drafts: Miranda Cumpston, Jamie Hartmann-Boyce, Tianjing Li, Rebecca Ryan and Hilary Thomson.

Funding: JEM is supported by an Australian National Health and Medical Research Council (NHMRC) Career Development Fellowship (1143429). SEB's position is supported by the NHMRC Cochrane Collaboration Funding Program.

12.6 References

Achana F, Hubbard S, Sutton A, Kendrick D, Cooper N. An exploration of synthesis methods in public health evaluations of interventions concludes that the use of modern statistical methods would be beneficial. *Journal of Clinical Epidemiology* 2014; **67**: 376–390.

Becker BJ. Combining significance levels. In: Cooper H, Hedges LV, editors. *A handbook of research synthesis*. New York (NY): Russell Sage; 1994. pp. 215–235.

Boonyasai RT, Windish DM, Chakraborti C, Feldman LS, Rubin HR, Bass EB. Effectiveness of teaching quality improvement to clinicians: a systematic review. *JAMA* 2007; **298**: 1023–1037.

Borenstein M, Hedges LV, Higgins JPT, Rothstein HR. Meta-Analysis methods based on direction and p-values. *Introduction to Meta-Analysis*. Chichester (UK): John Wiley & Sons, Ltd; 2009. pp. 325–330.

Brown LD, Cai TT, DasGupta A. Interval estimation for a binomial proportion. *Statistical Science* 2001; **16**: 101–117.

Bushman BJ, Wang MC. Vote-counting procedures in meta-analysis. In: Cooper H, Hedges LV, Valentine JC, editors. *Handbook of Research Synthesis and Meta-Analysis*. 2nd ed. New York (NY): Russell Sage Foundation; 2009. pp. 207–220.

Crowther M, Avenell A, MacLennan G, Mowatt G. A further use for the Harvest plot: a novel method for the presentation of data synthesis. *Research Synthesis Methods* 2011; **2**: 79–83.

Friedman L. Why vote-count reviews don't count. *Biological Psychiatry* 2001; **49**: 161–162.

Grimshaw J, McAuley LM, Bero LA, Grilli R, Oxman AD, Ramsay C, Vale L, Zwarenstein M. Systematic reviews of the effectiveness of quality improvement strategies and programmes. *Quality and Safety in Health Care* 2003; **12**: 298–303.

Harrison S, Jones HE, Martin RM, Lewis SJ, Higgins JPT. The albatross plot: a novel graphical tool for presenting results of diversely reported studies in a systematic review. *Research Synthesis Methods* 2017; **8**: 281–289.

Hedges L, Vevea J. Fixed- and random-effects models in meta-analysis. *Psychological Methods* 1998; **3**: 486–504.

Ioannidis JP, Patsopoulos NA, Rothstein HR. Reasons or excuses for avoiding meta-analysis in forest plots. *BMJ* 2008; **336**: 1413–1415.

Ivers N, Jamtvedt G, Flottorp S, Young JM, Odgaard-Jensen J, French SD, O'Brien MA, Johansen M, Grimshaw J, Oxman AD. Audit and feedback: effects on professional practice and healthcare outcomes. *Cochrane Database of Systematic Reviews* 2012; **6**: CD000259.

Jones DR. Meta-analysis: weighing the evidence. *Statistics in Medicine* 1995; **14**: 137–149.

Loughin TM. A systematic comparison of methods for combining p-values from independent tests. *Computational Statistics & Data Analysis* 2004; **47**: 467–485.

McGill R, Tukey JW, Larsen WA. Variations of box plots. *The American Statistician* 1978; **32**: 12–16.

McKenzie JE, Brennan SE. Complex reviews: methods and considerations for summarising and synthesising results in systematic reviews with complexity. Report to the Australian National Health and Medical Research Council. 2014.

O'Brien MA, Rogers S, Jamtvedt G, Oxman AD, Odgaard-Jensen J, Kristoffersen DT, Forsetlund L, Bainbridge D, Freemantle N, Davis DA, Haynes RB, Harvey EL. Educational outreach visits: effects on professional practice and health care outcomes. *Cochrane Database of Systematic Reviews* 2007; **4**: CD000409.

Ogilvie D, Fayter D, Petticrew M, Sowden A, Thomas S, Whitehead M, Worthy G. The harvest plot: a method for synthesising evidence about the differential effects of interventions. *BMC Medical Research Methodology* 2008; **8**: 8.

Riley RD, Higgins JP, Deeks JJ. Interpretation of random effects meta-analyses. *BMJ* 2011; **342**: d549.

Schriger DL, Sinha R, Schroter S, Liu PY, Altman DG. From submission to publication: a retrospective review of the tables and figures in a cohort of randomized controlled trials submitted to the British Medical Journal. *Annals of Emergency Medicine* 2006; **48**: 750–756, 756 e751–721.

Schriger DL, Altman DG, Vetter JA, Heafner T, Moher D. Forest plots in reports of systematic reviews: a cross-sectional study reviewing current practice. *International Journal of Epidemiology* 2010; **39**: 421–429.

ter Wee MM, Lems WF, Usan H, Gulpen A, Boonen A. The effect of biological agents on work participation in rheumatoid arthritis patients: a systematic review. *Annals of the Rheumatic Diseases* 2012; **71**: 161–171.

Thomson HJ, Thomas S. The effect direction plot: visual display of non-standardised effects across multiple outcome domains. *Research Synthesis Methods* 2013; **4**: 95–101.

Thornicroft G, Mehta N, Clement S, Evans-Lacko S, Doherty M, Rose D, Koschorke M, Shidhaye R, O'Reilly C, Henderson C. Evidence for effective interventions to reduce mental-health-related stigma and discrimination. *Lancet* 2016; **387**: 1123–1132.

Valentine JC, Pigott TD, Rothstein HR. How many studies do you need?: a primer on statistical power for meta-analysis. *Journal of Educational and Behavioral Statistics* 2010; **35**: 215–247.

13

Assessing risk of bias due to missing results in a synthesis

Matthew J Page, Julian PT Higgins, Jonathan AC Sterne

KEY POINTS

- Systematic reviews seek to identify all research that meets the eligibility criteria. However, this goal can be compromised by 'non-reporting bias': when decisions about how, when or where to report results of eligible studies are influenced by the P value, magnitude or direction of the results.
- There is convincing evidence for several types of non-reporting bias, reinforcing the need for review authors to search all possible sources where study reports and results may be located. It may be necessary to consult multiple bibliographic databases, trials registers, manufacturers, regulators and study authors or sponsors.
- Regardless of whether an entire study report or a particular study result is unavailable selectively (e.g. because the P value, magnitude or direction of the results were considered unfavourable by the investigators), the same consequence can arise: risk of bias in a synthesis because available results differ systematically from missing results.
- Several approaches for assessing risk of bias due to missing results have been suggested. A thorough assessment of selective non-reporting or under-reporting of results in the studies identified is likely to be the most valuable. Because the number of identified studies that have results missing for a given synthesis is known, the impact of selective non-reporting or under-reporting of results can be quantified more easily than the impact of selective non-publication of an unknown number of studies.
- Funnel plots (and the tests used for examining funnel plot asymmetry) may help review authors to identify evidence of non-reporting biases in cases where protocols or trials register records were unavailable for most studies. However, they have well-documented limitations.
- When there is evidence of funnel plot asymmetry, non-reporting biases should be considered as only one of a number of possible explanations. In these circumstances, review authors should attempt to understand the source(s) of the asymmetry, and consider their implications in the light of any qualitative signals that raise a suspicion of additional missing results, and other sensitivity analyses.

This chapter should be cited as: Page MJ, Higgins JPT, Sterne JAC. Chapter 13: Assessing risk of bias due to missing results in a synthesis. In: Higgins JPT, Thomas J, Chandler J, Cumpston M, Li T, Page MJ, Welch VA (editors). *Cochrane Handbook for Systematic Reviews of Interventions*. 2nd Edition. Chichester (UK): John Wiley & Sons, 2019: 349–374.

13.1 Introduction

Systematic reviews seek to identify all research that meets pre-specified eligibility criteria. This goal can be compromised if decisions about how, when or where to report results of eligible studies are influenced by the P value, magnitude or direction of the study's results. For example, 'statistically significant' results that suggest an intervention works are more likely than 'statistically non-significant' results to be available, available rapidly, available in high impact journals and cited by others, and hence more easily identifiable for systematic reviews. The term 'reporting bias' has often been used to describe this problem, but we prefer the term **non-reporting bias**.

Non-reporting biases lead to **bias due to missing results** in a systematic review. Syntheses such as meta-analyses are at risk of bias due to missing results when results of some eligible studies are unavailable because of the P value, magnitude or direction of the results. Bias due to missing results differs from a related source of bias – **bias in selection of the reported result** – where study authors select a result for reporting from among multiple measurements or analyses, on the basis of the P value, magnitude or direction of the results. In such cases, the study result that is available for inclusion in the synthesis is at risk of bias. Bias in selection of the reported result is described in more detail in Chapter 7, and addressed in the RoB 2 tool (Chapter 8) and ROBINS-I tool (Chapter 25).

Failure to consider the potential impact of non-reporting biases on the results of the review can lead to the uptake of ineffective and harmful interventions in clinical practice. For example, when unreported results were included in a systematic review of oseltamivir (Tamiflu) for influenza, the drug was not shown to reduce hospital admissions, had unclear effects on pneumonia and other complications of influenza, and increased the risk of harms such as nausea, vomiting and psychiatric adverse events. These findings were different from synthesized results based only on published study results (Jefferson et al 2014).

We structure the chapter as follows. We start by discussing approaches for avoiding or minimizing bias due to missing results in systematic reviews in Section 13.2, and provide guidance for assessing the risk of bias due to missing results in Section 13.3. For the purpose of discussing these biases, 'statistically significant' ($P < 0.05$) results are sometimes denoted as 'positive' results and 'statistically non-significant' or null results as 'negative' results. As explained in Chapter 15, Cochrane Review authors should not use any of these labels when reporting their review findings, since they are based on arbitrary thresholds and may not reflect the clinical or policy significance of the findings.

In this chapter, we use the term **result** to describe the combination of a point estimate (such as a mean difference or risk ratio) and a measure of its precision (such as a confidence interval) for a particular study outcome. We use the term **outcome** to refer to an event (such as mortality or a reduction in pain). When fully defined, an outcome for an individual participant includes the following elements: an outcome domain; a specific measure; a specific metric; and a time point (Zarin et al 2011). An example of a fully defined outcome is 'a 50% change from baseline to eight weeks on the Montgomery-Asberg Depression Rating Scale total score'. A corresponding result for this outcome additionally requires a method of aggregation across individuals: here it might be a risk ratio with 95% confidence interval, which estimates the between-group difference in the proportion of people with the outcome.

13.2 Minimizing risk of bias due to missing results

The convincing evidence for the presence of non-reporting biases, summarized in Chapter 7 (Section 7.2.3), should be of great concern to review authors. Regardless of whether an entire study report or a particular study result is unavailable selectively (e.g. because the P value, magnitude or direction of the results were considered unfavourable by the investigators), the same consequence can arise: risk of bias in a synthesis because available results differ systematically from missing results. We discuss two means of reducing, or potentially avoiding, bias due to missing results.

13.2.1 Inclusion of results from sources other than published reports

Eyding and colleagues provide a striking example of the value of searching beyond the published literature (Eyding et al 2010). They sought data from published trials of reboxetine versus placebo for major depression, as well as unpublished data from the manufacturer (Pfizer, Berlin). Of 13 trials identified, data for only 26% were published. Meta-analysis painted a far rosier picture of the effects of reboxetine when restricted to the published results (Figure 13.2.a). For example, the between-group difference in the number of patients with an important reduction in depression was much larger in the published trial compared with a meta-analysis of the published and unpublished trials. Similarly, a meta-analysis of two published trials suggested a negligible difference between reboxetine and placebo in the number of patients who withdrew because of adverse events. However, when six unpublished trials were

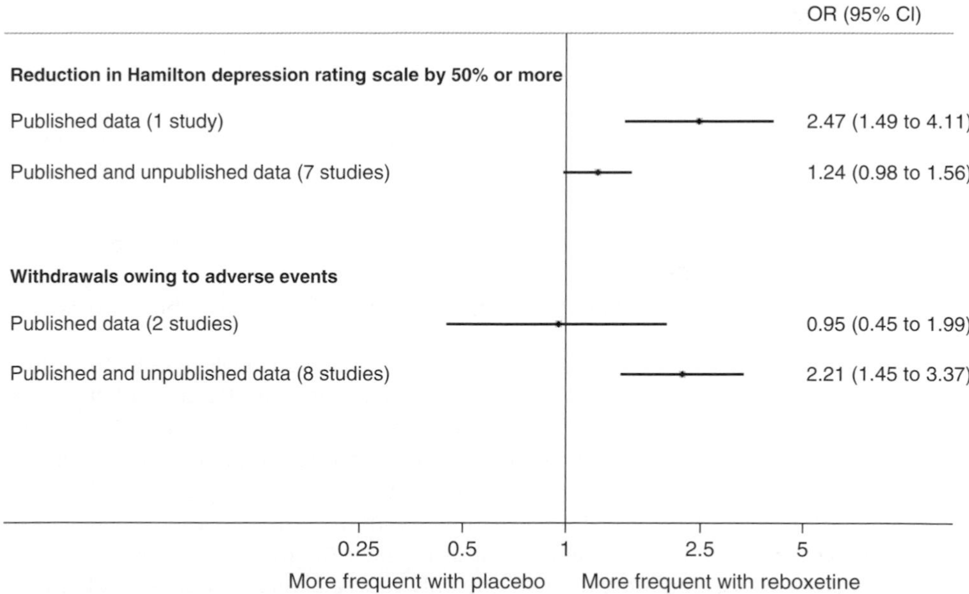

Figure 13.2.a Results of meta-analyses of reboxetine versus placebo for acute treatment of major depression, with or without unpublished data (data from Eyding et al 2010). Reproduced with permission of BMJ Publishing Group.

added, the summary estimate suggested that patients on reboxetine were more than twice as likely to withdraw (Eyding et al 2010).

Cases such as this illustrate how bias in a meta-analysis can be reduced by the inclusion of missing results. In other situations, the bias reduction may not be so dramatic. Schmucker and colleagues reviewed five methodological studies examining the difference in summary effect estimates of 173 meta-analyses that included or omitted results from sources other than journal articles (e.g. conference abstracts, theses, government reports, regulatory websites) (Schmucker et al 2017). They found that the direction and magnitude of the differences in summary estimates varied. While inclusion of unreported results may not change summary estimates markedly in all cases, doing so often leads to an increase in precision of the summary estimates (Schmucker et al 2017). Guidance on searching for unpublished sources is included in Chapter 4 (Section 4.3).

13.2.1.1 Inclusion of results from trials results registers

As outlined in Chapter 4 (Section 4.3.3), trials registers can be used to identify any initiated, ongoing or completed (but not necessarily published) studies that meet the eligibility criteria of a review. In 2008, ClinicalTrials.gov created data fields to accept summary results for any registered trial (see Chapter 5, Section 5.3.1) (Zarin et al 2011). A search of ClinicalTrials.gov in June 2019 retrieved over 305,000 studies, of which summary results were reported for around 36,000 (12%). Empirical evidence suggests that including results from ClinicalTrials.gov can lead to important changes in the results of some meta-analyses. When Baudard and colleagues searched trials registers for 95 systematic reviews of pharmaceutical interventions that had not already done so, they identified 122 trials that were eligible for inclusion in 41 (47%) of the reviews (Baudard et al 2017). Results for 45 of the 122 trials were available and could be included in a meta-analysis in 14 of the reviews. The percentage change in meta-analytic effects after including results from trials registers was greater than 10% for five of the 14 reviews and greater than 20% for two reviews; in almost all cases the revised meta-analysis showed decreased efficacy of the drug (Baudard et al 2017). Several initiatives are underway to increase results posting in ClinicalTrials.gov and the European Union Clinical Trials Register (DeVito et al 2018, Goldacre et al 2018), so searching these registers should continue to be an important way of minimizing bias in future systematic reviews.

13.2.1.2 Inclusion of results from clinical study reports and other regulatory documents

Another way to minimize risk of bias due to missing results in reviews of regulated interventions (e.g. drugs, biologics) is to seek clinical study reports (CSRs) and other regulatory documents, such as FDA Drug Approval Packages (see Chapter 4, Section 4.3.4). CSRs are comprehensive documents submitted by pharmaceutical companies in an application for regulatory approval of a product (Jefferson et al 2018), while FDA Drug Approval Packages (at the Drugs@FDA website) include summaries of CSRs and related documents, written by FDA staff (Ladanie et al 2018) (see Chapter 5, Sections 5.5.6 and 5.5.7). For some trials, regulatory data are the only source of information about the trial. Comparisons of the results available in regulatory documents with results available in corresponding journal articles have revealed that unfavourable results for benefit outcomes and adverse events are largely under-reported in journal articles (Wieseler et al

2013, Maund et al 2014, Schroll et al 2016). A few systematic reviews have found that conclusions about the benefits and harms of interventions changed after regulatory data were included in the review (Turner et al 2008, Rodgers et al 2013, Jefferson et al 2014).

CSRs and other regulatory documents have great potential for improving the credibility of systematic reviews of regulated interventions, but substantial resources are needed to access them and disentangle the data within them (Schroll et al 2015, Doshi and Jefferson 2016). Only limited guidance is currently available for review authors considering embarking on a review including regulatory data. Jefferson and colleagues provide criteria for assessing whether to include regulatory data for a drug or biologic in a systematic review (Jefferson et al 2018). The RIAT (Restoring Invisible and Abandoned Trials) Support Center website provides useful information, including a taxonomy of regulatory documents, a glossary of relevant terms, guidance on how to request CSRs from regulators and contact information for making requests (Doshi et al 2018). Also, Ladanie and colleagues provide guidance on how to access and use FDA Drug Approval Packages for evidence syntheses (Ladanie et al 2018).

13.2.2 Restriction of syntheses to inception cohorts

Review authors can sometimes reduce the risk of bias due to missing results by limiting the type of studies that are eligible for inclusion. Because systematic reviews traditionally search comprehensively for completed studies, non-reporting biases, poor indexing and other factors make it impossible to know whether all studies were in fact identified. An alternative approach is to review an **inception cohort** of studies. An inception cohort refers to a set of studies known to have been initiated, irrespective of their results (e.g. selecting studies only from trials registers) (Dwan et al 2013). This means there is a full accounting of which studies do and do not have results available.

There are various ways to assemble an inception cohort. Review authors could prespecify that studies will be included only if they were registered prospectively (e.g. registered before patient enrolment in public, industry or regulatory registers (Roberts et al 2015, Jørgensen et al 2018), or in grants databases such as NIH RePORTER (Driessen et al 2015). Or, review authors may obtain unabridged access to reports of all studies of a product conducted by a particular manufacturer (Simmonds et al 2013). Alternatively, a clinical trial collaborative group may prospectively plan to undertake multiple trials using similar designs, participants, interventions and outcomes, and synthesize the findings of all trials once completed ('prospective meta-analysis'; see Chapter 22) (Askie et al 2018). The benefit of these strategies is that review authors can identify all eligible studies regardless of the P value, magnitude or direction of any result.

Limiting inclusion to prospectively registered studies avoids the possibility of missing any eligible *studies*. However, there is still the potential for missing results in these studies. Therefore, review authors would need to assess the availability of results for each study identified (guidance on how to do so is provided in Section 13.3.3). If none of the prospectively registered studies suffer from selective non-reporting or under-reporting of results, then none of the syntheses will be at risk of bias due to missing results. Conversely, if some results are missing selectively, then there may be a risk of bias in the synthesis, particularly if the total amount of data missing is large (for more details see Section 13.3.4).

Reliance on trials registers to assemble an inception cohort may not be ideal in all instances. Prospective registration of trials started to increase only after 2004, when the International Committee of Medical Journal Editors announced that they would no longer publish trials that were not registered at inception (De Angelis et al 2004). For this reason, review authors are unlikely to identify any prospectively registered trials of interventions that were investigated only prior to this time. Also, until quite recently there have been fewer incentives to register prospectively trials of non-regulated interventions (Dal-Ré et al 2015), and unless registration rates increase, systematic reviews of such interventions are unlikely to identify many prospectively registered trials.

Restricting a synthesis to an inception cohort therefore involves a trade-off between bias, precision and applicability. For example, limiting inclusion to prospectively registered trials will avoid risk of bias due to missing results if no results are missing from a meta-analysis selectively. However, the precision of the meta-analysis may be low if there are only a few, small, prospectively registered trials. Also, the summary estimate from the meta-analysis may have limited applicability to the review question if the questions asked in the prospectively registered trials are narrower in scope than the questions asked in unregistered or retrospectively registered trials. Therefore, as with any synthesis, review authors will need to consider precision and applicability when interpreting the synthesis findings (methods for doing so are covered in Chapters 14 and 15).

13.3 A framework for assessing risk of bias due to missing results in a synthesis

The strategies outlined in Section 13.2 have a common goal: to prevent bias due to missing results in systematic reviews. However, neither strategy is infallible on its own. For example, review authors may have been able to include results from ClinicalTrials.gov for several unpublished trials, yet unable to obtain unreported results for other trials. Unless review authors can eliminate the potential for bias due to missing results (e.g. through prospective meta-analysis; see Chapter 22), they should formally assess the risk of this bias in their review.

Several methods are available for assessing non-reporting biases. For example, Page and colleagues identified 15 scales, checklists and domain-based tools designed for this purpose (Page et al 2018). In addition, many graphical and statistical approaches seeking to assess non-reporting biases have been developed (including funnel plots and statistical tests for funnel plot asymmetry) (Mueller et al 2016).

In this section we describe a framework for assessing the risk of bias due to missing results in a synthesis. This consolidates and extends existing guidance: a key feature is that review authors are prompted to consider whether a synthesis (e.g. meta-analysis) is missing any eligible results and, if so, whether the summary estimate can be trusted given the missing results. The framework consists of the following steps.

1) Select syntheses to assess for risk of bias due to missing results (Section 13.3.1).
2) Define which results are eligible for inclusion in each synthesis (Section 13.3.2).

3) Record whether any of the studies identified are missing from each synthesis because results known (or presumed) to have been generated by study investigators are unavailable: the 'known unknowns' (Section 13.3.3).
4) Consider whether each synthesis is likely to be biased because of the missing results in the studies identified (Section 13.3.4).
5) Consider whether results from additional studies are likely to be missing from each synthesis: the 'unknown unknowns' (Section 13.3.5).
6) Reach an overall judgement about risk of bias due to missing results in each synthesis (Section 13.3.6).

The framework is designed to assess risk of bias in syntheses of *quantitative* data about the effects of interventions, regardless of the type of synthesis (e.g. meta-analysis, or calculation of the median effect estimate across studies). The issue of non-reporting bias has received little attention in the context of qualitative research, so more work is needed to develop methods relevant to qualitative evidence syntheses (Toews et al 2017).

If review authors are unable to, or choose not to, generate a synthesized result (e.g. a meta-analytic effect estimate, or median effect across studies), then the complete framework cannot be applied. Nevertheless, review authors should not ignore any missing results when drawing conclusions in this situation (see Chapter 12). For example, the primary outcome in the Cochrane Review of latrepirdine for Alzheimer's disease (Chau et al 2015) was clinical global impression of change, measured by CIBIC-Plus (Clinician's Interview-Based Impression of Change Plus Caregiver Input). This was assessed in four trials, but results were available for only one, and review authors suspected selective non-reporting of results in the other three. After describing the mean difference in CIBIC-Plus from the trial with results available, the review authors concluded that they were uncertain about the efficacy of latrepirdine on clinical global impression of change, owing to the missing results from three trials.

13.3.1 Selecting syntheses to assess for risk of bias

It may not be feasible to assess risk of bias due to missing results in all syntheses in a review, particularly if many syntheses are conducted and many studies are eligible for inclusion in each. Review authors should therefore strive to assess risk of bias due to missing results in syntheses of outcomes that are most important to patients and health professionals. Such outcomes will typically be included in 'Summary of findings' tables (see Chapter 14). Ideally, review authors should pre-specify the syntheses for which they plan to assess the risk of bias due to missing results.

13.3.2 Defining eligible results for the synthesis

Review authors should consider what type of results are eligible for inclusion in each selected synthesis. Eligibility will depend on the specificity of the planned synthesis. For example, a highly specific approach may be to synthesize mean differences from trials measuring depression using a particular instrument (the Beck Depression Inventory (BDI)) at a particular time point (six weeks). A broader approach would be to synthesize mean differences from trials measuring depression using any instrument, at any time up to 12 weeks, while an even broader approach would be to synthesize mean differences from trials measuring any mental health outcome (e.g. depression or anxiety) at any time point (López-López et al 2018). The more specific the synthesis, the less likely it is that a given study result is eligible. For example, if a trial has results only for the BDI at two weeks, the result would be eligible for inclusion in a synthesis of 'Depression scores up to 12 weeks', but ineligible for inclusion in a synthesis of 'BDI scores *at* six weeks'.

Review authors should aim to define fully the results that are eligible for inclusion in each synthesis. This is achieved by specifying eligibility criteria for: outcome domain (e.g. depression), time points (e.g. up to six weeks) and measures/instruments (e.g. BDI or Hamilton Rating Scale for Depression) as discussed in Chapter 3 (Section 3.2.4.3) as well as how effect estimates will be computed in terms of metrics (e.g. post-intervention or change from baseline) and methods of aggregation (e.g. mean scores on depression scales or proportion of people with depression) as discussed in Chapter 6 (Mayo-Wilson et al 2017). It is best to pre-define eligibility criteria for all of these elements, although the measurement instruments, timing and analysis metrics used in studies identified can be difficult to predict, so plans may need to be refined. Failure to define fully which results are eligible makes it far more difficult to assess which results are missing.

How the synthesis is defined has implications both for the risk of bias due to missing results and the related risk of bias in selection of the reported result, which is addressed in the RoB 2 (Chapter 8) and ROBINS-I (Chapter 25) tools for assessing risk of bias in study results. For example, consider a trial where the BDI was administered at two and six weeks, but the six-week result was withheld because it was statistically non-significant. If the synthesis was defined as 'BDI scores up to eight weeks', the available two-week result would be eligible. If there were no missing results from other trials, there would be no risk of bias due to missing results in this synthesis, because each trial contributed an eligible result. However, the two-week result would be at high risk of bias in selection of the reported result. This example demonstrates that the risk of bias due to missing results in a synthesis depends not only on the availability of results in the eligible studies, but also on how review authors define the synthesis.

13.3.3 Recording whether any of the studies identified are missing from each synthesis because results known (or presumed) to have been generated by study investigators are unavailable: the 'known unknowns'

Once eligible results have been defined for each synthesis, review authors can investigate the availability of such results for all studies identified. Key questions to consider are as follows.

1) Are the particular results I am seeking unavailable for any study?
2) If so, are the results unavailable because of the P value, magnitude or direction of the results?

Review authors should try to identify results that are *completely* or *partially* unavailable because of the P value, magnitude or direction of the results (selective non-reporting or under-reporting of results, respectively). By completely unavailable, we mean that no information is available to estimate an intervention effect or to make any other inference (including a qualitative conclusion about the direction of effect) in any of the sources identified or from the study authors/sponsors. By partially unavailable, we mean that some, but not all, of the information necessary to include a result in a meta-analysis is available (e.g. study authors report only that results were 'non-significant' rather than providing summary statistics, or they provide a point estimate without any measure of precision) (Chan et al 2004).

There are several ways to detect selective non-reporting or under-reporting of results, although a thorough assessment is likely to be labour intensive. It is helpful to start by assembling all sources of information obtained about each study (see Chapter 4, Section 4.6.2). This may include the trial's register record, protocol, statistical analysis plan (SAP), reports of the results of the study (e.g. journal articles, CSRs) or any information obtained directly from the study authors or sponsor. The more sources of information sought, the more reliable the assessment is likely to be. Studies should be assessed regardless of whether a report of the results is available. For example, in some cases review authors may only know about a study because there is a registration record of it in ClinicalTrials.gov. If a long time has passed since the study was completed, it is possible that the results are not available because the investigators considered them unworthy of dissemination. Ignoring this registered study with no results available could lead to less concern about the risk of bias due to missing results than is warranted.

If study plans are available (e.g. in a trials register, protocol or statistical analysis plan), details of outcomes that were assessed can be compared with those for which results are available. Suspicion is raised if results are unavailable for any outcomes that were pre-specified in these sources. However, outcomes pre-specified in a trials register may differ from the outcomes pre-specified in a trial protocol (Chan et al 2017), and the latest version of a trials register record may differ from the initial version. Such differences may be explained by legitimate, yet undeclared, changes to the study plans: pre-specification of an outcome does not guarantee it was actually assessed. Further information should be sought from study authors or sponsors to resolve any unexplained discrepancies between sources.

If no study plans are available, then other approaches can be used to uncover missing results. Abstracts of presentations about the study may contain information about outcomes not subsequently mentioned in publications, or the methods section of a published article may list outcomes not subsequently mentioned in the results section.

Missing information that seems certain to have been recorded is of particular interest. For example, some measurements, such as systolic and diastolic blood pressure, are expected to appear together, so that if only one is reported we should wonder why. Williamson and Gamble give several examples, including a Cochrane Review in which all nine trials reported the outcome 'treatment failure' but only five reported mortality (Williamson and Gamble 2005). Since mortality was part of the definition of treatment failure, those data must have been collected in the other four trials. Searches of the Core Outcome Measures in Effectiveness Trials (COMET) database can help review authors identify core sets of outcomes that are expected to have been measured in all trials of particular conditions (Williamson and Clarke 2012), although review authors should keep in mind that trials conducted before the publication of a relevant core outcome set are less likely to have measured the relevant outcomes, and adoption of core outcome sets may not be complete even after they have been published.

If the particular results that review authors seek are not reported in any of the sources identified (e.g. journal article, trials results register, CSR), review authors should consider requesting the required result from the study authors or sponsors. Authors or sponsors may be able to calculate the result for the review authors or send the individual participant data for review authors to analyse themselves. Failure to obtain the results requested should be acknowledged when discussing the limitations of the review process. In some cases, review authors might be able to compute or impute missing details (e.g. imputing standard deviations; see Chapter 6, Section 6.5.2).

Once review authors have identified that a study result is *unavailable*, they must consider whether this is because of the P value, magnitude or direction of the result. The Outcome Reporting Bias In Trials (ORBIT) system for classifying reasons for missing results (Kirkham et al 2018) can be used to do this. Examples of scenarios where it may be reasonable to assume that a result is *not* unavailable because of the P value, magnitude or direction of the result include:

- it is clear (or very likely) that the outcome of interest was not measured in the study (based on examination of the study protocol or SAP, or correspondence with the authors/sponsors);
- the instrument or equipment needed to measure the outcome of interest was not available at the time the study was conducted; and
- the outcome of interest was measured but data were not analysed owing to a fault in the measurement instrument, or substantial missing data.

Examples of scenarios where it may be reasonable to suspect that a result *is* missing because of the P value, magnitude or direction of the result include:

- study authors claimed to have measured the outcome, but no results were available and no explanation for this is provided;
- the between-group difference for the result of interest was reported as being 'non-significant', whereas summary statistics (e.g. means and standard deviations) per intervention group were available for other outcomes in the study when the difference was statistically significant;
- results are missing for an outcome that tends to be measured together with another (e.g. results are available for cause-specific mortality and are favourable to the experimental intervention, yet results for all-cause mortality are missing);
- summary statistics (number of events, or mean scores) are available only globally across all groups (e.g. study authors claim that 10 of 100 participants in the trial experienced adverse events, but do not report the number of events by intervention group); and
- the outcome is expected to have been measured, and the study is conducted by authors or sponsored by an organization with a vested interest in the intervention who may be inclined to withhold results that are unfavourable to the intervention (guidance on assessing conflicts of interest is provided in Chapter 7).

Typically, selective non-reporting or under-reporting of results manifests as the suppression of results that are statistically non-significant or unfavourable to the experimental intervention. However, in some instances the opposite may occur. For example, a trialist who believes that an intervention is ineffective may choose not to report results indicating a difference in favour of the intervention over placebo. Therefore, review authors should consider the interventions being compared when considering reasons for missing results.

Review authors may find it useful to construct a matrix (with rows as studies and columns as syntheses) indicating the availability of study results for each synthesis to be assessed for risk of bias due to missing results. Table 13.3.a shows an example of a matrix indicating the availability of results for three syntheses in a Cochrane Review comparing selective serotonin reuptake inhibitors (SSRIs) with placebo for fibromyalgia (Walitt et al 2015). Results were available from all trials for the synthesis of 'number of patients with at least 30% pain reduction'. For the synthesis of 'mean fatigue scores', results were unavailable for two trials, but for a reason unrelated to the P value, magnitude or direction of the results (fatigue was not measured in these studies). For the synthesis of 'mean depression scores', results were unavailable for one study, likely on the basis of the P value (the trialists reported only that there was a 'non-significant' difference between groups, and review authors' attempts to obtain the necessary data for the synthesis were unsuccessful). Kirkham and colleagues have developed template

Table 13.3.a Matrix indicating availability of study results for three syntheses of trials comparing selective serotonin reuptake inhibitors (SSRIs) with placebo for fibromyalgia (Walitt et al 2015). Adapted from Kirkham et al (2018)

			Syntheses assessed for risk of bias		
Study ID	**Sample size (SSRI)**	**Sample size (placebo)**	**No. with at least 30% pain reduction**	**Mean fatigue scores (any scale)**	**Mean depression scores (any scale)**
Anderberg 2000	17	18	✓	✓	✓
Arnold 2002	25	26	✓	✓	✓
Goldenberg 1996	22	19	✓	✓	✓
GSK 2005	26	26	✓	–	✓
Norregaard 1995	20	21	✓	✓	✓
Patkar 2007	58	58	✓	–	X
Wolfe 1994	15	9	✓	✓	✓

Key:

✓ A study result is available for inclusion in the synthesis

X No study result is available for inclusion, (probably) because the P value, magnitude or direction of the results generated were considered unfavourable by the study investigators

– No study result is available for inclusion, (probably) because the outcome was not assessed, or for a reason unrelated to the P value, magnitude or direction of the results

? No study result is available for inclusion, and it is unclear if the outcome was assessed in the study

matrices that enable review authors to classify the reporting of results of clinical trials more specifically for both benefit and harm outcomes (Kirkham et al 2018).

13.3.4 Considering whether a synthesis is likely to be biased because of the missing results in the studies identified

If review authors suspect that some study results are unavailable because of the P value, magnitude or direction of the results, they should consider the potential impact of the missingness on the synthesis. Table 13.3.a shows that review authors suspected selective non-reporting of results for depression scores in the Patkar 2007 trial. A useful device is to draw readers' attention to this by displaying the trial in a forest plot, underneath a meta-analysis of the trials with available results (Figure 13.3.a). Examination of the sample sizes of the trials with available and missing results shows that nearly one-third of the total sample size across all eligible trials ((58 + 58)/(125 + 119 + 58 + 58) = 0.32) comes from the Patkar 2007 trial. Given that we know the result for the Patkar 2007 trial to be statistically non-significant, it would be reasonable to suspect that its inclusion in the synthesis would reduce the magnitude of the summary estimate. Thus, there is a risk of bias due to missing results in the synthesis of depression scores.

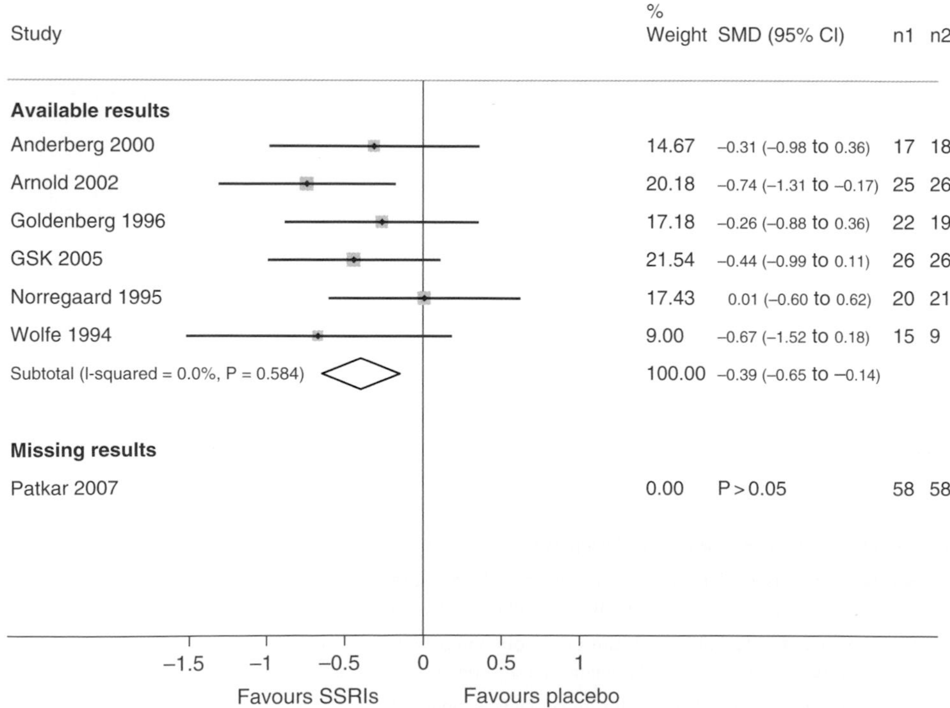

Figure 13.3.a Forest plot displaying available and missing results for a meta-analysis of depression scores (data from Walitt et al 2015). Reproduced with permission of John Wiley and Sons

In other cases, knowledge of the size of eligible studies may lead to reassurance that a meta-analysis is unlikely to be biased due to missing results. For example, López-López and colleagues performed a network meta-analysis of trials of oral anticoagulants for prevention of stroke in atrial fibrillation (López-López et al 2017). Among the five larger phase III trials comparing a direct acting oral anticoagulant with warfarin (each of which included thousands or tens of thousands of participants), results were fully available for important outcomes including stroke or systemic embolism, ischaemic stroke, myocardial infarction, all-cause mortality, major bleeding, intracranial bleeding and gastrointestinal bleeding. The review authors felt that the inability to include results for these outcomes from a few much smaller eligible trials (with at most a few hundred participants) was unlikely to change the summary estimates of these meta-analyses (López-López et al 2017).

Copas and colleagues have developed a more sophisticated model-based sensitivity analysis that explores the robustness of the meta-analytic estimate to the definitely missing results (Copas et al 2017). Its application requires that review authors use the ORBIT classification system (see Section 13.3.3). Review authors applying this method should always present the summary estimate from the sensitivity analysis alongside the primary estimate. Consultation with a statistician is recommended for its implementation.

When the amount of data missing from the synthesis due to selective non-reporting or under-reporting of results is very high, review authors may decide not to report a meta-analysis of the studies with results available, on the basis that such a synthesized estimate could be seriously biased. In other cases, review authors may be uncertain whether selective non-reporting or under-reporting of results occurred, because it was unclear whether the outcome of interest was even assessed. This uncertainty may arise when study plans (e.g. trials register record or protocol) were unavailable, and studies in the field are known to vary in what they assess. If outcome assessment was unclear for a large proportion of the studies identified, review authors might be wary when drawing conclusions about the synthesis, and alert users to the possibility that it could be missing additional results from these studies.

13.3.5 Assessing whether results from additional studies are likely to be missing from a synthesis: the 'unknown unknowns'

By this point, review authors may have judged that the synthesis they are assessing is likely to be biased because results are missing systematically from a considerable proportion of studies identified. It would be reasonable then to classify the synthesis as being at high risk of bias due to missing results and proceed to assess another synthesis.

Alternatively, it may be clear that results for some of the studies identified are definitely missing, but the potential impact on the synthesis might be considered to be minimal. This does not necessarily mean that the synthesis is free of bias due to missing results. It is possible that additional results are missing from the synthesis, particularly due to studies that have been undertaken but not reported at all, so that the review authors are unaware of them.

In this section, we describe methods that can be used to assess the possibility that such additional results – the 'unknown unknowns' – are missing from a synthesis.

13.3.5.1 Qualitative signals to raise suspicion of additional missing results

Whether results from additional studies are likely to be missing will depend on how studies are defined to be eligible for inclusion in the review. If only studies in an inception cohort (e.g. prospectively registered trials) are eligible, then by design none of the studies will have been missed. If studies outside an inception cohort are eligible, then review authors should consider how comprehensive their search was. A search of MEDLINE alone is unlikely to have captured all relevant studies, and failure to search specialized databases such as CINAHL and PsycINFO when the topic of the review is related to the focus of the database may increase the chances that eligible studies were missed (Bramer et al 2017). If evaluating an intervention that is more commonly delivered in countries speaking a language other than English (e.g. traditional Chinese medicine interventions), it may be reasonable to assume additional eligible studies are likely to have been missed if the search is limited to databases containing only English-language articles (Morrison et al 2012).

Further, if the research area is fast-moving, the availability of study information may be subject to time-lag bias, where studies with positive results are available more quickly than those with negative results (Hopewell et al 2007). If results of only a few, early studies are available, it may be reasonable to assume that a synthesis is missing results from additional studies that have been conducted but not yet disseminated. In addition, evidence suggests that phase III clinical trials (generally larger trials at a late stage of intervention development) are more likely to be published than phase II clinical trials (smaller trials at an earlier stage of intervention development): odds ratio 2.0 (95% CI 1.6 to 2.5) (Schmucker et al 2014). Therefore, review authors might be more concerned that there are additional missing studies when evaluating a new biomedical intervention that has not yet reached phase III testing.

The extent to which a study can be suppressed varies. For example, trials of population-wide screening programmes or mass media campaigns are often expensive, require many years of follow-up, and involve hundreds of thousands of participants. It is more difficult to hide such studies from the public than trials that can be conducted quickly and inexpensively. Therefore, review authors should consider the typical size and complexity of eligible studies when considering the likelihood of additional missing studies.

In all of these cases, a judgement is made by review authors on the basis of the limited information they have available. We now turn to graphical and statistical methods that may provide more information about the extent of missing results.

13.3.5.2 Funnel plots

Funnel plots have long been used to assess the possibility that results are missing from a meta-analysis in a manner that is related to their magnitude or P value. However, they require careful interpretation (Sterne et al 2011).

A funnel plot is a simple scatter plot of intervention effect estimates from individual studies against a measure of each study's size or precision. In common with forest plots, it is most common to plot the effect estimates on the horizontal scale, and thus the measure of study size on the vertical axis. This is the opposite of conventional graphical displays for scatter plots, in which the outcome (e.g. intervention effect) is plotted on the vertical axis and the covariate (e.g. study size) is plotted on the horizontal axis.

The name 'funnel plot' arises from the fact that precision of the estimated intervention effect increases as the size of the study increases. Effect estimates from small studies will therefore typically scatter more widely at the bottom of the graph, with the spread narrowing among larger studies. Ideally, the plot should approximately resemble a symmetrical (inverted) funnel. This is illustrated in Panel A of Figure 13.3.b in which the effect estimates in the larger studies are close to the true intervention odds ratio of 0.4. If there is bias due to missing results, for example because smaller studies without statistically significant effects (shown as open circles in Figure 13.3.b, Panel A) remain unpublished, this will lead to an asymmetrical appearance of the funnel plot with a gap at the bottom corner of the graph (Panel B). In this situation the summary estimate calculated in a meta-analysis will tend to over-estimate the intervention effect (Egger et al 1997). The more pronounced the asymmetry, the more likely it is that the amount of bias in the meta-analysis will be substantial.

We recommend that when generating funnel plots, effect estimates be plotted against the standard error of the effect estimate, rather than against the total sample size, on the vertical axis (Sterne and Egger 2001). This is because the statistical power of a trial is determined by factors in addition to sample size, such as the number of participants experiencing the event for dichotomous outcomes, and the standard deviation of responses for continuous outcomes. For example, a study with 100,000 participants and 10 events is less likely to show a statistically significant intervention effect than a study with 1000 participants and 100 events. The standard error summarizes these other factors. Plotting standard errors on a reversed scale places the larger, or most powerful, studies towards the top of the plot. Another advantage of using standard errors is that a simple triangular region can be plotted, within which 95% of studies would be expected to lie in the absence of both biases and heterogeneity. These regions are included in Figure 13.3.b. Funnel plots of effect estimates against their standard errors (on a reversed scale) can be created using RevMan and other statistical software. A triangular 95% confidence region based on a fixed-effect meta-analysis can be included in the plot, and different plotting symbols can be used to allow studies in different subgroups to be identified.

Ratio measures of intervention effect (such as odds ratios and risk ratios) should be plotted on a logarithmic scale. This ensures that effects of the same magnitude but opposite directions (e.g. odds ratios of 0.5 and 2) are equidistant from 1.0. For outcomes measured on a continuous (numerical) scale (e.g. blood pressure, depression score) intervention effects are measured as mean differences or standardized mean differences (SMDs), which should therefore be used as the horizontal axis in funnel plots.

Some authors have argued that visual interpretation of funnel plots is too subjective to be useful. In particular, Terrin and colleagues found that researchers had only a limited ability to identify correctly funnel plots for meta-analyses that were subject to bias due to missing results (Terrin et al 2005).

13.3.5.3 Different reasons for funnel plot asymmetry

Although funnel plot asymmetry has long been equated with non-reporting bias (Light and Pillemer 1984, Begg and Berlin 1988), the funnel plot should be seen as a generic means of displaying *small-study effects*: a tendency for the intervention effects estimated in smaller studies to differ from those estimated in larger studies (Sterne and Egger 2001). Small-study effects may be due to reasons other than non-reporting bias (Egger et al 1997, Sterne et al 2011), some of which are shown in Table 13.3.b.

A proposed amendment to the funnel plot is to include contour lines corresponding to perceived 'milestones' of statistical significance (P = 0.01, 0.05, 0.1, etc (Peters et al 2008)).

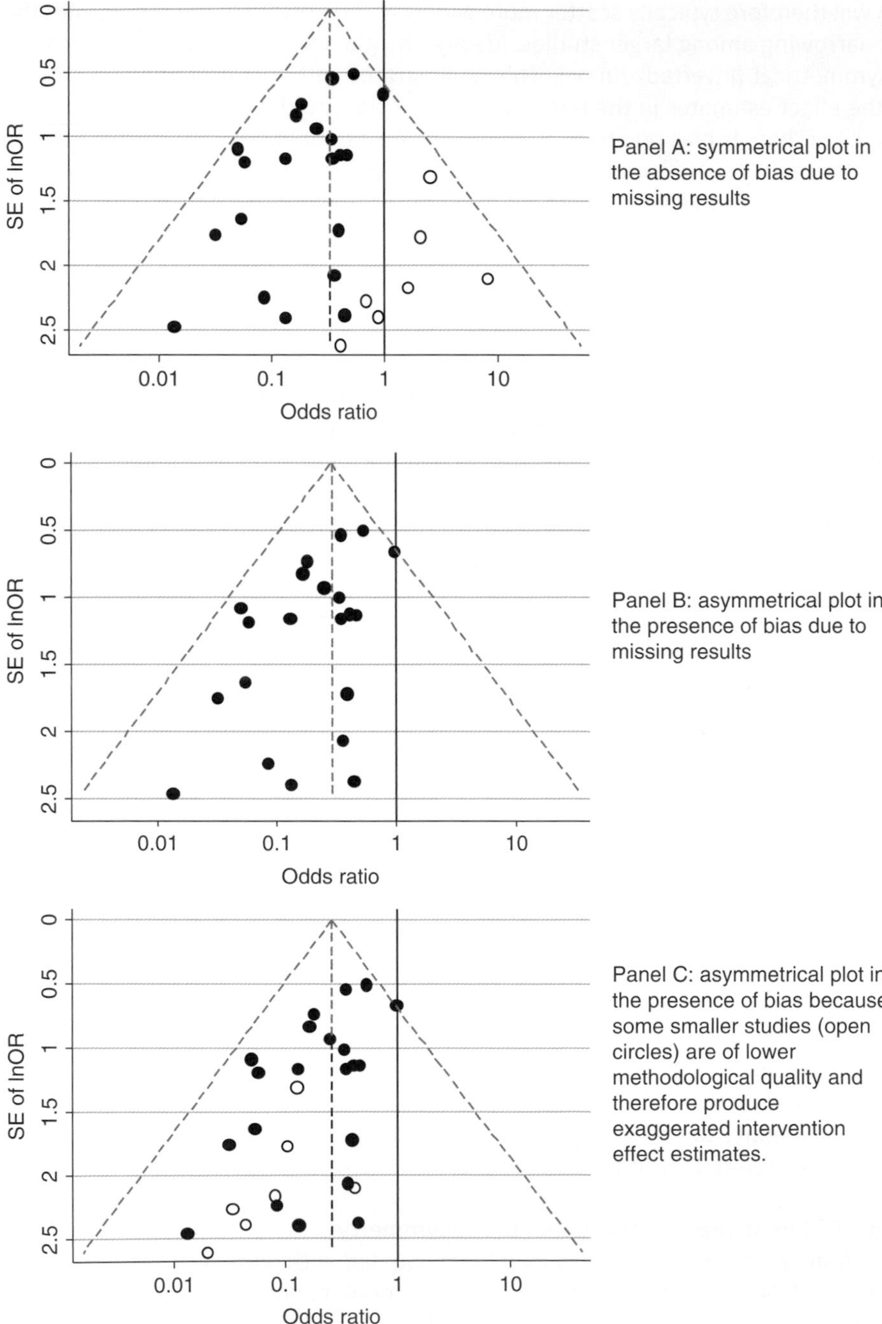
SE of lnOR
0
0.5
1
1.5
2
2.5
0.01
0.1
1
10
Odds ratio
Panel A: symmetrical plot in the absence of bias due to missing results
Panel B: asymmetrical plot in the presence of bias due to missing results
Panel C: asymmetrical plot in the presence of bias because some smaller studies (open circles) are of lower methodological quality and therefore produce exaggerated intervention effect estimates.

Figure 13.3.b Hypothetical funnel plots

Table 13.3.b Possible sources of asymmetry in funnel plots. Adapted from Egger et al (1997)

1) Non-reporting biases
• Entire study reports, or particular results, of smaller studies are unavailable because of the nature of the findings (e.g. statistical significance, direction of effect).
2) Poor methodological quality leading to spuriously inflated effects in smaller studies
• Trials with less methodological rigour tend to show larger intervention effects (Page et al 2016a). Therefore, trials that would have been 'negative', if conducted and analysed properly, may become 'positive'. Asymmetry can arise when some smaller studies are of lower methodological quality and therefore produce larger intervention effect estimates (Figure 13.3.b, Panel C).
3) True heterogeneity
• Substantial benefit may be seen only in patients at high risk for the outcome that is affected by the intervention, and usually these high-risk patients are more likely to be included in small, early studies (Davey Smith and Egger 1994).
• Some interventions may have been implemented less thoroughly in larger trials and may, therefore, have resulted in smaller estimates of the intervention effect (Stuck et al 1998).
4) Artefactual
• Some effect estimates (e.g. odds ratios and standardized mean differences) are naturally correlated with their standard errors, and this can produce spurious asymmetry in a funnel plot (Sterne et al 2011, Zwetsloot et al 2017).
5) Chance

This allows the statistical significance of study estimates, and areas in which studies are perceived to be missing, to be considered. Such **contour-enhanced funnel plots** may help review authors to differentiate asymmetry that is due to non-reporting biases from that due to other factors. For example, if studies appear to be missing in areas where results would be statistically non-significant and unfavourable to the experimental intervention (see Figure 13.3.c, Panel A) then this adds credence to the possibility that the asymmetry is due to non-reporting biases. Conversely, if the supposed missing studies are in areas where results would be statistically significant and favourable to the experimental intervention (see Figure 13.3.c, Panel B), this would suggest the cause of the asymmetry is more likely to be due to factors other than non-reporting biases (see Table 13.3.b).

13.3.5.4 Tests for funnel plot asymmetry

Tests for funnel plot asymmetry (small-study effects) examine whether the association between estimated intervention effects and a measure of study size is greater than expected to occur by chance (Sterne et al 2011). Several tests are available, the first and most well-known of which is the Egger test (Egger et al 1997). The tests typically have low power, which means that non-reporting biases cannot generally be excluded, and in practice they do not always lead to the same conclusions about the presence of small-study effects (Lin et al 2018).

After reviewing the results of simulation studies evaluating test characteristics, and based on theoretical considerations, Sterne and colleagues (Sterne et al 2011) made the following recommendations.

- As a rule of thumb, tests for funnel plot asymmetry should be used only when there are at least 10 studies included in the meta-analysis, because when there are fewer studies the power of the tests is low. Only 24% of a random sample of Cochrane Reviews indexed in 2014 included a meta-analysis with at least 10 studies

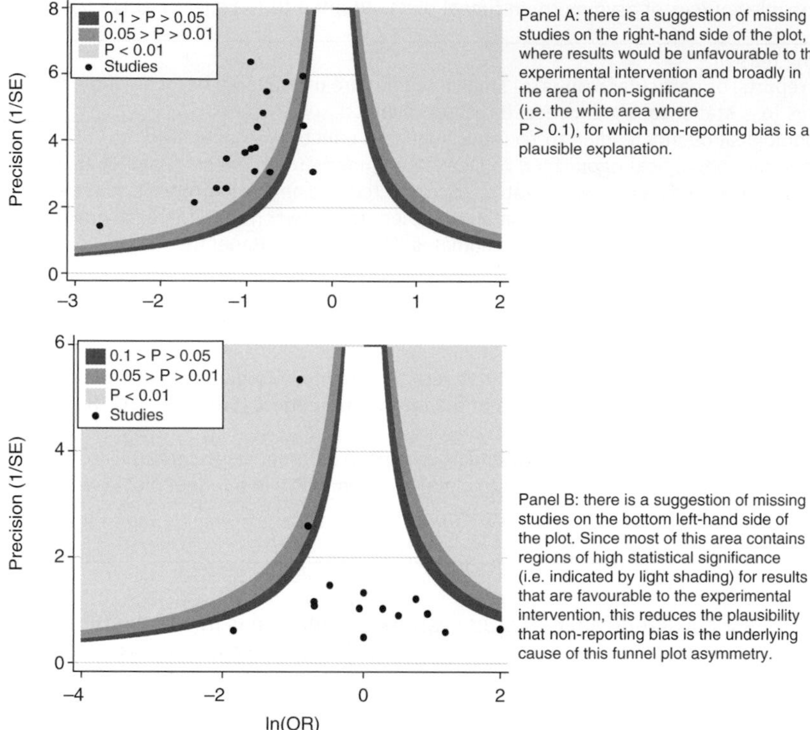

0.1 > P > 0.05
0.05 > P > 0.01
P < 0.01
Studies
Precision (1/SE)
Panel A: there is a suggestion of missing studies on the right-hand side of the plot, where results would be unfavourable to the experimental intervention and broadly in the area of non-significance (i.e. the white area where P > 0.1), for which non-reporting bias is a plausible explanation.
Panel B: there is a suggestion of missing studies on the bottom left-hand side of the plot. Since most of this area contains regions of high statistical significance (i.e. indicated by light shading) for results that are favourable to the experimental intervention, this reduces the plausibility that non-reporting bias is the underlying cause of this funnel plot asymmetry.
ln(OR)

Figure 13.3.c Contour-enhanced funnel plots

(Page et al 2016b), which implies that tests for funnel plot asymmetry are likely to be applicable in a minority of meta-analyses.

- Tests should not be used if studies are of similar size (similar standard errors of intervention effect estimates).
- Results of tests for funnel plot asymmetry should be interpreted in the light of visual inspection of the funnel plot (see Sections 13.3.5.2 and 13.3.5.3). Examining a contour-enhanced funnel plot may further aid interpretation (see Figure 13.3.c).
- When there is evidence of funnel plot asymmetry from a test, non-reporting biases should be considered as one of several possible explanations, and review authors should attempt to distinguish the different possible reasons for it (see Table 13.3.b).

Sterne and colleagues provided more detailed suggestions specific to intervention effects measured as mean differences, SMDs, odds ratios, risk ratios and risk differences (Sterne et al 2011). Some tests, including the original Egger test, are not recommended for application to odds ratios and SMDs because of artefactual correlations between the effect size and its standard error (Sterne et al 2011, Zwetsloot et al 2017). For odds ratios, methods proposed by Harbord and colleagues and Peters and colleagues overcome this problem (Harbord et al 2006, Peters et al 2006).

None of the recommended tests for funnel plot asymmetry is implemented in RevMan; Jin and colleagues describe other software available to implement them (Jin et al 2015).

13.3.5.5 Interpreting funnel plots: summary

To summarize, **funnel plot asymmetry should not be considered to be diagnostic for the presence of non-reporting bias**. Tests for funnel plot asymmetry are applicable only in the minority of meta-analyses for which their use is appropriate. If there is evidence of funnel plot asymmetry then review authors should attempt to distinguish the different possible reasons for it listed in Table 13.3.b. For example, considering the particular intervention, and the circumstances in which it was implemented in different studies can help identify true heterogeneity as a cause of funnel plot asymmetry. Nevertheless, a concern remains that visual interpretation of funnel plots is inherently subjective.

13.3.5.6 Sensitivity analyses

When review authors are concerned that small-study effects are influencing the results of a meta-analysis, they may want to conduct sensitivity analyses to explore the robustness of the meta-analysis conclusions to different assumptions about the causes of funnel plot asymmetry. The following approaches have been suggested. Ideally, these should be pre-specified.

Comparing fixed-effect and random-effects estimates In the presence of heterogeneity, a random-effects meta-analysis weights the studies relatively more equally than a fixed-effect analysis (see Chapter 10, Section 10.10.4.1). It follows that in the presence of small-study effects, in which the intervention effect is systematically different in the smaller compared with the larger studies, the random-effects estimate of the intervention effect will shift towards the results of the smaller studies. We recommend that when review authors are concerned about the influence of small-study effects on the results of a meta-analysis in which there is evidence of between-study heterogeneity ($I^2 > 0$), they compare the fixed-effect and random-effects estimates of the intervention effect. If the estimates are similar, then any small-study effects have little effect on the intervention effect estimate. If the random-effects estimate has shifted towards the results of the smaller studies, review authors should consider whether it is reasonable to conclude that the intervention was genuinely different in the smaller studies, or if results of smaller studies were disseminated selectively. Formal investigations of heterogeneity may reveal other explanations for funnel plot asymmetry, in which case presentation of results should focus on these. If the larger studies tend to be those conducted with more methodological rigour, or conducted in circumstances more typical of the use of the intervention in practice, then review authors should consider reporting the results of meta-analyses restricted to the larger, more rigorous studies.

Selection models Selection models were developed to estimate intervention effects 'corrected' for bias due to missing results (McShane et al 2016). The methods are based on the assumption that the size, direction and P value of study results and the size of studies influences the probability of their publication. For example, Copas proposed a model (different from that described in Section 13.3.4) in which the probability that a study is included in a meta-analysis depends on its standard error. Since it is not possible to estimate all model parameters precisely, he advocates sensitivity analyses in which the intervention effect is estimated under a range of assumptions about the severity of the selection bias (Copas 1999). These analyses show how the estimated intervention effect (and confidence interval) changes as the assumed amount of selection bias increases. If the estimates are relatively stable regardless of the selection model assumed, this suggests that the unadjusted estimate is unlikely to be influenced by non-reporting biases. On the other hand, if the estimates vary considerably depending on the selection model assumed, this suggests that non-reporting biases may well drive the unadjusted estimate (McShane et al 2016).

A major problem with selection models is that they assume that mechanisms leading to small-study effects other than non-reporting biases (see Table 13.3.b) are not operating, and may give misleading results if this assumption is not correct. Jin and colleagues summarize the advantages and disadvantages of eight selection models, indicate circumstances in which each can be used, and describe software available to implement them (Jin et al 2015). Given the complexity of the models, consultation with a statistician is recommended for their implementation.

Regression-based methods Moreno and colleagues propose an approach, based on tests for funnel plot asymmetry, in which a regression line to the funnel plot is extrapolated to estimate the effect of intervention in a very large study (Moreno et al 2009). They regress effect size on within-study variance, and incorporate heterogeneity as a multiplicative rather than additive component (Moreno et al 2012). This approach gives more weight to the larger studies than in either a standard fixed-effect or random-effects meta-analysis, so that the adjusted estimate will be closer to the effects observed in the larger studies. Rücker and colleagues combine a similar approach with a shrinkage procedure (Rücker et al 2011a, Rücker et al 2011b). The underlying model is an extended random-effects model, with an additional parameter representing the bias introduced by small-study effects.

In common with tests for funnel plot asymmetry, regression-based methods to estimate the effect of intervention in a large study should be used only when there are sufficient studies (at least 10) to allow appropriate estimation of the regression line. When all the studies are small, extrapolation to an infinitely sized study may produce effect estimates that are more extreme than any of the existing studies, and if the approach is used in such a situation it might be more appropriate to extrapolate only as far as the largest observed study.

13.3.6 Reaching an overall judgement about risk of bias due to missing results

We have described several approaches review authors can use to assess the risk of bias in a synthesis when entire studies or particular results within studies are missing selectively. These include comparison of protocols with published reports to detect selective non-reporting of results (Section 13.3.3), consideration of qualitative signals that suggest not all studies were identified (Section 13.3.5.1), and the use of funnel plots to identify small-study effects, for which non-reporting bias is one cause (Section 13.3.5.3).

Review authors should consider the findings of each approach when reaching an overall judgement about the risk of bias due to missing results in a synthesis. For example, selective non-reporting of results may not have been detected in any of the studies identified.

However, if the search for studies was not comprehensive, or if a contour-enhanced funnel plot or sensitivity analysis suggests results are missing systematically, then it would be reasonable to conclude that the synthesis is at risk of bias due to missing results. On the other hand, if the review is based on an inception cohort, such that all studies that have been conducted are known, and these studies were fully reported in line with their analysis plans, then there would be low risk of bias due to missing results in a synthesis. Indeed, such a low risk-of-bias judgement would carry even in the presence of asymmetry in a funnel plot; although it would be important to investigate the reason for this asymmetry (e.g. it might be due to systematic differences in the PICOs of smaller and larger studies, or to problems in the methodological conduct of the smaller studies).

13.4 Summary

There is clear evidence that selective dissemination of study reports and results leads to an over-estimate of the benefits and under-estimate of the harms of interventions in systematic reviews and meta-analyses. However, overcoming, detecting and correcting for bias due to missing results is difficult. Comprehensive searches are important, but are not on their own sufficient to prevent substantial potential biases. Review authors should therefore consider the risk of bias due to missing results in syntheses included in their review (see MECIR Box 13.4.a).

We have presented a framework for assessing risk of bias due to missing results in a synthesis. Of the approaches described, a thorough assessment of selective non-reporting or under-reporting of results in the studies identified (Section 13.3.3) is likely to be the most labour intensive, yet the most valuable. Because the number of identified studies with results missing for a given synthesis is known, the impact of selective non-reporting or under-reporting of results can be quantified more easily (see Section 13.3.4) than the impact of selective non-publication of an unknown number of studies.

MECIR Box 13.4.a Relevant expectations for conduct of intervention reviews	
C73: Investigating risk of bias due to missing results (**Highly desirable**)	
Consider the potential impact of non-reporting biases on the results of the review or the meta-analysis it contains.	There is overwhelming evidence of non-reporting biases of various types. These can be addressed at various points of the review. A thorough search, and attempts to obtain unpublished results, might minimize the risk. Analyses of the results of included studies, for example using funnel plots, can sometimes help determine the possible extent of the problem, as can attempts to identify study protocols, which should be a routine feature of Cochrane Reviews.

The value of the other methods described in the framework will depend on the circumstances of the review. For example, if review authors suspect that a synthesis is biased because results were missing selectively from a large proportion of the studies identified, then the graphical and statistical methods outlined in Section 13.3.5 (e.g. funnel plots) are unlikely to change their judgement. However, funnel plots, tests for funnel plot asymmetry and other sensitivity analyses may be useful in cases where protocols or records from trials registers were unavailable for most studies, making it difficult to assess selective non-reporting or under-reporting of results reliably. When there is evidence of funnel plot asymmetry, non-reporting biases should be considered as only one of a number of possible explanations: review authors should attempt to understand the sources of the asymmetry, and consider their implications in the light of any qualitative signals that raise a suspicion of additional missing results, and other sensitivity analyses.

13.5 Chapter information

Authors: Matthew J Page, Julian PT Higgins, Jonathan AC Sterne

Acknowledgments: We thank Douglas Altman, Isabelle Boutron, James Carpenter, Matthias Egger, Roger Harbord, David Jones, David Moher, Alex Sutton, Jennifer Tetzlaff and Lucy Turner for their contributions to previous versions of this chapter. We thank Isabelle Boutron, Sarah Dawson, Kay Dickersin, Kerry Dwan, Roy Elbers, Carl Heneghan, Asbjørn Hróbjartsson, Jamie Kirkham, Toby Lasserson, Tianjing Li, Andreas Lundh, Joanne McKenzie, Joerg Meerpohl, Hannah Rothstein, Lesley Stewart, Alex Sutton, James Thomas and Erick Turner for their contributions to the framework for assessing risk of bias due to missing results in a synthesis. We thank Evan Mayo-Wilson for his helpful comments on this chapter.

Funding: MJP is supported by an Australian National Health and Medical Research Council (NHMRC) Early Career Fellowship (1088535). JPTH and JACS received funding from Cochrane, UK Medical Research Council grant MR/M025209/1 and UK National Institute for Health Research Senior Investigator awards NF-SI-0617-10145 and NF-SI-0611-10168, respectively. The views expressed are those of the author(s) and not necessarily those of the NHS, the NIHR or the Department of Health.

Declarations of interest: Jonathan Sterne is an author on papers proposing tests for funnel plot asymmetry.

13.6 References

Askie LM, Darlow BA, Finer N, Schmidt B, Stenson B, Tarnow-Mordi W, Davis PG, Carlo WA, Brocklehurst P, Davies LC, Das A, Rich W, Gantz MG, Roberts RS, Whyte RK, Costantini L, Poets C, Asztalos E, Battin M, Halliday HL, Marlow N, Tin W, King A, Juszczak E, Morley CJ, Doyle LW, Gebski V, Hunter KE, Simes RJ. Association between oxygen saturation targeting and death or disability in extremely preterm infants in the Neonatal Oxygenation Prospective Meta-analysis Collaboration. *JAMA* 2018; **319**: 2190–2201.

Baudard M, Yavchitz A, Ravaud P, Perrodeau E, Boutron I. Impact of searching clinical trial registries in systematic reviews of pharmaceutical treatments: methodological systematic review and reanalysis of meta-analyses. *BMJ* 2017; **356**: j448.

Begg CB, Berlin JA. Publication bias: a problem in interpreting medical data. *Journal of the Royal Statistical Society: Series A (Statistics in Society)* 1988; **151**: 419–463.

Bramer WM, Rethlefsen ML, Kleijnen J, Franco OH. Optimal database combinations for literature searches in systematic reviews: a prospective exploratory study. *Systematic Reviews* 2017; **6**: 245.

Chan AW, Hróbjartsson A, Haahr MT, Gøtzsche PC, Altman DG. Empirical evidence for selective reporting of outcomes in randomized trials: comparison of protocols to published articles. *JAMA* 2004; **291**: 2457–2465.

Chan AW, Pello A, Kitchen J, Axentiev A, Virtanen JI, Liu A, Hemminki E. Association of trial registration with reporting of primary outcomes in protocols and publications. *JAMA* 2017; **318**: 1709–1711.

Chau S, Herrmann N, Ruthirakuhan MT, Chen JJ, Lanctot KL. Latrepirdine for Alzheimer's disease. *Cochrane Database of Systematic Reviews* 2015; **4**: CD009524.

Copas J. What works?: selectivity models and meta-analysis. *Journal of the Royal Statistical Society: Series A (Statistics in Society)* 1999; **162**: 95–109.

Copas J, Marson A, Williamson P, Kirkham J. Model-based sensitivity analysis for outcome reporting bias in the meta analysis of benefit and harm outcomes. *Statistical Methods in Medical Research* 2017; **28**: 889–903.

Dal-Ré R, Bracken MB, Ioannidis JPA. Call to improve transparency of trials of non-regulated interventions. *BMJ* 2015; **350**: h1323.

Davey Smith G, Egger M. Who benefits from medical interventions? Treating low risk patients can be a high risk strategy. *BMJ* 1994; **308**: 72–74.

De Angelis CD, Drazen JM, Frizelle FA, Haug C, Hoey J, Horton R, Kotzin S, Laine C, Marusic A, Overbeke AJ, Schroeder TV, Sox HC, Van der Weyden MB, International Committee of Medical Journal Editors. Clinical trial registration: a statement from the International Committee of Medical Journal Editors. *JAMA* 2004; **292**: 1363–1364.

DeVito NJ, Bacon S, Goldacre B. FDAAA TrialsTracker: a live informatics tool to monitor compliance with FDA requirements to report clinical trial results 2018. https://www.biorxiv.org/content/biorxiv/early/2018/02/16/266452.full.pdf.

Doshi P, Jefferson T. Open data 5 years on: a case series of 12 freedom of information requests for regulatory data to the European Medicines Agency. *Trials* 2016; **17**: 78.

Doshi P, Shamseer L, Jones M, Jefferson T. Restoring biomedical literature with RIAT. *BMJ* 2018; **361**: k1742.

Driessen E, Hollon SD, Bockting CL, Cuijpers P, Turner EH. Does publication bias inflate the apparent efficacy of psychological treatment for major depressive disorder? A systematic review and meta-analysis of US National Institutes of Health-Funded Trials. *PloS One* 2015; **10**: e0137864.

Dwan K, Gamble C, Williamson PR, Kirkham JJ, Reporting Bias Group. Systematic review of the empirical evidence of study publication bias and outcome reporting bias: an updated review. *PloS One* 2013; **8**: e66844.

Egger M, Davey Smith G, Schneider M, Minder C. Bias in meta-analysis detected by a simple, graphical test. *BMJ* 1997; **315**: 629–634.

Eyding D, Lelgemann M, Grouven U, Harter M, Kromp M, Kaiser T, Kerekes MF, Gerken M, Wieseler B. Reboxetine for acute treatment of major depression: systematic review and meta-analysis of published and unpublished placebo and selective serotonin reuptake inhibitor controlled trials. *BMJ* 2010; **341**: c4737.

Goldacre B, DeVito NJ, Heneghan C, Irving F, Bacon S, Fleminger J, Curtis H. Compliance with requirement to report results on the EU Clinical Trials Register: cohort study and web resource. *BMJ* 2018; **362**: k3218.

Harbord RM, Egger M, Sterne JA. A modified test for small-study effects in meta-analyses of controlled trials with binary endpoints. *Statistics in Medicine* 2006; **25**: 3443–3457.

Hopewell S, Clarke M, Stewart L, Tierney J. Time to publication for results of clinical trials. *Cochrane Database of Systematic Reviews* 2007; **2**: MR000011.

Jefferson T, Jones MA, Doshi P, Del Mar CB, Hama R, Thompson MJ, Spencer EA, Onakpoya I, Mahtani KR, Nunan D, Howick J, Heneghan CJ. Neuraminidase inhibitors for preventing and treating influenza in healthy adults and children. *Cochrane Database of Systematic Reviews* 2014; **4**: CD008965.

Jefferson T, Doshi P, Boutron I, Golder S, Heneghan C, Hodkinson A, Jones M, Lefebvre C, Stewart LA. When to include clinical study reports and regulatory documents in systematic reviews. *BMJ Evidence Based Medicine* 2018; **23**: 210–217.

Jin ZC, Zhou XH, He J. Statistical methods for dealing with publication bias in meta-analysis. *Statistics in Medicine* 2015; **34**: 343–360.

Jørgensen L, Gøtzsche PC, Jefferson T. Index of the human papillomavirus (HPV) vaccine industry clinical study programmes and non-industry funded studies: a necessary basis to address reporting bias in a systematic review. *Systematic Reviews* 2018; **7**: 8.

Kirkham JJ, Altman DG, Chan AW, Gamble C, Dwan KM, Williamson PR. Outcome reporting bias in trials: a methodological approach for assessment and adjustment in systematic reviews. *BMJ* 2018; **362**: k3802.

Ladanie A, Ewald H, Kasenda B, Hemkens LG. How to use FDA drug approval documents for evidence syntheses. *BMJ* 2018; **362**: k2815.

Light RJ, Pillemer DB. *Summing Up: The Science of Reviewing Research*. Cambridge (MA): Harvard University Press; 1984.

Lin L, Chu H, Murad MH, Hong C, Qu Z, Cole SR, Chen Y. Empirical comparison of publication bias tests in meta-analysis. *Journal of General Internal Medicine* 2018; **33**: 1260–1267.

López-López JA, Sterne JAC, Thom HHZ, Higgins JPT, Hingorani AD, Okoli GN, Davies PA, Bodalia PN, Bryden PA, Welton NJ, Hollingworth W, Caldwell DM, Savović J, Dias S, Salisbury C, Eaton D, Stephens-Boal A, Sofat R. Oral anticoagulants for prevention of stroke in atrial fibrillation: systematic review, network meta-analysis, and cost effectiveness analysis. *BMJ* 2017; **359**: j5058.

López-López JA, Page MJ, Lipsey MW, Higgins JPT. Dealing with effect size multiplicity in systematic reviews and meta-analyses. *Research Synthesis Methods* 2018; **9**: 336–351.

Maund E, Tendal B, Hróbjartsson A, Jørgensen KJ, Lundh A, Schroll J, Gøtzsche PC. Benefits and harms in clinical trials of duloxetine for treatment of major depressive disorder: comparison of clinical study reports, trial registries, and publications. *BMJ* 2014; **348**: g3510.

Mayo-Wilson E, Li T, Fusco N, Bertizzolo L, Canner JK, Cowley T, Doshi P, Ehmsen J, Gresham G, Guo N, Haythornthwaite JA, Heyward J, Hong H, Pham D, Payne JL, Rosman L, Stuart EA, Suarez-Cuervo C, Tolbert E, Twose C, Vedula S, Dickersin K. Cherry-picking by trialists and meta-analysts can drive conclusions about intervention efficacy. *Journal of Clinical Epidemiology* 2017; **91**: 95–110.

McShane BB, Bockenholt U, Hansen KT. Adjusting for publication bias in meta-analysis: an evaluation of selection methods and some cautionary notes. *Perspectives on Psychological Science* 2016; **11**: 730–749.

Moreno SG, Sutton AJ, Turner EH, Abrams KR, Cooper NJ, Palmer TM, Ades AE. Novel methods to deal with publication biases: secondary analysis of antidepressant trials in the FDA trial registry database and related journal publications. *BMJ* 2009; **339**: b2981.

Moreno SG, Sutton AJ, Thompson JR, Ades AE, Abrams KR, Cooper NJ. A generalized weighting regression-derived meta-analysis estimator robust to small-study effects and heterogeneity. *Statistics in Medicine* 2012; **31**: 1407–1417.

Morrison A, Polisena J, Husereau D, Moulton K, Clark M, Fiander M, Mierzwinski-Urban M, Clifford T, Hutton B, Rabb D. The effect of English-language restriction on systematic review-based meta-analyses: a systematic review of empirical studies. *International Journal of Technology Assessment in Health Care* 2012; **28**: 138–144.

Mueller KF, Meerpohl JJ, Briel M, Antes G, von Elm E, Lang B, Motschall E, Schwarzer G, Bassler D. Methods for detecting, quantifying and adjusting for dissemination bias in meta-analysis are described. *Journal of Clinical Epidemiology* 2016; **80**: 25–33.

Page MJ, Higgins JPT, Clayton G, Sterne JAC, Hróbjartsson A, Savović J. Empirical evidence of study design biases in randomized trials: systematic review of meta-epidemiological studies. *PloS One* 2016a; **11**: 7.

Page MJ, Shamseer L, Altman DG, Tetzlaff J, Sampson M, Tricco AC, Catala-Lopez F, Li L, Reid EK, Sarkis-Onofre R, Moher D. Epidemiology and reporting characteristics of systematic reviews of biomedical research: a cross-sectional study. *PLoS Medicine* 2016b; **13**: e1002028.

Page MJ, McKenzie JE, Higgins JPT. Tools for assessing risk of reporting biases in studies and syntheses of studies: a systematic review. *BMJ Open* 2018; **8**: e019703.

Peters JL, Sutton AJ, Jones DR, Abrams KR, Rushton L. Comparison of two methods to detect publication bias in meta-analysis. *JAMA* 2006; **295**: 676–680.

Peters JL, Sutton AJ, Jones DR, Abrams KR, Rushton L. Contour-enhanced meta-analysis funnel plots help distinguish publication bias from other causes of asymmetry. *Journal of Clinical Epidemiology* 2008; **61**: 991–996.

Roberts I, Ker K, Edwards P, Beecher D, Manno D, Sydenham E. The knowledge system underpinning healthcare is not fit for purpose and must change. *BMJ* 2015; **350**: h2463.

Rodgers MA, Brown JV, Heirs MK, Higgins JPT, Mannion RJ, Simmonds MC, Stewart LA. Reporting of industry funded study outcome data: comparison of confidential and published data on the safety and effectiveness of rhBMP-2 for spinal fusion. *BMJ* 2013; **346**: f3981.

Rücker G, Carpenter JR, Schwarzer G. Detecting and adjusting for small-study effects in meta-analysis. *Biometrical Journal* 2011a; **53**: 351–368.

Rücker G, Schwarzer G, Carpenter JR, Binder H, Schumacher M. Treatment-effect estimates adjusted for small-study effects via a limit meta-analysis. *Biostatistics* 2011b; **12**: 122–142.

Schmucker C, Schell LK, Portalupi S, Oeller P, Cabrera L, Bassler D, Schwarzer G, Scherer RW, Antes G, von Elm E, Meerpohl JJ. Extent of non-publication in cohorts of studies approved by research ethics committees or included in trial registries. *PloS One* 2014; **9**: e114023.

Schmucker CM, Blümle A, Schell LK, Schwarzer G, Oeller P, Cabrera L, von Elm E, Briel M, Meerpohl JJ. Systematic review finds that study data not published in full text articles have unclear impact on meta-analyses results in medical research. *PloS One* 2017; **12**: e0176210.

Schroll JB, Abdel-Sattar M, Bero L. The Food and Drug Administration reports provided more data but were more difficult to use than the European Medicines Agency reports. *Journal of Clinical Epidemiology* 2015; **68**: 102–107.

Schroll JB, Penninga EI, Gøtzsche PC. Assessment of adverse events in protocols, clinical study reports, and published papers of trials of orlistat: a document analysis. *PLoS Medicine* 2016; **13**: e1002101.

Simmonds MC, Brown JV, Heirs MK, Higgins JPT, Mannion RJ, Rodgers MA, Stewart LA. Safety and effectiveness of recombinant human bone morphogenetic protein-2 for spinal fusion: a meta-analysis of individual-participant data. *Annals of Internal Medicine* 2013; **158**: 877–889.

Sterne JAC, Egger M. Funnel plots for detecting bias in meta-analysis: guidelines on choice of axis. *Journal of Clinical Epidemiology* 2001; **54**: 1046–1055.

Sterne JAC, Sutton AJ, Ioannidis JPA, Terrin N, Jones DR, Lau J, Carpenter J, Rücker G, Harbord RM, Schmid CH, Tetzlaff J, Deeks JJ, Peters J, Macaskill P, Schwarzer G, Duval S, Altman DG, Moher D, Higgins JPT. Recommendations for examining and interpreting funnel plot asymmetry in meta-analyses of randomised controlled trials. *BMJ* 2011; **343**: d4002.

Stuck AE, Rubenstein LZ, Wieland D. Bias in meta-analysis detected by a simple, graphical test. Asymmetry detected in funnel plot was probably due to true heterogeneity. Letter. *BMJ* 1998; **316**: 469–471.

Terrin N, Schmid CH, Lau J. In an empirical evaluation of the funnel plot, researchers could not visually identify publication bias. *Journal of Clinical Epidemiology* 2005; **58**: 894–901.

Toews I, Booth A, Berg RC, Lewin S, Glenton C, Munthe-Kaas HM, Noyes J, Schroter S, Meerpohl JJ. Further exploration of dissemination bias in qualitative research required to facilitate assessment within qualitative evidence syntheses. *Journal of Clinical Epidemiology* 2017; **88**: 133–139.

Turner EH, Matthews AM, Linardatos E, Tell RA, Rosenthal R. Selective publication of antidepressant trials and its influence on apparent efficacy. *New England Journal of Medicine* 2008; **358**: 252–260.

Walitt B, Urrutia G, Nishishinya MB, Cantrell SE, Hauser W. Selective serotonin reuptake inhibitors for fibromyalgia syndrome. *Cochrane Database of Systematic Reviews* 2015; **6**: CD011735.

Wieseler B, Wolfram N, McGauran N, Kerekes MF, Vervolgyi V, Kohlepp P, Kamphuis M, Grouven U. Completeness of reporting of patient-relevant clinical trial outcomes: comparison of unpublished clinical study reports with publicly available data. *PLoS Medicine* 2013; **10**: e1001526.

Williamson P, Clarke M. The COMET (Core Outcome Measures in Effectiveness Trials) Initiative: its role in improving Cochrane Reviews. *Cochrane Database of Systematic Reviews* 2012; **5**: ED000041.

Williamson PR, Gamble C. Identification and impact of outcome selection bias in meta-analysis. *Statistics in Medicine* 2005; **24**: 1547–1561.

Zarin DA, Tse T, Williams RJ, Califf RM, Ide NC. The ClinicalTrials.gov results database: update and key issues. *New England Journal of Medicine* 2011; **364**: 852–860.

Zwetsloot P-P, Van Der Naald M, Sena ES, Howells DW, IntHout J, De Groot JAH, Chamuleau SAJ, MacLeod MR, Wever KE. Standardized mean differences cause funnel plot distortion in publication bias assessments. *eLife* 2017; **6**: e24260.

14

Completing 'Summary of findings' tables and grading the certainty of the evidence

Holger J Schünemann, Julian PT Higgins, Gunn E Vist, Paul Glasziou, Elie A Akl, Nicole Skoetz, Gordon H Guyatt; on behalf of the Cochrane GRADEing Methods Group (formerly Applicability and Recommendations Methods Group) and the Cochrane Statistical Methods Group

KEY POINTS

- A 'Summary of findings' table for a given comparison of interventions provides key information concerning the magnitudes of relative and absolute effects of the interventions examined, the amount of available evidence and the certainty (or quality) of available evidence.
- 'Summary of findings' tables include a row for each important outcome (up to a maximum of seven). Accepted formats of 'Summary of findings' tables and interactive 'Summary of findings' tables can be produced using GRADE's software GRADEpro GDT.
- Cochrane has adopted the GRADE approach (Grading of Recommendations Assessment, Development and Evaluation) for assessing certainty (or quality) of a body of evidence.
- The GRADE approach specifies four levels of the certainty for a body of evidence for a given outcome: high, moderate, low and very low.
- GRADE assessments of certainty are determined through consideration of five domains: risk of bias, inconsistency, indirectness, imprecision and publication bias. For evidence from non-randomized studies and rarely randomized studies, assessments can then be upgraded through consideration of three further domains.

14.1 'Summary of findings' tables

14.1.1 Introduction to 'Summary of findings' tables

'Summary of findings' tables present the main findings of a review in a transparent, structured and simple tabular format. In particular, they provide key information

This chapter should be cited as: Schünemann HJ, Higgins JPT, Vist GE, Glasziou P, Akl EA, Skoetz N, Guyatt GH. Chapter 14: Completing 'Summary of findings' tables and grading the certainty of the evidence. In: Higgins JPT, Thomas J, Chandler J, Cumpston M, Li T, Page MJ, Welch VA (editors). *Cochrane Handbook for Systematic Reviews of Interventions*. 2nd Edition. Chichester (UK): John Wiley & Sons, 2019: 375–402.

concerning the certainty or quality of evidence (i.e. the confidence or certainty in the range of an effect estimate or an association), the magnitude of effect of the interventions examined, and the sum of available data on the main outcomes. Cochrane Reviews should incorporate 'Summary of findings' tables during planning and publication, and should have at least one key 'Summary of findings' table representing the most important comparisons. Some reviews may include more than one 'Summary of findings' table, for example if the review addresses more than one major comparison, or includes substantially different populations that require separate tables (e.g. because the effects differ or it is important to show results separately). In the *Cochrane Database of Systematic Reviews (CDSR),* the principal 'Summary of findings' table of a review appears at the beginning, before the Background section. Other 'Summary of findings' tables appear between the Results and Discussion sections.

14.1.2 Selecting outcomes for 'Summary of findings' tables

Planning for the 'Summary of findings' table starts early in the systematic review, with the selection of the outcomes to be included in: (i) the review; and (ii) the 'Summary of findings' table. This is a crucial step, and one that review authors need to address carefully.

To ensure production of optimally useful information, Cochrane Reviews begin by developing a review question and by listing all main outcomes that are important to patients and other decision makers (see Chapters 2 and 3). The GRADE approach to assessing the certainty of the evidence (see Section 14.2) defines and operationalizes a rating process that helps separate outcomes into those that are critical, important or not important for decision making. Consultation and feedback on the review protocol, including from consumers and other decision makers, can enhance this process.

Critical outcomes are likely to include clearly important endpoints; typical examples include mortality and major morbidity (such as strokes and myocardial infarction). However, they may also represent frequent minor and rare major side effects, symptoms, quality of life, burdens associated with treatment, and resource issues (costs). Burdens represent the impact of healthcare workload on patient function and well-being, and include the demands of adhering to an intervention that patients or caregivers (e.g. family) may dislike, such as having to undergo more frequent tests, or the restrictions on lifestyle that certain interventions require (Spencer-Bonilla et al 2017).

Frequently, when formulating questions that include all patient-important outcomes for decision making, review authors will confront reports of studies that have not included all these outcomes. This is particularly true for adverse outcomes. For instance, randomized trials might contribute evidence on intended effects, and on frequent, relatively minor side effects, but not report on rare adverse outcomes such as suicide attempts. Chapter 19 discusses strategies for addressing adverse effects. To obtain data for all important outcomes it may be necessary to examine the results of non-randomized studies (see Chapter 24). Cochrane, in collaboration with others, has developed guidance for review authors to support their decision about when to look for and include non-randomized studies (Schünemann et al 2013).

If a review includes only randomized trials, these trials may not address all important outcomes and it may therefore not be possible to address these outcomes within the constraints of the review. Review authors should acknowledge these limitations and make them transparent to readers. Review authors are encouraged to include non-randomized studies to examine rare or long-term adverse effects that may not adequately be studied in randomized trials. This raises the possibility that harm outcomes may come from studies in which participants differ from those in studies used in the analysis of benefit. Review authors will then need to consider how much such differences are likely to impact on the findings, and this will influence the certainty of evidence because of concerns about indirectness related to the population (see Section 14.2.2).

Non-randomized studies can provide important information not only when randomized trials do not report on an outcome or randomized trials suffer from indirectness, but also when the evidence from randomized trials is rated as very low and non-randomized studies provide evidence of higher certainty. Further discussion of these issues appears also in Chapter 24.

14.1.3 General template for 'Summary of findings' tables

Several alternative standard versions of 'Summary of findings' tables have been developed to ensure consistency and ease of use across reviews, inclusion of the most important information needed by decision makers, and optimal presentation (see examples at Figures 14.1.a and 14.1.b). These formats are supported by research that focused on improved understanding of the information they intend to convey (Carrasco-Labra et al 2016, Langendam et al 2016, Santesso et al 2016). They are available through GRADE's official software package developed to support the GRADE approach: GRADEpro GDT (www.gradepro.org).

Standard Cochrane 'Summary of findings' tables include the following elements using one of the accepted formats. Further guidance on each of these is provided in Section 14.1.6.

1) A brief description of the population and setting addressed by the available evidence (which may be slightly different to or narrower than those defined by the review question).
2) A brief description of the comparison addressed in the 'Summary of findings' table, including both the experimental and comparison interventions.
3) A list of the most critical and/or important health outcomes, both desirable and undesirable, limited to seven or fewer outcomes.
4) A measure of the typical burden of each outcomes (e.g. illustrative risk, or illustrative mean, on comparator intervention).
5) The absolute and relative magnitude of effect measured for each (if both are appropriate).
6) The numbers of participants and studies contributing to the analysis of each outcomes.
7) A GRADE assessment of the overall certainty of the body of evidence for each outcome (which may vary by outcome).
8) Space for comments.
9) Explanations (formerly known as footnotes).

Ideally, 'Summary of findings' tables are supported by more detailed tables (known as 'evidence profiles') to which the review may be linked, which provide more detailed explanations. Evidence profiles include the same important health outcomes, and provide greater detail than 'Summary of findings' tables of both of the individual

Summary of findings (for an interactive version in GRADEpro, see http://bit.ly/2FI9SQI)

Compression stockings compared with no compression stockings for people taking long flights

Patients or population: anyone taking a long flight (lasting more than 6 hours)

Settings: international air travel

Intervention: compression stockings[a]

Comparison: without stockings

Outcomes	Illustrative comparative risks* (95% CI)		Relative effect (95% CI)	Number of participants (studies)	Certainty of the evidence (GRADE)	Comments
	Assumed risk	Corresponding risk				
	Without stockings	**With stockings**				
Symptomatic deep vein thrombosis (DVT)	See comment	See comment	Not estimable	2821 (9 studies)	See comment	0 participants developed symptomatic DVT in these studies
Symptomless DVT	**Low risk population[b]**		**RR 0.10** (0.04 to 0.26)	2637 (9 studies)	⊕⊕⊕⊕ **High**	
	10 per 1000	**1 per 1000** (0 to 3)				
	High risk population[b]					
	20 per 1000	**2 per 1000** (1 to 8)				
Superficial vein thrombosis	**13 per 1000**	**6 per 1000** (2 to 15)	**RR 0.45** (0.18 to 1.13)	1804 (8 studies)	⊕⊕⊕◯ **Moderate[c]**	
Oedema Post-flight values measured on a scale from 0, no oedema, to 10, maximum oedema	The mean oedema score ranged across control groups from **6 to 9**	The mean oedema score in the intervention groups was on average **4.7 lower** (95% CI −4.9 to −4.5)		1246 (6 studies)	⊕⊕◯◯ **Low[d]**	
Pulmonary embolus	See comment	See comment	Not estimable	2821 (9 studies)	See comment	0 participants developed pulmonary embolus in these studies[e]
Death	See comment	See comment	Not estimable	2821 (9 studies)	See comment	0 participants died in these studies
Adverse effects	See comment	See comment	Not estimable	1182 (4 studies)	See comment	The tolerability of the stockings was described as very good with no complaints of side effects in 4 studies[f]

*The basis for the **assumed risk** is provided in footnotes. The **corresponding risk** (and its 95% confidence interval) is based on the assumed risk in the intervention group and the **relative effect** of the intervention (and its 95% CI).
CI: confidence interval; RR: risk ratio; GRADE: GRADE Working Group grades of evidence (see explanations).

[a] All the stockings in the nine studies included in this review were below-knee compression stockings. In four studies the compression strength was 20 mmHg to 30 mmHg at the ankle. It was 10 mmHg to 20 mmHg in the other four studies. Stockings come in different sizes. If a stocking is too tight around the knee it can prevent essential venous return causing the blood to pool around the knee. Compression stockings should be fitted properly. A stocking that is too tight could cut into the skin on a long flight and potentially cause ulceration and increased risk of DVT. Some stockings can be slightly thicker than normal leg covering and can be potentially restrictive with tight foot wear. It is a good idea to wear stockings around the house prior to travel to ensure a good, comfortable fit. Participants put their stockings on two to three hours before the flight in most of the studies. The availability and cost of stockings can vary.

[b] Two studies recruited high risk participants defined as those with previous episodes of DVT, coagulation disorders, severe obesity, limited mobility due to bone or joint problems, neoplastic disease within the previous two years, large varicose veins or, in one of the studies, participants taller than 190 cm and heavier than 90 kg. The incidence for the seven studies that excluded high risk participants was 1.45% and the incidence for the two studies that recruited high-risk participants (with at least one risk factor) was 2.43%. We have used 10 and 30 per 1000 to express different risk strata, respectively.

[c] The confidence interval crosses no difference and does not rule out a small increase.

[d] The measurement of oedema was not validated (indirectness of the outcome) or blinded to the intervention (risk of bias).

[e] If there are very few or no events and the number of participants is large, judgement about the certainty of evidence (particularly judgements about imprecision) may be based on the absolute effect. Here the certainty rating may be considered 'high' if the outcome was appropriately assessed and the event, in fact, did not occur in 2821 studied participants.

[f] None of the other studies reported adverse effects, apart from four cases of superficial vein thrombosis in varicose veins in the knee region that were compressed by the upper edge of the stocking in one study.

Figure 14.1.a Example of a 'Summary of findings' table

Summary of findings (for an interactive version in GRADEpro, see http://bit.ly/2WQwVbJ)

Probiotics compared to no probiotics as an adjunct to antibiotics in children

Patient or population: children given antibiotics

Settings: inpatients and outpatient

Intervention: probiotics

Comparison: no probiotics

Outcomes No of participants (studies)	Relative effects (95% CI)	Anticipated absolute effects* (95% CI)			Certainty of the evidence (GRADE)	Comments
		Without probiotics	With probiotics	Difference		
Incidence of diarrhoea: Probiotic dose 5 billion CFU/day Follow-up: 10 days to 3 months					⊕⊕⊕⊖ **moderate**[b] Due to risk of bias	Probably decreases the incidence of diarrhoea.
Children < 5 years		**Children < 5 years**				
1474 (7 studies)	**RR 0.41** (0.29 to 0.55)	**22.3%**[a]	**8.9%** (6.5 to 12.2)	**13.4% fewer children**[a] (10.1 to 15.8 fewer)		
Children > 5 years		**Children > 5 years**			⊕⊕⊖⊖ **low**[b, c] Due to risk of bias and imprecision	May decrease the incidence of diarrhoea.
624 (4 studies)	**RR 0.81** (0.53 to 1.21)	**11.2%** [a]	**9%** (5.9 to 13.6)	**2.2% fewer children**[a] (5.3 fewer to 2.4 more)		
Adverse events[d] Follow-up: 10 to 44 days 1575 (11 studies)	-	**1.8%** [a]	**2.3%** (0.8 to 3.8)	**0.5% more adverse events**[e] (1 fewer to 2 more)	⊕⊕⊖⊖ **low**[f, g] Due to risk of bias and inconsistency	There may be little or no difference in adverse events.
Duration of diarrhoea Follow-up: 10 days to 3 months 897 (5 studies)	-	The mean duration of diarrhoea without probiotics was **4 days.**	-	**0.6 fewer days** (1.18 to 0.02 fewer days)	⊕⊕⊖⊖ **low**[h, i] Due to imprecision and inconsistency	May decrease the duration of diarrhoea.
Stools per day Follow-up: 10 days to 3 months 425 (4 studies)	-	The mean stools per day without probiotics was **2.5 stools per day.**	-	**0.3 fewer stools per day** (0.6 to 0 fewer)	⊕⊕⊖⊖ **low**[j, k] Due to imprecision and inconsistency	There may be little or no difference in stools per day.

*The basis for the **risk in the control group** (e.g. the median control group risk across studies) is provided in footnotes. The **risk in the intervention group** (and its 95% confidence interval) is based on the assumed risk in the comparison group and the **relative effect** of the intervention (and its 95% CI). **CI:** confidence interval; **RR:** risk ratio.

EXPLANATIONS

[a] Control group risk estimates come from pooled estimates of control groups. Relative effect based on available case analysis

[b] High risk of bias due to high loss to follow-up.

[c] Imprecision due to few events and confidence intervals include appreciable benefit or harm.

[d] Side effects: rash, nausea, flatulence, vomiting, increased phlegm, chest pain, constipation, taste disturbance and low appetite.

[e] Risks were calculated from pooled risk differences.

[f] High risk of bias. Only 11 of 16 trials reported on adverse events, suggesting a selective reporting bias.

[g] Serious inconsistency. Numerous probiotic agents and doses were evaluated amongst a relatively small number of trials, limiting our ability to draw conclusions on the safety of the many probiotics agents and doses administered.

[h] Serious unexplained inconsistency (large heterogeneity $I^2 = 79\%$, P value [P = 0.04], point estimates and confidence intervals vary considerably).

[i] Serious imprecision. The upper bound of 0.02 fewer days of diarrhoea is not considered patient important.

[j] Serious unexplained inconsistency (large heterogeneity $I^2 = 78\%$, P value [P = 0.05], point estimates and confidence intervals vary considerably).

[k] Serious imprecision. The 95% confidence interval includes no effect and lower bound of 0.60 stools per day is of questionable patient importance.

Figure 14.1.b Example of alternative 'Summary of findings' table

considerations feeding into the grading of certainty and of the results of the studies (Guyatt et al 2011a). They ensure that a structured approach is used to rating the certainty of evidence. Although they are rarely published in Cochrane Reviews, evidence profiles are often used, for example, by guideline developers in considering the certainty of the evidence to support guideline recommendations. Review authors will find it easier to develop the 'Summary of findings' table by completing the rating of the certainty of evidence in the evidence profile first in GRADEpro GDT. They can then automatically convert this to one of the 'Summary of findings' formats in GRADEpro GDT, including an interactive 'Summary of findings' for publication.

As a measure of the magnitude of effect for dichotomous outcomes, the 'Summary of findings' table should provide a relative measure of effect (e.g. risk ratio, odds ratio, hazard) and measures of absolute risk. For other types of data, an absolute measure alone (such as a difference in means for continuous data) might be sufficient. It is important that the magnitude of effect is presented in a meaningful way, which may require some transformation of the result of a meta-analysis (see also Chapter 15, Sections 15.4 and 15.5). Reviews with more than one main comparison should include a separate 'Summary of findings' table for each comparison.

Figure 14.1.a provides an example of a 'Summary of findings' table. Figure 14.1.b provides an alternative format that may further facilitate users' understanding and interpretation of the review's findings. Evidence evaluating different formats suggests that the 'Summary of findings' table should include a risk difference as a measure of the absolute effect and authors should preferably use a format that includes a risk difference (Carrasco-Labra et al 2016).

A detailed description of the contents of a 'Summary of findings' table appears in Section 14.1.6.

14.1.4 Producing 'Summary of findings' tables

The GRADE Working Group's software, GRADEpro GDT (www.gradepro.org), including GRADE's interactive handbook, is available to assist review authors in the preparation of 'Summary of findings' tables. GRADEpro can use data on the comparator group risk and the effect estimate (entered by the review authors or imported from files generated in RevMan) to produce the relative effects and absolute risks associated with experimental interventions. In addition, it leads the user through the process of a GRADE assessment, and produces a table that can be used as a standalone table in a review (including by direct import into software such as RevMan or integration with RevMan Web), or an interactive 'Summary of findings' table (see help resources in GRADEpro).

14.1.5 Statistical considerations in 'Summary of findings' tables

14.1.5.1 Dichotomous outcomes

'Summary of findings' tables should include both absolute and relative measures of effect for dichotomous outcomes. Risk ratios, odds ratios and risk differences are different ways of comparing two groups with dichotomous outcome data (see Chapter 6, Section 6.4.1). Furthermore, there are two distinct risk ratios, depending on which event (e.g. 'yes' or 'no') is the focus of the analysis (see Chapter 6, Section 6.4.1.5). In the presence of a non-zero intervention effect, any variation across studies in the comparator group risks (i.e. variation in the risk of the event occurring without the intervention of interest, for example in different populations) makes it impossible for more than one of these measures to be truly the same in every study.

It has long been assumed in epidemiology that relative measures of effect are more consistent than absolute measures of effect from one scenario to another. There is empirical evidence to support this assumption (Engels et al 2000, Deeks and Altman 2001, Furukawa et al 2002). For this reason, meta-analyses should generally use either a risk ratio or an odds ratio as a measure of effect (see Chapter 10, Section 10.4.3). Correspondingly, a single estimate of relative effect is likely to be a more appropriate summary than a single estimate of absolute effect. If a relative effect is indeed consistent across studies, then different comparator group risks will have different implications for absolute benefit. For instance, if the risk ratio is consistently 0.75, then the experimental intervention would reduce a comparator group risk of 80% to 60% in the intervention group (an absolute risk reduction of 20 percentage points), but would also reduce a comparator group risk of 20% to 15% in the intervention group (an absolute risk reduction of 5 percentage points).

'Summary of findings' tables are built around the assumption of a consistent relative effect. It is therefore important to consider the implications of this effect for different comparator group risks (these can be derived or estimated from a number of sources, see Section 14.1.6.3), which may require an assessment of the certainty of evidence for prognostic evidence (Spencer et al 2012, Iorio et al 2015). For any comparator group risk, it is possible to estimate a corresponding intervention group risk (i.e. the absolute risk with the intervention) from the meta-analytic risk ratio or odds ratio. Note that the numbers provided in the 'Corresponding risk' column are specific to the 'risks' in the adjacent column.

For the meta-analytic risk ratio (RR) and assumed comparator risk (ACR) the corresponding intervention risk is obtained as:

$$\text{Corresponding intervention risk per 1000} = 1000 \times \text{ACR} \times \text{RR}.$$

As an example, in Figure 14.1.a, the meta-analytic risk ratio for symptomless deep vein thrombosis (DVT) is RR = 0.10 (95% CI 0.04 to 0.26). Assuming a comparator risk of ACR = 10 per 1000 = 0.01, we obtain:

$$\text{Corresponding intervention risk per 1000} = 1000 \times 0.01 \times 0.10 = 1.$$

For the meta-analytic odds ratio (OR) and assumed comparator risk, ACR, the corresponding intervention risk is obtained as:

$$\text{Corresponding intervention risk per 1000} = 1000 \times \left(\frac{\text{OR} \times \text{ACR}}{1 - \text{ACR} + (\text{OR} \times \text{ACR})} \right).$$

Upper and lower confidence limits for the corresponding intervention risk are obtained by replacing RR or OR by their upper and lower confidence limits, respectively (e.g. replacing 0.10 with 0.04, then with 0.26, in the example). Such confidence intervals do not incorporate uncertainty in the assumed comparator risks.

When dealing with risk ratios, it is critical that the same definition of 'event' is used as was used for the meta-analysis. For example, if the meta-analysis focused on 'death' (as opposed to survival) as the event, then corresponding risks in the 'Summary of findings' table must also refer to 'death'.

In (rare) circumstances in which there is clear rationale to assume a consistent risk difference in the meta-analysis, in principle it is possible to present this for relevant 'assumed risks' and their corresponding risks, and to present the corresponding (different) relative effects for each assumed risk.

The risk difference expresses the difference between the ACR and the corresponding intervention risk (or the difference between the experimental and the comparator intervention).

For the meta-analytic risk ratio (RR) and assumed comparator risk (ACR) the corresponding risk difference is obtained as (note that risks can also be expressed using percentage or percentage points):

$$\text{Risk difference per 1000} = 1000 \times \text{ACR} \times (1 - \text{RR}),$$

$$\text{Risk difference in percentage points} = \text{ACR}\,\% \times (1 - \text{RR}).$$

As an example, in Figure 14.1.b the meta-analytic risk ratio is 0.41 (95% CI 0.29 to 0.55) for diarrhoea in children less than 5 years of age. Assuming a comparator group risk of 22.3% we obtain:

$$\text{Risk difference in percentage points} = 22.3\% \times (1 - 0.41) = 13.4\%.$$

For the meta-analytic odds ratio (OR) and assumed comparator risk (ACR) the absolute risk difference is obtained as (percentage points):

$$\text{Risk difference in percentage points} = \left(\frac{(1 - \text{OR}) \times \text{ACR}}{1-\text{ACR} + ((1-\text{OR}) \times \text{ACR})}\right).$$

Upper and lower confidence limits for the absolute risk difference are obtained by re-running the calculation above while replacing RR or OR by their upper and lower confidence limits, respectively (e.g. replacing 0.41 with 0.28, then with 0.55, in the example). Such confidence intervals do not incorporate uncertainty in the assumed comparator risks.

14.1.5.2 Time-to-event outcomes

Time-to-event outcomes measure whether and when a particular event (e.g. death) occurs (van Dalen et al 2007). The impact of the experimental intervention relative to the comparison group on time-to-event outcomes is usually measured using a hazard ratio (HR) (see Chapter 6, Section 6.8.1).

A hazard ratio expresses a relative effect estimate. It may be used in various ways to obtain absolute risks and other interpretable quantities for a specific population. Here we describe how to re-express hazard ratios in terms of: (i) absolute risk of event-free survival within a particular period of time; (ii) absolute risk of an event within a particular period of time; and (iii) median time to the event. All methods are built on an assumption of consistent relative effects (i.e. that the hazard ratio does not vary over time).

(i) *Absolute risk of event-free survival within a particular period of time* Event-free survival (e.g. overall survival) is commonly reported by individual studies. To obtain absolute effects for time-to-event outcomes measured as event-free survival, the summary HR can be used in conjunction with an assumed proportion of patients who are event-free in the comparator group (Tierney et al 2007). This proportion of patients will be specific to a period of time of observation. However, it is not strictly necessary to specify this period of time. For instance, a proportion of 50% of event-free patients might apply to patients with a high event rate observed over 1 year, or to patients with a low event rate observed over 2 years.

$$\text{Corresponding intervention risk, per 1000} \\ = \left(\exp\left[\ln\left(\text{proportion of patients event-free}\right) \times \text{HR}\right]\right) \times 1000.$$

As an example, suppose the meta-analytic hazard ratio is 0.42 (95% CI 0.25 to 0.72). Assuming a comparator group risk of event-free survival (e.g. for overall survival people being alive) at 2 years of ACR = 900 per 1000 = 0.9 we obtain:

$$\text{Corresponding intervention risk, per 1000} = \left(\exp\left[\ln(0.9) \times 0.42\right]\right) \times 1000 = 956$$

so that that 956 per 1000 people will be alive with the experimental intervention at 2 years. The derivation of the risk should be explained in a comment or footnote.

(ii) ***Absolute risk of an event within a particular period of time*** To obtain this absolute effect, again the summary HR can be used (Tierney et al 2007):

$$\text{Corresponding intervention risk per 1000} \\ = 1000 - \left(\left(\exp\left[\ln\left(1 - \text{proportion of patients with event}\right) \times \text{HR}\right]\right) \times 1000\right).$$

In the example, suppose we assume a comparator group risk of events (e.g. for mortality, people being dead) at 2 years of ACR = 100 per 1000 = 0.1. We obtain:

$$\text{Corresponding intervention risk, per 1000} \\ = 1000 - \left(\left(\exp\left[\ln(1 - 0.1) \times 0.42\right]\right) \times 1000\right) = 44$$

so that that 44 per 1000 people will be dead with the experimental intervention at 2 years.

(iii) ***Median time to the event*** Instead of absolute numbers, the time to the event in the intervention and comparison groups can be expressed as median survival time in months or years. To obtain median survival time the pooled HR can be applied to an assumed median survival time in the comparator group (Tierney et al 2007):

$$\text{Corresponding median survival, in months} = \text{comparator group median survival time, in months/HR.}$$

In the example, assuming a comparator group median survival time of 80 months, we obtain:

$$\text{Corresponding median survival, in months} = 80\ \text{months}/0.42 = 190\ \text{months.}$$

For all three of these options for re-expressing results of time-to-event analyses, upper and lower confidence limits for the corresponding intervention risk are obtained by replacing HR by its upper and lower confidence limits, respectively (e.g. replacing 0.42 with 0.25, then with 0.72, in the example). Again, as for dichotomous outcomes, such confidence intervals do not incorporate uncertainty in the assumed comparator group risks. This is of special concern for long-term survival with a low or moderate mortality rate and a corresponding high number of censored patients (i.e. a low number of patients under risk and a high censoring rate).

14.1.6 Detailed contents of a 'Summary of findings' table

14.1.6.1 Table title and header

The title of each 'Summary of findings' table should specify the healthcare question, framed in terms of the population and making it clear exactly what comparison of interventions are made. In Figure 14.1.a, the population is people taking long aeroplane flights, the intervention is compression stockings, and the control is no compression stockings.

The first rows of each 'Summary of findings' table should provide the following 'header' information:

Patients or population This further clarifies the population (and possibly the subpopulations) of interest and ideally the magnitude of risk of the most crucial adverse outcome at which an intervention is directed. For instance, people on a long-haul flight may be at different risks for DVT; those using selective serotonin reuptake inhibitors (SSRIs) might be at different risk for side effects; while those with atrial fibrillation may be at low (<1%), moderate (1% to 4%) or high (>4%) yearly risk of stroke.

Setting This should state any specific characteristics of the settings of the healthcare question that might limit the applicability of the summary of findings to other settings (e.g. primary care in Europe and North America).

Intervention The experimental intervention.

Comparison The comparator intervention (including no specific intervention).

14.1.6.2 Outcomes

The rows of a 'Summary of findings' table should include all desirable and undesirable health outcomes (listed in order of importance) that are essential for decision making, up to a maximum of *seven* outcomes. If there are more outcomes in the review, review authors will need to omit the less important outcomes from the table, and the decision selecting which outcomes are critical or important to the review should be made during protocol development (see Chapter 3). Review authors should provide time frames for the measurement of the outcomes (e.g. 90 days or 12 months) and the type of instrument scores (e.g. ranging from 0 to 100).

Note that review authors should include the pre-specified critical and important outcomes in the table *whether data are available or not.* However, they should be alert to the possibility that the importance of an outcome (e.g. a serious adverse effect) may only become known after the protocol was written or the analysis was carried out, and should take appropriate actions to include these in the 'Summary of findings' table.

The 'Summary of findings' table can include effects in subgroups of the population for different comparator risks and effect sizes separately. For instance, in Figure 14.1.b effects are presented for children younger and older than 5 years separately. Review authors may also opt to produce separate 'Summary of findings' tables for different populations.

Review authors should include serious adverse events, but it might be possible to combine minor adverse events as a single outcome, and describe this in an explanatory footnote (note that it is not appropriate to add events together unless they are independent, that is, a participant who has experienced one adverse event has an unaffected chance of experiencing the other adverse event).

Outcomes measured at multiple time points represent a particular problem. In general, to keep the table simple, review authors should present multiple time points only for outcomes critical to decision making, where either the result or the decision made are likely to vary over time. The remainder should be presented at a common time point where possible.

Review authors can present continuous outcome measures in the 'Summary of findings' table and should endeavour to make these interpretable to the target audience. This requires that the units are clear and readily interpretable, for example, days of pain, or frequency of headache, and the name and scale of any measurement tools used should be stated (e.g. a Visual Analogue Scale, ranging from 0 to 100). However, many measurement instruments are not readily interpretable by non-specialist clinicians or patients, for example, points on a Beck Depression Inventory or quality of life score. For these, a more interpretable presentation might involve converting a continuous to a dichotomous outcome, such as > 50% improvement (see Chapter 15, Section 15.5).

14.1.6.3 Best estimate of risk with comparator intervention

Review authors should provide up to three typical risks for participants receiving the comparator intervention. For dichotomous outcomes, we recommend that these be presented in the form of the number of people experiencing the event per 100 or 1000 people (natural frequency) depending on the frequency of the outcome. For continuous outcomes, this would be stated as a mean or median value of the outcome measured.

Estimated or assumed comparator intervention risks could be based on assessments of typical risks in different patient groups derived from the review itself, individual representative studies in the review, or risks derived from a systematic review of prognosis studies or other sources of evidence which may in turn require an assessment of the certainty for the prognostic evidence (Spencer et al 2012, Iorio et al 2015). Ideally, risks would reflect groups that clinicians can easily identify on the basis of their presenting features.

An explanatory footnote should specify the source or rationale for each comparator group risk, including the time period to which it corresponds where appropriate. In Figure 14.1.a, clinicians can easily differentiate individuals with risk factors for deep venous thrombosis from those without. If there is known to be little variation in baseline risk then review authors may use the median comparator group risk across studies. If typical risks are not known, an option is to choose the risk from the included studies, providing the second highest for a high and the second lowest for a low risk population.

14.1.6.4 Risk with intervention

For dichotomous outcomes, review authors should provide a corresponding absolute risk for each comparator group risk, along with a confidence interval. This absolute risk with the (experimental) intervention will usually be derived from the meta-analysis result presented in the relative effect column (see Section 14.1.6.6). Formulae are provided in Section 14.1.5. Review authors should present the absolute effect in the same format as the risks with comparator intervention (see Section 14.1.6.3), for example as the number of people experiencing the event per 1000 people.

For continuous outcomes, a difference in means or standardized difference in means should be presented with its confidence interval. These will typically be obtained directly from a meta-analysis. Explanatory text should be used to clarify the meaning, as in Figures 14.1.a and 14.1.b.

14.1.6.5 Risk difference

For dichotomous outcomes, the risk difference can be provided using one of the 'Summary of findings' table formats as an additional option (see Figure 14.1.b). This risk difference expresses the difference between the experimental and comparator intervention and will usually be derived from the meta-analysis result presented in the relative effect column (see Section 14.1.6.6). Formulae are provided in Section 14.1.5. Review authors should present the risk difference in the same format as assumed and corresponding risks with comparator intervention (see Section 14.1.6.3); for example, as the number of people experiencing the event per 1000 people or as percentage points if the assumed and corresponding risks are expressed in percentage.

For continuous outcomes, if the 'Summary of findings' table includes this option, the mean difference can be presented here and the 'corresponding risk' column left blank (see Figure 14.1.b).

14.1.6.6 Relative effect (95% CI)

The relative effect will typically be a risk ratio or odds ratio (or occasionally a hazard ratio) with its accompanying 95% confidence interval, obtained from a meta-analysis performed on the basis of the same effect measure. Risk ratios and odds ratios are similar when the comparator intervention risks are low and effects are small, but may differ considerably when comparator group risks increase. The meta-analysis may involve an assumption of either fixed or random effects, depending on what the review authors consider appropriate, and implying that the relative effect is either an estimate of the effect of the intervention, or an estimate of the average effect of the intervention across studies, respectively.

14.1.6.7 Number of participants (studies)

This column should include the number of participants assessed in the included studies for each outcome and the corresponding number of studies that contributed these participants.

14.1.6.8 Certainty of the evidence (GRADE)

Review authors should comment on the certainty of the evidence (also known as quality of the body of evidence or confidence in the effect estimates). Review authors should use the specific evidence grading system developed by the GRADE Working Group (Atkins et al 2004, Guyatt et al 2008, Guyatt et al 2011a), which is described in detail in Section 14.2. The GRADE approach categorizes the certainty in a body of evidence as 'high', 'moderate', 'low' or 'very low' by outcome. This is a result of judgement, but the judgement process operates within a transparent structure. As an example, the certainty would be 'high' if the summary were of several randomized trials with low risk of bias, but the rating of certainty becomes lower if there are concerns about risk of bias, inconsistency, indirectness, imprecision or publication bias. Judgements other than of 'high' certainty should be made transparent using explanatory footnotes or the 'Comments' column in the 'Summary of findings' table (see Section 14.1.6.10).

14.1.6.9 Comments

The aim of the 'Comments' field is to help interpret the information or data identified in the row. For example, this may be on the validity of the outcome measure or the presence of variables that are associated with the magnitude of effect. Important caveats about the results should be flagged here. Not all rows will need comments, and it is best to leave a blank if there is nothing warranting a comment.

14.1.6.10 Explanations

Detailed explanations should be included as footnotes to support the judgements in the 'Summary of findings' table, such as the overall GRADE assessment. The explanations should describe the rationale for important aspects of the content. Table 14.1.a lists guidance for useful explanations. Explanations should be concise, informative, relevant, easy to understand and accurate. If explanations cannot be sufficiently described in footnotes, review authors should provide further details of the issues in the Results and Discussion sections of the review.

Table 14.1.a Guidance for providing useful explanations in 'Summary of findings' (SoF) tables. Adapted from Santesso et al (2016)

General guidance

1) Enter the information for readers directly into the table if possible (e.g. information about the duration of follow-up or the scale used).
2) Generally, do not cite references in the explanations section, unless there are specific reasons, for example, for providing information about sources of baseline risks (see point 3).
3) Provide the source of information about the baseline risks used to calculate absolute effects.
4) On completion of the table, review all explanations to determine if some could be referenced multiple times if reworded or combined.
5) Provide reasons for upgrading and downgrading the evidence (see domain-specific guidance below) and use GRADEpro GDT software to adhere to GRADE guidance.
6) The body of evidence for a particular outcome may be determined to have serious or very serious issues for the affected domain (or critically serious for risk of bias when ROBINS-I is used). Thus, it may be useful to indicate the number of levels for downgrading (e.g. downgraded by one level for risk of bias), but avoid repetition of what is in the table (and the impression of formulaic or algorithmic reporting). In evidence profiles, this information is already in the cells of the table.
7) Although explanations about the certainty in the evidence are primarily required when they alter the certainty, consider adding an explanation when the certainty in the evidence has not been altered but when this decision may be questioned by others. This will help with understanding reasons for disagreement.

(*Continued*)

Table 14.1.a (Continued)

8) Ensure that the table is not used as a description of the methods of the review (e.g. do not describe the reasons for the statistical analysis).
9) Enter results for outcomes that could not be combined statistically in a meta-analysis (i.e. narrative outcomes) directly into the SoF table in the results columns. An explanation may not be necessary to communicate those results. If considered beneficial to the intended audience, add complementary estimates of intervention effects (e.g. number needed to treat for benefit and harm, risk difference expressed as percentage, continuous outcome expressed in minimal important difference units) in the Comments column.
10) Use the information presented in the explanations about the GRADE process to inform other key parts of the review, including summary versions and the discussion.

Domain-specific guidance for writing useful explanations

Risk of bias

1) Describe the number of studies, or the amount of information that they provide in the meta-analysis, that were at high risk of bias and for which criterion.
   a) Use terms such as majority, minority, all, some or none; or the number of studies as X/X studies.
   b) For randomized trials, mention the specific criteria including allocation sequence concealment, selective outcome reporting, etc.
      For non-randomized studies, describe the criterion in the tool used (e.g. using the ROBINS-I tool).
   c) Indicate if the effect of the risk of bias was examined in a sensitivity analysis. When appropriate, mention the contribution of the studies at high risk of bias to the estimates.
2) Information about study design may be included in the explanations, in particular, in SoF when different study designs are included.

Inconsistency

1) Indicate the measure used to judge inconsistency, such as the statistical test or measure (I^2, Chi^2, Tau), or the overlap of confidence intervals, or similarity of point estimates.
2) If inconsistency is based on I^2, describe it as considerable, substantial, moderate or not important.
3) If applicable, mention if heterogeneity was explored in subgroup analyses by PICO (patients, intervention, comparison, outcome), and if there are other potential reasons for the heterogeneity.
4) In the case of a single study for an outcome, say that there is 'none' rather than 'not applicable'.

Indirectness

1) Indicate where indirectness is due to the elements of PICO (see Table 14.2.b).

Imprecision

1) Indicate where the sample size or number of events does not meet the optimal information size as calculated, or the 'rules of thumb' (e.g. 400 events). Avoid reference to the number of studies as a reason for imprecision.
2) Indicate whether the confidence intervals include the possibility of a small or no effect AND important benefit or harm. If known, provide the numerical value of the threshold of important benefit.
3) Avoid reporting the result as statistically or non-statistically significant.

Publication bias

1) Indicate the reason or methods used to detect publication bias (e.g. asymmetrical funnel plot, small studies with positive results, suspected selective availability of data from published or unpublished studies).

Upgrading

1) Mention the reason for upgrading: due to large effect; a dose-response gradient; or plausible residual opposing confounding increases the certainty of evidence.
2) For large effects, report if the relative effect is > 2 or > 5. For dose-response gradients, provide the level of intervention and effect on the outcome. For the domain 'plausible residual opposing confounding', describe the effect of the confounding factor on the estimate.

14.2 Assessing the certainty or quality of a body of evidence

14.2.1 The GRADE approach

The Grades of Recommendation, Assessment, Development and Evaluation Working Group (GRADE Working Group) has developed a system for grading the certainty of evidence (Schünemann et al 2003, Atkins et al 2004, Schünemann et al 2006, Guyatt et al 2008, Guyatt et al 2011a). Over 100 organizations including the World Health Organization (WHO), the American College of Physicians, the American Society of Hematology (ASH), the Canadian Agency for Drugs and Technology in Health (CADTH) and the National Institutes of Health and Clinical Excellence (NICE) in the UK have adopted the GRADE system (www.gradeworkinggroup.org).

Cochrane has also formally adopted this approach, and all Cochrane Reviews should use GRADE to evaluate the certainty of evidence for important outcomes (see MECIR Box 14.2.a).

MECIR Box 14.2.a Relevant expectations for conduct of intervention reviews	
C74: Assessing the certainty of the body of evidence (**Mandatory**)	
Use the five GRADE considerations (risk of bias, consistency of effect, imprecision, indirectness and publication bias) to assess the certainty of the body of evidence for each outcome, and to draw conclusions about the certainty of evidence within the text of the review.	GRADE is the most widely used approach for summarizing confidence in effects of interventions by outcome across studies. It is preferable to use the online GRADEpro tool, and to use it as described in the help system of the software. This should help to ensure that author teams are accessing the same information to inform their judgements. Ideally, two people working independently should assess the certainty of the body of evidence and reach a consensus view on any downgrading decisions. The five GRADE considerations should be addressed irrespective of whether the review includes a 'Summary of findings' table. It is helpful to draw on this information in the Discussion, in the Authors' conclusions and to convey the certainty in the evidence in the Abstract and Plain language summary.
C75: Justifying assessments of the certainty of the body of evidence (**Mandatory**)	
Justify and document all assessments of the certainty of the body of evidence (e.g. downgrading or upgrading using GRADE).	The adoption of a structured approach ensures transparency in formulating an interpretation of the evidence, and the result is more informative to the user.

For systematic reviews, the GRADE approach defines the certainty of a body of evidence as the extent to which one can be confident that an estimate of effect or association is close to the quantity of specific interest. Assessing the certainty of a body of evidence involves consideration of within- and across-study risk of bias (limitations in study design and execution or methodological quality), inconsistency (or heterogeneity), indirectness of evidence, imprecision of the effect estimates and risk of publication bias (see Section 14.2.2), as well as domains that may increase our confidence in the effect estimate (as described in Section 14.2.3). The GRADE system entails an assessment of the certainty of a body of evidence for each individual outcome. Judgements about the domains that determine the certainty of evidence should be described in the results or discussion section and as part of the 'Summary of findings' table.

The GRADE approach specifies four levels of certainty (Figure 14.2.a). For interventions, including diagnostic and other tests that are evaluated as interventions (Schünemann et al 2008b, Schünemann et al 2008a, Balshem et al 2011, Schünemann et al 2012), the starting point for rating the certainty of evidence is categorized into two types:

- randomized trials; and
- non-randomized studies of interventions (NRSI), including observational studies (including but not limited to cohort studies, and case-control studies, cross-sectional studies, case series and case reports, although not all of these designs are usually included in Cochrane Reviews).

There are many instances in which review authors rely on information from NRSI, in particular to evaluate potential harms (see Chapter 24). In addition, review authors can obtain relevant data from both randomized trials and NRSI, with each type of evidence complementing the other (Schünemann et al 2013).

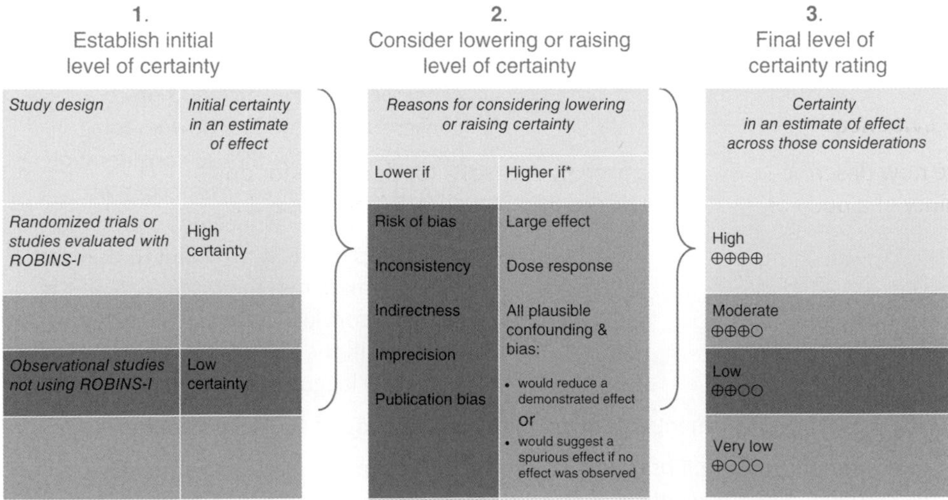

Figure 14.2a Levels of the certainty of a body of evidence in the GRADE approach. *Upgrading criteria are usually applicable to non-randomized studies only (but exceptions exist).

In GRADE, a body of evidence from randomized trials begins with a high-certainty rating while a body of evidence from NRSI begins with a low-certainty rating. The lower rating with NRSI is the result of the potential bias induced by the lack of randomization (i.e. confounding and selection bias).

However, when using the new Risk Of Bias In Non-randomized Studies of Interventions (ROBINS-I) tool (Sterne et al 2016), an assessment tool that covers the risk of bias due to lack of randomization, all studies may start as high certainty of the evidence (Schünemann et al 2018). The approach of starting all study designs (including NRSI) as high certainty does not conflict with the initial GRADE approach of starting the rating of NRSI as low certainty evidence. This is because a body of evidence from NRSI should generally be downgraded by two levels due to the inherent risk of bias associated with the lack of randomization, namely confounding and selection bias. Not downgrading NRSI from high to low certainty needs transparent and detailed justification for what mitigates concerns about confounding and selection bias (Schünemann et al 2018). Very few examples of where not rating down by two levels is appropriate currently exist.

The highest certainty rating is a body of evidence when there are no concerns in any of the GRADE factors listed in Figure 14.2.a. Review authors often downgrade evidence to moderate, low or even very low certainty evidence, depending on the presence of the five factors in Figure 14.2.a. Usually, certainty rating will fall by one level for each factor, up to a maximum of three levels for all factors. If there are very severe problems for any one domain (e.g. when assessing risk of bias, all studies were unconcealed, unblinded and lost over 50% of their patients to follow-up), evidence may fall by two levels due to that factor alone. It is not possible to rate lower than 'very low certainty' evidence.

Review authors will generally grade evidence from sound non-randomized studies as low certainty, even if ROBINS-I is used. If, however, such studies yield large effects and there is no obvious bias explaining those effects, review authors may rate the evidence as moderate or – if the effect is large enough – even as high certainty (Figure 14.2.a). The very low certainty level is appropriate for, but is not limited to, studies with critical problems and unsystematic clinical observations (e.g. case series or case reports).

14.2.2 Domains that can lead to decreasing the certainty level of a body of evidence

We now describe in more detail the five reasons (or domains) for downgrading the certainty of a body of evidence for a specific outcome. In each case, if a reason is found for downgrading the evidence, it should be classified as 'no limitation' (not important enough to warrant downgrading), 'serious' (downgrading the certainty rating by one level) or 'very serious' (downgrading the certainty grade by two levels). For non-randomized studies assessed with ROBINS-I, rating down by three levels should be classified as 'extremely' serious.

1) **Risk of bias or limitations in the detailed design and implementation**

Our confidence in an estimate of effect decreases if studies suffer from major limitations that are likely to result in a biased assessment of the intervention effect. For randomized trials, these methodological limitations include failure to generate a random sequence, lack of allocation sequence concealment, lack of blinding (particularly with subjective outcomes that are highly susceptible to biased assessment), a large loss to follow-up or selective reporting of outcomes. Chapter 8 provides a discussion of study-level assessments of risk of bias in the context of a Cochrane Review, and proposes an approach to assessing the risk of bias for an outcome across studies as 'Low' risk of bias, 'Some concerns' and 'High' risk of bias for randomized trials. Levels of 'Low'. 'Moderate', 'Serious' and 'Critical' risk of bias arise for non-randomized studies assessed with ROBINS-I (Chapter 25). These assessments should feed directly into this GRADE domain. In particular, 'Low' risk of bias would indicate 'no limitation'; 'Some concerns' would indicate either 'no limitation' or 'serious limitation'; and 'High' risk of bias would indicate either 'serious limitation' or 'very serious limitation'. 'Critical' risk of bias on ROBINS-I would indicate extremely serious limitations in GRADE. Review authors should use their judgement to decide between alternative categories, depending on the likely magnitude of the potential biases.

Every study addressing a particular outcome will differ, to some degree, in the risk of bias. Review authors should make an overall judgement on whether the certainty of evidence for an outcome warrants downgrading on the basis of study limitations. The assessment of study limitations should apply to the studies contributing to the results in the 'Summary of findings' table, rather than to all studies that could potentially be included in the analysis. We have argued in Chapter 7 (Section 7.6.2) that the primary analysis should be restricted to studies at low (or low and unclear) risk of bias where possible.

Table 14.2.a presents the judgements that must be made in going from assessments of the risk of bias to judgements about study limitations for each outcome included in a 'Summary of findings' table. A rating of high certainty evidence can be achieved only when most evidence comes from studies that met the criteria for low risk of bias. For example, of the 22 studies addressing the impact of beta-blockers on mortality in patients with heart failure, most probably or certainly used concealed allocation of the sequence, all blinded at least some key groups and follow-up of randomized patients was almost complete (Brophy et al 2001). The certainty of evidence might be downgraded by one level when most of the evidence comes from individual studies either with a crucial limitation for one item, or with some limitations for multiple items. An example of very serious limitations, warranting downgrading by two levels, is provided by evidence on surgery versus conservative treatment in the management of patients with lumbar disc prolapse (Gibson and Waddell 2007). We are uncertain of the benefit of surgery in reducing symptoms after one year or longer, because the one study included in the analysis had inadequate concealment of the allocation sequence and the outcome was assessed using a crude rating by the surgeon without blinding.

2) **Unexplained heterogeneity or inconsistency of results**

When studies yield widely differing estimates of effect (heterogeneity or variability in results), investigators should look for robust explanations for that heterogeneity. For instance, drugs may have larger relative effects in sicker populations or when given in larger doses. A detailed discussion of heterogeneity and its investigation is provided in Chapter 10 (Sections 10.10 and 10.11). If an important modifier exists, with good evidence that important outcomes are different in different subgroups (which would ideally be pre-specified), then a separate 'Summary of findings' table may be considered for a separate population. For instance, a separate 'Summary of findings' table would

Table 14.2.a Further guidelines for domain 1 (of 5) in a GRADE assessment: going from assessments of risk of bias in studies to judgements about study limitations for main outcomes across studies

Risk of bias	Across studies	Interpretation	Considerations	GRADE assessment of risk of bias or study limitations of study limitations
Low risk of bias	Most information is from results at low risk of bias.	Plausible bias unlikely to seriously alter the results.	No apparent limitations.	No serious limitations, do not downgrade.
Some concerns	Most information is from results at low risk of bias or with some concerns.	Plausible bias that raises some doubt about the results.	Potential limitations are unlikely to lower confidence in the estimate of effect.	No serious limitations, do not downgrade.
			Potential limitations are likely to lower confidence in the estimate of effect.	Serious limitations, downgrade one level.
High risk of bias	The proportion of information from results at high risk of bias is sufficient to affect the interpretation of results.	Plausible bias that seriously weakens confidence in the results.	Crucial limitation for one criterion, or some limitations for multiple criteria, sufficient to lower confidence in the estimate of effect.	Serious limitations, downgrade one level.
			Crucial limitation for one or more criteria sufficient to substantially lower confidence in the estimate of effect.	Very serious limitations, downgrade two levels.

be used for carotid endarterectomy in symptomatic patients with high grade stenosis (70% to 99%) in which the intervention is, in the hands of the right surgeons, beneficial, and another (if review authors considered it relevant) for asymptomatic patients with low grade stenosis (less than 30%) in which surgery appears harmful (Orrapin and Rerkasem 2017). When heterogeneity exists and affects the interpretation of results, but review authors are unable to identify a plausible explanation with the data available, the certainty of the evidence decreases.

3) **Indirectness of evidence**

Two types of indirectness are relevant. First, a review comparing the effectiveness of alternative interventions (say A and B) may find that randomized trials are available, but they have compared A with placebo and B with placebo. Thus, the evidence is restricted to indirect comparisons between A and B. Where indirect comparisons are undertaken within a network meta-analysis context, GRADE for network meta-analysis should be used (see Chapter 11, Section 11.5).

Second, a review may find randomized trials that meet eligibility criteria but address a restricted version of the main review question in terms of population, intervention, comparator or outcomes. For example, suppose that in a review addressing an intervention for secondary prevention of coronary heart disease, most identified studies happened to be in people who also had diabetes. Then the evidence may be regarded as indirect in relation to the broader question of interest because the population is primarily related to people with diabetes. The opposite scenario can equally apply: a review addressing the effect of a preventive strategy for coronary heart disease in people with diabetes may consider studies in people without diabetes to provide relevant, albeit indirect, evidence. This would be particularly likely if investigators had conducted few if any randomized trials in the target population (e.g. people with diabetes). Other sources of indirectness may arise from interventions studied (e.g. if in all included studies a technical intervention was implemented by expert, highly trained specialists in specialist centres, then evidence on the effects of the intervention outside these centres may be indirect), comparators used (e.g. if the comparator groups received an intervention that is less effective than standard treatment in most settings) and outcomes assessed (e.g. indirectness due to surrogate outcomes when data on patient-important outcomes are not available, or when investigators seek data on quality of life but only symptoms are reported). Review authors should make judgements transparent when they believe downgrading is justified, based on differences in anticipated effects in the group of primary interest. Review authors may be aided and increase transparency of their judgements about indirectness if they use Table 14.2.b available in the GRADEpro GDT software (Schünemann et al 2013).

4) **Imprecision of results**

When studies include few participants or few events, and thus have wide confidence intervals, review authors can lower their rating of the certainty of the evidence. The confidence intervals included in the 'Summary of findings' table will provide readers with information that allows them to make, to some extent, their own rating of precision. Review authors can use a calculation of the optimal information size (OIS) or review information size (RIS), similar to sample size calculations, to make judgements about imprecision (Guyatt et al 2011b, Schünemann 2016). The OIS or RIS is calculated on the basis of the number of participants required for an adequately powered individual study. If the 95% confidence interval excludes a risk ratio (RR) of 1.0, and the total number of events or patients exceeds the OIS criterion, precision is adequate. If the 95% CI includes appreciable benefit or harm (an RR of under 0.75 or over 1.25 is often suggested as a very rough guide) downgrading for imprecision may be appropriate even if OIS criteria are met (Guyatt et al 2011b, Schünemann 2016).

5) **High probability of publication bias**

The certainty of evidence level may be downgraded if investigators fail to report studies on the basis of results (typically those that show no effect: publication bias) or outcomes (typically those that may be harmful or for which no effect was observed: selective outcome non-reporting bias). Selective reporting of outcomes from among multiple outcomes measured is assessed at the study level as part of the assessment

Table 14.2.b Judgements about indirectness by outcome (available in GRADEpro GDT)

Outcome: …						
Domain (original question asked)	**Description (evidence found and included, including evidence from other studies) – consider the domains of study design and study limitation, inconsistency, imprecision and publication bias**	**Judgement – is the evidence sufficiently direct?**				
Population:		Yes	Probably yes	Probably no	No	
		☐	☐	☐	☐	
Intervention:		Yes	Probably yes	Probably no	No	
		☐	☐	☐	☐	
Comparator:		Yes	Probably yes	Probably no	No	
		☐	☐	☐	☐	
Direct comparison:		Yes	Probably yes	Probably no	No	
		☐	☐	☐	☐	
Outcome:		Yes	Probably yes	Probably no	No	
		☐	☐	☐	☐	
Final judgement about indirectness across domains:		**☐ No indirectness**	**☐ Serious indirectness**		**☐ Very serious indirectness**	

of risk of bias (see Chapter 8, Section 8.7), so for the studies contributing to the outcome in the 'Summary of findings' table this is addressed by domain 1 above (limitations in the design and implementation). If a large number of studies included in the review do not contribute to an outcome, or if there is evidence of publication bias, the certainty of the evidence may be downgraded. Chapter 13 provides a detailed discussion of reporting biases, including publication bias, and how it may be tackled in a Cochrane Review. A prototypical situation that may elicit suspicion of publication bias is when published evidence includes a number of small studies, all of which are industry-funded (Bhandari et al 2004). For example, 14 studies of flavanoids in patients with haemorrhoids have shown apparent large benefits, but enrolled a total of only

1432 patients (i.e. each study enrolled relatively few patients) (Alonso-Coello et al 2006). The heavy involvement of sponsors in most of these studies raises questions of whether unpublished studies that suggest no benefit exist (publication bias).

A particular body of evidence can suffer from problems associated with more than one of the five factors listed here, and the greater the problems, the lower the certainty of evidence rating that should result. One could imagine a situation in which randomized trials were available, but all or virtually all of these limitations would be present, and in serious form. A very low certainty of evidence rating would result.

14.2.3 Domains that may lead to increasing the certainty level of a body of evidence

Although NRSI and downgraded randomized trials will generally yield a low rating for certainty of evidence, there will be unusual circumstances in which review authors could 'upgrade' such evidence to moderate or even high certainty (Table 14.3.a).

1) ***Large effects*** On rare occasions when methodologically well-done observational studies yield large, consistent and precise estimates of the magnitude of an intervention effect, one may be particularly confident in the results. A large estimated effect (e.g. RR > 2 or RR < 0.5) in the absence of plausible confounders, or a very large effect (e.g. RR > 5 or RR < 0.2) in studies with no major threats to validity, might qualify for this. In these situations, while the NRSI may possibly have provided an over-estimate of the true effect, the weak study design may not explain all of the apparent observed benefit. Thus, despite reservations based on the observational study design, review authors are confident that the effect exists. The magnitude of the effect in these studies may move the assigned certainty of evidence from low to moderate (if the effect is large in the absence of other methodological limitations). For example, a meta-analysis of observational studies showed that bicycle helmets reduce the risk of head injuries in cyclists by a large margin (odds ratio (OR) 0.31, 95% CI 0.26 to 0.37) (Thompson et al 2000). This large effect, in the absence of obvious bias that could create the association, suggests a rating of moderate-certainty evidence.

   Note: GRADE guidance suggests the possibility of rating up one level for a large effect if the relative effect is greater than 2.0. However, if the point estimate of the relative effect is greater than 2.0, but the confidence interval is appreciably below 2.0, then some hesitation would be appropriate in the decision to rate up for a large effect. Another situation allows inference of a strong association without a formal comparative study. Consider the question of the impact of routine colonoscopy versus no screening for colon cancer on the rate of perforation associated with colonoscopy. Here, a large series of representative patients undergoing colonoscopy may provide high certainty evidence about the risk of perforation associated with colonoscopy. When the risk of the event among patients receiving the relevant comparator is known to be near 0 (i.e. we are certain that the incidence of spontaneous colon perforation in patients not undergoing colonoscopy is extremely low), case series or cohort studies of representative patients can provide high certainty evidence of adverse effects associated with an intervention, thereby allowing us to infer a strong association from even a limited number of events.

2) ***Dose-response*** The presence of a dose-response gradient may increase our confidence in the findings of observational studies and thereby enhance the assigned certainty of evidence. For example, our confidence in the result of observational studies that show an increased risk of bleeding in patients who have supratherapeutic anticoagulation levels is increased by the observation that there is a dose-response gradient between the length of time needed for blood to clot (as measured by the international normalized ratio (INR)) and an increased risk of bleeding (Levine et al 2004). A systematic review of NRSI investigating the effect of cyclooxygenase-2 inhibitors on cardiovascular events found that the summary estimate (RR) with rofecoxib was 1.33 (95% CI 1.00 to 1.79) with doses less than 25 mg/d, and 2.19 (95% CI 1.64 to 2.91) with doses more than 25 mg/d. Although residual confounding is likely to exist in the NRSI that address this issue, the existence of a dose-response gradient and the large apparent effect of higher doses of rofecoxib markedly increase our strength of inference that the association cannot be explained by residual confounding, and is therefore likely to be both causal and, at high levels of exposure, substantial.

   Note: GRADE guidance suggests the possibility of rating up one level for a large effect if the relative effect is greater than 2.0. Here, the fact that the point estimate of the relative effect is greater than 2.0, but the confidence interval is appreciably below 2.0 might make some hesitate in the decision to rate up for a large effect
3) ***Plausible confounding*** On occasion, all plausible biases from randomized or non-randomized studies may be working to under-estimate an apparent intervention effect. For example, if only sicker patients receive an experimental intervention or exposure, yet they still fare better, it is likely that the actual intervention or exposure effect is larger than the data suggest. For instance, a rigorous systematic review of observational studies including a total of 38 million patients demonstrated higher death rates in private for-profit versus private not-for-profit hospitals (Devereaux et al 2002). One possible bias relates to different disease severity in patients in the two hospital types. It is likely, however, that patients in the not-for-profit hospitals were sicker than those in the for-profit hospitals. Thus, to the extent that residual confounding existed, it would bias results against the not-for-profit hospitals. The second likely bias was the possibility that higher numbers of patients with excellent private insurance coverage could lead to a hospital having more resources and a spill-over effect that would benefit those without such coverage. Since for-profit hospitals are likely to admit a larger proportion of such well-insured patients than not-for-profit hospitals, the bias is once again against the not-for-profit hospitals. Since the plausible biases would all diminish the demonstrated intervention effect, one might consider the evidence from these observational studies as moderate rather than low certainty. A parallel situation exists when observational studies have failed to demonstrate an association, but all plausible biases would have increased an intervention effect. This situation will usually arise in the exploration of apparent harmful effects. For example, because the hypoglycaemic drug phenformin causes lactic acidosis, the related agent metformin was under suspicion for the same toxicity. Nevertheless, very large observational studies have failed to demonstrate an association (Salpeter et al 2007). Given the likelihood that clinicians would be more alert to lactic acidosis in the presence of the agent and over-report its occurrence, one might consider this moderate, or even high certainty, evidence refuting a causal relationship between typical therapeutic doses of metformin and lactic acidosis.

14.3 Describing the assessment of the certainty of a body of evidence using the GRADE framework

Review authors should report the grading of the certainty of evidence in the Results section for each outcome for which this has been performed, providing the rationale for downgrading or upgrading the evidence, and referring to the 'Summary of findings' table where applicable.

Table 14.3.a provides a framework and examples for how review authors can justify their judgements about the certainty of evidence in each domain. These justifications should also be included in explanatory notes to the 'Summary of findings' table (see Section 14.1.6.10).

Table 14.3.a Framework for describing the certainty of evidence and justifying downgrading or upgrading

Domains for assessing certainty of evidence by outcome	Results section	Examples of reasons for lowering or increasing the certainty of evidence
Risk of bias	Describe the risk of bias based on the criteria used in the risk-of-bias table.	Downgraded because of 10 randomized trials, five did not blind patients and caretakers.
Inconsistency	Describe the degree of inconsistency by outcome using one or more indicators (e.g. I^2 and P value), confidence interval overlap, difference in point estimate, between-study variance.	Not downgraded because the proportion of the variability in effect estimates that is due to true heterogeneity rather than chance is not important ($I^2 = 0\%$).
Indirectness	Describe if the majority of studies address the PICO – were they similar to the question posed?	Downgraded because the included studies were restricted to patients with advanced cancer.
Imprecision	Describe the number of events, and width of the confidence intervals.	The confidence intervals for the effect on mortality are consistent with both an appreciable benefit and appreciable harm and we lowered the certainty.
Publication bias	Describe the possible degree of publication bias.	1) The funnel plot of 14 randomized trials indicated that there were several small studies that showed a small positive effect, but small studies that showed no effect or harm may have been unpublished. The certainty of the evidence was lowered. 2) There are only three small positive studies, it appears that studies showing no effect or harm have not been published. There also is for-profit interest in the intervention. The certainty of the evidence was lowered.

Table 14.3.a (Continued)

Domains for assessing certainty of evidence by outcome	Results section	Examples of reasons for lowering or increasing the certainty of evidence
Large effects (upgrading)	Describe the magnitude of the effect and the widths of the associate confidence intervals.	Upgraded because the RR is large: 0.3 (95% CI 0.2 to 0.4), with a sufficient number of events to be precise.
Dose response (upgrading)	The studies show a clear relation with increases in the outcome of an outcome (e.g. lung cancer) with higher exposure levels.	Upgraded because the dose-response relation shows a relative risk increase of 10% in never smokers, 15% in smokers of 10 pack years and 20% in smokers of 15 pack years.
Opposing plausible residual bias and confounding (upgrading)	Describe which opposing plausible biases and confounders may have not been considered.	The estimate of effect is not controlled for the following possible confounders: smoking, degree of education, but the distribution of these factors in the studies is likely to lead to an under-estimate of the true effect. The certainty of the evidence was increased.

Chapter 15 (Section 15.6) describes in more detail how the overall GRADE assessment across all domains can be used to draw conclusions about the effects of the intervention, as well as providing implications for future research.

14.4 Chapter information

Authors: Holger J Schünemann, Julian PT Higgins, Gunn E Vist, Paul Glasziou, Elie A Akl, Nicole Skoetz, Gordon H Guyatt; on behalf of the Cochrane GRADEing Methods Group (formerly Applicability and Recommendations Methods Group) and the Cochrane Statistical Methods Group

Acknowledgements: Andrew D Oxman contributed to earlier versions. Professor Penny Hawe contributed to the text on adverse effects in earlier versions. Jon Deeks provided helpful contributions on an earlier version of this chapter. For details of previous authors and editors of the *Handbook*, please refer to the Preface.

Funding: This work was in part supported by funding from the Michael G DeGroote Cochrane Canada Centre and the Ontario Ministry of Health.

14.5 References

Alonso-Coello P, Zhou Q, Martinez-Zapata MJ, Mills E, Heels-Ansdell D, Johanson JF, Guyatt G. Meta-analysis of flavonoids for the treatment of haemorrhoids. *British Journal of Surgery* 2006; **93**: 909–920.

Atkins D, Best D, Briss PA, Eccles M, Falck-Ytter Y, Flottorp S, Guyatt GH, Harbour RT, Haugh MC, Henry D, Hill S, Jaeschke R, Leng G, Liberati A, Magrini N, Mason J, Middleton P, Mrukowicz J, O'Connell D, Oxman AD, Phillips B, Schünemann HJ, Edejer TT, Varonen H, Vist GE, Williams JW, Jr., Zaza S. Grading quality of evidence and strength of recommendations. *BMJ* 2004; **328**: 1490.

Balshem H, Helfand M, Schünemann HJ, Oxman AD, Kunz R, Brozek J, Vist GE, Falck-Ytter Y, Meerpohl J, Norris S, Guyatt GH. GRADE guidelines: 3. Rating the quality of evidence. *Journal of Clinical Epidemiology* 2011; **64**: 401–406.

Bhandari M, Busse JW, Jackowski D, Montori VM, Schünemann H, Sprague S, Mears D, Schemitsch EH, Heels-Ansdell D, Devereaux PJ. Association between industry funding and statistically significant pro-industry findings in medical and surgical randomized trials. *Canadian Medical Association Journal* 2004; **170**: 477–480.

Brophy JM, Joseph L, Rouleau JL. Beta-blockers in congestive heart failure: a Bayesian meta-analysis. *Annals of Internal Medicine* 2001; **134**: 550–560.

Carrasco-Labra A, Brignardello-Petersen R, Santesso N, Neumann I, Mustafa RA, Mbuagbaw L, Etxeandia Ikobaltzeta I, De Stio C, McCullagh LJ, Alonso-Coello P, Meerpohl JJ, Vandvik PO, Brozek JL, Akl EA, Bossuyt P, Churchill R, Glenton C, Rosenbaum S, Tugwell P, Welch V, Garner P, Guyatt G, Schünemann HJ. Improving GRADE evidence tables part 1: a randomized trial shows improved understanding of content in summary of findings tables with a new format. *Journal of Clinical Epidemiology* 2016; **74**: 7–18.

Deeks JJ, Altman DG. Effect measures for meta-analysis of trials with binary outcomes. In: Egger M, Davey Smith G, Altman DG, editors. *Systematic Reviews in Health Care: Meta-analysis in Context*. 2nd ed. London (UK): BMJ Publication Group; 2001. pp. 313–335.

Devereaux PJ, Choi PT, Lacchetti C, Weaver B, Schünemann HJ, Haines T, Lavis JN, Grant BJ, Haslam DR, Bhandari M, Sullivan T, Cook DJ, Walter SD, Meade M, Khan H, Bhatnagar N, Guyatt GH. A systematic review and meta-analysis of studies comparing mortality rates of private for-profit and private not-for-profit hospitals. *Canadian Medical Association Journal* 2002; **166**: 1399–1406.

Engels EA, Schmid CH, Terrin N, Olkin I, Lau J. Heterogeneity and statistical significance in meta-analysis: an empirical study of 125 meta-analyses. *Statistics in Medicine* 2000; **19**: 1707–1728.

Furukawa TA, Guyatt GH, Griffith LE. Can we individualize the 'number needed to treat'? An empirical study of summary effect measures in meta-analyses. *International Journal of Epidemiology* 2002; **31**: 72–76.

Gibson JN, Waddell G. Surgical interventions for lumbar disc prolapse: updated Cochrane Review. *Spine* 2007; **32**: 1735–1747.

Guyatt G, Oxman A, Vist G, Kunz R, Falck-Ytter Y, Alonso-Coello P, Schünemann H. GRADE: an emerging consensus on rating quality of evidence and strength of recommendations. *BMJ* 2008; **336**: 3.

Guyatt G, Oxman AD, Akl EA, Kunz R, Vist G, Brozek J, Norris S, Falck-Ytter Y, Glasziou P, DeBeer H, Jaeschke R, Rind D, Meerpohl J, Dahm P, Schünemann HJ. GRADE guidelines: 1. Introduction-GRADE evidence profiles and summary of findings tables. *Journal of Clinical Epidemiology* 2011a; **64**: 383–394.

Guyatt GH, Oxman AD, Kunz R, Brozek J, Alonso-Coello P, Rind D, Devereaux PJ, Montori VM, Freyschuss B, Vist G, Jaeschke R, Williams JW, Jr., Murad MH, Sinclair D, Falck-Ytter Y, Meerpohl J, Whittington C, Thorlund K, Andrews J, Schünemann HJ. GRADE guidelines 6. Rating the quality of evidence–imprecision. *Journal of Clinical Epidemiology* 2011b; **64**: 1283–1293.

Iorio A, Spencer FA, Falavigna M, Alba C, Lang E, Burnand B, McGinn T, Hayden J, Williams K, Shea B, Wolff R, Kujpers T, Perel P, Vandvik PO, Glasziou P, Schünemann H, Guyatt G. Use of GRADE for assessment of evidence about prognosis: rating confidence in estimates of event rates in broad categories of patients. *BMJ* 2015; **350**: h870.

Langendam M, Carrasco-Labra A, Santesso N, Mustafa RA, Brignardello-Petersen R, Ventresca M, Heus P, Lasserson T, Moustgaard R, Brozek J, Schünemann HJ. Improving GRADE evidence tables part 2: a systematic survey of explanatory notes shows more guidance is needed. *Journal of Clinical Epidemiology* 2016; **74**: 19–27.

Levine MN, Raskob G, Landefeld S, Kearon C, Schulman S. Hemorrhagic complications of anticoagulant treatment: the Seventh ACCP Conference on Antithrombotic and Thrombolytic Therapy. *Chest* 2004; **126**: 287S–310S.

Orrapin S, Rerkasem K. Carotid endarterectomy for symptomatic carotid stenosis. *Cochrane Database of Systematic Reviews* 2017; **6**: CD001081.

Salpeter S, Greyber E, Pasternak G, Salpeter E. Risk of fatal and nonfatal lactic acidosis with metformin use in type 2 diabetes mellitus. *Cochrane Database of Systematic Reviews* 2007; **4**: CD002967.

Santesso N, Carrasco-Labra A, Langendam M, Brignardello-Petersen R, Mustafa RA, Heus P, Lasserson T, Opiyo N, Kunnamo I, Sinclair D, Garner P, Treweek S, Tovey D, Akl EA, Tugwell P, Brozek JL, Guyatt G, Schünemann HJ. Improving GRADE evidence tables part 3: detailed guidance for explanatory footnotes supports creating and understanding GRADE certainty in the evidence judgments. *Journal of Clinical Epidemiology* 2016; **74**: 28–39.

Schünemann HJ, Best D, Vist G, Oxman AD, Group GW. Letters, numbers, symbols and words: how to communicate grades of evidence and recommendations. *Canadian Medical Association Journal* 2003; **169**: 677–680.

Schünemann HJ, Jaeschke R, Cook DJ, Bria WF, El-Solh AA, Ernst A, Fahy BF, Gould MK, Horan KL, Krishnan JA, Manthous CA, Maurer JR, McNicholas WT, Oxman AD, Rubenfeld G, Turino GM, Guyatt G. An official ATS statement: grading the quality of evidence and strength of recommendations in ATS guidelines and recommendations. *American Journal of Respiratory and Critical Care Medicine* 2006; **174**: 605–614.

Schünemann HJ, Oxman AD, Brozek J, Glasziou P, Jaeschke R, Vist GE, Williams JW Jr, Kunz R, Craig J, Montori VM, Bossuyt P, Guyatt GH. Grading quality of evidence and strength of recommendations for diagnostic tests and strategies. *BMJ* 2008a; **336**: 1106–1110.

Schünemann HJ, Oxman AD, Brozek J, Glasziou P, Bossuyt P, Chang S, Muti P, Jaeschke R, Guyatt GH. GRADE: assessing the quality of evidence for diagnostic recommendations. *ACP Journal Club* 2008b; **149**: 2.

Schünemann HJ, Mustafa R, Brozek J. [Diagnostic accuracy and linked evidence–testing the chain.] *Zeitschrift für Evidenz, Fortbildung und Qualität im Gesundheitswesen* 2012; **106**: 153–160.

Schünemann HJ, Tugwell P, Reeves BC, Akl EA, Santesso N, Spencer FA, Shea B, Wells G, Helfand M. Non-randomized studies as a source of complementary, sequential or replacement evidence for randomized controlled trials in systematic reviews on the effects of interventions. *Research Synthesis Methods* 2013; **4**: 49–62.

Schünemann HJ. Interpreting GRADE's levels of certainty or quality of the evidence: GRADE for statisticians, considering review information size or less emphasis on imprecision? *Journal of Clinical Epidemiology* 2016; **75**: 6–15.

Schünemann HJ, Cuello C, Akl EA, Mustafa RA, Meerpohl JJ, Thayer K, Morgan RL, Gartlehner G, Kunz R, Katikireddi SV, Sterne J, Higgins JPT, Guyatt G; GRADE Working Group. GRADE guidelines: 18. How ROBINS-I and other tools to assess risk of bias in nonrandomized studies should be used to rate the certainty of a body of evidence. *Journal of Clinical Epidemiology* 2018.

Spencer-Bonilla G, Quinones AR, Montori VM, International Minimally Disruptive Medicine Workgroup. Assessing the burden of treatment. *Journal of General Internal Medicine* 2017; **32**: 1141–1145.

Spencer FA, Iorio A, You J, Murad MH, Schünemann HJ, Vandvik PO, Crowther MA, Pottie K, Lang ES, Meerpohl JJ, Falck-Ytter Y, Alonso-Coello P, Guyatt GH. Uncertainties in baseline risk estimates and confidence in treatment effects. *BMJ* 2012; **345**: e7401.

Sterne JAC, Hernán MA, Reeves BC, Savović J, Berkman ND, Viswanathan M, Henry D, Altman DG, Ansari MT, Boutron I, Carpenter JR, Chan AW, Churchill R, Deeks JJ, Hróbjartsson A, Kirkham J, Jüni P, Loke YK, Pigott TD, Ramsay CR, Regidor D, Rothstein HR, Sandhu L, Santaguida PL, Schünemann HJ, Shea B, Shrier I, Tugwell P, Turner L, Valentine JC, Waddington H, Waters E, Wells GA, Whiting PF, Higgins JPT. ROBINS-I: a tool for assessing risk of bias in non-randomised studies of interventions. *BMJ* 2016; **355**: i4919.

Thompson DC, Rivara FP, Thompson R. Helmets for preventing head and facial injuries in bicyclists. *Cochrane Database of Systematic Reviews* 2000; **2**: CD001855.

Tierney JF, Stewart LA, Ghersi D, Burdett S, Sydes MR. Practical methods for incorporating summary time-to-event data into meta-analysis. *Trials* 2007; **8**: 16.

van Dalen EC, Tierney JF, Kremer LCM. Tips and tricks for understanding and using SR results. No. 7: time-to-event data. *Evidence-Based Child Health* 2007; **2**: 1089–1090.

15

Interpreting results and drawing conclusions

Holger J Schünemann, Gunn E Vist, Julian PT Higgins, Nancy Santesso, Jonathan J Deeks, Paul Glasziou, Elie A Akl, Gordon H Guyatt; on behalf of the Cochrane GRADEing Methods Group

KEY POINTS

- This chapter provides guidance on interpreting the results of synthesis in order to communicate the conclusions of the review effectively.
- Methods are presented for computing, presenting and interpreting relative and absolute effects for dichotomous outcome data, including the number needed to treat (NNT).
- For continuous outcome measures, review authors can present summary results for studies using natural units of measurement or as minimal important differences when all studies use the same scale. When studies measure the same construct but with different scales, review authors will need to find a way to interpret the standardized mean difference, or to use an alternative effect measure for the meta-analysis such as the ratio of means.
- Review authors should not describe results as 'statistically significant', 'not statistically significant' or 'non-significant' or unduly rely on thresholds for P values, but report the confidence interval together with the exact P value.
- Review authors should not make recommendations about healthcare decisions, but they can – after describing the certainty of evidence and the balance of benefits and harms – highlight different actions that might be consistent with particular patterns of values and preferences and other factors that determine a decision such as cost.

15.1 Introduction

The purpose of Cochrane Reviews is to facilitate healthcare decisions by patients and the general public, clinicians, guideline developers, administrators and policy makers. They also inform future research. A clear statement of findings, a considered discussion

This chapter should be cited as: Schünemann HJ, Vist GE, Higgins JPT, Santesso N, Deeks JJ, Glasziou P, Akl EA, Guyatt GH. Chapter 15: Interpreting results and drawing conclusions. In: Higgins JPT, Thomas J, Chandler J, Cumpston M, Li T, Page MJ, Welch VA (editors). *Cochrane Handbook for Systematic Reviews of Interventions*. 2nd Edition. Chichester (UK): John Wiley & Sons, 2019: 403–432.

and a clear presentation of the authors' conclusions are, therefore, important parts of the review. In particular, the following issues can help people make better informed decisions and increase the usability of Cochrane Reviews:

- information on all important outcomes, including adverse outcomes;
- the certainty of the evidence for each of these outcomes, as it applies to specific populations and specific interventions; and
- clarification of the manner in which particular values and preferences may bear on the desirable and undesirable consequences of the intervention.

A 'Summary of findings' table, described in Chapter 14 (Section 14.1), provides key pieces of information about health benefits and harms in a quick and accessible format. It is highly desirable that review authors include a 'Summary of findings' table in Cochrane Reviews alongside a sufficient description of the studies and meta-analyses to support its contents. This description includes the rating of the certainty of evidence, also called the quality of the evidence or confidence in the estimates of the effects, which is expected in all Cochrane Reviews.

'Summary of findings' tables are usually supported by full evidence profiles which include the detailed ratings of the evidence (Guyatt et al 2011a, Guyatt et al 2013a, Guyatt et al 2013b, Santesso et al 2016). The Discussion section of the text of the review provides space to reflect and consider the implications of these aspects of the review's findings. Cochrane Reviews include five standard subheadings to ensure the Discussion section places the review in an appropriate context: 'Summary of main results (benefits and harms)'; 'Potential biases in the review process'; 'Overall completeness and applicability of evidence'; 'Certainty of the evidence'; and 'Agreements and disagreements with other studies or reviews'. Following the Discussion, the Authors' conclusions section is divided into two standard subsections: 'Implications for practice' and 'Implications for research'. The assessment of the certainty of evidence facilitates a structured description of the implications for practice and research.

Because Cochrane Reviews have an international audience, the Discussion and Authors' conclusions should, so far as possible, assume a broad international perspective and provide guidance for how the results could be applied in different settings, rather than being restricted to specific national or local circumstances. Cultural differences and economic differences may both play an important role in determining the best course of action based on the results of a Cochrane Review. Furthermore, individuals within societies have widely varying values and preferences regarding health states, and use of societal resources to achieve particular health states. For all these reasons, and because information that goes beyond that included in a Cochrane Review is required to make fully informed decisions, different people will often make different decisions based on the same evidence presented in a review.

Thus, review authors should avoid specific recommendations that inevitably depend on assumptions about available resources, values and preferences, and other factors such as equity considerations, feasibility and acceptability of an intervention. The purpose of the review should be to present information and aid interpretation rather than to offer recommendations. The discussion and conclusions should help people understand the implications of the evidence in relation to practical decisions and apply the results to their specific situation. Review authors can aid this understanding of the implications by laying out different scenarios that describe certain value structures.

In this chapter, we address first one of the key aspects of interpreting findings that is also fundamental in completing a 'Summary of findings' table: the certainty of evidence related to each of the outcomes. We then provide a more detailed consideration of issues around applicability and around interpretation of numerical results, and provide suggestions for presenting authors' conclusions.

15.2 Issues of indirectness and applicability

15.2.1 The role of the review author

"A leap of faith is always required when applying any study findings to the population at large" or to a specific person. "In making that jump, one must always strike a balance between making justifiable broad generalizations and being too conservative in one's conclusions" (Friedman et al 1985). In addition to issues about risk of bias and other domains determining the certainty of evidence, this leap of faith is related to how well the identified body of evidence matches the posed PICO (Population, Intervention, Comparator(s) and Outcome) question. As to the population, no individual can be entirely matched to the population included in research studies. At the time of decision, there will always be differences between the study population and the person or population to whom the evidence is applied; sometimes these differences are slight, sometimes large.

The terms applicability, generalizability, external validity and transferability are related, sometimes used interchangeably and have in common that they lack a clear and consistent definition in the classic epidemiological literature (Schünemann et al 2013). However, all of the terms describe one overarching theme: whether or not available research evidence can be directly used to answer the health and healthcare question at hand, ideally supported by a judgement about the degree of confidence in this use (Schünemann et al 2013). GRADE's certainty domains include a judgement about 'indirectness' to describe all of these aspects including the concept of direct versus indirect comparisons of different interventions (Atkins et al 2004, Guyatt et al 2008, Guyatt et al 2011b).

To address adequately the extent to which a review is relevant for the purpose to which it is being put, there are certain things the review author must do, and certain things the user of the review must do to assess the degree of indirectness. Cochrane and the GRADE Working Group suggest using a very structured framework to address indirectness. We discuss here and in Chapter 14 what the review author can do to help the user. Cochrane Review authors must be extremely clear on the population, intervention and outcomes that they intend to address. Chapter 14 (Section 14.1.2) also emphasizes a crucial step: the specification of all patient-important outcomes relevant to the intervention strategies under comparison.

In considering whether the effect of an intervention applies equally to all participants, and whether different variations on the intervention have similar effects, review authors need to make a priori hypotheses about possible effect modifiers, and then examine those hypotheses (see Chapter 10, Sections 10.10 and 10.11). If they find apparent subgroup effects, they must ultimately decide whether or not these effects are credible (Sun et al 2012). Differences between subgroups, particularly those that correspond to differences between studies, should be interpreted cautiously. Some chance variation between subgroups is inevitable so, unless there is good reason to believe that there is an interaction, review authors should not assume that the subgroup effect exists. If, despite due caution, review authors judge subgroup effects in terms of relative effect estimates as credible (i.e. the effects differ credibly), they should conduct separate meta-analyses for the relevant subgroups, and produce separate 'Summary of findings' tables for those subgroups.

The user of the review will be challenged with 'individualization' of the findings, whether they seek to apply the findings to an individual patient or a policy decision in a specific context. For example, even if relative effects are similar across subgroups, absolute effects will differ according to baseline risk. Review authors can help provide this information by identifying identifiable groups of people with varying baseline risks in the 'Summary of findings' tables, as discussed in Chapter 14 (Section 14.1.3). Users can then identify their specific case or population as belonging to a particular risk group, if relevant, and assess their likely magnitude of benefit or harm accordingly. A description of the identifying prognostic or baseline risk factors in a brief scenario (e.g. age or gender) will help users of a review further.

Another decision users must make is whether their individual case or population of interest is so different from those included in the studies that they cannot use the results of the systematic review and meta-analysis at all. Rather than rigidly applying the inclusion and exclusion criteria of studies, it is better to ask whether or not there are compelling reasons why the evidence should not be applied to a particular patient. Review authors can sometimes help decision makers by identifying important variation where divergence might limit the applicability of results (Rothwell 2005, Schünemann et al 2006, Guyatt et al 2011b, Schünemann et al 2013), including biologic and cultural variation, and variation in adherence to an intervention.

In addressing these issues, review authors cannot be aware of, or address, the myriad of differences in circumstances around the world. They can, however, address differences of known importance to many people and, importantly, they should avoid assuming that other people's circumstances are the same as their own in discussing the results and drawing conclusions.

15.2.2 Biological variation

Issues of biological variation that may affect the applicability of a result to a reader or population include divergence in pathophysiology (e.g. biological differences between women and men that may affect responsiveness to an intervention) and divergence in a causative agent (e.g. for infectious diseases such as malaria, which may be caused by several different parasites). The discussion of the results in the review should make clear whether the included studies addressed all or only some of these groups, and whether any important subgroup effects were found.

15.2.3 Variation in context

Some interventions, particularly non-pharmacological interventions, may work in some contexts but not in others; the situation has been described as program by context interaction (Hawe et al 2004). Contextual factors might pertain to the host organization in which an intervention is offered, such as the expertise, experience and morale of the staff expected to carry out the intervention, the competing priorities for the clinician's or staff's attention, the local resources such as service and facilities made available to the program and the status or importance given to the program by the host organization. Broader context issues might include aspects of the system within which the host organization operates, such as the fee or payment structure for healthcare providers and the local insurance system. Some interventions, in particular complex interventions (see Chapter 17), can be only partially implemented in some contexts, and this requires judgements about indirectness of the intervention and its components for readers in that context (Schünemann 2013).

Contextual factors may also pertain to the characteristics of the target group or population, such as cultural and linguistic diversity, socio-economic position, rural/urban setting. These factors may mean that a particular style of care or relationship evolves between service providers and consumers that may or may not match the values and technology of the program.

For many years these aspects have been acknowledged when decision makers have argued that results of evidence reviews from other countries do not apply in their own country or setting. Whilst some programmes/interventions have been successfully transferred from one context to another, others have not (Resnicow et al 1993, Lumley et al 2004, Coleman et al 2015). Review authors should be cautious when making generalizations from one context to another. They should report on the presence (or otherwise) of context-related information in intervention studies, where this information is available.

15.2.4 Variation in adherence

Variation in the adherence of the recipients and providers of care can limit the certainty in the applicability of results. Predictable differences in adherence can be due to divergence in how recipients of care perceive the intervention (e.g. the importance of side effects), economic conditions or attitudes that make some forms of care inaccessible in some settings, such as in low-income countries (Dans et al 2007). It should not be assumed that high levels of adherence in closely monitored randomized trials will translate into similar levels of adherence in normal practice.

15.2.5 Variation in values and preferences

Decisions about healthcare management strategies and options involve trading off health benefits and harms. The right choice may differ for people with different values and preferences (i.e. the importance people place on the outcomes and interventions), and it is important that decision makers ensure that decisions are consistent with a patient or population's values and preferences. The importance placed on outcomes, together with other factors, will influence whether the recipients of care will or will not accept an option that is offered (Alonso-Coello et al 2016) and, thus, can be one factor influencing adherence. In Section 15.6, we describe how the review author can help this process and the limits of supporting decision making based on intervention reviews.

15.3 Interpreting results of statistical analyses

15.3.1 Confidence intervals

Results for both individual studies and meta-analyses are reported with a point estimate together with an associated confidence interval. For example, 'The odds ratio was 0.75 with a 95% confidence interval of 0.70 to 0.80'. The point estimate (0.75) is the best estimate of the magnitude and direction of the experimental intervention's effect compared with the comparator intervention. The confidence interval describes the uncertainty inherent in any estimate, and describes a range of values within which we can be reasonably sure that the true effect actually lies. If the confidence interval is relatively narrow (e.g. 0.70 to 0.80), the effect size is known precisely. If the interval is wider (e.g. 0.60 to 0.93) the uncertainty is greater, although there may still be enough precision to make decisions about the utility of the intervention. Intervals that are very wide (e.g. 0.50 to 1.10) indicate that we have little knowledge about the effect and this imprecision affects our certainty in the evidence, and that further information would be needed before we could draw a more certain conclusion.

A 95% confidence interval is often interpreted as indicating a range within which we can be 95% certain that the true effect lies. This statement is a loose interpretation, but is useful as a rough guide. The strictly correct interpretation of a confidence interval is based on the hypothetical notion of considering the results that would be obtained if the study were repeated many times. If a study were repeated infinitely often, and on each occasion a 95% confidence interval calculated, then 95% of these intervals would contain the true effect (see Section 15.3.3 for further explanation).

The width of the confidence interval for an individual study depends to a large extent on the sample size. Larger studies tend to give more precise estimates of effects (and hence have narrower confidence intervals) than smaller studies. For continuous outcomes, precision depends also on the variability in the outcome measurements (i.e. how widely individual results vary between people in the study, measured as the standard deviation); for dichotomous outcomes it depends on the risk of the event (more frequent events allow more precision, and narrower confidence intervals), and for time-to-event outcomes it also depends on the number of events observed. All these quantities are used in computation of the standard errors of effect estimates from which the confidence interval is derived.

The width of a confidence interval for a meta-analysis depends on the precision of the individual study estimates and on the number of studies combined. In addition, for random-effects models, precision will decrease with increasing heterogeneity and confidence intervals will widen correspondingly (see Chapter 10, Section 10.10.4). As more studies are added to a meta-analysis the width of the confidence interval usually decreases. However, if the additional studies increase the heterogeneity in the meta-analysis and a random-effects model is used, it is possible that the confidence interval width will increase.

Confidence intervals and point estimates have different interpretations in fixed-effect and random-effects models. While the fixed-effect estimate and its confidence interval address the question 'what is the best (single) estimate of the effect?', the random-effects estimate assumes there to be a distribution of effects, and the estimate and its confidence interval address the question 'what is the best estimate of the average effect?' A confidence interval may be reported for any level of confidence (although they are most commonly reported for 95%, and sometimes 90% or 99%). For example, the odds ratio of 0.80 could be reported with an 80% confidence interval of 0.73 to 0.88; a 90% interval of 0.72 to 0.89; and a 95% interval of 0.70 to 0.92. As the confidence level increases, the confidence interval widens.

There is logical correspondence between the confidence interval and the P value (see Section 15.3.3). The 95% confidence interval for an effect will exclude the null value (such as an odds ratio of 1.0 or a risk difference of 0) if and only if the test of significance yields a P value of less than 0.05. If the P value is exactly 0.05, then either the upper or lower limit of the 95% confidence interval will be at the null value. Similarly, the 99% confidence interval will exclude the null if and only if the test of significance yields a P value of less than 0.01.

Together, the point estimate and confidence interval provide information to assess the effects of the intervention on the outcome. For example, suppose that we are evaluating an intervention that reduces the risk of an event and we decide that it would be useful only if it reduced the risk of an event from 30% by at least 5 percentage points to 25% (these values will depend on the specific clinical scenario and outcomes, including the anticipated harms). If the meta-analysis yielded an effect estimate of a reduction of 10 percentage points with a tight 95% confidence interval, say, from 7% to 13%, we would be able to conclude that the intervention was useful since both the point estimate and the entire range of the interval exceed our criterion of a reduction of 5% for net health benefit. However, if the meta-analysis reported the same risk reduction of 10% but with a wider interval, say, from 2% to 18%, although we would still conclude that our best estimate of the intervention effect is that it provides net benefit, we could not be so confident as we still entertain the possibility that the effect could be between 2% and 5%. If the confidence interval was wider still, and included the null value of a difference of 0%, we would still consider the possibility that the intervention has no effect on the outcome whatsoever, and would need to be even more sceptical in our conclusions.

Review authors may use the same general approach to conclude that an intervention is *not* useful. Continuing with the above example where the criterion for an important difference that should be achieved to provide more benefit than harm is a 5% risk difference, an effect estimate of 2% with a 95% confidence interval of 1% to 4% suggests that the intervention does not provide net health benefit.

15.3.2 P values and statistical significance

A P value is the standard result of a statistical test, and is the probability of obtaining the observed effect (or larger) under a 'null hypothesis'. In the context of Cochrane Reviews there are two commonly used statistical tests. The first is a test of overall effect (a Z-test), and its null hypothesis is that there is no overall effect of the experimental intervention compared with the comparator on the outcome of interest. The second is the (Chi^2) test for heterogeneity, and its null hypothesis is that there are no differences in the intervention effects across studies.

A P value that is very small indicates that the observed effect is very unlikely to have arisen purely by chance, and therefore provides evidence against the null hypothesis. It has been common practice to interpret a P value by examining whether it is smaller than particular threshold values. In particular, P values less than 0.05 are often reported as 'statistically significant', and interpreted as being small enough to justify rejection of the null hypothesis. However, the 0.05 threshold is an arbitrary one that became commonly used in medical and psychological research largely because P values were determined by comparing the test statistic against tabulations of specific percentage points of statistical distributions. If review authors decide to present a P value with the results of a meta-analysis, they should report a precise P value (as calculated by most statistical software), together with the 95% confidence interval. **Review authors should not describe results as 'statistically significant', 'not statistically significant' or 'non-significant' or unduly rely on thresholds for P values**, but report the confidence interval together with the exact P value (see MECIR Box 15.3.a).

We discuss interpretation of the test for heterogeneity in Chapter 10 (Section 10.10.2); the remainder of this section refers mainly to tests for an overall effect. For tests of an overall effect, the computation of P involves both the effect estimate and precision of the effect estimate (driven largely by sample size). As precision increases, the range of plausible effects that could occur by chance is reduced. Correspondingly, the statistical significance of an effect of a particular magnitude will usually be greater (the P value will be smaller) in a larger study than in a smaller study.

P values are commonly misinterpreted in two ways. First, a moderate or large P value (e.g. greater than 0.05) may be misinterpreted as evidence that the intervention has no effect on the outcome. There is an important difference between this statement and the correct interpretation that there is a high probability that the observed effect on the outcome is due to chance alone. To avoid such a misinterpretation, review authors should always examine the effect estimate and its 95% confidence interval.

The second misinterpretation is to assume that a result with a small P value for the summary effect estimate implies that an experimental intervention has an important benefit. Such a misinterpretation is more likely to occur in large studies and meta-analyses that accumulate data over dozens of studies and thousands of participants. The P value addresses the question of whether the experimental intervention effect is precisely nil; it does not examine whether the effect is of a magnitude of importance to potential recipients of the intervention. In a large study, a small P value may represent the detection of a trivial effect that may not lead to net health benefit when compared with the potential harms (i.e. harmful effects on other important outcomes). Again, inspection of the point estimate and confidence interval helps correct interpretations (see Section 15.3.1).

MECIR Box 15.3.a Relevant expectations for conduct of intervention reviews	
C72: Interpreting results (**Mandatory**)	
Do not describe results as statistically significant or non-significant. Interpret the confidence intervals and their width.	Authors commonly mistake a lack of evidence of effect as evidence of a lack of effect.

15.3.3 Relation between confidence intervals, statistical significance and certainty of evidence

The confidence interval (and imprecision) is only one domain that influences overall uncertainty about effect estimates. Uncertainty resulting from imprecision (i.e. statistical uncertainty) may be no less important than uncertainty from indirectness, or any other GRADE domain, in the context of decision making (Schünemann 2016). Thus, the extent to which interpretations of the confidence interval described in Sections 15.3.1 and 15.3.2 correspond to conclusions about overall certainty of the evidence for the outcome of interest depends on these other domains. If there are no concerns about other domains that determine the certainty of the evidence (i.e. risk of bias, inconsistency, indirectness or publication bias), then the interpretation in Sections 15.3.1 and 15.3.2. about the relation of the confidence interval to the true effect may be carried forward to the overall certainty. However, if there are concerns about the other domains that affect the certainty of the evidence, the interpretation about the true effect needs to be seen in the context of further uncertainty resulting from those concerns.

For example, nine randomized controlled trials in almost 6000 cancer patients indicated that the administration of heparin reduces the risk of venous thromboembolism (VTE), with a risk ratio of 43% (95% CI 19% to 60%) (Akl et al 2011a). For patients with a plausible baseline risk of approximately 4.6% per year, this relative effect suggests that heparin leads to an absolute risk reduction of 20 fewer VTEs (95% CI 9 fewer to 27 fewer) per 1000 people per year (Akl et al 2011a). Now consider that the review authors or those applying the evidence in a guideline have lowered the certainty in the evidence as a result of indirectness. While the confidence intervals would remain unchanged, the certainty in that confidence interval and in the point estimate as reflecting the truth for the question of interest will be lowered. In fact, the certainty range will have unknown width so there will be unknown likelihood of a result within that range because of this indirectness. The lower the certainty in the evidence, the less we know about the width of the certainty range, although methods for quantifying risk of bias and understanding potential direction of bias may offer insight when lowered certainty is due to risk of bias. Nevertheless, decision makers must consider this uncertainty, and must do so in relation to the effect measure that is being evaluated (e.g. a relative or absolute measure). We will describe the impact on interpretations for dichotomous outcomes in Section 15.4.

15.4 Interpreting results from dichotomous outcomes (including numbers needed to treat)

15.4.1 Relative and absolute risk reductions

Clinicians may be more inclined to prescribe an intervention that reduces the relative risk of death by 25% than one that reduces the risk of death by 1 percentage point, although both presentations of the evidence may relate to the same benefit (i.e. a reduction in risk from 4% to 3%). The former refers to the *relative* reduction in risk and the latter to the *absolute* reduction in risk. As described in Chapter 6

(Section 6.4.1), there are several measures for comparing dichotomous outcomes in two groups. Meta-analyses are usually undertaken using risk ratios (RR), odds ratios (OR) or risk differences (RD), but there are several alternative ways of expressing results.

Relative risk reduction (RRR) is a convenient way of re-expressing a risk ratio as a percentage reduction:

$$\text{RRR} = 100\% \times (1 - \text{RR}).$$

For example, a risk ratio of 0.75 translates to a relative risk reduction of 25%, as in the example above.

The risk difference is often referred to as the **absolute risk reduction** (ARR) or absolute risk increase (ARI), and may be presented as a percentage (e.g. 1%), as a decimal (e.g. 0.01), or as account (e.g. 10 out of 1000). We consider different choices for presenting absolute effects in Section 15.4.3. We then describe computations for obtaining these numbers from the results of individual studies and of meta-analyses in Section 15.4.4.

15.4.2 Number needed to treat (NNT)

The **number needed to treat** (NNT) is a common alternative way of presenting information on the effect of an intervention. The NNT is defined as the expected number of people who need to receive the experimental rather than the comparator intervention for one additional person to either incur or avoid an event (depending on the direction of the result) in a given time frame. Thus, for example, an NNT of 10 can be interpreted as 'it is expected that one additional (or less) person will incur an event for every 10 participants receiving the experimental intervention rather than comparator over a given time frame'. It is important to be clear that:

1) since the NNT is derived from the risk difference, it is still a *comparative* measure of effect (experimental versus a specific comparator) and not a general property of a single intervention; and
2) the NNT gives an 'expected value'. For example, NNT = 10 does not imply that one additional event *will* occur in each and every group of 10 people.

NNTs can be computed for both beneficial and detrimental events, and for interventions that cause both improvements and deteriorations in outcomes. In all instances NNTs are expressed as positive whole numbers. Some authors use the term 'number needed to harm' (NNH) when an intervention leads to an adverse outcome, or a decrease in a positive outcome, rather than improvement. However, this phrase can be misleading (most notably, it can easily be read to imply the number of people who will experience a harmful outcome if given the intervention), and it is strongly recommended that 'number needed to harm' and 'NNH' are avoided. The preferred alternative is to use phrases such as 'number needed to treat for an additional beneficial outcome' (NNTB) and 'number needed to treat for an additional harmful outcome' (NNTH) to indicate direction of effect.

As NNTs refer to events, their interpretation needs to be worded carefully when the binary outcome is a dichotomization of a scale-based outcome. For example, if the outcome is pain measured on a 'none, mild, moderate or severe' scale it may have been dichotomized as 'none or mild' versus 'moderate or severe'. It would be inappropriate for an NNT from these data to be referred to as an 'NNT for pain'. It is an 'NNT for moderate or severe pain'.

We consider different choices for presenting absolute effects in Section 15.4.3. We then describe computations for obtaining these numbers from the results of individual studies and of meta-analyses in Section 15.4.4.

15.4.3 Expressing risk differences

Users of reviews are liable to be influenced by the choice of statistical presentations of the evidence. Hoffrage and colleagues suggest that physicians' inferences about statistical outcomes are more appropriate when they deal with 'natural frequencies' – whole numbers of people, both treated and untreated (e.g. treatment results in a drop from 20 out of 1000 to 10 out of 1000 women having breast cancer) – than when effects are presented as percentages (e.g. 1% absolute reduction in breast cancer risk) (Hoffrage et al 2000). Probabilities may be more difficult to understand than frequencies, particularly when events are rare. While standardization may be important in improving the presentation of research evidence (and participation in healthcare decisions), current evidence suggests that the presentation of natural frequencies for expressing differences in absolute risk is best understood by consumers of healthcare information (Akl et al 2011b). This evidence provides the rationale for presenting absolute risks in 'Summary of findings' tables as numbers of people with events per 1000 people receiving the intervention (see Chapter 14).

RRs and RRRs remain crucial because relative effects tend to be substantially more stable across risk groups than absolute effects (see Chapter 10, Section 10.4.3). Review authors can use their own data to study this consistency (Cates 1999, Smeeth et al 1999). Risk differences from studies are least likely to be consistent across baseline event rates; thus, they are rarely appropriate for computing numbers needed to treat in systematic reviews. If a relative effect measure (OR or RR) is chosen for meta-analysis, then a comparator group risk needs to be specified as part of the calculation of an RD or NNT. In addition, if there are several different groups of participants with different levels of risk, it is crucial to express absolute benefit for each clinically identifiable risk group, clarifying the time period to which this applies. Studies in patients with differing severity of disease, or studies with different lengths of follow-up will almost certainly have different comparator group risks. In these cases, different comparator group risks lead to different RDs and NNTs (except when the intervention has no effect). A recommended approach is to re-express an odds ratio or a risk ratio as a variety of RD or NNTs across a range of assumed comparator risks (ACRs) (McQuay and Moore 1997, Smeeth et al 1999). Review authors should bear these considerations in mind not only when constructing their 'Summary of findings' table, but also in the text of their review.

For example, a review of oral anticoagulants to prevent stroke presented information to users by describing absolute benefits for various baseline risks (Aguilar and Hart 2005, Aguilar et al 2007). They presented their principal findings as "The inherent risk of stroke should be considered in the decision to use oral anticoagulants in atrial fibrillation patients, selecting those who stand to benefit most for this therapy" (Aguilar and

Hart 2005). Among high-risk atrial fibrillation patients with prior stroke or transient ischaemic attack who have stroke rates of about 12% (120 per 1000) per year, warfarin prevents about 70 strokes yearly per 1000 patients, whereas for low-risk atrial fibrillation patients (with a stroke rate of about 2% per year or 20 per 1000), warfarin prevents only 12 strokes. This presentation helps users to understand the important impact that typical baseline risks have on the absolute benefit that they can expect.

15.4.4 Computations

Direct computation of risk difference (RD) or a number needed to treat (NNT) depends on the summary statistic (odds ratio, risk ratio or risk differences) available from the study or meta-analysis. When expressing results of meta-analyses, review authors should use, in the computations, whatever statistic they determined to be the most appropriate summary for meta-analysis (see Chapter 10, Section 10.4.3). Here we present calculations to obtain RD as a reduction in the number of participants per 1000. For example, a risk difference of –0.133 corresponds to 133 *fewer* participants with the event per 1000.

RDs and NNTs should not be computed from the aggregated total numbers of participants and events across the trials. This approach ignores the randomization within studies, and may produce seriously misleading results if there is unbalanced randomization in any of the studies. Using the pooled result of a meta-analysis is more appropriate. When computing NNTs, the values obtained are by convention always rounded up to the next whole number.

15.4.4.1 Computing NNT from a risk difference (RD)

A NNT may be computed from a risk difference as

$$\text{NNT} = \frac{1}{\text{absolute value of risk difference}} = \frac{1}{|\text{RD}|},$$

where the vertical bars ('absolute value of') in the denominator indicate that any minus sign should be ignored. It is convention to round the NNT up to the nearest whole number. For example, if the risk difference is –0.12 the NNT is 9; if the risk difference is –0.22 the NNT is 5. Cochrane Review authors should qualify the NNT as referring to benefit (improvement) or harm by denoting the NNT as NNTB or NNTH. Note that this approach, although feasible, should be used only for the results of a meta-analysis of risk differences. In most cases meta-analyses will be undertaken using a relative measure of effect (RR or OR), and those statistics should be used to calculate the NNT (see Section 15.4.4.2 and 15.4.4.3).

15.4.4.2 Computing risk differences or NNT from a risk ratio

To aid interpretation of the results of a meta-analysis of risk ratios, review authors may compute an absolute risk reduction or NNT. In order to do this, an assumed comparator risk (ACR) (otherwise known as a baseline risk, or risk that the outcome of interest would occur with the comparator intervention) is required. It will usually be appropriate to do this for a range of different ACRs. The computation proceeds as follows:

$$\text{number fewer per 1000 (ARR)} = 1000 \times \text{ACR} \times (1 - \text{RR}),$$

$$\text{NNT} = \left| \frac{1}{\text{ACR} \times (1 - \text{RR})} \right|.$$

As an example, suppose the risk ratio is RR = 0.92, and an ACR = 0.3 (300 per 1000) is assumed. Then the effect on risk is 24 fewer per 1000:

$$\text{number fewer per 1000} = 1000 \times 0.3 \times (1 - 0.92) = 24.$$

The NNT is 42:

$$\text{NNT} = \left| \frac{1}{0.3 \times (1 - 0.92)} \right| = \left| \frac{1}{0.3 \times 0.08} \right| = 41.67.$$

15.4.4.3 Computing risk differences or NNT from an odds ratio

Review authors may wish to compute a risk difference or NNT from the results of a meta-analysis of odds ratios. In order to do this, an ACR is required. It will usually be appropriate to do this for a range of different ACRs. The computation proceeds as follows:

$$\text{number fewer per 1000} = 1000 \times \left(\text{ACR} - \frac{\text{OR} \times \text{ACR}}{1 - \text{ACR} + \text{OR} \times \text{ACR}} \right)$$

$$\text{NNT} = \frac{1}{\left| \left(\text{ACR} - \frac{\text{OR} \times \text{ACR}}{1 - \text{ACR} + \text{OR} \times \text{ACR}} \right) \right|}.$$

As an example, suppose the odds ratio is OR = 0.73, and a comparator risk of ACR = 0.3 is assumed. Then the effect on risk is 62 fewer per 1000:

$$\begin{aligned} \text{number fewer per 1000} &= 1000 \times \left(0.3 - \frac{0.73 \times 0.3}{1 - 0.3 + 0.73 \times 0.3} \right) \\ &= 1000 \times \left(0.3 - \frac{0.219}{1 - 0.3 + 0.219} \right) \\ &= 1000 \times (0.3 - 0.238) = 61.7. \end{aligned}$$

The NNT is 17:

$$\begin{aligned} \text{NNT} &= \frac{1}{\left| \left(0.3 - \frac{0.73 \times 0.3}{1 - 0.3 + 0.73 \times 0.3} \right) \right|} \\ &= \frac{1}{\left| \left(0.3 - \frac{0.219}{1 - 0.3 + 0.219} \right) \right|} \\ &= \frac{1}{|0.3 - 0.238|} = 16.2. \end{aligned}$$

15.4.4.4 Computing risk ratio from an odds ratio

Because risk ratios are easier to interpret than odds ratios, but odds ratios have favourable mathematical properties, a review author may decide to undertake a meta-analysis based on odds ratios, but to express the result as a summary risk ratio (or relative risk reduction). This requires an ACR. Then

$$\mathrm{RR} = \frac{\mathrm{OR}}{1 - \mathrm{ACR} \times (1 - \mathrm{OR})}.$$

It will often be reasonable to perform this transformation using the median comparator group risk from the studies in the meta-analysis.

15.4.4.5 Computing confidence limits

Confidence limits for RDs and NNTs may be calculated by applying the above formulae to the upper and lower confidence limits for the summary statistic (RD, RR or OR) (Altman 1998). Note that this confidence interval does not incorporate uncertainty around the ACR.

If the 95% confidence interval of OR or RR includes the value 1, one of the confidence limits will indicate benefit and the other harm. Thus, appropriate use of the words 'fewer' and 'more' is required for each limit when presenting results in terms of events. For NNTs, the two confidence limits should be labelled as NNTB and NNTH to indicate the direction of effect in each case. The confidence interval for the NNT will include a 'discontinuity', because increasingly smaller risk differences that approach zero will lead to NNTs approaching infinity. Thus, the confidence interval will include both an infinitely large NNTB and an infinitely large NNTH.

15.5 Interpreting results from continuous outcomes (including standardized mean differences)

15.5.1 Meta-analyses with continuous outcomes

Review authors should describe in the study protocol how they plan to interpret results for continuous outcomes. When outcomes are continuous, review authors have a number of options to present summary results. These options differ if studies report the same measure that is familiar to the target audiences, studies report the same or very similar measures that are less familiar to the target audiences, or studies report different measures.

15.5.2 Meta-analyses with continuous outcomes using the same measure

If all studies have used the same familiar units, for instance, results are expressed as durations of events, such as symptoms for conditions including diarrhoea, sore throat, otitis media, influenza or duration of hospitalization, a meta-analysis may generate a summary estimate in those units, as a difference in mean response (see, for instance, the row summarizing results for duration of diarrhoea in Chapter 14, Figure 14.1.b and the row summarizing oedema in Chapter 14, Figure 14.1.a). For such outcomes, the 'Summary of findings' table should include a difference of means between the two interventions. However, when units of such outcomes may be difficult to interpret, particularly when they relate to rating scales (again, see the oedema row of Chapter 14, Figure 14.1.a). 'Summary of findings' tables should include the minimum and maximum of the scale of measurement, and the direction. Knowledge of the smallest change in instrument score that patients perceive is important – the minimal important difference (MID) – and can greatly facilitate the interpretation of results (Guyatt et al 1998, Schünemann and Guyatt 2005). Knowing the MID allows review authors and users to place results in context. Review authors should state the MID – if known – in the Comments column of their 'Summary of findings' table. For example, the chronic respiratory questionnaire has possible scores in health-related quality of life ranging from 1 to 7 and 0.5 represents a well-established MID (Jaeschke et al 1989, Schünemann et al 2005).

15.5.3 Meta-analyses with continuous outcomes using different measures

When studies have used different instruments to measure the same construct, a standardized mean difference (SMD) may be used in meta-analysis for combining continuous data. Without guidance, clinicians and patients may have little idea how to interpret results presented as SMDs. Review authors should therefore consider issues of interpretability when planning their analysis at the protocol stage and should consider whether there will be suitable ways to re-express the SMD or whether alternative effect measures, such as a ratio of means, or possibly as minimal important difference units (Guyatt et al 2013b) should be used. Table 15.5.a and the following sections describe these options.

Table 15.5.a Approaches and their implications to presenting results of continuous variables when primary studies have used different instruments to measure the same construct. Adapted from Guyatt et al (2013b)

Approach	Observations about using the approach	Recommendation
Options for interpreting SMDs		
1a. Generic standard deviation (SD) units and guiding rules	It is widely used, but the interpretation is challenging. It can be misleading depending on whether the population is very homogenous or heterogeneous (i.e. how variable the outcome was in the population of each included study, and therefore how applicable a standard SD is likely to be). See Section 15.5.3.1.	Use together with other approaches below.
1b. Re-express and present as units of a familiar measure	Presenting data with this approach may be viewed by users as closer to the primary data. However, few	When the units and measures are familiar to the decision makers (e.g. healthcare providers and patients),

(Continued)

Table 15.5.a (Continued)

Approach	Observations about using the approach	Recommendation
	instruments are sufficiently used in clinical practice to make many of the presented units easily interpretable. See Section 15.5.3.2.	this presentation should be seriously considered. *Note:* Conversion to natural units is also an option for expressing results using the MID approach below (row 3).
1c. Re-express as result for a dichotomous outcome	Dichotomous outcomes are very familiar to clinical audiences and may facilitate understanding. However, this approach involves assumptions that may not always be valid (e.g. it assumes that distributions in intervention and comparator group are roughly normally distributed and variances are similar). It allows applying GRADE guidance for large and very large effects. See Section 15.5.3.3.	Consider this approach if the assumptions appear reasonable. If the minimal important difference for an instrument is known describing the probability of individuals achieving this difference may be more intuitive. Review authors should always seriously consider this option. *Note:* Re-expressing SMDs is not the only way of expressing results as dichotomous outcomes. For example, the actual outcomes in the studies can be dichotomized, either directly or using assumptions, prior to meta-analysis.
Options based on other effect measures		
2. Ratio of means	This approach may be easily interpretable to clinical audiences and involves fewer assumptions than some other approaches. It allows applying GRADE guidance for large and very large effects. It cannot be applied when measure is a change from baseline and therefore negative values possible and the interpretation requires knowledge and interpretation of comparator group mean. See Section 15.5.3.4	Consider as complementing other approaches, particularly the presentation of relative and absolute effects.
3. Minimal important difference units	This approach may be easily interpretable for audiences but is applicable only when minimal important differences are known. See Section 15.5.3.5.	Consider as complementing other approaches, particularly the presentation of relative and absolute effects.

15.5.3.1 Presenting and interpreting SMDs using generic effect size estimates

The SMD expresses the intervention effect in standard units rather than the original units of measurement. The SMD is the difference in mean effects between the experimental and comparator groups divided by the pooled standard deviation of participants' outcomes, or external SDs when studies are very small (see Chapter 6,

Section 6.5.1.2). The value of a SMD thus depends on both the size of the effect (the difference between means) and the standard deviation of the outcomes (the inherent variability among participants or based on an external SD).

If review authors use the SMD, they might choose to present the results directly as SMDs (row 1a, Table 15.5.a and Table 15.5.b). However, absolute values of the intervention and comparison groups are typically not useful because studies have used different measurement instruments with different units. Guiding rules for interpreting SMDs (or 'Cohen's effect sizes') exist, and have arisen mainly from researchers in the social sciences (Cohen 1988). One example is as follows: 0.2 represents a small effect, 0.5 a moderate effect and 0.8 a large effect (Cohen 1988). Variations exist (e.g. < 0.40 = small, 0.40 to 0.70 = moderate, > 0.70 = large). Review authors might consider including such a guiding rule in interpreting the SMD in the text of the review, and in summary versions such as the Comments column of a 'Summary of findings' table. However, some methodologists believe that such interpretations are problematic because *patient* importance of a finding is context-dependent and not amenable to generic statements.

15.5.3.2 Re-expressing SMDs using a familiar instrument

The second possibility for interpreting the SMD is to express it in the units of one or more of the specific measurement instruments used by the included studies (row 1b, Table 15.5.a and Table 15.5.b). The approach is to calculate an absolute difference in means by multiplying the SMD by an estimate of the SD associated with the most familiar instrument. To obtain this SD, a reasonable option is to calculate a weighted average across all intervention groups of all studies that used the selected instrument (preferably a pre-intervention or post-intervention SD as discussed in Chapter 10, Section 10.5.2). To better reflect among-person variation in practice, or to use an instrument not represented in the meta-analysis, it may be preferable to use a standard deviation from a representative observational study. The summary effect is thus re-expressed in the original units of that particular instrument and the clinical relevance and impact of the intervention effect can be interpreted using that familiar instrument.

The same approach of re-expressing the results for a familiar instrument can also be used for other standardized effect measures such as when standardizing by MIDs (Guyatt et al 2013b): see Section 15.5.3.5.

15.5.3.3 Re-expressing SMDs through dichotomization and transformation to relative and absolute measures

A third approach (row 1c, Table 15.5.a and Table 15.5.b) relies on converting the continuous measure into a dichotomy and thus allows calculation of relative and absolute effects on a binary scale. A transformation of a SMD to a (log) odds ratio is available, based on the assumption that an underlying continuous variable has a logistic distribution with equal standard deviation in the two intervention groups, as discussed in Chapter 10 (Section 10.6) (Furukawa 1999, Guyatt et al 2013b). The assumption is unlikely to hold exactly and the results must be regarded as an approximation. The log odds ratio is estimated as

$$\ln(\mathrm{OR}) = \frac{\pi}{\sqrt{3}}\mathrm{SMD},$$

Table 15.5.b Application of approaches when studies have used different measures: effects of dexamethasone for pain after laparoscopic cholecystectomy (Karanicolas et al 2008). Reproduced with permission of Wolters Kluwer

Options for presenting information about the outcome post-operative pain and suggested description of the measure	Estimated risk or estimated score/ value with placebo	Risk difference or relative reduction in score/value with dexamethasone	Relative effect (95% CI)	Number of participants (studies)	Certainty of evidence[1]	Comments
1a. Post-operative pain, standard deviation units Investigators measured pain using different instruments. Lower scores mean less pain.	The pain score in the dexamethasone groups was on average **0.79 SDs (1.41 to 0.17) lower** than in the placebo groups).		–	539 (5)	⊕⊕OO[2,3] Low	As a rule of thumb, 0.2 SD represents a small difference, 0.5 a moderate and 0.8 a large.
1b. Post-operative pain Measured on a scale from 0, no pain, to 100, worst pain imaginable.	The mean post-operative pain scores with placebo ranged from 43 to 54.	The mean pain score in the intervention groups was on average **8.1 (1.8 to 14.5) lower.**	–	539 (5)	⊕⊕OO Low[2,3]	Scores calculated based on an SMD of 0.79 (95% CI –1.41 to –0.17) and rescaled to a 0 to 100 pain scale. The minimal important difference on the 0 to 100 pain scale is approximately 10.
1c. Substantial post-operative pain, dichotomized Investigators measured pain using different instruments.	20 per 100[4]	15 more (4 more to 18 more) per 100 patients in dexamethasone group achieved important improvement in the pain score.	RR = 0.25 (95% CI 0.05 to 0.75)	539 (5)	⊕⊕OO[2,3] Low	Scores estimated based on an SMD of 0.79 (95% CI –1.41 to –0.17).
2. Post-operative pain Investigators measured pain using different instruments. Lower scores mean less pain.	The mean post-operative pain scores with placebo was 28.1.[5]	On average a 3.7 lower pain score (0.6 to 6.1 lower)	Ratio of means 0.87 (0.78 to 0.98)	539 (5)	⊕⊕OO[2,3] Low	Weighted average of the mean pain score in dexamethasone group divided by mean pain score in placebo.
3. Post-operative pain Investigators measured pain using different instruments.	The pain score in the dexamethasone groups was on average **0.40 (95% CI 0.74 to 0.07) minimal important difference units** less than the control group.		–	539 (5)	⊕⊕OO[2,3] Low	An effect less than half the minimal important difference suggests a small or very small effect.

[1] Certainty rated according to GRADE from very low to high certainty.
[2] Substantial unexplained heterogeneity in study results.
[3] Imprecision due to wide confidence intervals.
[4] The 20% comes from the proportion in the control group requiring rescue analgesia.
[5] Crude (arithmetic) means of the post-operative pain mean responses across all five trials when transformed to a 100-point scale.

Table 15.5.c Risk difference derived for specific SMDs for various given 'proportions improved' in the comparator group (Furukawa 1999, Guyatt et al 2013b). Reproduced with permission of Elsevier

Comparator group response proportion	**0.1**	**0.2**	**0.3**	**0.4**	**0.5**	**0.6**	**0.7**	**0.8**	**0.9**
Situations in which the event is undesirable, reduction (or increase if intervention harmful) in adverse events with the intervention									
SMD = −0.2	**−3%**	**−5%**	**−7%**	**−8%**	**−8%**	**−8%**	**−7%**	**−6%**	**−40%**
SMD = −0.5	**−6%**	**−11%**	**−15%**	**−17%**	**−19%**	**−20%**	**−20%**	**−17%**	**−12%**
SMD = −0.8	**−8%**	**−15%**	**−21%**	**−25%**	**−29%**	**−31%**	**−31%**	**−28%**	**−22%**
SMD = −1.0	**−9%**	**−17%**	**−24%**	**−23%**	**−34%**	**−37%**	**−38%**	**−36%**	**−29%**
Situations in which the event is desirable, increase (or decrease if intervention harmful) in positive responses to the intervention									
SMD = 0.2	**4%**	**61%**	**7%**	**8%**	**8%**	**8%**	**7%**	**5%**	**3%**
SMD = 0.5	**12%**	**17%**	**19%**	**20%**	**19%**	**17%**	**15%**	**11%**	**6%**
SMD = 0.8	**22%**	**28%**	**31%**	**31%**	**29%**	**25%**	**21%**	**15%**	**8%**
SMD = 1.0	**29%**	**36%**	**38%**	**38%**	**34%**	**30%**	**24%**	**17%**	**9%**

(or approximately 1.81 × SMD). The resulting odds ratio can then be presented as normal, and in a 'Summary of findings' table, combined with an assumed comparator group risk to be expressed as an absolute risk difference. The comparator group risk in this case would refer to the proportion of people who have achieved a specific value of the continuous outcome. In randomized trials this can be interpreted as the proportion who have improved by some (specified) amount (responders), for instance by 5 points on a 0 to 100 scale. Table 15.5.c shows some illustrative results from this method. The risk differences can then be converted to NNTs or to people per thousand using methods described in Section 15.4.4.

15.5.3.4 Ratio of means

A more frequently used approach is based on calculation of a ratio of means between the intervention and comparator groups (Friedrich et al 2008) as discussed in Chapter 6 (Section 6.5.1.3). Interpretational advantages of this approach include the ability to pool studies with outcomes expressed in different units directly, to avoid the vulnerability of heterogeneous populations that limits approaches that rely on SD units, and for ease of clinical interpretation (row 2, Table 15.5.a and Table 15.5.b). This method is currently designed for post-intervention scores only. However, it is possible to calculate a ratio of change scores if both intervention and comparator groups change in the same direction in each relevant study, and this ratio may sometimes be informative.

Limitations to this approach include its limited applicability to change scores (since it is unlikely that both intervention and comparator group changes are in the same direction in all studies) and the possibility of misleading results if the comparator group mean is very small, in which case even a modest difference from the intervention group will yield a large and therefore misleading ratio of means. It also requires that separate ratios of means be calculated for each included study, and then entered into a generic inverse variance meta-analysis (see Chapter 10, Section 10.3).

The ratio of means approach illustrated in Table 15.5.b suggests a relative reduction in pain of only 13%, meaning that those receiving steroids have a pain severity 87% of those in the comparator group, an effect that might be considered modest.

15.5.3.5 Presenting continuous results as minimally important difference units

To express results in MID units, review authors have two options. First, they can be combined across studies in the same way as the SMD, but instead of dividing the mean difference of each study by its SD, review authors divide by the MID associated with that outcome (Johnston et al 2010, Guyatt et al 2013b). Instead of SD units, the pooled results represent MID units (row 3, Table 15.5.a and Table 15.5.b), and may be more easily interpretable. This approach avoids the problem of varying SDs across studies that may distort estimates of effect in approaches that rely on the SMD. The approach, however, relies on having well-established MIDs. The approach is also risky in that a difference less than the MID may be interpreted as trivial when a substantial proportion of patients may have achieved an important benefit.

The other approach makes a simple conversion (not shown in Table 15.5.b), before undertaking the meta-analysis, of the means and SDs from each study to means and SDs on the scale of a particular familiar instrument whose MID is known. For example, one can rescale the mean and SD of other chronic respiratory disease instruments (e.g. rescaling a 0 to 100 score of an instrument) to a the 1 to 7 score in Chronic Respiratory Disease Questionnaire (CRQ) units (by assuming 0 equals 1 and 100 equals 7 on the CRQ). Given the MID of the CRQ of 0.5, a mean difference in change of 0.71 after rescaling of all studies suggests a substantial effect of the intervention (Guyatt et al 2013b). This approach, presenting in units of the most familiar instrument, may be the most desirable when the target audiences have extensive experience with that instrument, particularly if the MID is well established.

15.6 Drawing conclusions

15.6.1 Conclusions sections of a Cochrane Review

Authors' conclusions in a Cochrane Review are divided into implications for practice and implications for research. While Cochrane Reviews about interventions can provide meaningful information and guidance for practice, decisions about the desirable and undesirable consequences of healthcare options require evidence and judgements for criteria that most Cochrane Reviews do not provide (Alonso-Coello et al 2016). In describing the implications for practice and the development of recommendations, however, review authors may consider the certainty of the evidence, the balance of benefits and harms, and assumed values and preferences.

15.6.2 Implications for practice

Drawing conclusions about the practical usefulness of an intervention entails making trade-offs, either implicitly or explicitly, between the estimated benefits, harms and the values and preferences. Making such trade-offs, and thus making specific recommendations for an action in a specific context, goes beyond a Cochrane Review and requires additional evidence and informed judgements that most Cochrane Reviews do not provide (Alonso-Coello et al 2016). Such judgements are typically the domain of clinical practice guideline developers for which Cochrane Reviews will provide crucial information (Graham et al 2011, Schünemann et al 2014, Zhang et al 2018a). Thus, authors of Cochrane Reviews should not make recommendations.

If review authors feel compelled to lay out actions that clinicians and patients could take, they should – after describing the certainty of evidence and the balance of benefits and harms – highlight different actions that might be consistent with particular patterns of values and preferences. Other factors that might influence a decision should also be highlighted, including any known factors that would be expected to modify the effects of the intervention, the baseline risk or status of the patient, costs and who bears those costs, and the availability of resources. Review authors should ensure they consider all patient-important outcomes, including those for which limited data may be available. In the context of public health reviews the focus may be on population-important outcomes as the target may be an entire (non-diseased) population and include outcomes that are not measured in the population receiving an intervention (e.g. a reduction of transmission of infections from those receiving an intervention). This process implies a high level of explicitness in judgements about values or preferences attached to different outcomes and the certainty of the related evidence (Zhang et al 2018b, Zhang et al 2018c); this and a full cost-effectiveness analysis is beyond the scope of most Cochrane Reviews (although they might well be used for such analyses; see Chapter 20).

A review on the use of anticoagulation in cancer patients to increase survival (Akl et al 2011a) provides an example for laying out clinical implications for situations where there are important trade-offs between desirable and undesirable effects of the intervention: "The decision for a patient with cancer to start heparin therapy for survival benefit should balance the benefits and downsides and integrate the patient's values and preferences. Patients with a high preference for a potential survival prolongation, limited aversion to potential bleeding, and who do not consider heparin (both UFH or LMWH) therapy a burden may opt to use heparin, while those with aversion to bleeding may not."

15.6.3 Implications for research

The second category for authors' conclusions in a Cochrane Review is implications for research. To help people make well-informed decisions about future healthcare research, the 'Implications for research' section should comment on the need for further research, and the nature of the further research that would be most desirable. It is helpful to consider the population, intervention, comparison and outcomes that could be addressed, or addressed more effectively in the future, in the context of the certainty of the evidence in the current review (Brown et al 2006):

- P (Population): diagnosis, disease stage, comorbidity, risk factor, sex, age, ethnic group, specific inclusion or exclusion criteria, clinical setting;
- I (Intervention): type, frequency, dose, duration, prognostic factor;
- C (Comparison): placebo, routine care, alternative treatment/management;
- O (Outcome): which clinical or patient-related outcomes will the researcher need to measure, improve, influence or accomplish? Which methods of measurement should be used?

While Cochrane Review authors will find the PICO domains helpful, the domains of the GRADE certainty framework further support understanding and describing what additional research will improve the certainty in the available evidence. Note that as the certainty of the evidence is likely to vary by outcome, these implications will be specific to certain outcomes in the review. Table 15.6.a shows how review authors may be aided in their interpretation of the body of evidence and drawing conclusions about future research and practice.

The review of compression stockings for prevention of deep vein thrombosis (DVT) in airline passengers described in Chapter 14 provides an example where there is some convincing evidence of a benefit of the intervention: "This review shows that the question of the effects on symptomless DVT of wearing versus not wearing compression stockings in the types of people studied in these trials should now be regarded as answered. Further research may be justified to investigate the relative effects of different strengths of stockings or of stockings compared to other preventative strategies. Further randomised trials to address the remaining uncertainty about the effects of wearing versus not wearing compression stockings on outcomes such as death, pulmonary embolism and symptomatic DVT would need to be large." (Clarke et al 2016).

A review of therapeutic touch for anxiety disorder provides an example of the implications for research when no eligible studies had been found: "This review highlights the need for randomized controlled trials to evaluate the effectiveness of therapeutic touch in reducing anxiety symptoms in people diagnosed with anxiety disorders. Future trials need to be rigorous in design and delivery, with subsequent reporting to include high quality descriptions of all aspects of methodology to enable appraisal and interpretation of results." (Robinson et al 2007).

15.6.4 Reaching conclusions

A common mistake is to confuse 'no evidence of an effect' with 'evidence of no effect'. When the confidence intervals are too wide (e.g. including no effect), it is wrong to claim that the experimental intervention has 'no effect' or is 'no different' from the comparator intervention. Review authors may also incorrectly 'positively' frame results for some effects but not others. For example, when the effect estimate is positive for a beneficial outcome but confidence intervals are wide, review authors may describe the effect as promising. However, when the effect estimate is negative for an outcome that is considered harmful but the confidence intervals include no effect, review authors report no effect. Another mistake is to frame the conclusion in wishful terms. For example, review authors might write, "there were too few people in the analysis to detect a reduction in mortality" when the included studies showed a reduction or even increase in mortality that was not 'statistically significant'. One way of avoiding errors such as

Table 15.6.a Implications for research and practice suggested by individual GRADE domains

Domain	Implications for research	Examples for research statements	Implications for practice
Risk of bias	Need for methodologically better designed and executed studies.	All studies suffered from lack of blinding of outcome assessors. Trials of this type are required.	The estimates of effect may be biased because of a lack of blinding of the assessors of the outcome.
Inconsistency	Unexplained inconsistency: need for individual participant data meta-analysis; need for studies in relevant subgroups.	Studies in patients with small cell lung cancer are needed to understand if the effects differ from those in patients with pancreatic cancer.	Unexplained inconsistency: consider and interpret overall effect estimates as for the overall certainty of a body of evidence. Explained inconsistency (if results are not presented in strata): consider and interpret effects estimates by subgroup.
Indirectness	Need for studies that better fit the PICO question of interest.	Studies in patients with early cancer are needed because the evidence is from studies in patients with advanced cancer.	It is uncertain if the results directly apply to the patients or the way that the intervention is applied in a particular setting.
Imprecision	Need for more studies with more participants to reach optimal information size.	Studies with approximately 200 more events in the experimental intervention group and the comparator intervention group are required.	Same uncertainty interpretation as for certainty of a body of evidence: e.g. the true effect may be substantially different.
Publication bias	Need to investigate and identify unpublished data; large studies might help resolve this issue.	Large studies are required.	Same uncertainty interpretation as for certainty of a body of evidence (e.g. the true effect may be substantially different).
Large effects	No direct implications.	Not applicable.	The effect is large in the populations that were included in the studies and the true effect is likely going to cross important thresholds.
Dose effects	No direct implications.	Not applicable.	The greater the reduction in the exposure the larger is the expected harm (or benefit).
Opposing bias and confounding	Studies controlling for the residual bias and confounding are needed.	Studies controlling for possible confounders such as smoking and degree of education are required.	The effect could be even larger or smaller (depending on the direction of the results) than the one that is observed in the studies presented here.

these is to consider the results blinded; that is, consider how the results would be presented and framed in the conclusions if the direction of the results was reversed. If the confidence interval for the estimate of the difference in the effects of the interventions overlaps with no effect, the analysis is compatible with both a true beneficial effect and a true harmful effect. If one of the possibilities is mentioned in the conclusion, the other possibility should be mentioned as well. Table 15.6.b suggests narrative statements for drawing conclusions based on the effect estimate from the meta-analysis and the certainty of the evidence.

Table 15.6.b Suggested narrative statements for phrasing conclusions

Size of the effect estimate	**Suggested statements for conclusions** *(replace X with intervention, choose 'reduce' or 'increase' depending on the direction of the effect, replace 'outcome' with name of outcome, include 'when compared with Y' when needed)*
High certainty of the evidence	
Large effect	X results in a large reduction/increase in outcome
Moderate effect	X reduces/increases outcome X results in a reduction/increase in outcome
Small important effect	X reduces/increases outcome slightly X results in a slight reduction/increase in outcome
Trivial, small unimportant effect or no effect	X results in little to no difference in outcome X does not reduce/increase outcome
Moderate certainty of the evidence	
Large effect	X likely results in a large reduction/increase in outcome X probably results in a large reduction/increase in outcome
Moderate effect	X likely reduces/increases outcome X probably reduces/increases outcome X likely results in a reduction/increase in outcome X probably results in a reduction/increase in outcome
Small important effect	X probably reduces/increases outcome slightly X likely reduces/increases outcome slightly X probably results in a slight reduction/increase in outcome X likely results in a slight reduction/increase in outcome
Trivial, small unimportant effect or no effect	X likely results in little to no difference in outcome X probably results in little to no difference in outcome X likely does not reduce/increase outcome X probably does not reduce/increase outcome
Low certainty of the evidence	
Large effect	X may result in a large reduction/increase in outcome The evidence suggests X results in a large reduction/increase in outcome
Moderate effect	X may reduce/increase outcome The evidence suggests X reduces/increases outcome X may result in a reduction/increase in outcome The evidence suggests X results in a reduction/increase in outcome
Small important effect	X may reduce/increase outcome slightly The evidence suggests X reduces/increases outcome slightly X may result in a slight reduction/increase in outcome

Table 15.6.b (Continued)

Size of the effect estimate	**Suggested statements for conclusions** *(replace X with intervention, choose 'reduce' or 'increase' depending on the direction of the effect, replace 'outcome' with name of outcome, include 'when compared with Y' when needed)*
Trivial, small unimportant effect or no effect	The evidence suggests X results in a slight reduction/increase in outcome X may result in little to no difference in outcome The evidence suggests that X results in little to no difference in outcome X may not reduce/increase outcome The evidence suggests that X does not reduce/increase outcome
Very low certainty of the evidence	
Any effect	The evidence is very uncertain about the effect of X on outcome X may reduce/increase/have little to no effect on outcome but the evidence is very uncertain

Another common mistake is to reach conclusions that go beyond the evidence. Often this is done implicitly, without referring to the additional information or judgements that are used in reaching conclusions about the implications of a review for practice. Even when additional information and explicit judgements support conclusions about the implications of a review for practice, review authors rarely conduct systematic reviews of the additional information. Furthermore, implications for practice are often dependent on specific circumstances and values that must be taken into consideration. As we have noted, review authors should always be cautious when drawing conclusions about implications for practice and they should not make recommendations.

15.7 Chapter information

Authors: Holger J Schünemann, Gunn E Vist, Julian PT Higgins, Nancy Santesso, Jonathan J Deeks, Paul Glasziou, Elie Akl, Gordon H Guyatt; on behalf of the Cochrane GRADEing Methods Group

Acknowledgements: Andrew Oxman, Jonathan Sterne, Michael Borenstein and Rob Scholten contributed text to earlier versions of this chapter.

Funding: This work was in part supported by funding from the Michael G DeGroote Cochrane Canada Centre and the Ontario Ministry of Health. JJD receives support from the National Institute for Health Research (NIHR) Birmingham Biomedical Research Centre at the University Hospitals Birmingham NHS Foundation Trust and the University of Birmingham. JPTH receives support from the NIHR Biomedical Research Centre at University Hospitals Bristol NHS Foundation Trust and the University of Bristol. The views expressed are those of the author(s) and not necessarily those of the NHS, the NIHR or the Department of Health.

15.8 References

Aguilar MI, Hart R. Oral anticoagulants for preventing stroke in patients with non-valvular atrial fibrillation and no previous history of stroke or transient ischemic attacks. *Cochrane Database of Systematic Reviews* 2005; **3**: CD001927.

Aguilar MI, Hart R, Pearce LA. Oral anticoagulants versus antiplatelet therapy for preventing stroke in patients with non-valvular atrial fibrillation and no history of stroke or transient ischemic attacks. *Cochrane Database of Systematic Reviews* 2007; **3**: CD006186.

Akl EA, Gunukula S, Barba M, Yosuico VE, van Doormaal FF, Kuipers S, Middeldorp S, Dickinson HO, Bryant A, Schünemann H. Parenteral anticoagulation in patients with cancer who have no therapeutic or prophylactic indication for anticoagulation. *Cochrane Database of Systematic Reviews* 2011a; **1**: CD006652.

Akl EA, Oxman AD, Herrin J, Vist GE, Terrenato I, Sperati F, Costiniuk C, Blank D, Schünemann H. Using alternative statistical formats for presenting risks and risk reductions. *Cochrane Database of Systematic Reviews* 2011b; **3**: CD006776.

Alonso-Coello P, Schünemann HJ, Moberg J, Brignardello-Petersen R, Akl EA, Davoli M, Treweek S, Mustafa RA, Rada G, Rosenbaum S, Morelli A, Guyatt GH, Oxman AD, GRADE Working Group. GRADE Evidence to Decision (EtD) frameworks: a systematic and transparent approach to making well informed healthcare choices. 1: Introduction. *BMJ* 2016; **353**: i2016.

Altman DG. Confidence intervals for the number needed to treat. *BMJ* 1998; **317**: 1309–1312.

Atkins D, Best D, Briss PA, Eccles M, Falck-Ytter Y, Flottorp S, Guyatt GH, Harbour RT, Haugh MC, Henry D, Hill S, Jaeschke R, Leng G, Liberati A, Magrini N, Mason J, Middleton P, Mrukowicz J, O'Connell D, Oxman AD, Phillips B, Schünemann HJ, Edejer TT, Varonen H, Vist GE, Williams JW, Jr., Zaza S. Grading quality of evidence and strength of recommendations. *BMJ* 2004; **328**: 1490.

Brown P, Brunnhuber K, Chalkidou K, Chalmers I, Clarke M, Fenton M, Forbes C, Glanville J, Hicks NJ, Moody J, Twaddle S, Timimi H, Young P. How to formulate research recommendations. *BMJ* 2006; **333**: 804–806.

Cates C. Confidence intervals for the number needed to treat: pooling numbers needed to treat may not be reliable. *BMJ* 1999; **318**: 1764–1765.

Clarke MJ, Broderick C, Hopewell S, Juszczak E, Eisinga A. Compression stockings for preventing deep vein thrombosis in airline passengers. *Cochrane Database of Systematic Reviews* 2016; **9**: CD004002.

Cohen J. *Statistical Power Analysis in the Behavioral Sciences*. 2nd ed. Hillsdale (NJ): Lawrence Erlbaum Associates, Inc.; 1988.

Coleman T, Chamberlain C, Davey MA, Cooper SE, Leonardi-Bee J. Pharmacological interventions for promoting smoking cessation during pregnancy. *Cochrane Database of Systematic Reviews* 2015; **12**: CD010078.

Dans AM, Dans L, Oxman AD, Robinson V, Acuin J, Tugwell P, Dennis R, Kang D. Assessing equity in clinical practice guidelines. *Journal of Clinical Epidemiology* 2007; **60**: 540–546.

Friedman LM, Furberg CD, DeMets DL. *Fundamentals of Clinical Trials*. 2nd ed. Littleton (MA): John Wright PSG, Inc.; 1985.

Friedrich JO, Adhikari NK, Beyene J. The ratio of means method as an alternative to mean differences for analyzing continuous outcome variables in meta-analysis: a simulation study. *BMC Medical Research Methodology* 2008; **8**: 32.

Furukawa T. From effect size into number needed to treat. *Lancet* 1999; **353**: 1680.

Graham R, Mancher M, Wolman DM, Greenfield S, Steinberg E. Committee on Standards for Developing Trustworthy Clinical Practice Guidelines, Board on Health Care Services: Clinical Practice Guidelines We Can Trust. Washington, DC: National Academies Press; 2011.

Guyatt G, Oxman AD, Akl EA, Kunz R, Vist G, Brozek J, Norris S, Falck-Ytter Y, Glasziou P, DeBeer H, Jaeschke R, Rind D, Meerpohl J, Dahm P, Schünemann HJ. GRADE guidelines: 1. Introduction-GRADE evidence profiles and summary of findings tables. *Journal of Clinical Epidemiology* 2011a; **64**: 383–394.

Guyatt GH, Juniper EF, Walter SD, Griffith LE, Goldstein RS. Interpreting treatment effects in randomised trials. *BMJ* 1998; **316**: 690–693.

Guyatt GH, Oxman AD, Vist GE, Kunz R, Falck-Ytter Y, Alonso-Coello P, Schünemann HJ. GRADE: an emerging consensus on rating quality of evidence and strength of recommendations. *BMJ* 2008; **336**: 924–926.

Guyatt GH, Oxman AD, Kunz R, Woodcock J, Brozek J, Helfand M, Alonso-Coello P, Falck-Ytter Y, Jaeschke R, Vist G, Akl EA, Post PN, Norris S, Meerpohl J, Shukla VK, Nasser M, Schünemann HJ. GRADE guidelines: 8. Rating the quality of evidence–indirectness. *Journal of Clinical Epidemiology* 2011b; **64**: 1303–1310.

Guyatt GH, Oxman AD, Santesso N, Helfand M, Vist G, Kunz R, Brozek J, Norris S, Meerpohl J, Djulbegovic B, Alonso-Coello P, Post PN, Busse JW, Glasziou P, Christensen R, Schünemann HJ. GRADE guidelines: 12. Preparing summary of findings tables-binary outcomes. *Journal of Clinical Epidemiology* 2013a; **66**: 158–172.

Guyatt GH, Thorlund K, Oxman AD, Walter SD, Patrick D, Furukawa TA, Johnston BC, Karanicolas P, Akl EA, Vist G, Kunz R, Brozek J, Kupper LL, Martin SL, Meerpohl JJ, Alonso-Coello P, Christensen R, Schünemann HJ. GRADE guidelines: 13. Preparing summary of findings tables and evidence profiles-continuous outcomes. *Journal of Clinical Epidemiology* 2013b; **66**: 173–183.

Hawe P, Shiell A, Riley T, Gold L. Methods for exploring implementation variation and local context within a cluster randomised community intervention trial. *Journal of Epidemiology and Community Health* 2004; **58**: 788–793.

Hoffrage U, Lindsey S, Hertwig R, Gigerenzer G. Medicine. Communicating statistical information. *Science* 2000; **290**: 2261–2262.

Jaeschke R, Singer J, Guyatt GH. Measurement of health status. Ascertaining the minimal clinically important difference. *Controlled Clinical Trials* 1989; **10**: 407–415.

Johnston B, Thorlund K, Schünemann H, Xie F, Murad M, Montori V, Guyatt G. Improving the interpretation of health-related quality of life evidence in meta-analysis: the application of minimal important difference units. *Health Outcomes and Qualithy of Life* 2010; **11**: 116.

Karanicolas PJ, Smith SE, Kanbur B, Davies E, Guyatt GH. The impact of prophylactic dexamethasone on nausea and vomiting after laparoscopic cholecystectomy: a systematic review and meta-analysis. *Annals of Surgery* 2008; **248**: 751–762.

Lumley J, Oliver SS, Chamberlain C, Oakley L. Interventions for promoting smoking cessation during pregnancy. *Cochrane Database of Systematic Reviews* 2004; **4**: CD001055.

McQuay HJ, Moore RA. Using numerical results from systematic reviews in clinical practice. *Annals of Internal Medicine* 1997; **126**: 712–720.

Resnicow K, Cross D, Wynder E. The Know Your Body program: a review of evaluation studies. *Bulletin of the New York Academy of Medicine* 1993; **70**: 188–207.

Robinson J, Biley FC, Dolk H. Therapeutic touch for anxiety disorders. *Cochrane Database of Systematic Reviews* 2007; **3**: CD006240.

Rothwell PM. External validity of randomised controlled trials: "to whom do the results of this trial apply?" *Lancet* 2005; **365**: 82–93.

Santesso N, Carrasco-Labra A, Langendam M, Brignardello-Petersen R, Mustafa RA, Heus P, Lasserson T, Opiyo N, Kunnamo I, Sinclair D, Garner P, Treweek S, Tovey D, Akl EA, Tugwell P, Brozek JL, Guyatt G, Schünemann HJ. Improving GRADE evidence tables part 3: detailed guidance for explanatory footnotes supports creating and understanding GRADE certainty in the evidence judgments. *Journal of Clinical Epidemiology* 2016; **74**: 28–39.

Schünemann HJ, Guyatt GH. Commentary-goodbye M(C)ID! Hello MID, where do you come from? *Health Services Research* 2005; **40**: 593–597.

Schünemann HJ, Puhan M, Goldstein R, Jaeschke R, Guyatt GH. Measurement properties and interpretability of the Chronic respiratory disease questionnaire (CRQ). *COPD: Journal of Chronic Obstructive Pulmonary Disease* 2005; **2**: 81–89.

Schünemann HJ, Fretheim A, Oxman AD. Improving the use of research evidence in guideline development: 13. Applicability, transferability and adaptation. *Health Research Policy and Systems* 2006; **4**: 25.

Schünemann HJ. Methodological idiosyncracies, frameworks and challenges of non-pharmaceutical and non-technical treatment interventions. *Zeitschrift für Evidenz, Fortbildung und Qualität im Gesundheitswesen* 2013; **107**: 214–220.

Schünemann HJ, Tugwell P, Reeves BC, Akl EA, Santesso N, Spencer FA, Shea B, Wells G, Helfand M. Non-randomized studies as a source of complementary, sequential or replacement evidence for randomized controlled trials in systematic reviews on the effects of interventions. *Research Synthesis Methods* 2013; **4**: 49–62.

Schünemann HJ, Wiercioch W, Etxeandia I, Falavigna M, Santesso N, Mustafa R, Ventresca M, Brignardello-Petersen R, Laisaar KT, Kowalski S, Baldeh T, Zhang Y, Raid U, Neumann I, Norris SL, Thornton J, Harbour R, Treweek S, Guyatt G, Alonso-Coello P, Reinap M, Brozek J, Oxman A, Akl EA. Guidelines 2.0: systematic development of a comprehensive checklist for a successful guideline enterprise. *CMAJ: Canadian Medical Association Journal* 2014; **186**: E123–142.

Schünemann HJ. Interpreting GRADE's levels of certainty or quality of the evidence: GRADE for statisticians, considering review information size or less emphasis on imprecision? *Journal of Clinical Epidemiology* 2016; **75**: 6–15.

Smeeth L, Haines A, Ebrahim S. Numbers needed to treat derived from meta-analyses–sometimes informative, usually misleading. *BMJ* 1999; **318**: 1548–1551.

Sun X, Briel M, Busse JW, You JJ, Akl EA, Mejza F, Bala MM, Bassler D, Mertz D, Diaz-Granados N, Vandvik PO, Malaga G, Srinathan SK, Dahm P, Johnston B, Alonso-Coello P, Hassouneh B, Walter SD, Heels-Ansdell D, Bhatnagar N, Altman DG, Guyatt GH. Credibility of claims of subgroup effects in randomised controlled trials: systematic review. *BMJ* 2012; **344**: e1553.

Zhang Y, Akl EA, Schünemann HJ. Using systematic reviews in guideline development: the GRADE approach. *Research Synthesis Methods* 2018a; doi: 10.1002/jrsm.1313.

Zhang Y, Alonso-Coello P, Guyatt GH, Yepes-Nuñez JJ, Akl EA, Hazlewood G, Pardo-Hernandez H, Etxeandia-Ikobaltzeta I, Qaseem A, Williams JW, Jr., Tugwell P, Flottorp S, Chang Y, Zhang Y, Mustafa RA, Rojas MX, Schünemann HJ. GRADE Guidelines: 19. Assessing the certainty of evidence in the importance of outcomes or values and preferences-Risk of bias and indirectness. *Journal of Clinical Epidemiology* 2018b; doi: 10.1016/j.jclinepi.2018.01.013.

Zhang Y, Alonso Coello P, Guyatt G, Yepes-Nuñez JJ, Akl EA, Hazlewood G, Pardo-Hernandez H, Etxeandia-Ikobaltzeta I, Qaseem A, Williams JW, Jr., Tugwell P, Flottorp S, Chang Y, Zhang Y, Mustafa RA, Rojas MX, Xie F, Schünemann HJ. GRADE Guidelines: 20. Assessing the certainty of evidence in the importance of outcomes or values and preferences – Inconsistency, Imprecision, and other Domains. *Journal of Clinical Epidemiology* 2018c; doi: 10.1016/j.jclinepi.2018.05.011.

Zhang Y, Alonso-Coello P, Guyatt G, Yepes-Nuñez JJ, Akl EA, Hazlewood G, Pardo-Hernandez H, Etxeandia-Ikobaltzeta I, Qaseem A, Williams JW Jr, Tugwell P, Flottorp S, Chang Y, Zhang Y, Mustafa RA, Rojas MX, Xie F, Schünemann HJ. GRADE Guidelines: 20. Assessing the certainty of evidence in the importance of outcomes or values and preferences – inconsistency, imprecision, and other domains. *Journal of Clinical Epidemiology* 2019; doi: 10.1016/j.jclinepi.2018.05.011.

Part Two

Specific perspectives in reviews

16

Equity and specific populations

Vivian A Welch, Jennifer Petkovic, Janet Jull, Lisa Hartling, Terry Klassen, Elizabeth Kristjansson, Jordi Pardo Pardo, Mark Petticrew, David J Stott, Denise Thomson, Erin Ueffing, Katrina Williams, Camilla Young, Peter Tugwell

KEY POINTS

- Health equity is the absence of avoidable and unfair differences in health.
- Health inequity may be experienced across characteristics defined by PROGRESS-Plus (Place of residence, Race/ethnicity/culture/language, Occupation, Gender/sex, Religion, Education, Socio-economic status, Social capital and other characteristics ('Plus') such as sexual orientation, age and disability).
- Cochrane Reviews can inform decision making by considering the distribution of effects in the population and implications for equity.
- To address health equity in Cochrane Reviews, review authors may: consider health equity at the question formulation stage, possibly using a logic model; decide what methods will be used to identify and appraise evidence related to equity and specific populations; consider implications for 'Summary of findings' tables (e.g. separate tables for disadvantaged populations, separate rows for differences in risk of events); and interpret findings related to health equity in the discussion.

16.1 Introduction to equity in systematic reviews

Health equity reflects a concern for social justice (Braveman 2006, Krieger 2008, Marmot et al 2008, Frieden 2011, Marmot et al 2012). When differences in health are avoidable, remediable and considered unjust and unfair, they are considered health inequities (Whitehead 1992). Not all health differences are considered inequitable. For example, sickle cell disease is more common in some populations defined by ethnicity due to

This chapter should be cited as: Welch VA, Petkovic J, Jull J, Hartling L, Klassen T, Kristjansson E, Pardo Pardo J, Petticrew M, Stott DJ, Thomson D, Ueffing E, Williams K, Young C, Tugwell P. Chapter 16: Equity and specific populations. In: Higgins JPT, Thomas J, Chandler J, Cumpston M, Li T, Page MJ, Welch VA (editors). *Cochrane Handbook for Systematic Reviews of Interventions*. 2nd Edition. Chichester (UK): John Wiley & Sons, 2019: 435–450.

genetic differences and is not likely to be considered unfair. However, socio-economic differences in childhood asthma rates due to differential distribution of air pollutants would be considered an inequity. Reducing health inequities is considered an important public policy objective for social justice (i.e. moral grounds), social cohesion (for utilitarian reasons) and inter-generational solidarity (for sustainability).

We use the term 'disadvantaged' to denote disadvantage created by social, political and legal structures and processes (Welch et al 2015). Axes of potential disadvantage can be defined by the acronym PROGRESS-Plus (place of residence, race/ethnicity/culture/language, occupation, gender/sex, religion, education, socio-economic status and social capital) and 'Plus' refers to additional categories such as age, sexual orientation and disability which may influence opportunities for health of individuals and populations (O'Neill et al 2013). Other lists of characteristics may be helpful, depending on the intended audience of the review, such as the social determinants of health or SCRAP (sex, comorbidities, race, age and pathophysiology) (Dans et al 2008). The degree to which these factors are associated with disadvantage depends on time, place and interaction between the determinants (Lorenc et al 2013).

Review authors and decision makers increasingly recognize the importance of the impact of interventions on health equity. Some populations may not benefit from interventions to the same extent as others, which could lead to unintentional intervention-generated inequities (Lorenc et al 2013). Policy makers report that the lack of health equity considerations in systematic reviews limits their usefulness for decision making (Petticrew et al 2004).

Average results hide differences in effects between different populations. Therefore, review authors should consider not only what works on average, but also consider intervention impacts on health inequities. Systematic reviews may assess effects on health equity according to three types of interventions (Welch et al 2012):

1) interventions aimed at the general population, where it is important to understand the distribution of effects across one or more PROGRESS-Plus characteristics;
2) interventions focused on disadvantaged or at-risk populations in which there may not be equity outcomes but that may provide evidence about reducing inequities; and
3) interventions aimed at reducing social gradients across populations or among subgroups of the population.

Trials often exclude populations that are disadvantaged or those above or below a certain age. The exclusion of these populations may influence the applicability of results beyond the trial settings. Review authors should report on the characteristics of the populations according to relevant PROGRESS-Plus factors as well as whether there are population subgroups with a higher risk of the condition or problem or if there are differences in factors that influence access to care. Such factors include values, preferences, affordability and feasibility from the patient/public perspective and conscious or unconscious bias by practitioners. Wait times for total joint arthroplasty provide an example of practitioner bias and gender differences in access to care (Pederson and Armstrong 2015). These factors may vary according to context.

It is usually not feasible to assess all PROGRESS-Plus characteristics. Thus, in choosing characteristics to assess, review authors should consider the perspective of the intended beneficiaries of the interventions and the intended users of the evidence.

16.2 Formulation of the review

Five issues are important for formulating the review question: (i) defining health equity; (ii) hypotheses related to equity and logic models; (iii) appropriate study designs; (iv) appropriate outcomes; and (v) context.

16.2.1 Defining health equity

As health equity implies a judgement about fairness, the first step for review authors is to define which populations experience health inequity with respect to the condition/problem or intervention being assessed. For example, in a Cochrane Review of school meals, socio-economic status, gender and rurality were considered important factors associated with health inequity, but proxy measures were also used: baseline nutritional status was used as a proxy measure for socio-economic disadvantage (Kristjansson et al 2007). Justification for the use of proxies should be given, their use should be transparent and their limitations should be clearly reported.

Review authors may need to consider specific populations separately, either within a broader review or in a focused review, depending on the question and the intended recipients of the intervention. For example, it may be important to consider a separate review for indigenous peoples such as a review on family-centred interventions for indigenous childhood well-being (McCalman et al 2017). For interventions delivered to diverse populations, review authors should assess the primary studies for transparent reporting of participant demographics. It is also important to assess the need for sensitivity or subgroup analyses to explore potential differences in effects. Equity reviews can consider these differences across populations defined by one or more PROGRESS-Plus factors (e.g. migrants, linguistic minorities, homeless); however, they likely cannot address all PROGRESS-Plus factors. Thus, at the question formulation stage, review authors should explicitly consider which factors are most important and how they will be addressed in the methods of the review. Box 16.2.a provides information related to considerations for deciding whether there may be differences in the relevance or appropriateness of an intervention based on whether it is being implemented in low- and middle- and/or high-income countries. Box 16.2.b provides resources that may be helpful when planning systematic reviews of studies including children and youth.

Moreover, rather than using one category to describe people's experiences, intersectionality illuminates the complex ways a person experiences discrimination simultaneously – across ageism, sexism, racism, and other forms of institutionalized discrimination (Hankivsky 2014).

For example, a Cochrane Review of school feeding for improving the physical and psychosocial health of disadvantaged students reported: "children were classified as 'predominantly disadvantaged' by …the following criteria: 1) Living in a rural area or village; 2) Living in an urban area and described as socio-economically disadvantaged (e.g. poor or low-income) or from poor areas (e.g. slums); 3) if statistics were presented showing that 30% or more of the children in the sample were underweight, or stunted (nutritionist judgement) or that the average weight, height, and Body Mass Index (BMI) were low (nutritionist judgement) and 4) studies were implicitly or explicitly aimed at disadvantaged children, and indicators of disadvantage were provided in the paper."(Kristjansson et al 2007)

Box 16.2.a Low- and middle-income countries (LMICs)

It is important to consider whether the functioning of an intervention or its relevance may differ among high-, middle- or low-income country settings and populations. For example, health systems may vary in financing, regulation, organization, and mechanisms of care delivery. There may also be differences in the wider context, e.g. economy and geography, and the relative importance of health issues. It may be appropriate to include only studies conducted in LMICs when:

1) the intervention(s) that the review addresses is highly relevant in LMICs and of little or no relevance in high-income countries (HICs);
2) there are compelling reasons to believe that the problem or the intervention(s) are different in LMICs;
3) the outcomes of interest are different;
4) the intervention(s) would be expected to function differently, so that the evidence would be unlikely to be transferrable between LMICs and HICs; or
5) the researchers or review commissioners are particularly interested in evidence from LMICs.

Focusing solely on LMICs because the intervention is uncommon in HICs is not sufficient unless the problem or outcomes of interest are different in LMICs and HICs, and the intervention is expected to function differently.

For reviews that include studies from all countries, and where the topic is particularly important for LMICs but relevant for HICs, the Background of the review should address why the same intervention might have different absolute and/or relative effects in LMICs and HICs. Where appropriate, review authors should include subgroup analyses for LMICs and HICs and consider the applicability of the evidence for LMICs and HICs in the discussion.

For all reviews, review authors should consider (Oxman et al 2009):

- if LMIC populations are likely to be disadvantaged by the intervention delivered;
- whether there is evidence of differences in baseline conditions across LMIC and HICs, or for groups within these settings, which would result in differences in the absolute effectiveness of the intervention;
- whether there is evidence of differences in access to care or the quality of care across LMIC and HICs; and
- the implications of these differences for implementing the intervention to ensure that inequities are reduced if possible and they are not increased.

16.2.2 Logic models and theories of change to articulate hypotheses about equity

Analytic frameworks such as logic models, causal chains and funnels of attrition are increasingly being used in systematic reviews to identify key questions across the population, intervention, comparison group and outcomes (PICO) of interest (Chapter 2, Section 2.4). Funnel-of-attrition or equity-effectiveness frameworks explain why effect sizes decrease along the causal chain and allow for identification of the various factors

Box 16.2.b Systematic reviews including children and youth

Differences between children and adults, and amongst children and youth of disparate ages, mean that questions often arise around defining the population and planning subgroup analyses. Tools from the STAR Child initiative can be useful in planning a review (Sinha et al 2012, Williams et al 2012).

For reviews of conditions that are relevant to both children and adults, review authors should be aware of and document potential differences in:

- the nature or course of the condition;
- the intervention when delivered to adults and children;
- the efficacy, effectiveness or safety profile of the intervention; and
- important outcomes, measurement of outcomes, and clinically important differences (Sinha et al 2012, Williams et al 2012).

Note: Differences across sex/gender and other elements of PROGRESS-Plus may be relevant to consider.

such as coverage and uptake that may impact the implementation of an intervention (Tugwell et al 2008, White 2014). Logic models, which show the relationships between inputs and results, can help identify the key questions that are relevant to assessing effects on health equity by predicting likely differences in response, differences in baseline risk, applicability and also factors that may mediate effects. These factors and differences can guide the methods of the review. They can help scope the review question, identify eligibility criteria, focus the search strategy, design a process evaluation and consider relevance to policy and/or practice (Anderson et al 2011, O'Connor et al 2011). For example, a Cochrane Review of food supplementation for improving the physical and psychosocial health of socio-economically disadvantaged children included a logic model showing how socio-economic factors and family structure might modify effectiveness of supplementary feeding (Kristjansson et al 2015).

Theories of change provide a comprehensive description and illustration of how and why a desired change is expected to happen in a particular context (Mackinnon et al 2006, Kneale et al 2015). Pathways to change may be uncovered in the process of doing the review, therefore, theories of change may need to be updated and revised during the review process to incorporate discoveries about the processes and barriers and facilitators to implementation.

16.2.3 Appropriate study designs to assess equity

Eligible study designs should be chosen according to their fitness for purpose (Tugwell et al 2010), and the rationale should be clearly explained (see Chapter 3). Review authors need to consider whether non-randomized studies may provide relevant and meaningful evidence about the impact of the intervention in populations and settings that they consider important (Tugwell et al 2010). These different study designs need different assessment of potential bias (see Chapter 24).

16.2.4 Appropriate outcomes for equity

Outcomes need to be selected based on the stakeholder/user groups. A framework may be helpful in defining the relevant groups. For example, these could include the 9 'P's: patients, practitioners, the public, policy makers, press, product makers (e.g. drug and devices manufacturers), payers (e.g. medical insurers), purchasers (e.g. employers, governments) and principal investigators (Concannon et al 2012, Rader et al 2014). Outcomes to be considered include benefits and harms (and their trade-off): mortality (general/condition specific), impact (symptoms, physical/emotional/social/spiritual function, quality of life, utility, inconvenience, financial burden) and intermediate/surrogate outcomes/biomarkers (Boers et al 2014). See Box 16.2.c for specific considerations for outcomes of importance for children and youth and older adults.

The relative importance of health and social outcomes may differ for populations who experience health inequity. For example, maternal employment, family income and education are important outcomes in a Cochrane Review of day care for preschool children of disadvantaged mothers (Zoritch et al 2000). These outcomes may be less important for mothers with higher socio-economic status. A similar analysis of relative importance could be applied to older adults with pension or other forms of social security, in contrast to those without. The importance of outcomes for different settings and populations needs to be rated when selecting outcomes for 'Summary of

Box 16.2.c Outcomes for child health or ageing

There may be differences among children, adults, and older adults in disease pathogenesis, clinical features and natural history, physiological and psychological outcomes, and contrasting roles within the contexts of families and society in general. Across age groups, appropriate doses and likelihood of compliance will vary.

For children and youth:

- developmental outcomes and growth will be important;
- autonomy and independence may be important for youth; and
- outcomes for parents and carers can have direct relevance for children.

For older adults:

- appropriate outcomes should consider well-being, frailty, a continuum of abilities and disabilities, physical and cognitive decline, social participation and low mood;
- outcomes are often measured in decades rather than years, in terms of trajectories over the life course; and
- adverse effects are particularly common in later life, often presenting non-specifically, for example falls, immobility, cognitive problems (delirium and dementia) and incontinence. Other adverse events include loss of ability to live independently (e.g. requiring home care, community services or a move to residential care home) and impacts on informal carers (who may also be older adults), including caregiver stress and depression) (Jull 2010).

Note: Differences across sex/gender and other elements of PROGRESS-Plus may be relevant to consider.

findings' tables (Chapter 14, Section 14.1.2). Context should be considered in rating importance of outcomes (Section 16.2.5). Additionally, inconvenience, burden (e.g. out-of-pocket costs, travel time) and stigma need to be considered as potential outcomes even if they are not commonly reported in primary studies since they may be of utmost importance to the intended recipients of the intervention.

16.2.5 Context and equity

Review authors should consider the social, cultural and political contexts in which interventions are planned and implemented (Marmot et al 2008). Primary research on health and social interventions is conducted within particular temporal, cultural, geographical, political and organizational settings (Pope et al 2007), and these may influence intervention effectiveness (Hawe et al 2004).

'Taking context into account' means understanding the important aspects of context, how these may influence the intervention (e.g. implementation), and describing, stratifying and exploring the extent to which they influence outcomes (Lewin et al 2017). For example, for reviews including older adults, multimorbidity without integrated care, and overall declines in capacities are an important contextual issue. One aspect can be assessed with the number of prescribed medicines and therefore review authors may wish to report this indicator. Some tools have been developed to collect and extract data on context, including the Context and Implementation of Complex Interventions (CICI) framework (Pfadenhauer et al 2017).

Review authors may wish to assess and document whether research procedures in included studies meet international ethical standards, since populations experiencing health inequities may be vulnerable in research and need additional protections (Welch et al 2017a). Systematic reviews can reinforce ethical practices by identifying ethical concerns in included studies.

Variations in context between studies can be assessed qualitatively and/or quantitatively. Context may be described in different sections of the primary studies or in accompanying papers, reports, policies or historical documents; finding these descriptions may need expert knowledge (Noyes et al 2013). Thus, the full team and advisory board (if the review has one) or other key stakeholders should be involved in interpretation to ensure that the review is useful, relevant and applicable. For example, a Cochrane Review on environmental interventions to reduce the consumption of sugar-sweetened beverages reported: "the context in which included studies were done can therefore be essential for assessing the transferability and applicability of their results… We will therefore extract contextual data, using the categories defined by the CICI (Context and Implementation of Complex Interventions) framework." (von Philipsborn et al 2016).

16.3 Identification of evidence

Searches for equity-focused reviews should follow the general guidance (Chapter 4), but should ensure there is enough coverage of populations of interest. Searches related to health equity are likely to address perspectives beyond the biomedical lens. Thus, potentially relevant studies may be found in a wider range of literature sources and may be unreliably categorized. This may influence the databases and search terms chosen. A Cochrane Review of interventions for promoting reintegration and reducing harmful behaviour and lifestyles in street-connected children and young people searched a broad range of websites and grey literature sources (Coren et al 2016).

16.3.1 Databases to consider

Non-health databases may be relevant if the outcomes of interest include, for example, labour productivity or educational, economic or social outcomes. The information retrieval guidance of the Campbell Collaboration is an excellent resource for searches related to social outcomes (Kugley et al 2017), while the Norwegian Satellite of the Effective Practice and Organisation of Care (EPOC) Group maintains a list of databases relevant for low- and middle-income countries (EPOC 2013). For example, a Cochrane EPOC review of strategies to increase the ownership and use of insecticide-treated nets to prevent malaria searched multiple databases in addition to MEDLINE and EMBASE, including: CINAHL, Web of Science, Dissertations and Theses, African Index Medicus, LILACS and WHOLIS (Augustincic Polec et al 2015).

16.3.2 Term selection and use of search filters for equity

Using standard search filters (i.e. those available in the search interface of a database) for equity-related content carries significant risks, as many of the words describing PROGRESS-Plus categories are not indexed in the major databases (MEDLINE/Pubmed added a new MeSH term, 'health equity', in 2016). Paediatric studies are also often poorly indexed. Authors of studies on children-specific conditions may fail to use paediatric terms explicitly in the title, abstract, or even within the manuscript. Therefore, when searching electronic databases, we recommend using a paediatric search filter (a combination of the subject headings, age limits [if available], and free text terms) rather than indexing or age limits alone. Searching for studies related to older people may consider available search filters for relevance (van de Glind et al 2012). When validated filters are available, their use will save time in building the search and in reducing the number of articles to screen. For example, validated search filters have been developed for sex and gender specific outcome data (Lorenzetti and Lin 2017) and for equity-focused studies (Prady et al 2018) may be helpful in designing searches. Additional filters can be found on the ISSG search filters resource (ISSG 2018).

16.3.3 Practical advice

Appropriate retrieval strategies vary, depending on the research question and the specific populations and settings included. Practical suggestions include the following.

- Use expert advice on planning and executing the search strategy, given the anticipated complexity of the searches (Chapter 4). Experts might know of unpublished, non-indexed or hard-to-locate evidence.

- Identify validated filters, considering sensitivity and specificity, and trying to correct known limitations. If the filter is not validated, consider carefully the risk of missing vital information.
- Look beyond traditional databases: small and specific databases addressing the research topic may be more relevant (Ogilvie et al 2005, Augustincic Polec et al 2015).
- Develop logic models to make explicit the decisions on the search strategy.
- Conduct iterative searches: language changes over time and varies by place.

16.4 Appraisal of evidence

For equity questions, baseline imbalance across PROGRESS-Plus factors may be important to assess by checking for poor randomization. Further, equity factors may be considered as potential confounders in non-randomized studies. Authors should document whether losses occurred differentially from specific populations defined by PROGRESS-Plus. Otherwise, the critical appraisal of evidence is similar to other reviews (discussed in Chapter 8 and Chapter 25).

16.5 Synthesis of evidence

Equity analysis involves three steps: first, identifying in the protocol which populations are likely to experience health inequity; second, assessing whether the intervention results in important improvement; and third, assessing whether the identified populations achieve the same improvement in both absolute and relative effects as other populations. Methods for assessing gradients of effects and gaps in absolute and relative effects are described by Evans et al (2001).

A Cochrane Review on culturally appropriate health education for type 2 diabetes mellitus in ethnic minority groups included equity considerations in the synthesis of the data: "we anticipated the need to stratify participants in age groups, as it can be an important effect modifier of outcomes; the effect of gender of participants, matched with gender of educators, were also analysed; … we tried to explore difference between different literacy subgroups, ability to speak language of the majority population and countries where the interventions take place; we stratified participants by ethnic groups." Differences by age, gender and education were not explored because of insufficient data (Hawthorne et al 2008).

16.5.1 Subgroup analyses

For interventions provided to a broad population, equity may be considered through subgroup analyses across one or more PROGRESS-Plus factors, as pre-specified in the logic model and protocol (Chapter 2, Section 2.5.1).

Any subgroup analyses should be pre-specified and justified (Chapter 10, Section 10.11). In the process of doing the review, other important factors influencing outcomes may be uncovered. Authors should be open to this and all post-hoc decisions should be documented.

Meta-regression (Chapter 10, Section 10.11.4) may also be feasible to assess the role of explanatory variables such as population, context or process factors (Hollands et al 2015).

16.5.2 'Summary of findings' tables

Authors may want to consider one of five methods to incorporate findings about health inequities in 'Summary of findings' tables (Welch et al 2017b):

1) include health equity as an outcome;
2) consider patient-important outcomes relevant to health equity;
3) present separate tables for populations who experience health inequity to highlight important differences in relative effectiveness;
4) create different rows within a single table to highlight differences in baseline risk for specific populations; and
5) assess indirectness of evidence for populations that are predefined as important who experience health inequity.

16.6 Interpretation of evidence

Interpretation of evidence for specific populations defined across PROGRESS-Plus should focus on those populations identified at the protocol stage as important recipients of the intervention. Interpretation should consider the questions: Are findings likely to be applicable in those populations, even if they did not make up a large proportion of the participant populations in included studies? Why or why not? This section should be transparent and rely on details in the 'Summary of findings' table for specific populations. Any subgroup analyses should be interpreted with caution (Chapter 10, Section 10.11.6). See Box 16.6.a for specific examples of issues with interpretation for reviews including older adults.

Box 16.6.a Issues with interpretation for reviews including older adults

It is often difficult to determine applicability to all older people, including those who are frail and dependent. Frailty is an important concept, but it is of limited use as there are no widely adopted operational criteria. However, the following reported data can be useful:

- type of residence, for example the proportion of patients living long-term in a care home (can be a proxy measure for those who are frail, disabled or have chronic cognitive impairment or dementia);
- ability to perform basic activities of daily living (allows interpretation of whether results are applicable to older people living with disability); and
- number and proportion of those with dementia, or whether dementia was a study exclusion criterion (allows consideration of whether results are generalizable to older people with major chronic cognitive impairment).

Box 16.7.a Checklists for review authors

Several published checklists can help review authors to work through and consider issues of equity:

1) Cochrane and Campbell Equity Checklist for Systematic Review Authors for protocol planning (Ueffing et al 2009);
2) PRISMA-Equity Checklist to report findings from equity-focused systematic reviews (Welch et al 2012);
3) Sex and gender assessment tool (Doull et al 2010); and
4) Sex/gender analysis briefing notes (Doull et al 2014)

For more information see the websites of the Campbell and Cochrane Equity Methods Group, the Sex/Gender Methods Group, Cochrane Child Health and Cochrane Global Ageing.

16.7 Concluding remarks

We recommend that review authors explicitly consider the relevance of health equity to their review at the title and protocol stages using tools such as the Equity Checklist (Ueffing et al 2009), then design their methods accordingly to assess effects on health equity and/or discuss generalizability and applicability. Checklists for review authors are listed in Box 16.7.a.

16.8 Chapter information

Authors: Vivian A Welch, Jennifer Petkovic, Janet Jull, Lisa Hartling, Terry Klassen, Elizabeth Kristjansson, Jordi Pardo Pardo, Mark Petticrew, David J Stott, Denise Thomson, Erin Ueffing, Katrina Williams, Camilla Young, Peter Tugwell

Acknowledgements: We would like to acknowledge Sari Tudiver and the Sex/Gender Methods Group whose work helped to inform this chapter and Ritu Sadana for useful comments. We acknowledge Simon Lewin for contributions to the equity concepts related to LMIC.

Funding: VAW holds an Early Researcher Award (2014–2019) from the Ontario Government. PT holds a Canada Research Chair in Health Equity (Tier 1), 2016–2024.

16.9 References

Anderson LM, Petticrew M, Rehfuess E, Armstrong R, Ueffing E, Baker P, Francis D, Tugwell P. Using logic models to capture complexity in systematic reviews. *Research Synthesis Methods* 2011; **2**: 33–42.

Augustincic Polec L, Petkovic J, Welch V, Ueffing E, Tanjong Ghogomu E, Pardo Pardo J, Grabowsky M, Attaran A, Wells GA, Tugwell P. Strategies to increase the ownership and use of insecticide-treated bednets to prevent malaria. *Cochrane Database of Systematic Reviews* 2015; **3**: CD009186.

Boers M, Kirwan JR, Wells G, Beaton D, Gossec L, d'Agostino MA, Conaghan PG, Bingham CO, 3rd, Brooks P, Landewe R, March L, Simon LS, Singh JA, Strand V, Tugwell P. Developing core outcome measurement sets for clinical trials: OMERACT filter 2.0. *Journal of Clinical Epidemiology* 2014; **67**: 745–753.

Braveman P. Health disparities and health equity: concepts and measurement. *Annual Review of Public Health* 2006; **27**: 167–194.

Concannon TW, Meissner P, Grunbaum JA, McElwee N, Guise J-M, Santa J, Conway PH, Daudelin D, Morrato EH, Leslie LK. A New Taxonomy for Stakeholder Engagement in Patient-Centered Outcomes Research. *Journal of General Internal Medicine* 2012; **27**: 985–991.

Coren E, Hossain R, Pardo Pardo J, Bakker B. Interventions for promoting reintegration and reducing harmful behaviour and lifestyles in street-connected children and young people. *Cochrane Database of Systematic Reviews* 2016; **1**: CD009823.

Dans A, Dans L, Guyatt G. Applying results to individual patients. In: Guyatt G, Rennie D, Meade M, Coon J, editors. *Part B Therapy*. New York (NY): McGraw-Hill Companies; 2008. p. 273–289.

Doull M, Runnels VE, Tudiver S, Boscoe M. Appraising the evidence: applying sex- and gender-based analysis (SGBA) to Cochrane systematic reviews on cardiovascular diseases. *Journal of Women's Health* 2010; **19**: 997–1003.

Doull M, Welch V, Puil L, Runnels V, Coen SE, Shea B, O'Neill J, Borkhoff C, Tudiver S, Boscoe M. Development and evaluation of 'briefing notes' as a novel knowledge translation tool to aid the implementation of sex/gender analysis in systematic reviews: a pilot study. *PloS One* 2014; **9**: e110786–e110786.

EPOC. LMIC Databases: Effective Practice and Organisation of Care; 2013. http://epoc.cochrane.org/lmic-databases.

Evans T, Whitehead M, Diderichsen F, Bhuya A, Wirth M. *Challenging Inequities in Health: from Ethics to Action*. New York (NY): Oxford University Press; 2001.

Frieden TR. Forward: CDC Health Disparities and Inequalities Report – United States, 2011. *MMWR Supplements* 2011; **60**: 1–2.

Hankivsky O. Intersectionality 101 Vancouver (BC): Institute for Intersectionality Research & Policy, Simon Fraser University; 2014. https://docplayer.net/4773103-Intersectionality-101-olena-hankivsky-phd.html.

Hawe P, Shiell A, Riley T. Complex interventions: how "out of control" can a randomised controlled trial be? *BMJ* 2004; **328**: 1561–1563.

Hawthorne K, Robles Y, Cannings-John R, Edwards AG. Culturally appropriate health education for type 2 diabetes mellitus in ethnic minority groups. *Cochrane Database of Systematic Reviews* 2008; **3**: CD006424.

Hollands GJ, Shemilt I, Marteau TM, Jebb SA, Lewis HB, Wei Y, Higgins JPT, Ogilvie D. Portion, package or tableware size for changing selection and consumption of food, alcohol and tobacco. *Cochrane Database of Systematic Reviews* 2015; **9**: CD011045.

ISSG. The InterTASC Information Specialists' Sub-Group Search Filter Resource 2018. https://sites.google.com/a/york.ac.uk/issg-search-filters-resource/home.

Jull J. Seniors caring for seniors: examining the literature on injuries and contributing factors affecting the health and well-being of older adult care-givers. Ottawa (ON): Public Health Agency of Canada; 2010.

Kneale D, Thomas J, Harris K. Developing and optimising the use of logic models in systematic reviews: exploring practice and good practice in the use of programme theory in reviews. *PLoS ONE* 2015; **10**: e0142187.

Krieger N. Proximal, distal, and the politics of causation: what's level got to do with it? *American Journal of Public Health* 2008; **98**: 221–230.

Kristjansson E, Francis DK, Liberato S, Benkhalti Jandu M, Welch V, Batal M, Greenhalgh T, Rader T, Noonan E, Shea B, Janzen L, Wells GA, Petticrew M. Food supplementation for improving the physical and psychosocial health of socio-economically disadvantaged children aged three months to five years. *Cochrane Database of Systematic Reviews* 2015; **3**: CD009924.

Kristjansson EA, Robinson V, Petticrew M, MacDonald B, Krasevec J, Janzen L, Greenhalgh T, Wells G, MacGowan J, Farmer A, Shea BJ, Mayhew A, Tugwell P. School feeding for improving the physical and psychosocial health of disadvantaged elementary school children. *Cochrane Database of Systematic Reviews* 2007; **1**: CD004676.

Kugley S, Wade A, Thomas J, Mahood Q, Jørgensen AMK, Hammerstrom K, Sathe N. Searching for studies: a guide to information retrieval for Campbell systematic reviews. Campbell Collboration; 2017. Version 1.1 https://www.campbellcollaboration.org/library/searching-for-studies-information-retrieval-guide-campbell-reviews.html

Lewin S, Hendry M, Chandler J, Oxman AD, Michie S, Shepperd S, Reeves BC, Tugwell P, Hannes K, Rehfuess EA, Welch V, McKenzie JE, Burford B, Petkovic J, Anderson LM, Harris J, Noyes J. Assessing the complexity of interventions within systematic reviews: development, content and use of a new tool (iCAT_SR). *BMC Medical Research Methodology* 2017; **17**: 76.

Lorenc T, Petticrew M, Welch V, Tugwell P. What types of interventions generate inequalities? Evidence from systematic reviews. *Journal of Epidemiology and Community Health* 2013; **67**: 190–193.

Lorenzetti DL, Lin Y. Locating sex- and gender-specific data in health promotion research: evaluating the sensitivity and precision of published filters. *Journal of the Medical Library Association* 2017; **105**: 216–225.

Mackinnon A, Amott N, McGarvey C. Mapping change: using a theory of change to guide planning and evaluation 2006. http://www.grantcraft.org/index.cfm.

Marmot M, Friel S, Bell R, Houweling T, Taylor S, Commission on Social Determinants of Health. Closing the gap in a generation: health equity through action on the social determinants of health. *Lancet* 2008; **372**: 1661–1669.

Marmot M, Allen J, Bell R, Goldblatt P. Building of the global movement for health equity: from Santiago to Rio and beyond. *Lancet* 2012; **379**: 181–188.

McCalman J, Heyeres M, Campbell S, Bainbridge R, Chamberlain C, Strobel N, Ruben A. Family-centred interventions by primary healthcare services for Indigenous early childhood wellbeing in Australia, Canada, New Zealand and the United States: a systematic scoping review. *BMC Pregnancy and Childbirth* 2017; **17**: 71.

Noyes J, Gough D, Lewin S, Mayhew A, Michie S, Pantoja T, Petticrew M, Pottie K, Rehfuess E, Shemilt I, Shepperd S, Sowden A, Tugwell P, Welch V. A research and development agenda for systematic reviews that ask complex questions about complex interventions. *Journal of Clinical Epidemiology* 2013; **66**: 1262–1270.

O'Neill J, Tabish H, Welch V, Petticrew M, Pottie K, Clarke M, Evans T, Pardo Pardo J, Waters E, White H, Tugwell P. Applying an Equity Lens to interventions: Using PROGRESS to ensure consideration of socially stratifying factors to illuminate inequities in health. *Journal of Clinical Epidemiology* 2013; **67**: 56–64.

O'Connor D, Green S, Higgins JPT, editors. Chapter 5: Defining the review question and developing criteria for including studies. In: Higgins JPT, Green S, editors. *Cochrane Handbook for Systematic Reviews of Interventions*. Version 5.1.0 (updated March 2011): The Cochrane Collaboration; 2011.

Ogilvie D, Hamilton V, Egan M, Petticrew M. Systematic reviews of health effects of social interventions: 1. Finding the evidence: how far should you go? *Journal of Epidemiology and Community Health* 2005; **59**: 804–808.

Oxman AD, Lavis JN, Lewin S, Fretheim A. SUPPORT Tools for evidence-informed health Policymaking (STP) 10: Taking equity into consideration when assessing the findings of a systematic review. *Health Research Policy and Systems* 2009; **7** Suppl 1: S10.

Pederson A, Armstrong P. Sex, gender and systematic reviews: the example of wait times for hip and knee replacements. In: Armstrong P, Pederson A, editors. *Women's Health: Intersections of Policy, Research and Practice*. Toronto: Women's Press; 2015. pp. 56–72.

Petticrew M, Whitehead M, Macintyre SJ, Graham H, Egan M. Evidence for public health policy on inequalities: 1: The reality according to policymakers. *Journal of Epidemiology and Community Health* 2004; **58**: 811.

Pfadenhauer LM, Gerhardus A, Mozygemba K, Lysdahl KB, Booth A, Hofmann B, Wahlster P, Polus S, Burns J, Brereton L, Rehfuess E. Making sense of complexity in context and implementation: the Context and Implementation of Complex Interventions (CICI) framework. *Implementation Science* 2017; **12**: 21.

Pope C, Mays N, Popay J. *Synthesising qualitative and quantitative health evidence: A guide to methods: A guide to methods*. McGraw-Hill Education (UK); 2007.

Prady SL, Uphoff EP, Power M, Golder S. Development and validation of a search filter to identify equity-focused studies: reducing the number needed to screen. *BMC Medical Research Methodology* 2018; **18**: 106.

Rader T, Pardo Pardo J, Stacey D, Ghogomu E, Maxwell LJ, Welch VA, Singh JA, Buchbinder R, Legare F, Santesso N, Toupin April K, O'Connor AM, Wells GA, Winzenberg TM, Johnston R, Tugwell P. Update of strategies to translate evidence from Cochrane Musculoskeletal Group systematic reviews for use by various audiences. *Journal of Rheumatology* 2014; **41**: 206–215.

Sinha IP, Altman DG, Beresford MW, Boers M, Clarke M, Craig J, Alberighi OD, Fernandes RM, Hartling L, Johnston BC, Lux A, Plint A, Tugwell P, Turner M, van der Lee JH, Offringa M, Williamson PR, Smyth RL. Standard 5: selection, measurement, and reporting of outcomes in clinical trials in children. *Pediatrics* 2012; **129** Suppl 3: S146–152.

Tugwell P, Maxwell L, Welch V, Kristjansson E, Petticrew M, Wells G, Buchbinder R, Suarez-Almazor ME, Nowlan MA, Ueffing E, Khan M, Shea B, Tsikata S. Is health equity considered in systematic reviews of the Cochrane Musculoskeletal Group? *Arthritis and Rheumatism* 2008; **59**: 1603–1610.

Tugwell P, Petticrew M, Kristjansson E, Welch V, Ueffing E, Waters E, Bonnefoy J, Morgan A, Doohan E, Kelly MP. Assessing equity in systematic reviews: realising the recommendations of the Commission on Social Determinants of Health. *BMJ* 2010; **341**: c4739.

Ueffing E, Tugwell P, Welch V, Petticrew M, Kristjansson E. C1, C2 Equity Checklist for Systematic Review Authors. Version 2009-05-28. 2009. http://equity.cochrane.org/sites/equity.cochrane.org/files/uploads/equitychecklist.pdf

van de Glind EM, van Munster BC, Spijker R, Scholten RJ, Hooft L. Search filters to identify geriatric medicine in Medline. *Journal of the American Medical Informatics Association* 2012; **19**: 468–472.

von Philipsborn P, Stratil JM, Burns J, Busert LK, Pfadenhauer LM, Polus S, Holzapfel C, Hauner H, Rehfuess E. Environmental interventions to reduce the consumption of sugar-sweetened beverages and their effects on health. *Cochrane Database of Systematic Reviews* 2016; **7**: CD012292.

Welch V, Petticrew M, Tugwell P, Moher D, O'Neill J, Waters E, White H. PRISMA-Equity 2012 extension: reporting guidelines for systematic reviews with a focus on health equity. *PLoS Medicine* 2012; **9**: e1001333.

Welch V, Jull J, Petkovic J, Armstrong R4, Boyer Y, Cuervo LG, Edwards S, Lydiatt A, Gough D, Grimshaw J, Kristjansson E, Mbuagbaw L, McGowan J, Moher D, Pantoja T, Petticrew M, Pottie K, Rader T, Shea B, Taljaard M, Waters E, Weijer C, Wells GA, White H, Whitehead M, Tugwell P. Protocol for the development of a CONSORT-equity guideline to improve reporting of health equity in randomized trials. *Implement Science* 2015; **10**: 146.

Welch VA, Norheim OF, Jull J, Cookson R, Sommerfelt H, Tugwell P. CONSORT-Equity 2017 extension and elaboration for better reporting of health equity in randomised trials. *BMJ* 2017a; **359**: j5085.

Welch VA, Akl EA, Pottie K, Ansari MT, Briel M, Christensen R, Dans A, Dans L, Eslava-Schmalbach J, Guyatt G, Hultcrantz M, Jull J, Katikireddi SV, Lang E, Matovinovic E, Meerpohl JJ, Morton RL, Mosdol A, Murad MH, Petkovic J, Schünemann H, Sharaf R, Shea B, Singh JA, Sola I, Stanev R, Stein A, Thabaneii L, Tonia T, Tristan M, Vitols S, Watine J, Tugwell P. GRADE equity guidelines 3: considering health equity in GRADE guideline development: rating the certainty of synthesized evidence. *Journal of Clinical Epidemiology* 2017b; **90**: 76–83.

White H. Current challenges in impact evaluation. *European Journal of Development Research* 2014; **26**: 18–30.

Whitehead M. The concepts and principles of equity and health. *International Journal of Health Services* 1992; **22**: 429–445.

Williams K, Thomson D, Seto I, Contopoulos-Ioannidis DG, Ioannidis JP, Curtis S, Constantin E, Batmanabane G, Hartling L, Klassen T. Standard 6: age groups for pediatric trials. *Pediatrics* 2012; **129** Suppl 3: S153–160.

Zoritch B, Roberts I, Oakley A. Day care for pre-school children. *Cochrane Database of Systematic Reviews* 2000; **3**: CD000564.

17

Intervention complexity

James Thomas, Mark Petticrew, Jane Noyes, Jacqueline Chandler, Eva Rehfuess, Peter Tugwell, Vivian A Welch

KEY POINTS

- We refer to 'intervention complexity', rather than 'complex intervention', because no intervention is simple, and many review authors will need to consider some aspects of complexity.
- There are three ways of understanding intervention complexity:
  i) in terms of the number of components in the intervention;
  ii) in terms of interactions between intervention components or interactions between the intervention and its context, or both; and
  iii) in terms of the wider system within which the intervention is introduced.
- Of most relevance to Cochrane Review authors are (i) and (ii), and the chapter focuses mainly on these understandings of intervention complexity.

17.1 Introduction

This chapter introduces how to conceptualize and consider intervention complexity within systematic reviews. Advice available on this subject can appear contradictory and there is a risk that accounting for intervention complexity can make the review itself overly complex and less comprehensible to users. The key issue is how to identify an approach that assists in a specific systematic review. The chapter aims to signpost review authors to advice that helps them make decisions on when and in which circumstances to apply that advice. It does not aim to cover all aspects of complexity but advises review authors on how to frame review questions to address issues of intervention complexity and directs them to other sources for further reference. Other parts of this *Handbook* have been expanded to support considerations of intervention complexity, and this chapter provides cross-references where appropriate. Most of the methods

This chapter should be cited as: Thomas J, Petticrew M, Noyes J, Chandler J, Rehfuess E, Tugwell P, Welch VA. Chapter 17: Intervention complexity. In: Higgins JPT, Thomas J, Chandler J, Cumpston M, Li T, Page MJ, Welch VA (editors). *Cochrane Handbook for Systematic Reviews of Interventions*. 2nd Edition. Chichester (UK): John Wiley & Sons, 2019: 451–478.

discussed in this chapter have been thoroughly tested and published elsewhere. Some are still relatively new and under development. These new and emerging methods are flagged as such when they are discussed.

17.1.1 Conceptualizing intervention complexity

The terms 'simple' and 'complex' interventions are common in many texts addressing intervention complexity. We will refer to **intervention complexity** specifically because 'simplicity' and 'complexity' are not physical properties that separate interventions into simple and complex binary categories. Drugs – often characterized as simple – can equally be conceptualized as 'complex interventions' if we analyse them in their wider context (e.g. as part of the patient–clinician relationship, or as part of the health or other system through which the drug is provided, or both). Even the apparently simple intervention of *taking* a drug becomes complex if we consider the pharmacokinetics and pharmacodynamics of the drug within the body. Considering complexity as a multidimensional continuum, where there may be higher or lower levels of complexity across different aspects of the intervention and those involved in delivering or receiving it, can help review authors to decide what aspects of complexity are most important to focus on in their review.

There are three broad ways to think about intervention complexity, which offer alternative perspectives on the intervention and its wider context. The first two perspectives are focused on the intervention in question: (i) on how the intervention itself may be complex; and (ii) on how its implementation in specific situations may result in complex interactions. The third perspective shifts the focus of analysis from an individual intervention to (iii) the wider context within which it is implemented.

In the first, and simplest, understanding of intervention complexity, interventions with more than one component are described as 'complex'. This is because it can be difficult to understand which components are most important, and which are responsible for intervention effects (if any). Analysis methods are often based on the assumption that multiple components act in an additive way.

The second perspective of intervention complexity focuses on interactions, which may be between components of the intervention, between the intervention and study participants, with the intervention context, or a combination of these aspects. Understanding complexity in these terms has two important implications: (1) considering more complex interactions may require different methods of analysis (e.g. where the dose or intensity of one component needs to reach a given threshold before another is activated); and (2) while the intervention may appear quite 'simple' (e.g. in the prescription of a single drug), complexity arises when other issues are considered, such as patient adherence to treatment.

In the third perspective, the analysis can shift focus from the consideration of a specific intervention and outcome(s), towards the wider context (understood as a 'system') within which the intervention is introduced. Here the analysis might examine the impact of the intervention on the system, or the effect of the system on the intervention. This approach attempts to address the bi-directional feedback that occurs in systems that can impact on the intervention's effectiveness by either reducing or enhancing its effect.

This chapter focuses mainly on addressing the first two perspectives of intervention complexity, rather than the systems perspective, because these are most commonly used in Cochrane Reviews. The next section introduces the first two aspects of complexity in more detail, and the following section outlines some implications when the analysis is focused on the wider system.

17.1.2 Perspectives 1 and 2: intervention complexity arising from multiple components and/or interactions inside and outside the intervention

Systematic reviews often adopt an approach whereby effects of interventions, and (combinations of) their components, are seen to be additive (which of course they often are), without fully considering the implications of complexity. These reviews have appraised the primary studies on their ability to isolate components of interventions effectively from their context (see Section 17.2.4). However, intervention components may often have synergistic (as opposed to additive) and dis-synergistic effects, and this is one often-cited characteristic of intervention complexity (Pigott et al 2017).

The UK Medical Research Council has produced guidance which highlights specific difficulties for evaluating "complex" interventions (as defined by the MRC):

> There are specific difficulties in defining, developing, documenting, and reproducing complex interventions that are subject to more variation than a drug. A typical example would be the design of a trial to evaluate the benefits of specialist stroke units. Such a trial would have to consider the expertise of various health professionals as well as investigations, drugs, treatment guidelines, and arrangements for discharge and follow up. Stroke units may also vary in terms of organization, management, and skill mix. The active components of the stroke unit may be difficult to specify, making it difficult to replicate the intervention.
>
> (Campbell et al 2000)

Further elaboration describes key aspects of intervention complexity (Craig et al 2008, Petticrew et al 2019):

- whether there are multiple components within the experimental and control interventions, and whether they may interact with one another;
- the range of behaviours required by those delivering or receiving the intervention, and how difficult or variable they may be;
- whether the intervention, or its components, result in non-linear effects;
- the number of groups or organizational levels targeted by the intervention;
- the number and variability of outcomes; and
- the degree of flexibility or tailoring of the intervention permitted.

17.1.2.1 Context, implementation and mechanisms of action

Context is usually described as a key concept in the complexity literature, but it is difficult to define in isolation, and is often combined with related issues concerning how interventions are implemented and how they might work. Oxford Dictionaries define 'context' as:

> the circumstances that form the setting for an event, statement, or idea, and in terms of which it can be fully understood.

When defined in these terms, knowing the context of an intervention, and thus, 'fully understanding' how it gave rise to its outcomes, is both a highly desirable and an extremely challenging objective for review authors.

A further challenge is that defining 'context' is itself a matter of judgement. The ROBINS-I tool for appraisal of non-randomized studies (see Chapter 25) defines context broadly as "characteristics of the healthcare setting (e.g. public outpatient versus hospital outpatient), organizational service structure (e.g. managed care or publicly funded program), geographical setting (e.g. rural vs urban), and cultural setting and the legal environment where the intervention is implemented".

Pfadenhauer and colleagues concur that the physical and social setting of the intervention needs to be considered as part of the context but, in line with the guidance in Section 17.1.1 on 'conceptualizing intervention complexity', expand this understanding to acknowledge the potential for interactions between intervention, participants and the setting within which the intervention is introduced:

> *Context* reflects a set of characteristics and circumstances that consist of active and unique factors, within which the implementation is embedded. As such, context is not [just] a backdrop for implementation, but interacts, influences, modifies and facilitates or constrains the intervention and its implementation. Context is usually considered in relation to an intervention, with which it actively interacts. It is an overarching concept, comprising not only a physical location but also roles, interactions and relationships at multiple levels.
>
> (Pfadenhauer et al 2017)

An intervention may be planned as a specific set of procedures to be followed, but careful thought should also be given to **implementation**. Pfadenhauer and colleagues define **intervention implementation** as:

> an actively planned and deliberately initiated effort with the intention to bring a given intervention into policy and practice within a particular setting. These actions are undertaken by agents who either actively promote the use of the intervention or adopt the newly appraised practices. Usually, a structured implementation process consisting of specific implementation strategies is used being underpinned by an implementation theory.
>
> (Pfadenhauer et al 2017)

Important aspects to consider include complexity in implementation (i.e. situations in which we expect the effects of an intervention to be modified by variation in implementation processes from study to study) and complexity in participant responses (i.e. situations in which we expect the effects of an intervention to be modified by variation between the participants receiving an intervention from study to study) (Noyes et al 2013). Sometimes intervention adaptations occur for implementation in different contexts (Evans et al 2019). Some adaptations and their implementation will work and some will not; it may even be possible to compare these different intervention adaptations and their implementations within the systematic review. To understand what has happened, it will be necessary to unpack the intended 'function' of the intervention that underlies variations in form.

> With most (simple) interventions, integrity is defined as having the 'dose' delivered at an optimal level and in the same way in each site. Complex intervention thinking defines integrity of interventions differently. The issue is to allow the form to be adapted while standardising the process and function.
>
> (Hawe et al 2004).

Separating what is meant by intervention form as opposed to its function is illustrated by a cluster-randomized trial of a whole-community educational intervention to prevent depression. To maintain the 'form' of the intervention across clusters, the evaluators might want to ensure that the same written information was being given to every patient. On the other hand, to ensure that 'function' was consistent across clusters, they might want to support each site in devising a way to communicate the intervention which was tailored to "local literacy, language, culture and learning styles" (Hawe et al 2004). In this example, it was necessary to adapt the 'form' of part of the original intervention in order to ensure fidelity to its 'function' (or mechanism).

It can also be difficult to separate 'context' from 'setting' and 'implementation'. For example, variations to context may also be influenced by the types and characteristics of participants receiving and delivering the intervention (and their responses), which may subsequently alter the context or the intervention (Hawe et al 2004).

To understand and explain the anticipated **mechanisms of action** by which the intervention is expected to work it is advised, when addressing intervention complexity, to have an understanding of the theoretical basis of the intervention (Craig et al 2008). In some situations, there is a relatively well-understood (or perhaps just well-accepted) causal pathway between the intervention and its outcomes. This may derive from basic science – for example, the physiological pathways between specific medical interventions and changes in outcomes. For other more complex situations (such as those in which the intervention interacts with and adapts to its context) such pathways may be less well understood, less predictable and, crucially, non-linear (Petticrew et al 2019). Setting out the theoretical basis at the start of a review can help to clarify initial assumptions (e.g. among evidence users, or among the review team) about how the intervention is expected to work, and through what mechanisms. The results of the systematic review will inform and develop the intervention theory, as well as test its validity. The 2015 MRC guidance on designing complex intervention process evaluations is a helpful resource to inform this stage (Moore et al 2015). Advice is also available on appropriate use of mechanistic reasoning (Howick et al 2010), and on some of its limitations (Howick et al 2013).

To understand how an intervention works requires identifying its individual components and how these exert their effect, either separately or in combination. Further consideration will also need to be given to the implementation context and the processes involved in implementing an intervention (Campbell et al 2000, Craig et al 2008). The implication of this is that the situations in which we expect the effects of an intervention to be modified by variation in the implementation processes may vary from study to study in a review. Further, situations in which we expect the effects of an intervention to be modified by variation between the participants receiving an intervention may also vary from study to study (Noyes et al 2013). Logic models and the use of theory in systematic reviews (Noyes et al 2016a) are described in Section 17.2.1, and elsewhere in the *Handbook* (see also Chapter 2, Section 2.5.1, Chapter 3, Section 3.2 and Chapter 21, Section 21.6.1.)

Example review An exemplar multicomponent Cochrane Review of school-based self-management interventions for asthma in children and adolescents is used throughout this chapter to illustrate aspects of complexity and its management in a systematic review (see Box 17.1.a). This review was interested in addressing both intervention effectiveness and understanding how the intervention was implemented, and whether implementation in different groups might explain differences in observed impact.

Box 17.1.a A published example of a Cochrane Review assessing a multi-component intervention and how the interpretation of the effectiveness data is enhanced by an additional analysis (Harris et al 2018). Reproduced with permission of John Wiley & Sons

School-based self-management interventions for asthma in children and adolescents: a mixed methods systematic review

The problem	Asthma is a common chronic respiratory condition in children characterized by symptoms including wheeze, shortness of breath, chest tightness and cough. Improving the inhaler technique of children with asthma in response to recognizing their worsening symptoms may enable children to manage their condition more effectively. Schools are an opportunity to engage with these children to improve self-management of their asthma care because: • they offer a potentially supportive environment; • the educational environment aligns with skill and knowledge acquisition; and • they may reach children who do not regularly engage with primary care. Self-management interventions have multiple components, which vary across studies, so the review needs to consider the combination of intervention components that are associated with successful delivery of the intervention with in the school context.

Participant	School aged children and young people (5 to 18 years) with asthma who participated in an intervention in their school
Intervention	School-based asthma self-management programmes
Comparison	Usual care
Outcome (primary)	Asthma symptoms or exacerbations leading to admission to hospital
Review questions	1) To identify the intervention components and processes that are aligned with successful school-based asthma self-management intervention implementation. 2) To assess the effectiveness of school-based interventions for improvement of asthma self-management on children's outcomes.
Types of data	1) Studies that measured process elements (mechanisms, context, implementation) using qualitative or quantitative methods. 2) Individual or cluster randomized parallel-group designs.
Review design and methods used	1) Implementation success was measured through process evaluation reports of attrition, intervention dosage and adherence, irrespective of the effect of the intervention. To identify intervention features that lead to successful implementation of asthma self-management interventions qualitative comparative analysis (QCA) (Thomas et al 2014) was used. 2) To measure the effects of interventions, data from eligible studies were combined using meta-analysis and meta-regression. Review author certainty in the evidence was rated with GRADE.
Intervention description and dimensions of complexity	Self-management is the process of educating and enabling patients to control their asthma symptoms to prevent acute episodes warranting medical intervention. These might include the following intervention, implementation and context aspects: *More than one active component included in the intervention delivered across included studies*, such as

	• Materials to deliver information techniques for self-management: face-to-face lessons or groups. Video and other media, computer programs, training manuals, breathing techniques.
	• Practitioners to deliver the information and instruction on the techniques, e.g. promote:
	  ∘ regular lung function monitoring and instruction on inhaler technique;
	  ∘ appropriate use of reliever therapies; and
	  ∘ regular contact with health practitioners; and tackle risky behaviour e.g. smoking.
	
	Usual care: Standard asthma education
	
	Behaviour or actions of intervention recipients or participants to which the intervention is directed: good inhaler technique, being able to recognize and respond to asthma symptoms.
	
	Organizational levels in the school context targeted by the intervention: disseminating self-management education through schools to improve school attendance. Health care is managed through the education system, from health policy to school policy on asthma management.
	
	The degree of intervention adaption expected, or flexibility permitted, within the studies across schools applying or implementing the intervention.
	
	The level of skill required by those delivering the intervention in order to meet the intervention objectives, such as the knowledge to instruct children in self-management of asthma (e.g. teacher, healthcare practitioner).
	
	The level of skill required for the targeted behaviour when entering the included studies by those receiving the intervention, in order to meet the intervention objectives: the child's capacity to learn.

Intervention mechanisms	*How the intervention might work* is outlined in the pre-analysis logic model (see Figure 17.2.a) to theorize the causal chain necessary to lead to outcomes of interest from school-based self-management interventions.

	The post-analysis logic model presents the components of the actual interventions modelled where evidence or impact was observed in the data and where it was not. The model maps moderators, intermediate outcomes, proximal and distal outcomes and notes review gaps.
Results	Thirty-three studies provided information for the QCA analysis and 33 randomized trials measured the effects of interventions. In summary, the review authors concluded school-based asthma self-management interventions probably reduce hospital admission and may slightly reduce children's emergency department attendance, although their impact on school attendance could not be measured reliably. They probably reduce the number of days where children experience asthma symptoms, but their effects on asthma-related quality of life are small. Interventions that had a theoretical framework, engaged parents and were run outside of children's free time were associated with successful implementation. QCA results highlighted the importance of an intervention being theory-driven along with additional factors, such as parental involvement, child satisfaction and running the intervention outside of children's own time as being drivers of successful implementation. School-based self-management interventions were shown to be likely to reduce mean hospitalizations, reduce unplanned visits to hospitals or primary care, reduce the number of days of restricted activity by just under half a day over a two-week period and may reduce the number of children who visit emergency departments. However, there is insufficient evidence to determine whether requirement of reliever medications is affected by these interventions. See study for further details on results.

There is a socio-economic gradient in educational impacts due to asthma, with children from lower socio-economic groups and ethnic minorities being more likely than others to report asthma-related hospitalization. One of the reasons for this may be differential effects in school-based self-management interventions. Given that socio-economic inequalities are manifest in the environment, these issues cannot be understood purely in terms of individual participant characteristics, and the review needed to take account of the external context and school characteristics. It did not, however, attempt a 'full systems' perspective on the intervention as outlined in Section 17.1.1.

17.1.3 Perspective 3: interventions within complex (adaptive) systems

The systems perspective sees the intervention not as an isolated event or as a package of components, but as a part of, or an 'event' within, an interconnected system (Hawe et al 2009). Thus, the intervention interacts with and within a pre-existing system and the review aims to understand the intervention within this wider context, examining how it changes the system, how the system affects the intervention, or both. When doing a review using this perspective, authors not only need to consider the components of the intervention (as in Section 17.1.2), but will also need to define the system within which the intervention is introduced. For example, the introduction of a new vaccine (including its precise timing) in a low- or middle-income country needs to take many factors into account including: supplies of the vaccine (possibly including agreements between governments and international companies); maintenance of the cold chain by upgrading healthcare facilities (e.g. fridges); training of health workers; and delivery of the vaccine through the normal health system as opposed to parallel vaccination systems (e.g. to deliver standard childhood vaccinations). This may have positive or negative impacts on the system as a whole, by using synergies and investing in better infrastructure or human capacities or by over-burdening an already overstretched health system and affecting other services and interventions in unintended (and sometimes unanticipated) ways.

In a systems perspective, complexity arises not only from interactions between components, but also from the relationships and interactions between a system's agents (e.g. people, or groups that interact with each other and their environment), and its context (Section 17.2.4) (Petticrew et al 2019). One of the implications for systematic reviews is that the intervention itself may be defined very broadly: as a change in a system, or a set of processes, compared to a package of interacting components, or both. Also, reviews taking a systems perspective may aim to answer a wide range of questions about the functioning of the system and how it changes over time, and about the contribution of interventions to those system changes (Garside et al 2010, Petticrew 2015). A full description is beyond the scope of this chapter and the role of complex systems perspectives in systematic reviews is still evolving.

Review authors should refer to Petticrew and colleagues (Petticrew et al 2019) when deciding whether a systems perspective will add value to a review. The following questions should be considered when deciding whether a systems perspective might be helpful.

- What do my review users want to know about? The intervention, the system, or both?
- At what level is the intervention delivered? Is the intervention likely to have anticipated effects of interest to users at levels above the individual level? If the implementation and effects spill over into the family, community, or beyond, then taking a systems perspective may be helpful.
- Is the intervention: (i) a discrete, identifiable intervention, or package of interventions; or (ii) a more diffuse change within an existing system?

Review authors should also take account of the resources available to conduct the review. A large scale, theoretically informed review of an intervention within its wider system may be time-consuming, expensive and require a large multidisciplinary team. It may also produce complex answers that are beyond the needs of many users.

17.1.4 Summary of main points in this section

There are three ways of understanding intervention complexity: (i) in terms of the number of components in the intervention; (ii) in terms of interactions between intervention components or interactions between the intervention and its context, or both; and (iii) in terms of the wider system within which the intervention is introduced. When considering intervention complexity review authors may need to pay particular attention to the intervention's mechanisms of action, the contexts(s) within which it is introduced, and issues relating to implementation.

A review team should consider which perspective on complexity might be relevant to their review:

- Is the review dealing with interventions comprising multiple components?
- Are interventions of interest likely to interact with the context in which they are implemented, and is intervention adaptation likely to be taking place?
- Which analytical methods will need to be used (e.g. those suitable for modelling interactions and/or non-linear effects)?
- How are the core concepts of mechanisms of action, context and implementation defined?

e.g. For further information on logic models and defining interventions see Chapter 2 (Section 2.5.1), Chapter 3 (Section 3.2) and Chapter 21 (Section 21.6.1). See the following for key references on the topics discussed in this section. On understanding intervention complexity: Campbell et al (2000), Craig et al (2008), Kelly et al (2017), Petticrew et al (2019); on mechanisms of action: Howick et al (2010), Fletcher et al (2016), Noyes et al (2016a); on context and implementation: Hawe et al (2009), Noyes et al (2013), Moore et al (2015), Pfadenhauer et al (2017).

17.2 Formulation of the review

Addressing complexity in a review frequently involves asking questions about issues other than effectiveness, such as the following.

- Under what circumstances does the intervention work (Thomas et al 2004, Squires et al 2013)?
- What is the relative importance of, and synergy between, different components of multicomponent interventions?
- What are the mechanisms of action by which the intervention achieves an effect?
- What are the factors that impact on implementation and participant responses?
- What is the feasibility and acceptability of the intervention in different contexts?
- What are the dynamics of the wider system?

Broadly, therefore, systematic reviews can consider complexity in terms of the intervention (e.g. how the components of the intervention interact), and also in terms of how it is implemented. In this situation, systematic reviews can use the concept of complexity to help develop theories of implementation, and inform strategies to improve implementation (Nilsen 2015).

As Chapters 2 and 3 outline, addressing broader review questions has implications for the search strategy, the types of evidence, the eligibility criteria, the evidence appraisal, and the review design and synthesis methods (Squires et al 2013). Sometimes more than one type of study design may be required to address the questions of interest, the products of which might subsequently be integrated in a third synthesis (see Chapter 21 and Glenton et al 2013, Harris et al 2018).

17.2.1 The role of theory and logic models

As outlined in Chapter 2, review authors should set out in their protocol how they expect the intervention of interest to work. When the causal pathways are well accepted, as they are in many reviews, this can be a relatively straightforward process which simply references the appropriate literature. In reviews where there is a lot of complexity or diversity between interventions, logic models are used to provide schematic representations of causal pathways that illustrate the potential mechanisms of action – and their mediators and moderators – underlying interventions (Anderson et al 2011), as discussed in Chapter 2 (Section 2.5.1).

The example Cochrane Review in Box 17.1.a illustrates the benefits of using a logic model with both pre- and post-synthesis versions (Harris et al 2018). Figure 17.2.a presents the pre-synthesis version of the review logic model that starts to model the interventions' core elements and expected outcomes in changes of behaviour on delivery of the intervention. The model also identifies contextual and individual participant aspects that might modify intervention delivery. The model also introduces the identification of process measures to inform the expected function of the intervention.

17.2.2 Formulating questions to address intervention complexity

We emphasize the importance of having a clear objective when starting a review, observing that it is often more useful to address questions that seek to identify the circumstances where particular approaches to intervention might be more appropriate than others, rather than simply asking 'does this intervention work?' (Higgins et al 2019). Chapter 2 outlines the issues that should be considered when formulating review questions and Petticrew and colleagues outline how to refine review questions through drawing on existing theoretical models, emphasizing it is important to prioritize which contextual factors to examine (Booth et al 2019b, Petticrew et al 2019). In situations of greater intervention complexity, review authors should consider how consumers and other stakeholders might help identify which contextual factors might need detailed examination in the review. It is possible that different groups of people will have quite diverse needs and taking them all into account in a single review may be impossible. Detailed advice is available, however, on ways to engage interested parties in the development of review questions, including formal methods for question prioritization. (See Chapter 2, Section 2.4, and Oliver et al 2017, Booth et al 2019b for further information

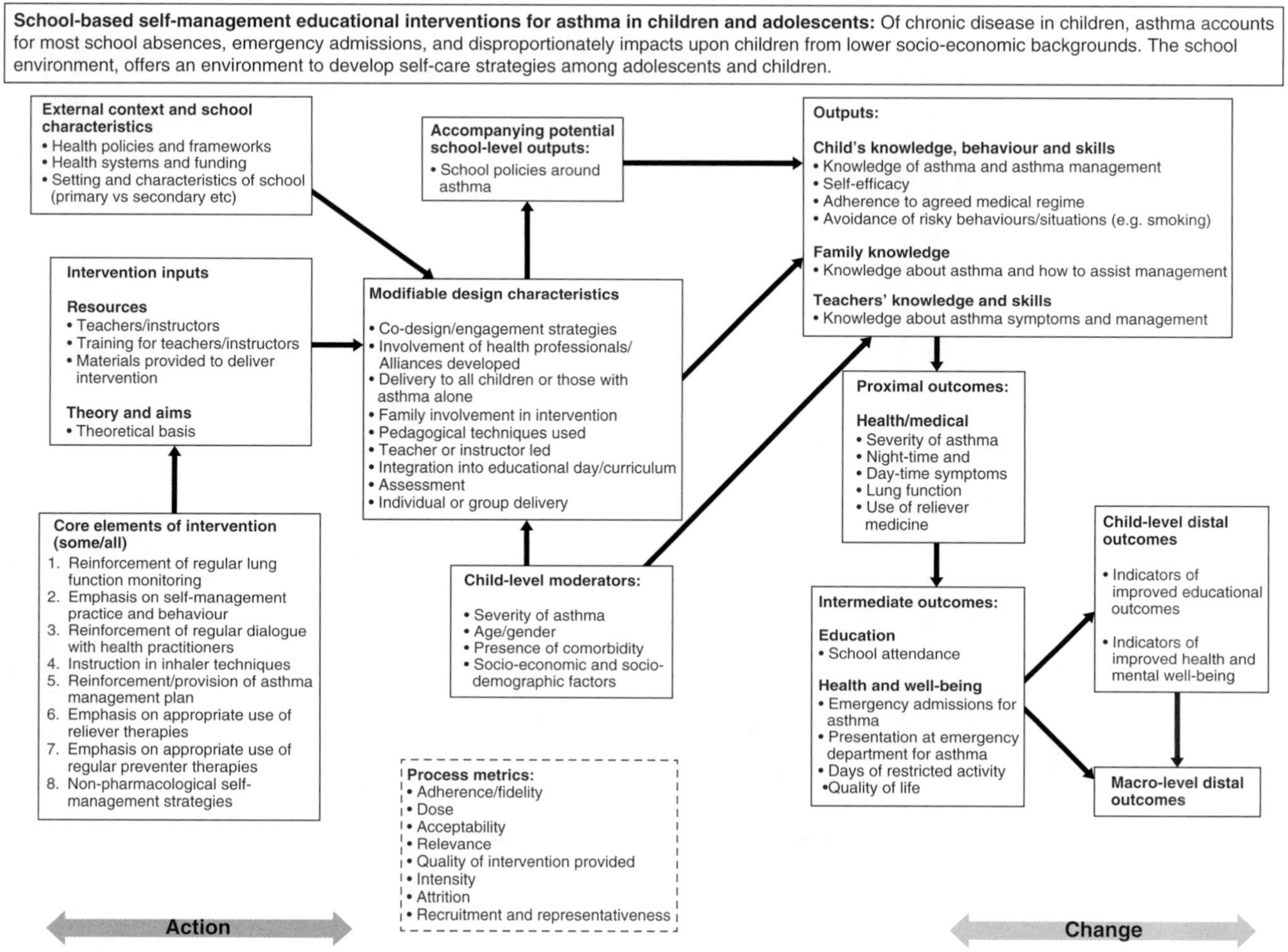

School-based self-management educational interventions for asthma in children and adolescents: Of chronic disease in children, asthma accounts for most school absences, emergency admissions, and disproportionately impacts upon children from lower socio-economic backgrounds. The school environment, offers an environment to develop self-care strategies among adolescents and children.

External context and school characteristics
- Health policies and frameworks
- Health systems and funding
- Setting and characteristics of school (primary vs secondary etc)

Intervention inputs

Resources
- Teachers/instructors
- Training for teachers/instructors
- Materials provided to deliver intervention

Theory and aims
- Theoretical basis

Core elements of intervention (some/all)
1. Reinforcement of regular lung function monitoring
2. Emphasis on self-management practice and behaviour
3. Reinforcement of regular dialogue with health practitioners
4. Instruction in inhaler techniques
5. Reinforcement/provision of asthma management plan
6. Emphasis on appropriate use of reliever therapies
7. Emphasis on appropriate use of regular preventer therapies
8. Non-pharmacological self-management strategies

Accompanying potential school-level outputs:
- School policies around asthma

Modifiable design characteristics
- Co-design/engagement strategies
- Involvement of health professionals/ Alliances developed
- Delivery to all children or those with asthma alone
- Family involvement in intervention
- Pedagogical techniques used
- Teacher or instructor led
- Integration into educational day/curriculum
- Assessment
- Individual or group delivery

Child-level moderators:
- Severity of asthma
- Age/gender
- Presence of comorbidity
- Socio-economic and socio-demographic factors

Process metrics:
- Adherence/fidelity
- Dose
- Acceptability
- Relevance
- Quality of intervention provided
- Intensity
- Attrition
- Recruitment and representativeness

Outputs:

Child's knowledge, behaviour and skills
- Knowledge of asthma and asthma management
- Self-efficacy
- Adherence to agreed medical regime
- Avoidance of risky behaviours/situations (e.g. smoking)

Family knowledge
- Knowledge about asthma and how to assist management

Teachers' knowledge and skills
- Knowledge about asthma symptoms and management

Proximal outcomes:

Health/medical
- Severity of asthma
- Night-time and
- Day-time symptoms
- Lung function
- Use of reliever medicine

Intermediate outcomes:

Education
- School attendance

Health and well-being
- Emergency admissions for asthma
- Presentation at emergency department for asthma
- Days of restricted activity
- Quality of life

Child-level distal outcomes
- Indicators of improved educational outcomes
- Indicators of improved health and mental well-being

Macro-level distal outcomes

Action

Change

Figure 17.2.a Logic model of school-based asthma interventions (Harris et al 2018). Reproduced with permission of John Wiley & Sons

on consumer and stakeholder involvement in formulating review questions.) Review authors may find guidance given in Chapter 3 helpful to prioritize which comparisons to examine and, thus, which questions to answer. Sometimes review authors may find that they need to undertake a formal scoping review in order to understand fully how the intervention is defined in the literature (Squires et al 2013).

When considering which aspects of the intervention or its implementation and wider context might be important, review authors should remember that some variation is often inevitable and investigating every conceivable difference will be impossible. In particular, not all aspects of intervention complexity should be detailed in the review question; it may be sufficient to consider these within the logic model and any subgroups identified for synthesis. The review question simply specifies which sources of variation in outcomes will be investigated. In the review example detailed in Box 17.1.a, there were two overall objectives: (1) to identify the intervention features that are aligned with successful intervention implementation; and (2) to assess the effectiveness of school-based interventions for improvement of asthma self-management on children's outcomes. The ways in which these objectives shaped the review's eligibility criteria and analytical methods will be described in the following sections.

17.2.3 PICO and complexity

The PICO framework (population, intervention, comparator(s) and outcomes, see Chapter 3) is widely used by systematic review authors to help think through the framing of research questions. The PICO elements may become more complex in reviews where significant intervention complexity is anticipated.

The population considered in a review is commonly described in terms of aspects of a health condition (e.g. patients with osteoporosis) or behaviour (e.g. adolescents who smoke) as well as relevant demographic factors and features of the setting of the study. In complex health and social research that focuses on changes in populations, the definition of a population may be contested. Crucially, populations are not just aggregates of individual characteristics, but social (and physical) relations may also shape population health distributions, as shown in analysis of the spread of obesity through social networks (Christakis and Fowler 2007, Krieger 2012). Review authors are often interested in both the population as a whole, and how the intervention differentially affects different groups within the population (see also Chapter 16 on equity).

With respect to the intervention, the key challenge lies in defining the intervention, for reasons described in detail in the previous sections. When considering intervention complexity, review authors should consider the wide range of ways in which an intervention may be implemented and be wary of excluding primary evaluations of the intervention simply because the form appears different, even if the function is similar (see Section 17.1.2).

The comparisons in the review may require careful consideration. Identifying a suitable comparator can be difficult, particularly where structural interventions, such as taxation, regulation or environmental change, are being evaluated (Blankenship et al 2006), or where each intervention arm is complex. Review authors should be particularly mindful of possible confounding due to systems effects, where wider contextual factors might reduce, or enhance, the effects of an intervention in particular circumstances (see Sections 17.1.1 and 17.1.3). For a detailed discussion of planning comparisons for synthesis, see Chapters 3 and 9.

Outcomes of interest are likely to include a range of intended and unintended health and non-health effects of interest to review users. The choice of outcomes to prioritize is a matter of judgement and perspective, and the rationale for selection decisions should be explicitly reported. Review authors should note that the prioritization of outcomes varies culturally, and according to the perspective of those directly affected by an intervention (e.g. patients, an at-risk population), those delivering the intervention (e.g. clinicians, staff working for healthcare or public health institutions), or policy makers or others deciding on or financing an intervention and the general public. However, the answer is not simply to include any plausible outcome: a plausible theoretical case can probably be made for most outcomes, but that does not mean they are meaningful. Worse, including a wide range of speculative outcomes raises the risk of data dredging and vastly increases the complexity of the analysis and interpretation (see Chapter 9, Section 9.3.3 on multiplicity of outcomes and Chapter 3, Section 3.4.4). Again, an understanding of the intervention theory can help select the outcomes for which the strongest plausible a priori case can be made for inclusion – perhaps those outcomes for which there is prior evidence of an important association with the intervention. As the illustrative logic model (Figure 17.2.a) shows, there can be numerous intermediate outcomes between the intervention and the final outcome of interest. Guidance is available on how to select the most important outcomes from the list of all plausible outcomes (Chapter 3, Section 2.4.4 and Guyatt et al 2011). It will also be important to determine the availability of core outcome sets within the review context (see www.comet-initiative.org). Core outcome sets are now becoming available for more complex interventions and may help to guide outcome selection (e.g. see Kaufman et al 2017).

17.2.4 Addressing context and implementation

One key aspect of intervention complexity is that intervention effects are often strongly context-dependent, with context acting as a moderator of the effect (i.e. influencing its strength or direction) as well as a mediator of the effect (i.e. explaining why an effect is observed). This has implications for judging the wider applicability of review findings when applying GRADE assessment (see Chapter 14). One of the most common challenges is that interventions have different effects in different contexts, and so the review authors will need to take a view (in consultation with review stakeholders and review users) about whether it is more meaningful to restrict the review's focus to one particular context or setting (e.g. studies carried out in schools, or studies conducted in specific geographical areas), or to include evidence from a range of contexts (a variant of the 'lumping' and 'splitting' argument (Chapter 2, Section 2.3.2)). For some reviews, understanding how the intervention and its effects change across different contexts is often a key reason for doing the review, and in such cases review authors will need to take account of context in planning and conducting their review. Booth and colleagues provide guidance on how to do this, noting that there are a range of contexts to be considered, including: (i) the context of the review question; (ii) the contexts of the included studies; and (iii) the implementation context into which the findings or recommendations arising from the review are to be introduced (Booth et al 2019a). Note, however, that Cochrane Reviews are rarely written with a specific context in mind although some systematic reviews may be undertaken for a specific setting (see Pantoja et al 2017 for an example of an overview of reviews which examines specifically issues from a low-income country perspective). When a review aims to inform decisions in a specific situation, consideration should be given to the 'directness' of the evidence (the extent to which the participants, interventions and outcome measures are similar to those of interest); this is a core feature of GRADE assessment, discussed in Chapter 14 (GRADE Working Group 2004).

The TIDieR framework (Hoffman et al 2014) refers to "*the type(s) of location(s) where the intervention occurred, including any necessary infrastructure or relevant features*", and the iCAT_SR tool notes that "*the effects of an intervention may be dependent on the societal, political, economic, health systems or environmental context in which the intervention is delivered*" (Lewin et al 2017). Finally, the PRECIS-2 tool, while written to support the design of trials, also contains useful information for review authors when considering how to address issues relating to context and implementation (Loudon et al 2015).

These are important considerations because for social and public health (and perhaps *any* intervention), the political context is often an important determinant of whether interventions can be implemented or not; regulatory interventions (e.g. alcohol or tobacco control policies) may be less politically acceptable within certain jurisdictions, even if such interventions are likely to be effective. Historical and cultural contexts are also often important moderators of the effects and acceptability of public health interventions (Craig et al 2018). It is therefore impossible (and probably misleading) to attempt to specify what 'is' or 'isn't' context, as this depends on the intervention and the review question, as well as how the intervention and its effects are theorized (implicitly or explicitly) by the review authors. Booth and colleagues suggest that a supplementary framework (e.g. the Context and Implementation of Complex Interventions (CICI) Framework (Pfadenhauer et al 2017); see Section 17.1.2.1) can help to understand and explore contextual issues: for example, helping to decide whether to 'lump' or 'split' studies by context, and how to frame the review question and subsequent stages of the review (Booth et al 2019a).

17.2.5 Which types of study address intervention complexity?

As always, the decision about which study designs to include should be led by the review questions, and the 'fitness for purpose' of those studies for answering the review question(s) (Tugwell et al 2010). As Chapter 3, Section 3.3 outlines, most Cochrane Reviews focus on synthesizing the results from randomized trials, because of the strength of this study design in establishing a causal relationship between an intervention and its outcome(s). However, as it is not always feasible to conduct randomized trials of all types of intervention (e.g. the 'structural' interventions mentioned in Section 17.2.3), it is also accepted that evidence about the effects of interventions, and interactions between components of interventions, may be derived from randomized, quasi-experimental or non-randomized designs (see also Chapter 24). Large-scale and policy-based interventions (such as area-based regeneration programmes) may not be able to use closely comparable control populations, or may not use separate control groups at all, and may use uncontrolled before and after or interrupted time series designs or a range of quasi-experimental approaches. Excluding non-randomized and uncontrolled studies may mean excluding the few evaluations that exist, and in some cases such designs can provide adequate evidence of effect (Craig et al 2012). For example, when evaluating the impact of a smoking ban on hospital admissions for coronary heart disease, Khuder and colleagues employed a quasi-experimental design with interrupted time series (Khuder et al 2007).

As outlined in Section 17.2.2, the questions asked in systematic reviews that address complexity often go beyond asking whether a given intervention works, to ask how it might work, in which circumstances and for whom. Addressing these questions can require the inclusion of a range of different research designs. In particular, when evidence about the processes by which an intervention influences intermediate and final outcomes, as well as evidence on intervention acceptability and implementation, qualitative evidence is often included. Qualitative evidence can also identify evidence of unintended adverse effects which may not be reported in the main quantitative evaluation studies (Thomas and Harden 2008). Petticrew and colleagues' Table 1 summarizes each aspect of complexity and suggests which types of evidence might be most useful to address each issue. For example, when aiming to understand interactions between intervention and context, multicentre trials with stratified reporting, observational studies which provide evidence of mediators and moderators, and qualitative studies which observe behaviours and ask people about their understandings and experiences are suggested as being helpful study designs to include (Petticrew et al 2019). See also Noyes et al (2019) and Rehfuess et al (2019) for further information on matching study designs to research questions to address intervention complexity.

17.2.6 Summary of main points in this section

In systematic reviews addressing intervention complexity it may be more useful to address questions that seek to identify the circumstances where particular approaches to intervention might be more appropriate, effective and feasible than others, rather than simply asking 'does this intervention work?'

Logic models represent graphically the way that the intervention is thought to result in its outcomes and the range of interactions between it and its context.

Definitions of population, intervention and outcomes (i.e. the review and comparison PICOs) are sometimes quite broad, and need to consider how interventions and their effects can change across contexts.

Review authors need to consider whether and how to review evidence across multiple contexts, and in particular whether it makes sense, scientifically and practically (in terms of value to decision makers), to integrate them within the same review.

A range of different types of study may be relevant in systematic reviews addressing intervention complexity. Review authors should specify their questions in detail, identifying which types of study are needed for different aspects of their question(s).

For example, Chapter 3 contains detailed information on specifying review and comparison PICOs that is essential reading for review authors addressing intervention complexity. The illustration of a logic model in Figure 17.2.a should be read alongside the introduction to logic models in Chapter 2, Section 2.5.1. See also Chapter 2, Section 2.3 for discussion about breadth and depth in review questions. See the following for key references on the topics discussed in this section. On theory and logic models:

Anderson et al (2011), Kneale et al (2015), Rohwer et al (2017); on question formulation: Squires et al (2013), Higgins et al (2019), Petticrew et al (2019); on the TIDieR framework: Hoffman et al (2014); on the iCAT_SR tool: Lewin et al (2017); on the PRECIS-2 tool: Loudon et al (2015); on the CICI framework: Pfadenhauer et al (2017); on which types of study to include: Noyes et al (2019), Petticrew et al (2019), Rehfuess et al (2019).

17.3 Identification of evidence

There is relatively little detailed guidance on searching for evidence to include in reviews that focus on exploring intervention complexity (though see Chapter 4 and associated supplementary information (Noyes et al 2019)). A key challenge is that, as outlined in Sections 17.2.5 and 17.5, such reviews may include a wide range of qualitative and quantitative evidence to answer a range of questions. Searches for information on theory, context, processes and mechanisms (see Section 17.1.2) by which interventions are implemented and outcomes achieved may also be needed.

This requires some consideration of the location of such data sources (e.g. including sources outside the standard health literature), likely study designs, and the role of theory in guiding the review searches and methodological decisions. Policy documents, qualitative data, sources outside the standard health literature and discussion with a knowledgeable advisory group may also provide useful information. Kelly and colleagues outline in more detail the scoping and refining stages that are required for reviews that need to encompass intervention complexity (Kelly et al 2017). Indeed, including a separate 'mapping' phase within a systematic review, where a broader search is carried out to understand the extent of research activity, can be a highly valuable additional phase to add into the review process (Gough et al 2012). Some preparatory examination of this evidence may help to determine what form the intervention takes, what levels or structures it is aimed at changing, what its objectives are and how it is expected to bring about change (in effect, what is the underlying logic model). The iCAT_SR tool, which can help with characterizing the main dimensions of intervention complexity can also help here to determine what type of evidence needs to be located (see Box 17.1.a; Lewin et al 2017).

Booth and colleagues provide useful pointers on the value of 'cluster searching', which they define as a "systematic attempt, using a variety of search techniques, to identify papers or other research outputs that relate to a single study" (Booth et al 2013; p. 4). This means that a cluster of studies both directly and indirectly related to a 'core' effectiveness study are located to inform, for example, context, acceptability, feasibility and the processes by which the intervention influences the outcomes of interest (Booth et al 2013). Consideration of these issues is often critical for understanding intervention complexity, so review authors need to take account of all relevant information about included studies, even though it may be scattered between multiple publications. Beyond cluster searching, a wider search for qualitative and process evaluation studies that are unrelated to the included trials of interventions may help to create a bigger pool of evidence to synthesize, enabling review authors to address broader aspects such as intervention implementation (Noyes et al 2016b).

While this kind of search can inform the design and framing of the review, a comprehensive search is required to identify as much as possible of the body of evidence relevant to the review (see Chapter 4). As for any review, the search should be led by the review question, a detailed understanding of the PICO elements, and the review's eligibility criteria (Chapter 3).

17.3.1 Summary of main points in this section

Addressing intervention complexity in systematic reviews may involve searching for evidence on a range of issues other than effectiveness; it may involve searching for evidence on processes, mechanisms and theory.

The identification of relevant evidence should be driven by the review questions, and should consider the 'fitness for purpose' of different types of qualitative and quantitative evidence for answering those questions.

For further information see Chapter 4 and also the supplementary information associated with Noyes et al (2019). Table 1 in Petticrew et al (2019) also describes the relationship between different types of review questions, and the sort of evidence that might be sought to answer them. See the following for key references on the topics discussed in this section: Booth et al (2013), Brunton et al (2017).

17.4 Appraisal of evidence

It was noted in Section 17.2.5 that reviews addressing intervention complexity need to be focused on the concept of 'fitness for purpose' of evidence – that is, they need to consider what type of evidence is best suited to answer the research question(s). As previously described, these include questions about the implementation, feasibility and acceptability of interventions, and questions about the processes and mechanisms by which interventions bring about change. This has implications for the appraisal of evidence in a systematic review, and appropriate tools should be used for each type of evidence included, assessing the risk of bias for the way in which it is used in each review. When appraising studies that evaluate the effectiveness of an intervention, the Cochrane risk-of-bias tool should be used for trials (Chapter 8) and the ROBINS-I tool for non-randomized study designs (Chapter 25). Chapter 21 contains guidance on evaluating qualitative and implementation evidence.

17.5 Synthesis of evidence

Many useful sources provide further guidance on how to choose an analytic approach that takes account of intervention complexity. This section highlights texts for further reading in terms of which types of questions different methods might enable review authors to answer.

Higgins and colleagues separate synthesis methods into three levels: (i) those that are essentially descriptive, and help to compare and contrast studies and interventions with one another; (ii) those that might be considered 'standard' methods of meta-analysis – including meta-regression (see Chapter 10) – which enable review authors to examine possible moderators of effect at the study level; and (iii) more advanced methods, which include network meta-analysis (see Chapter 11), but go beyond this and encompass methods that enable review authors to examine intervention components, mechanisms of action, and complexities of the system into which the intervention is introduced (Higgins et al 2019).

At the outset, even when a statistical synthesis is planned, it is usually useful to begin the synthesis using non-quantitative methods, understanding the characteristics of the populations and interventions included in the review, and reviewing the outcome data from the available studies in a structured way. Informative tables and graphical tools can play an important role in this regard, assisting review authors to visualize and explore complexity. These include harvest plots, box-and-whisker plots, bubble plots, network diagrams and forest plots. See Chapters 9 and 12 for further discussion of these approaches.

Standard meta-analytic methods may not always be appropriate, since they do depend on reasonable comparability of both interventions and comparators – something that may not apply when synthesizing evidence with high heterogeneity. Chapter 3 considers in detail how to think about the comparability of, and categories within, interventions, populations and outcomes. However, where interventions and populations are judged sufficiently similar to answer questions which aggregate the findings from similar studies, then approaches such as standard meta-analysis, meta-regression or network meta-analysis may be appropriate, particularly when the mechanism of action is clearly understood (Viswanathana et al 2017).

Questions concerning the circumstances in which the intervention might work and the relative importance of different components of interventions require methods that explore between-study heterogeneity. Subgroup analysis and meta-regression enable review authors to investigate effect moderators with the usual caveats that pertain to such observational analyses (see Chapter 10). Caldwell and Welton describe alternative quantitative approaches to synthesis, which include 'component-based' meta-analysis where individual intervention components (or meaningful combinations of components) are modelled explicitly, thus enabling review authors to identify those components most (or least) associated with intervention success (Caldwell and Welton 2016).

When the review questions ask review authors to consider *how* interventions achieve their effect, other types of evidence, other than randomized trials, are vital to provide theory that identifies causal connections between intervention(s) and outcome(s). Logic models (see Section 17.2.1 and Chapter 2) can provide some rationale for the selection of factors to include in analysis, but the review may require an additional synthesis of qualitative evidence to elucidate the complexity adequately. This is especially the case when understanding differential intervention effects that require review authors to consider the perspectives and experiences of those receiving the intervention. See Chapter 21 for a detailed exploration of the methods available. While logic models aim to summarize how the interactions between intervention, participant and context may produce outcomes, specific causal pathways may be identified for testing. Causal chain analysis encompasses a range of methods that help review authors to do this (Kneale et al 2018), including meta-analytic path analysis and structural equation modelling (Tanner-Smith and Grant 2018), and model-based meta-analysis (Becker 2009). These types of analyses are rare in Cochrane Reviews, as methods are still developing and require relatively large datasets.

Integrating different types of data within the same analysis can be a challenging but powerful approach, often enabling the theories generated in synthesis of qualitative literature to be used to explore and explain heterogeneity between quantitative studies (Thomas et al 2004). Reviews with multiple components and analyses can address different questions relating to complexity often in a sequential way, with each component building on the findings of the previous one. Methods used include: mixed-methods synthesis (involving qualitative thematic synthesis, meta-analysis and cross-study synthesis); Bayesian synthesis (where qualitative studies are used to generate informative priors); and qualitative comparative analysis (QCA: a set-based method which uses Boolean algebra to juxtapose intervention components in configurational patterns; see Chapter 21 (Section 21.13) and (Thomas et al 2014)). Such analyses are *explanatory* analyses, to identify differential intervention effect, and also to explain *why* it occurs (Cook et al 1994). The example review given in Box 17.1.a is a multi-component review, which integrates different types of data in order better to understand differential intervention effects. It uses qualitative data from process evaluations to identify which intervention features were associated with successful implementation. It then uses the inferences generated in this analysis to explore heterogeneity between the results of randomized trials, using what might be considered 'standard' meta-analytic and meta-regression methods. It is important to bear in mind that the review question always comes first in these multi-component reviews: the decision to use process evaluation data in this way was driven by an understanding of the context within which these interventions are implemented. A different mix of data will be appropriate in different situations.

Finally, review authors may want to synthesize research to reach a better understanding of the dynamics of the wider system in which the intervention is introduced. Analytical methods can include some of those already mentioned – for combining diverse types of data – but may also include methods developed in systems science such as systems dynamics models and agent-based modelling (Luke and Stamatakis 2012).

17.5.1 Summary of main points in this section

Methods of synthesis can be understood at three levels: (i) those that help review authors describe studies and understand their similarities and differences; (ii) those that can be used to combine study findings in fairly standard ways; and (iii) more advanced approaches that include network meta-analysis for combining results across different interventions, but also enable review authors to examine intervention components, mechanisms of action and complexities of the system within which the intervention is introduced.

For further information about steps to follow before results are combined, review authors should consider the guidance in Chapter 9 to summarize studies and prepare for synthesis. Standard meta-analytical methods are outlined in Chapter 10, with Section 10.10 on investigating heterogeneity particularly relevant. Methods for undertaking network meta-analysis are outlined in Chapter 11.

17.6 Interpretation of evidence

As with other systematic reviews, reviews with a complexity focus are also aimed at helping decision makers. They therefore need a clear statement of findings and clear conclusions, taking account of the quality of the body of evidence. In this, it is important to refer to Chapters 14 and 15 and (Montgomery et al 2019) for further guidance on the use of GRADE when assessing intervention effects, and Chapter 21 when using CERQual to consider the confidence in synthesized qualitative findings.

For any review, consideration of how the review findings might apply in different contexts and settings is also important, and probably even more so when addressing intervention complexity. As noted in Section 17.1.3, the effects of an intervention may be significantly moderated by its context, and a review author may be able to describe which are the key aspects of context that the decision maker needs to consider, when deciding whether and how to implement the intervention in their setting. This can be done explicitly in the review by describing different scenarios (see Chapter 3) and by clearly describing the reasons for heterogeneity in results across the studies. One potential risk for reviews with a significant focus on complexity is that every implemention of every intervention can look different (although see the discussion on intervention function and form in Section 17.1.2.1); it is easy for a decision maker to conclude that, because there is no identical intervention or setting to the one in which they are interested, there is no evidence at all. However, as for any other review, it will be helpful to think about whether there are compelling reasons that the evidence from the review *cannot* be used to inform a new decision. In short, because of complexity (in interventions, and in their implementation) there will always be contextual differences, but this does not render the evidence unusable. Rather, review authors need to consider how this review-level evidence (about the effects of the intervention across different contexts) can be used to inform a new decision. For example, the review can show the range of effect size estimates, or how the types of anticipated and unanticipated outcomes vary, across settings in previous studies, thus giving the decision maker an idea of the range of responses that may be possible, as well as the possible moderating factors, in future implementations.

17.6.1 Reporting guidelines and systematic reviews

Systematic reviews that consider intervention complexity are themselves complex, integrating a wide range of different types of evidence using a range of methods. An extension of the PRISMA reporting guideline for systematic reviews has been developed with specific guidance for reporting the methods and results of 'complex interventions' (Guise et al 2017b, Guise et al 2017a), known as PRISMA-CI, which primarily focuses on quantitative evidence and complementing the TIDieR checklist for describing interventions (Hoffman et al 2014). The relevant extended items relate to clearly identifying the review as one covering 'complex interventions', providing justification for the specific elements of complexity under consideration in the review, and describing aspects of the complexity of the intervention or its context. The ENTREQ and eMERGe reporting guidelines are for reporting qualitative evidence syntheses and meta-ethnography (Tong et al 2012, France et al 2019). For mixed-method reviews no guidelines currently exist, but Flemming and colleagues suggest a 'pick and mix' approach to incorporate the appropriate reporting criteria from existing quantitative and qualitative reporting guidelines (see Chapter 21 for further details) (Flemming et al 2018). One of the challenges that review authors may meet when addressing complexity through incorporating a range of study designs beyond randomized trials is that GRADE assessments of evidence can generally turn out to be 'low', offering little assistance to readers in terms of understanding the relative confidence in the different studies included. See Montgomery et al (2019) for practical advice in this situation.

Increasing the quantity and range of evidence synthesized in a systematic review can make reports quite challenging (and lengthy) to read. Preparing a report that is sufficiently clear in its conclusions can take many rounds of redrafting, and it is also useful to obtain feedback from consumers and other stakeholders involved in the review (Chapter 1, Section 1.3.1). Intervention complexity can thus increase the resources needed at this phase of the review too, and it is essential to plan for this if the reporting of the review is to be sufficiently clear for it to be used to inform decisions. (See also Chapter 15 and online Chapter III.)

17.6.2 Summary of main points in this section

Synopsis It is important (as with any review) to consider decision makers' needs when conducting a review with a complexity focus. In practice, this means ensuring that there is a clear summary of how the findings vary across different contexts, and setting out the potential implications for decision making.

Involving users in the review process – particularly at the stage of defining the review question(s) – will help with producing a review that meets their needs.

Relevant reporting guidelines should be consulted to ensure that the methods and findings are accurately and transparently reported.

Further information in this **Handbook** Chapter 2 on question formulation; Chapters 14 and 15 on completing 'Summary of findings' tables, and drawing conclusions. See also Section 17.2.2 of this chapter for information on engagement with key users of the review in formulating its questions.

17.7 Chapter information

Authors: James Thomas, Mark Petticrew, Jane Noyes, Jacqueline Chandler, Eva Rehfuess, Peter Tugwell, Vivian A Welch

Acknowledgements: This chapter replaces Chapter 21 in the first edition of this *Handbook* (2008) and subsequent version 5.2. We would like to thank the previous chapter authors Rebecca Armstrong, Jodie Doyle, Helen Morgan and Elizabeth Waters.

Funding: VAW holds an Early Researcher Award (2014–2019) from the Ontario Government. JT is supported by the National Institute for Health Research (NIHR) Collaboration for Leadership in Applied Health Research and Care North Thames at Barts Health NHS Trust. The views expressed are those of the author(s) and not necessarily those of the NHS, the NIHR or the Department of Health.

17.8 References

Anderson L, Petticrew M, Rehfuess E, Armstrong R, Ueffing E, Baker P, Francis D, Tugwell P. Using logic models to capture complexity in systematic reviews. *Research Synthesis Methods* 2011; **2**: 33–42.

Becker B. Model-based meta-analysis. In: Cooper H, Hedges L, Valentine J, editors. *The Handbook of Research Synthesis and Meta-Analysis*. New York (NY): Russell Sage Foundation; 2009. pp. 377–395.

Blankenship KM, Friedman SR, Dworkin S, Mantell JE. Structural interventions: concepts, challenges and opportunities for research. *Journal of Urban Health* 2006; **83**: 59–72.

Booth A, Harris J, Croot E, Springett J, Campbell F, Wilkins E. Towards a methodology for cluster searching to provide conceptual and contextual "richness" for systematic reviews of complex interventions: case study (CLUSTER). *BMC Medical Research Methodology* 2013; **13**: 118.

Booth A, Moore G, Flemming K, Garside R, Rollins N, Tuncalp Ö, Noyes J. Taking account of context in systematic reviews and guidelines considering a complexity perspective. *BMJ Global Health* 2019a; **4**: e000840.

Booth A, Noyes J, Flemming K, Moore G, Tuncalp Ö, Shakibazadeh E. Formulating questions to explore complex interventions within qualitative evidence synthesis. *BMJ Global Health* 2019b; **4**: e001107.

Brunton G, Stansfield C, Caird J, Thomas J. Finding relevant studies. In: Gough D, Oliver S, Thomas J, editors. *An Introduction to Systematic Reviews*. 2nd ed. London: Sage; 2017.

Caldwell D, Welton N. Approaches for synthesising complex mental health interventions in meta-analysis. *Evidence-Based Mental Health* 2016; **19**: 16–21.

Campbell M, Fitzpatrick R, Haines A, Kinmonth A, Sandercock P, Spiegelhalter D, Tyrer P. Framework for design and evaluation of complex interventions to improve health. *BMJ* 2000; **321**: 694–696.

Christakis N, Fowler J. The spread of obesity in a large social network over 32 years. *New England Journal of Medicine* 2007; **357**: 370–379.

Cook TD, Cooper H, Cordray DS, Hartmann H, Hedges LV, Light RJ, Louis TA, Mosteller F. *Meta-Analysis for Explanation: A Casebook*. New York (NY): Russell Sage Foundation; 1994.

Craig P, Dieppe P, Macintyre S, Michie S, Petticrew M, Nazareth I. Developing and evaluating complex interventions: the new Medical Research Council guidance. *BMJ* 2008; **337**: a1655.

Craig P, Cooper C, Gunnell D, Haw S, Lawson K, Macintyre S, Ogilvie D, Petticrew M, Reeves B, Sutton M, Thompson S. Using natural experiments to evaluate population health interventions: new MRC guidance. *Journal of Epidemiology and Community Health* 2012; **66**: 1182–1186.

Craig P, Di Ruggiero E, Frohlich K, Mykhalovskiy E, White M, on behalf of the Canadian Institutes of Health Research (CIHR)–National Institute for Health Research (NIHR) Context Guidance Authors Group. Taking account of context in population health intervention research: guidance for producers, users and funders of research. Southampton; 2018.

Evans RE, Craig P, Hoddinott P, Littlecott H, Moore L, Murphy S, O'Cathain A, Pfadenhauer L, Rehfuess E, Segrott J, Moore G. When and how do 'effective' interventions need to be adapted and/or re-evaluated in new contexts? The need for guidance. *Journal of Epidemiology and Community Health* 2019; **73**: 481–482.

Flemming K, Booth A, Hannes K, Cargo M, Noyes J. Cochrane Qualitative and Implementation Methods Group guidance series-paper 6: reporting guidelines for qualitative, implementation, and process evaluation evidence syntheses. *Journal of Clinical Epidemiology* 2018; **97**: 79–85.

Fletcher A, Jamal F, Moore G, Evans RE, Murphy S, Bonell C. Realist complex intervention science: applying realist principles across all phases of the Medical Research Council framework for developing and evaluating complex interventions. *Evaluation (London, England : 1995)* 2016; **22**: 286–303.

France E, Cunningham M, Ring N, Uny I, Duncan E, Jepson R, Maxwell M, Roberts R, Turley R, Booth A, Britten N, Flemming K, Gallagher I, Garside R, Hannes K, Lewin S, Noblit G, Pope C, Thomas J, Vanstone M, Higginbottom GMA, Noyes J. Improving reporting of meta-ethnography: the eMERGe Reporting Guidance. *Journal of Advanced Nursing* 2019; **75**: 1126–1139.

Garside R, Pearson M, Hunt H, Moxham T, Anderson R. Identifying the key elements and interactions of a whole system approach to obesity prevention. London: National Institute for Health and Care Excellence; 2010.

Glenton C, Colvin CJ, Carlsen B, Swartz A, Lewin S, Noyes J, Rashidian A. Barriers and facilitators to the implementation of lay health worker programmes to improve access to maternal and child health: qualitative evidence synthesis. *Cochrane Database of Systematic Reviews* 2013; **10**: CD010414.

Gough D, Thomas J, Oliver S. Clarifying differences between review designs and methods. *Systematic Reviews* 2012; **1**: 28.

GRADE Working Group. Grading quality of evidence and strength of recommendations. *BMJ* 2004; **328**: 1490–1494.

Guise JM, Butler ME, Chang C, Viswanathan M, Pigott T, Tugwell P. AHRQ series on complex intervention systematic reviews paper 6: PRISMA-CI extension. *Journal of Clinical Epidemiololgy* 2017a; **90**: 43–50.

Guise JM, Butler M, Chang C, Viswanathan M, Pigott T, Tugwell P. AHRQ series on complex intervention systematic reviewsdpaper 7: PRISMA-CI elaboration and explanation. *Journal of Clinical Epidemiology* 2017b; **90**: 51–58.

Guyatt G, Oxman AD, Kunz R, Atkins D, Brozek J, Vist G, Alderson P, Glasziou P, Falck-Ytter Y, Schünemann HJ. GRADE guidelines: 2. Framing the question and deciding on important outcomes. *Journal of Clinical Epidemiology* 2011; **64**: 395–400.

Harris K, Kneale D, Lasserson T, McDonald V, Grigg J, Thomas J. School-based self management interventions for asthma in children and adolescents: amixed methods systematic review. *Cochrane Database of Systematic Reviews* 2018; **6**: CD011651.

Hawe P, Shiell A, Riley T. Complex interventions: how 'out of control' can a randomised controlled trial be? *BMJ* 2004; **328**: 1561–1563.

Hawe P, Shiell A, Riley T. Theorising interventions as events in systems. *American Journal of Community Psychology* 2009; **43**: 267–276.

Higgins JPT, López-López JA, Becker BJ, Davies SR, Dawson S, Grimshaw JM, McGuinness LA, Moore THM, Rehfuess E, Thomas J, Caldwell DM. Synthesizing quantitative evidence in systematic reviews of complex health interventions. *BMJ Global Health* 2019; **4**: e000858.

Hoffman T, Glasziou P, Boutron I, Milne R, Perera R, Moher D, Altman D, Barbour V, Macdonald H, Johnston M, Lamb S, Dixon-Woods M, McCulloch P, Wyatt J, Chan A-W, Michie S. Better reporting of interventions: template for intervention description and replication (TIDieR) checklist and guide. *BMJ* 2014; **348**: g1687.

Howick J, Glasziou P, Aronson JK. Evidence-based mechanistic reasoning. *Journal of the Royal Society of Medicine* 2010; **103**: 433–441.

Howick J, Glasziou P, Aronson JK. Problems with using mechanisms to solve the problem of extrapolation. *Theoretical Medicine and Bioethics* 2013; **34**: 275–291.

Kaufman J, Ryan R, Glenton C, Lewin S, Bosch-Capblanch X, Cartier Y, Cliff J, Oyo-Ita A, Ames H, Muloliwa AM, Oku A, Rada G, Hill S. Childhood vaccination communication outcomes unpacked and organized in a taxonomy to facilitate core outcome establishment. *Journal of Clinical Epidemiology* 2017; **84**: 173–184.

Kelly M, Noyes J, Kane R, Chang C, Uhl S, Robinson K, Springs S, Butler M, Guise J. AHRQ series on complex intervention systematic reviews-paper 2: defining complexity, formulating scope, and questions. *Journal of Clinical Epidemiology* 2017; **90**: 11–18.

Khuder SA, Milz S, Jordan T, Price J, Silvestri K, Butler P. The impact of a smoking ban on hospital admissions for coronary heart disease. *Preventive Medicine* 2007; **45**: 3–8.

Kneale D, Thomas J, Harris K. Developing and optimising the use of logic models in systematic reviews: exploring practice and good practice in the use of programme theory in reviews. *PloS One* 2015; **10**: e0142187.

Kneale D, Thomas J, Bangpan M, Waddington H, Gough D. Conceptualising causal pathways in systematic reviews of international development interventions through adopting a causal chain analysis approach. *Journal of Development Effectiveness* 2018; **10**: 422–437.

Krieger N. Who and what is a 'population'? Historical debates, current controversies, and implications for understanding "Population Health" and rectifying health inequities. *Milbank Quarterly* 2012; **90**: 634–681.

Lewin S, Hendry M, Chandler J, Oxman A, Michie S, Shepperd S, Reeves B, Tugwell P, Hannes K, Rehfuess E, Welch V, Mckenzie J, Burford B, Petkovic J, Anderson L, Harris J, Noyes J. Assessing the complexity of interventions within systematic reviews: development, content and use of a new tool (iCAT_SR). *BMC Medical Research Methodology* 2017; **17**: 76.

Loudon K, Treweek S, Sullivan F, Donnan P, Thorpe KE, Zwarenstein M. The PRECIS-2 tool: designing trials that are fit for purpose. *BMJ* 2015; **350**: h2147.

Luke D, Stamatakis K. Systems science methods in public health: dynamics, networks, and agents. *Annual Review of Public Health* 2012; **33**: 357–376.

Montgomery M, Movsisyan A, Grant S. Considerations of complexity in rating certainty of evidence in systematic reviews: a primer on using the GRADE approach in global health. *BMJ Global Health* 2019; **4**: e000848.

Moore G, Audrey S, Barker M, Bond L, Bonell C, Hardeman W, Moore L, O'Cathain A, Tinati T, Wight D, Baird J. Process evaluation of complex interventions: Medical Research Council guidance. *BMJ* 2015; **350**: h1258.

Nilsen P. Making sense of implementation theories, models and frameworks. *Implementation Science* 2015; **10**: 53.

Noyes J, Gough D, Lewin S, Mayhew A, Welch V. A research and development agenda for systematic reviews that ask complex questions about complex interventions. *Journal of Clinical Epidemiology* 2013; **66**: 1262–1270.

Noyes J, Hendry M, Booth A, Chandler J, Lewin S, Glenton C, Garside R. Current use was established and Cochrane guidance on selection of social theories for systematic reviews of complex interventions was developed. *Journal of Clinical Epidemiology* 2016a; **75**: 78–92.

Noyes J, Hendry M, Lewin S, Glenton C, Chandler J, Rashidian A. Qualitative 'trial-sibling' studies and 'unrelated' qualitative studies contributed to complex intervention reviews. *Journal of Clinical Epidemiology* 2016b; **74**: 133–143.

Noyes J, Booth A, Moore G, Flemming K, Tuncalp Ö, Shakibazadeh E. Synthesising quantitative and qualitative evidence to inform guidelines on complex interventions:

clarifying the purposes, designs and outlining some methods. *BMJ Global Health* 2019; **4** (Suppl 1): e000893.

Oliver S, Dickson K, Bangpan M, Newman M. Getting started with a review. In: Gough D, Oliver S, Thomas J, editors. *An Introduction to Systematic Reviews*. London: Sage Publications Ltd.; 2017. pp. 71–92

Pantoja T, Opiyo N, Lewin S, Paulsen E, Ciapponi A, Wiysonge CS, Herrera CA, Rada G, Peñaloza B, Dudley L, Gagnon MP, Garcia Marti S, Oxman AD. Implementation strategies for health systems in low-income countries: an overview of systematic reviews. *Cochrane Database of Systematic Reviews* 2017; **9**: CD011086.

Petticrew M. Time to rethink the systematic review catechism. *Systematic Reviews* 2015; **4**: 1.

Petticrew M, Knai C, Thomas J, Rehfuess E, Noyes J, Gerhardus A, Grimshaw J, Rutter H, McGill E. Implications of a complex systems perspective perspective for systematic reviews and guideline development in health decision-making. *BMJ Global Health* 2019; **4** (Suppl 1): e000899.

Pfadenhauer L, Gerhardus A, Mozygemba K, Bakke Lysdahl K, Booth A, Hofmann B, Wahlster P, Polus S, Burns J, Brereton L, Rehfuess E. Making sense of complexity in context and implementation: the Context and Implementation of Complex Interventions (CICI) framework. *Implementation Science* 2017; **12**: 21.

Pigott T, Noyes J, Umscheid CA, Myers E, Morton SC, Fu R, Sanders-Schmidler GD, Devine B, Murad MH, Kelly MP, Fonnesbeck C, Kahwati L, Beretvas SN. AHRQ series on complex intervention systematic reviews-paper 5: advanced analytic methods. *Journal of Clinical Epidemiology* 2017; **90**: 37–42.

Rehfuess EA, Stratil JM, Scheel IB, Portela A, Norris SL, Baltussen R. Integrating WHO norms and values into guideline and other health decisions: the WHO-INTEGRATE evidence to decision framework version 1.0. *BMJ Global Health* 2019; **4**: e000844.

Rohwer A, Pfadenhauer L, Burns J, Brereton L, Gerhardus A, Booth A, Oortwijn W, Rehfuess E. Series: Clinical Epidemiology in South Africa. Paper 3: Logic models help make sense of complexity in systematic reviews and health technology assessments. *Journal of Clinical Epidemiology* 2017; **83**: 37–47.

Squires J, Valentine J, Grimshaw J. Systematic reviews of complex interventions: framing the review question. *Journal of Clinical Epidemiology* 2013; **66**: 1215–1222.

Tanner-Smith E, Grant S. Meta-analysis of complex interventions. *Annual Review of Public Health* 2018; **391617**: 1–16.

Thomas J, Harden A, Oakley A, Sutcliffe K, Rees R, Brunton G, Kavanagh K. Integrating qualitative research with trials in systematic reviews. *BMJ* 2004; **328**: 1010–1012.

Thomas J, Harden A. Methods for the thematic synthesis of qualitative research in systematic reviews. *BMC Medical Research Methodology* 2008; **8**: 45.

Thomas J, O'Mara-Eves A, Brunton G. Using qualitative comparative analysis (QCA) in systematic reviews of complex interventions: a worked example. *Systematic Reviews* 2014; **3**: 67.

Tong A, Flemming K, McInnes E, Oliver S, Craig J. Enhancing transparency in reporting the synthesis of qualitative research: ENTREQ. *BMC Medical Research Methodology* 2012; **12**: 181.

Tugwell P, Petticrew M, Kristjansson E, Welch V, Ueffing E, Waters E, Bonnefoy J, Morgan A, Doohan E, Kelly M. Assessing equity in systematic reviews: realising the recommendations of the Commission on Social Determinants of Health. *BMJ* 2010; **341**: c4739.

Viswanathana M, McPheeters M, Hassan Murad M, Butler M, Devine E, Dyson M, Guise J, Kahwatia L, Milesh J, Morton S. AHRQ series on complex intervention systematic reviews paper 4: selecting analytic approaches. *Journal of Clinical Epidemiology* 2017; **90**: 28–36.

18

Patient-reported outcomes

Bradley C Johnston, Donald L Patrick, Tahira Devji, Lara J Maxwell, Clifton O Bingham III, Dorcas E Beaton, Maarten Boers, Matthias Briel, Jason W Busse, Alonso Carrasco-Labra, Robin Christensen, Bruno R da Costa, Regina El Dib, Anne Lyddiatt, Raymond W Ostelo, Beverley Shea, Jasvinder Singh, Caroline B Terwee, Paula R Williamson, Joel J Gagnier, Peter Tugwell, Gordon H Guyatt

KEY POINTS

- Summary data on patient-reported outcomes (PROs) are important to ensure health-care decision makers are informed about the outcomes most meaningful to patients.
- Authors of systematic reviews that include PROs should have a good understanding of how patient-reported outcome measures (PROMs) are developed, including the constructs they are intended to measure, their reliability, validity and responsiveness.
- Authors should pre-specify at the protocol stage a hierarchy of preferred PROMs to measure the outcomes of interest.

18.1 Introduction to patient-reported outcomes

18.1.1 What are patient-reported outcomes?

A **patient-reported outcome** (PRO) is "any report of the status of a patient's health condition that comes directly from the patient without interpretation of the patient's response by a clinician or anyone else" (FDA 2009). PROs are one of several clinical outcome assessment methods that complement biomarkers, measures of morbidity (e.g. stroke, myocardial infarction), burden (e.g. hospitalization), and survival used and reported in clinical trials and non-randomized studies (FDA 2018).

Patient-reported outcome measures (PROMs) are instruments that are used to measure the PROs, most often self-report questionnaires. Although investigators

This chapter should be cited as: Johnston BC, Patrick DL, Devji T, Maxwell LJ, Bingham III CO, Beaton D, Boers M, Briel M, Busse JW, Carrasco-Labra A, Christensen R, da Costa BR, El Dib R, Lyddiatt A, Ostelo RW, Shea B, Singh J, Terwee CB, Williamson PR, Gagnier JJ, Tugwell P, Guyatt GH. Chapter 18: Patient-reported outcomes. In: Higgins JPT, Thomas J, Chandler J, Cumpston M, Li T, Page MJ, Welch VA (editors). *Cochrane Handbook for Systematic Reviews of Interventions*. 2nd Edition. Chichester (UK): John Wiley & Sons, 2019: 479–492.

may address patient-relevant outcomes via proxy reports or observations from caregivers, health professionals, or parents and guardians, these are not PROMs but rather clinician-reported or observer-reported outcomes (Powers et al 2017).

PROs provide crucial information for patients and clinicians facing choices in health care. Conducting systematic reviews and meta-analyses including PROMs and interpreting their results is not straightforward, and guidance can help review authors address the challenges.

The objectives of this chapter are to: (i) describe the category of outcomes known as PROs and their importance for healthcare decision making; (ii) illustrate the key issues related to reliability, validity and responsiveness that systematic review authors should consider when including PROs; and (iii) address the structure and content (domains, items) of PROs and provide guidance for combining information from different PROs. This chapter outlines a step-by-step approach to addressing each of these elements in the systematic review process. The focus is on the use of PROs in randomized trials, and what is crucial in this context when selecting PROs to include in a meta-analysis. The principles also apply to systematic reviews of non-randomized studies addressing PROs (e.g. dealing with adverse drug reactions).

18.1.2 Why patient-reported outcomes?

PROs provide patients' perspectives regarding treatment benefit and harm, directly measure treatment benefit and harm beyond survival, major morbid events and biomarkers, and are often the outcomes of most importance to patients and families.

Self-reported outcomes often correlate poorly with physiological and other outcomes such as performance-related outcomes, clinician-reported outcomes, or biomarkers. In asthma, Yohannes and colleagues (Yohannes et al 1998) found that variability in exercise capacity contributed to only 3% of the variability in breathing problems on a patient self-report questionnaire. In chronic obstructive pulmonary disease (COPD), the reported correlations between forced expiratory volume (FEV1) and quality of life (QoL) are weak ($r = 0.14$ to 0.41) (Jones 2001). In peripheral arterial occlusive disease, correlations between haemodynamic variables and QoL are low (e.g. $r = -0.17$ for QoL pain subscale and Doppler sonographic ankle/brachial pressure index) (Müller-Bühl et al 2003). In osteoarthritis, there is discordance between radiographic arthritis and patient-reported pain (Hannan et al 2000). These findings emphasize the often important limitations of biomarkers for informing the impact of interventions on the patient experience or the patient's perspective of disease (Bucher et al 2014).

PROs are essential when externally observable patient-important outcomes are rare or unavailable. They provide the only reasonable strategy for evaluating treatment impact of many conditions including pain syndromes, fatigue, disorders such as irritable bowel syndrome, sexual dysfunction, and emotional function and adverse effects such as nausea and anxiety for which physiological measurements are limited or unavailable.

18.2 Formulation of the review

In this section we describe PROMs in more detail and discuss some issues to consider when deciding which PROMs to address in a review.

A common term used in the health status measurement literature is **construct**. Construct refers to what PROMs are trying to measure, the concept that defines the PROM such as pain, physical function or depressive mood. Constructs are the postulated attributes of the person that investigators hope to capture with the PROM (Cronbach and Meehl 1955).

Many different ways exist to label and classify PROMs and the constructs they measure. For instance, reports from patients include signs (observable manifestations of a condition), sensations (most commonly classified as symptoms that may be attributable to disease and/or treatment), behaviours and abilities (commonly classified as functional status), general perceptions or feelings of well-being, general health, satisfaction with treatment, reports of adverse effects, adherence to treatment, and participation in social or community events and health-related quality of life (HRQoL).

Investigators can use different approaches to capture patient perspectives, including interviews, self-completed questionnaires, diaries, and via different interfaces such as hand-held devices or computers. Review authors must identify the postulated constructs that are important to patients, and then determine the extent to which the PROMs used and reported in the trials address those constructs, the characteristics (measurement properties) of the PROMs used, and communicate this information to the reader (Calvert et al 2013).

Focusing now on HRQoL, an important PRO, some approaches attempt to cover the full range of health-related patient experience – including, for instance, self-care, and physical, emotional and social function – and thus enable comparisons between the impact of treatments on HRQoL across diseases or conditions. Authors often call these approaches **generic instruments** (Guyatt et al 1989, Patrick and Deyo 1989). These include utility measures such as the EuroQol five dimensions questionnaire (EQ-5D) or the Health Utilities Index (HUI). They also include health profiles such as the Short Form 36-item (SF-36) or the SF-12; these have come to dominate the field of health profiles (Tarlov et al 1989, Ware et al 1995, Ware et al 1996). An alternative approach to measuring PROs is to focus on much more specific constructs: PROMs may be specific to function (e.g. sleep, sexual function), to a disease (e.g. asthma, heart failure), to a population (e.g. the frail elderly) or to a symptom (pain, fatigue) (Guyatt et al 1989, Patrick and Deyo 1989). Another domain-specific measurement system now receiving attention is Patient-Reported Outcomes Measurement Instruments System (PROMIS). PROMIS is a National Institutes of Health funded PROM programme using computerized adaptive testing from large item banks for over 70 domains (e.g. anxiety, depression, pain, social function) relevant to wide variety of chronic diseases (Cella et al 2007, Witter 2016, PROMIS 2018).

Authors often use the terms 'quality of life', 'health status', 'functional status', 'HRQoL' and 'well-being' loosely and interchangeably. Systematic review authors must therefore consider carefully the constructs that the PROMs have actually measured. To do so, they may need to examine the items or questions included in a PROM.

Another issue to consider is whether and how the individual items of instruments are weighted. A number of approaches can be used to arrive at weights (Wainer 1976). Utility instruments designed for economic analysis put greater emphasis on item weighting, attempting ultimately to present HRQoL as a continuum anchored between death and full health. Many PROMs weight items equally in the calculation of the overall score, a reasonable approach. Readers can refer to a helpful overview of classical test theory

Table 18.2.a Checklist for describing and assessing PROMs in clinical trials. Adapted from Guyatt et al (1997)

1) **What were the PROMs assessing?**
   1.1. What concepts or constructs were the PROMs used in the study assessing?
   1.2. What rationale (if any) for selection of concepts or constructs did the authors provide?
   1.3. Were patients involved in the development (e.g. focus groups, surveys) of PROMs?
2) **Omissions**
   2.1. Were there any important aspects of patient's health (e.g. symptoms, function, perceptions) or quality of life (e.g. overall evaluation, satisfaction with life) that were not reported in this study? A search for 'Core Outcome Sets' for condition would be helpful (see Section 18.4.1).
3) **What were the measurement strategies?**
   3.1. Did investigators use instruments that yield a single indicator or index number, or a profile, or a battery of instruments?
   3.2. Did investigators use specific or generic measures, or both?
4) **Did the instruments work in the way they were supposed to work – validity?**
   4.1. Was evidence of prior validation for use in the current population presented?
5) **Did the instruments work in the way they were supposed to work – responsiveness?**
   5.1 Are the PROMs able to detect important change in patient status, even if those changes are small?
6) **Can you make the magnitude of effect (if any) understandable to readers – interpretability?**
   6.1 If the intervention has had an apparent impact on a PROM, can you provide users with a sense of whether that effect is trivial, small but important, moderate, or large?

and item response theory to understand better the merits and limitations of weighting (Cappelleri et al 2014).

Table 18.2.a presents a framework for considering and reporting PROMs in clinical trials, including their constructs and how they were measured. A good understanding of the PROMs identified in the included studies for a review is essential to appropriate analysis of outcomes across studies, and appraisal of the certainty of the evidence.

18.3 Appraisal of evidence

18.3.1 Measurement of PROs: single versus multiple time-points

To be useful, instruments must be able to distinguish between situations of interest (Boers et al 1998). When results are available for only one time-point (e.g. for classification), the key issue for PROMs is to be able to distinguish individuals with more desirable scores from those whose scores are less desirable. The key measurement issues in such contexts are reliability and cross-sectional construct validity (Kirshner and Guyatt 1985, Beaton et al 2016).

In longitudinal studies such as randomized trials, investigators usually obtain measurements at multiple time-points, for example at the beginning of the trial and again following administration of the interventions. In this context, PROMs must be able to distinguish those who have experienced positive changes over time from those who have experienced negative changes, those who experienced less positive change, or those who experienced no change at all, and to estimate accurately the magnitude of those changes. The key measurement issues in these contexts – sometimes referred to as evaluative – are responsiveness and longitudinal construct validity (Kirshner and Guyatt 1985, Beaton et al 2016).

18.3.2 Reliability

Intuitively, many think of reliability as obtaining the same scores on repeated administration of an instrument in stable respondents. That stability (or lack of measurement error) is important, but not sufficient. Satisfactory instruments must be able to distinguish between individuals despite measurement error.

Reliability statistics therefore look at the ratio of the variability between respondents (typically the numerator of a reliability statistic) and the total variability (the variability between respondents and the variability within respondents). The most commonly used statistics to measure reliability is a kappa coefficient for categorical data, a weighted kappa coefficient for ordered categorical data, and an intraclass correlation coefficient for continuous data (de Vet et al 2011).

Limitations in reliability will be of most concern for the review author when randomized trials have failed to establish the superiority of an experimental intervention over a comparator intervention. The reason is that lack of reliability cannot create intervention effects that are not present, but can obscure true intervention effects as a result of random error. When a systematic review does not find evidence that an intervention affects a PROM, review authors should consider whether this may be due to poor reliability (e.g. if reliability coefficients are less than 0.7) rather than lack of an effect.

18.3.3 Validity

Validity has to do with whether the instrument is measuring what it is intended to measure. *Content validity* assessment involves patient and clinician evaluation of the relevance and comprehensiveness of the content contained in the measures, usually obtained through qualitative research with patients and families (Johnston et al 2012). Guidance is available on the assessment of content validity for PROMs used in clinical trials (Patrick et al 2011a, Patrick et al 2011b).

Construct validity involves examining the logical relationships that should exist between assessment measures. For example, in patients with COPD, we would expect that patients with lower treadmill exercise capacity generally will have more dyspnoea (shortness of breath) in daily life than those with higher exercise capacity, and we would expect to see substantial correlations between a new measure of emotional function and existing emotional function questionnaires.

When we are interested in evaluating change over time – that is, in the context of evaluation when measures are available both before and after an intervention – we examine correlations of change scores. For example, patients with COPD who deteriorate in their treadmill exercise capacity should, in general, show increases in dyspnea, while those whose exercise capacity improves should experience less dyspnea. Similarly, a new emotional function instrument should show concurrent improvement in patients who improve on existing measures of emotional function. The technical term for this process is testing an instrument's longitudinal construct validity. Review authors should look for evidence of the validity of PROMs used in clinical studies. Unfortunately, reports of randomized trials using PROMs seldom review or report evidence of the validity of the instruments they use, but when these are available review authors can gain some reassurance from statements (backed by citations) that the questionnaires have been previously validated, or could seek additional published information on named PROMs. Ideally, review authors should look for systematic reviews of the measurement properties of the instruments in question. The Consensus-based standards for the selection of health measurement instruments (COSMIN) website offers a database of such reviews (COSMIN Database of Systematic Reviews). In addition, the Patient-Reported Outcomes and Quality of Life Instruments Database (PROQOLID) provides documentation of the measurement properties for over 1000 PROs.

If the validity of the PROMs used in a systematic review remains unclear, review authors should consider whether the PROM is an appropriate measure of the review's planned outcomes, or whether it should be excluded (ideally, this would be considered at the protocol stage), and any included results should be interpreted with appropriate caution. For instance, in a review of flavonoids for haemorrhoids, authors of primary trials used PROMs to ascertain patients' experience with pain and bleeding (Alonso-Coello et al 2006). Although the wording of these PROMs was simple and made intuitive sense, the absence of formal validation raises concerns over whether these measures can give meaningful data to distinguish between the intervention and its comparators.

A final concern about validity arises if the measurement instrument is used with a different population, or in a culturally and linguistically different environment from the one in which it was developed. Ideally, PROMs should be re-validated in each study, but systematic review authors should be careful not to be too critical on this basis alone.

18.3.4 Responsiveness

In the evaluative context, randomized trial participant measurements are typically available before and after the intervention. PROMs must therefore be able to distinguish among patients who remain the same, improve or deteriorate over the course of the trial (Guyatt et al 1987, Revicki et al 2008). Authors often refer to this measurement property as responsiveness; alternatives are sensitivity to change or ability to detect change.

As with reliability, responsiveness becomes an issue when a meta-analysis suggests no evidence of a difference between an intervention and control. An instrument with a poor ability to measure change can result in false-negative results, in which the intervention improves how patients feel, yet the instrument fails to detect the improvement. This problem may be particularly salient for generic questionnaires that have the advantage of covering all relevant areas of HRQoL, but the disadvantage of covering each area superficially or without the detail required for the particular context of use (Wiebe et al 2003, Johnston et al 2016a). Thus, in studies that show no difference in PROMs between intervention and control, lack of instrument responsiveness is one possible reason. Review authors should look for published evidence of responsiveness. If there is an absence of prior evidence of responsiveness, this represents a potential reason for being less certain about evidence from a series of randomized trials. For instance, a systematic review of respiratory muscle training in COPD found no effect on patients' function. However, two of the four studies that assessed a PROM used instruments without established responsiveness (Smith et al 1992).

18.3.5 Reporting bias

Studies focusing on PROs often use a number of PROMs to measure the same or similar constructs. This situation creates a risk of selective outcome reporting bias, in which trial authors select for publication a subset of the PROMs on the basis of the results; that is, those that indicate larger intervention effects or statistically significant P values (Kirkham et al 2010). Further detailed discussion of selective outcome reporting is presented in Chapter 7 (Section 7.2.3.3); see also Chapter 8 (Section 8.7).

Systematic reviews focusing on PROs should be alert to this problem. When only a small number of eligible studies have reported results for a particular PROM, particularly if the PROM is mentioned in a study protocol or methods section, or if it is a salient outcome that one would expect conscientious investigators to measure, review authors should note the possibility of reporting bias and consider rating down certainty in evidence as part of their GRADE assessment (see Chapter 14) (Guyatt et al 2011). For instance, authors of a systematic review evaluating the responsiveness of PROs among patients with rare lysosomal storage diseases encountered eligible studies in which the use of a PRO was described in the methods, but there were either no data or limited PRO data in the results. When authors did present some information about results, the reports sometimes included only interim or end-of-study results. Such instances are likely to be an indication of selective outcome reporting bias: it seems implausible that, if results showed apparent benefit on PROs, investigators would mention a PRO in the methods and subsequently fail to report results (Johnston et al 2016b).

18.4 Synthesis and interpretation of evidence

18.4.1 Selecting from multiple PROMs

The definition of a particular PRO may vary between studies, and this may justify use of different instruments (i.e. different PROMs). Even if the definitions are similar (or if, as happens more commonly, the investigators do not define the PRO), the investigators may choose different instruments to measure the PROs, especially if there is a lack of consensus on which instrument to use (Prinsen et al 2016).

When trials report results for more than one instrument, authors should – independent of knowledge of the results and ideally at the protocol stage – create a hierarchy based on reported measurement properties of PROMs (Tendal et al 2011, Christensen et al 2015), considering a detailed understanding of what each PROM measures (see Table 18.2.a), and its demonstrated reliability, validity, responsiveness and interpretability (see Section 18.3). This will allow authors to decide which instruments will be used for data extraction and synthesis. For example, the following instruments are all validated, patient-reported pain instruments that an investigator may use in a primary study to assess an intervention's usefulness for treating pain:

- 7-item Integrated Pain Score;
- 10-point Visual Analogue Scale for Pain;
- 20-item McGill Pain Questionnaire; and
- 56-item Brief Pain Inventory (PROQOLID 2018).

In some clinical fields core outcome sets are available to guide the use of appropriate PROs (COMET 2018). Only rarely do these include specific guidance on which PROMs are preferable, although methods have been proposed for this (Prinsen et al 2016). Within the field of rheumatology, the Outcome Measures in Rheumatology (OMERACT) initiative has developed a conceptual framework known as OMERACT Filter 2.0 to identify both core domain sets (what outcome should be measured) and core outcome measurement sets (how the outcome should be measured, i.e. which PROM to use) (Boers et al 2014). This is a generic framework and applicable to those developing core outcome sets outside the field of rheumatology.

As an example of a pre-defined hierarchy, for knee osteoarthritis, OMERACT has used a published hierarchy based on responsiveness for extraction of PROMs evaluating pain and physical function for performing systematic reviews (Juhl et al 2012).

Authors should decide in advance whether to exclude PROMs not included in the hierarchy, or to include additional measures where none of the preferred measures are available.

18.4.2 Synthesizing data from multiple PROMs

While a hierarchy can be helpful in identifying the review authors' preferred measures, and excluding some measures considered inappropriate, it remains likely that authors will encounter studies using several different PROMs to measure a given construct, either within one study or across multiple studies. Authors must then decide how to approach synthesis of multiple measures, and among them, consider which measures to include in a single meta-analysis on a particular construct (Tendal et al 2011, Christensen et al 2015).

When deciding if statistical synthesis is appropriate, review authors will often find themselves reading between the lines to try and get a precise notion of the underlying construct for the PROMs used. They may have to consult the articles that describe the development and prior use of PROMs included in the primary studies, or look at the instruments to understand the concepts being measured.

For example, authors of a Cochrane Review of cognitive behavioural therapy (CBT) for tinnitus included HRQoL as a PRO (Martinez-Devesa et al 2007), assessed with different PROMs: four trials using the Tinnitus Handicap Questionnaire; one trial the Tinnitus Questionnaire; and one trial the Tinnitus Reaction Questionnaire. Review authors compared the content of the PROMs and concluded that statistical pooling was appropriate.

The most compelling evidence regarding the appropriateness of including different PROMs in the same meta-analysis would come from a finding of substantial correlations between the instruments. For example, the two major instruments used to measure HRQoL in patients with COPD are the Chronic Respiratory Questionnaire (CRQ) and the St. George's Respiratory Questionnaire (SGRQ). Correlations between the two questionnaires in individual studies have varied from 0.3 to 0.6 in both cross-sectional (correlations at a point in time) and longitudinal (correlations of change) comparisons (Rutten-van Mölken et al 1999, Singh et al 2001, Schünemann et al 2003, Schünemann et al 2005). In one study, investigators examined the correlations between group mean changes in the CRQ and SGRQ in 15 studies including 23 patient groups and found a correlation of 0.88 (Puhan et al 2006).

Ideally, the decision to combine scores from different PROMs would be based not only on their measuring similar constructs but also on their satisfactory validity, and, depending on whether before and after intervention or only after intervention measurements were available, and on their responsiveness or reliability. For example, extensive evidence of validity is available for both CRQ and the SGRQ. The CRQ has, however, proved more responsive than the SGRQ: in an investigation that included 15 studies using both instruments, standardized response means of the CRQ (median 0.51, interquartile range (IQR) 0.19 to 0.98) were significantly higher ($P < 0.001$) than those associated with the SGRQ (median 0.26, IQR −0.03 to 0.40) (Puhan et al 2006). As a result, pooling results from trials using these two instruments could lead to underestimates of intervention effect in studies using the SGRQ (Puhan et al 2006, Johnston et al 2010). This can be tested using a sensitivity analysis of studies using the more responsive versus less responsive instrument.

Usually, detailed data such as those described above will be unavailable. Investigators must then fall back on intuitive decisions about the extent to which different instruments are measuring the same underlying concept. For example, the authors of a meta-analysis of psychosocial interventions in the treatment of pre-menstrual syndrome faced a profusion of outcome measures, with 25 PROMs used in their nine eligible studies (Busse et al 2009).

Table 18.4.a Examples of potentially combinable PROMs measuring similar constructs from a review of psychosocial interventions in the treatment of pre-menstrual syndrome (Busse et al 2009). Reproduced with permission of Karger

Anxiety
Beck Anxiety Inventory
Menstrual Symptom Diary-Anxiety domain
State and Trait Anxiety Scale-State Anxiety domain
Behavioural Changes
Menstrual Distress Questionnaire-Behavioural Changes domain
Pre-Menstrual Assessment Form-Social Withdrawal domain
Depression
Beck Depression Inventory
Depression Adjective Checklist State-Depression domain
General Contentment Scale-Depression and Well-being domain
Menstrual Symptom Diary-Depression domain
Menstrual Distress Questionnaire-Negative Affect domain
Interference
Global Rating of Interference Daily Record of Menstrual Complaints-Interference domain
Sexual Relations
Martial Satisfaction Inventory-Sexual Dissatisfaction domain
Social Adjustment Scale-Sexual Relationship domain
Water Retention and Oedema
Menstrual Distress Questionnaire-Water Retention domain
Menstrual Symptom Diary-Oedema domain

They dealt with this problem by having two experienced clinical researchers, knowledgeable to the study area and not otherwise involved in the review, independently examine each instrument – including all domains – and group 16 PROMs into six discrete conceptual categories. Any discrepancies were resolved by discussion to achieve consensus. Table 18.4.a details the categories and the included instruments within each category.

Authors should follow the guidance elsewhere in this *Handbook* on appropriate methods of synthesizing different outcome measures in a single analysis (Chapter 10) and interpreting these results in a way that is most meaningful for decision makers (Chapter 15).

Having decided which PROs and subsequently PROMs to include in a meta-analysis, review authors face the challenge of ensuring the results they present are interpretable to their target audiences. For instance, if told that the mean difference between rehabilitation and standard care in a series of randomized trials using the CRQ was 1.0 (95% CI 0.6 to 1.5), many readers would be uncertain whether this represents a trivial, small but important, moderate, or large effect (Guyatt et al 1998, Brozek et al 2006, Schünemann et al 2006). Similarly, the interpretation of a standardized mean difference is challenging for most (Johnston et al 2016b). Chapter 15 summarizes the various statistical presentation approaches that can be used to improve the interpretability of summary estimates. Further, for those interested in additional guidance, the GRADE working group summarizes five presentation approaches to enhancing the interpretability of pooled estimates of PROs when preparing 'Summary of findings' tables (Thorlund et al 2011, Guyatt et al 2013, Johnston et al 2013).

18.5 Chapter information

Authors: Bradley C Johnston, Donald L Patrick, Tahira Devji, Lara J Maxwell, Clifton O Bingham III, Dorcas Beaton, Maarten Boers, Matthias Briel, Jason W Busse, Alonso Carrasco-Labra, Robin Christensen, Bruno R da Costa, Regina El Dib, Anne Lyddiatt, Raymond W Ostelo, Beverley Shea, Jasvinder Singh, Caroline B Terwee, Paula R Williamson, Joel J Gagnier, Peter Tugwell, Gordon H Guyatt

Funding: DB is on the executive of OMERACT (Outcome Measurement in Rheumatology) (unpaid position). OMERACT is supported through partnership with multiple industries and OMERACT funds support staff to assist in the development of methods and materials around core outcome set development that influenced this chapter. The Parker Institute, Bispebjerg and Frederiksberg Hospital (RC) is supported by a core grant from the Oak Foundation (OCAY-13-309). TD has received funding from the Canadian Institutes of Health Research for research related to patient-reported outcomes and minimal important differences. RWO received research grants (paid to the Institute) from Netherlands Organisation Scientific Research (NWO); Netherlands Organisation for Health Research and Development (ZonMw); Wetenschappelijk College Fysiotherapie/KNGF Ned Ver Manuele Therapie; European Chiropractors' Union; Amsterdam Movement Sciences; National Health Care Institute (ZiN); De Friesland Zorgverzekeraar. PRW's work within the COMET Initiative is funded through grant NIHR Senior Investigator Award (NF-SI_0513-10025).

18.6 References

Alonso-Coello P, Zhou Q, Martinez-Zapata MJ, Mills E, Heels-Ansdell D, Johanson JF, Guyatt G. Meta-analysis of flavonoids for the treatment of haemorrhoids. *British Journal of Surgery* 2006; **93**: 909–920.

Beaton D, Boers M, Tugwell P. Assessment of health outcomes. In: Firestein G, Budd R, Gabriel SE, McInnes IB, O'Dell J, editors. *Kelley and Firestein's Textbook of Rheumatology*. 10th ed. Philadelphia (PA): Elsevier; 2016. pp. 496–508.

Boers M, Brooks P, Strand CV, Tugwell P. The OMERACT filter for Outcome Measures in Rheumatology. *Journal of Rheumatology* 1998; **25**: 198–199.

Boers M, Kirwan JR, Wells G, Beaton D, Gossec L, d'Agostino MA, Conaghan PG, Bingham CO, 3rd, Brooks P, Landewe R, March L, Simon LS, Singh JA, Strand V, Tugwell P. Developing core outcome measurement sets for clinical trials: OMERACT filter 2.0. *Journal of Clinical Epidemiology* 2014; **67**: 745–753.

Brozek JL, Guyatt GH, Schünemann HJ. How a well-grounded minimal important difference can enhance transparency of labelling claims and improve interpretation of a patient reported outcome measure. *Health and Quality of Life Outcomes* 2006; **4**: 69.

Bucher HC, Cook DJ, Holbrook AM, Guyatt G. Chapter 13.4: Surrogate outcomes. In: Guyatt G, Rennie D, Meade MO, Cook DJ, editors. *Users' Guides to the Medical Literature: A Manual for Evidence-Based Clinical Practice*. 3rd ed. New York: McGraw-Hill Education; 2014.

Busse JW, Montori VM, Krasnik C, Patelis-Siotis I, Guyatt GH. Psychological intervention for premenstrual syndrome: a meta-analysis of randomized controlled trials. *Psychotherapy and Psychosomatics* 2009; **78**: 6–15.

Calvert M, Blazeby J, Altman DG, Revicki DA, Moher D, Brundage MD. Reporting of patient-reported outcomes in randomized trials: the CONSORT PRO extension. *JAMA* 2013; **309**: 814–822.

Cappelleri JC, Jason Lundy J, Hays RD. Overview of classical test theory and item response theory for the quantitative assessment of items in developing patient-reported outcomes measures. *Clinical Therapeutics* 2014; **36**: 648–662.

Cella D, Yount S, Rothrock N, Gershon R, Cook K, Reeve B, Ader D, Fries JF, Bruce B, Rose M. The Patient-Reported Outcomes Measurement Information System (PROMIS): progress of an NIH Roadmap cooperative group during its first two years. *Medical Care* 2007; **45**: S3–S11.

Christensen R, Maxwell LJ, Jüni P, Tovey D, Williamson PR, Boers M, Goel N, Buchbinder R, March L, Terwee CB, Singh JA, Tugwell P. Consensus on the need for a hierarchical list of patient-reported pain outcomes for metaanalyses of knee osteoarthritis trials: an OMERACT objective. *Journal of Rheumatology* 2015; **42**: 1971–1975.

COMET. Core Outcome Measures in Effectiveness Trials 2018. http://www.comet-initiative.org.

Cronbach LJ, Meehl PE. Construct validity in psychological tests. *Psychological Bulletin* 1955; **52**: 281–302.

de Vet HCW, Terwee CB, Mokkink LB, Knol DL. *Measurement in Medicine: A Practical Guide*. Cambridge: Cambridge University Press; 2011.

FDA. Guidance for Industry: Patient-Reported Outcome Measures: Use in Medical Product Development to Support Labeling Claims. Rockville, MD; 2009. http://www.fda.gov/downloads/Drugs/GuidanceComplianceRegulatoryInformation/Guidances/UCM193282.pdf

FDA. Clinical Outcome Assessment Program Silver Spring, MD: US Food and Drug Administration; 2018. https://www.fda.gov/Drugs/DevelopmentApprovalProcess/DrugDevelopmentToolsQualificationProgram/ucm284077.htm.

Guyatt G, Walter S, Norman G. Measuring change over time: assessing the usefulness of evaluative instruments. *Journal of Chronic Diseases* 1987; **40**: 171–178.

Guyatt G, Oxman AD, Akl EA, Kunz R, Vist G, Brozek J, Norris S, Falck-Ytter Y, Glasziou P, DeBeer H, Jaeschke R, Rind D, Meerpohl J, Dahm P, Schünemann HJ. GRADE guidelines: 1. Introduction-GRADE evidence profiles and summary of findings tables. *Journal of Clinical Epidemiology* 2011; **64**: 383–394.

Guyatt GH, Veldhuyzen Van Zanten SJ, Feeny DH, Patrick DL. Measuring quality of life in clinical trials: a taxonomy and review. *CMAJ: Canadian Medical Association Journal* 1989; **140**: 1441–1448.

Guyatt GH, Naylor CD, Juniper E, Heyland DK, Jaeschke R, Cook DJ. Users' guides to the medical literature. XII. How to use articles about health-related quality of life. Evidence-Based Medicine Working Group. *JAMA* 1997; **277**: 1232–1237.

Guyatt GH, Juniper EF, Walter SD, Griffith LE, Goldstein RS. Interpreting treatment effects in randomised trials. *BMJ* 1998; **316**: 690–693.

Guyatt GH, Thorlund K, Oxman AD, Walter SD, Patrick D, Furukawa TA, Johnston BC, Karanicolas P, Akl EA, Vist G, Kunz R, Brozek J, Kupper LL, Martin SL, Meerpohl JJ, Alonso-Coello P, Christensen R, Schünemann HJ. GRADE guidelines: 13. Preparing summary of findings tables and evidence profiles-continuous outcomes. *Journal of Clinical Epidemiology* 2013; **66**: 173–183.

Hannan MT, Felson DT, Pincus T. Analysis of the discordance between radiographic changes and knee pain in osteoarthritis of the knee. *Journal of Rheumatology* 2000; **27**: 1513–1517.

Johnston BC, Thorlund K, Schünemann HJ, Xie F, Murad MH, Montori VM, Guyatt GH. Improving the interpretation of quality of life evidence in meta-analyses: the application of minimal important difference units. *Health and Quality of Life Outcomes* 2010; **8**: 116.

Johnston BC, Thorlund K, da Costa BR, Furukawa TA, Guyatt GH. New methods can extend the use of minimal important difference units in meta-analyses of continuous outcome measures. *Journal of Clinical Epidemiology* 2012; **65**: 817–826.

Johnston BC, Patrick DL, Thorlund K, Busse JW, da Costa BR, Schünemann HJ, Guyatt GH. Patient-reported outcomes in meta-analyses-part 2: methods for improving interpretability for decision-makers. *Health and Quality of Life Outcomes* 2013; **11**: 211.

Johnston BC, Miller PA, Agarwal A, Mulla S, Khokhar R, De Oliveira K, Hitchcock CL, Sadeghirad B, Mohiuddin M, Sekercioglu N, Seweryn M, Koperny M, Bala MM, Adams-Webber T, Granados A, Hamed A, Crawford MW, van der Ploeg AT, Guyatt GH. Limited responsiveness related to the minimal important difference of patient-reported outcomes in rare diseases. *Journal of Clinical Epidemiology* 2016a; **79**: 10–21.

Johnston BC, Alonso-Coello P, Friedrich JO, Mustafa RA, Tikkinen KA, Neumann I, Vandvik PO, Akl EA, da Costa BR, Adhikari NK, Dalmau GM, Kosunen E, Mustonen J, Crawford MW, Thabane L, Guyatt GH. Do clinicians understand the size of treatment effects? A randomized survey across 8 countries. *CMAJ: Canadian Medical Association Journal* 2016b; **188**: 25–32.

Jones PW. Health status measurement in chronic obstructive pulmonary disease. *Thorax* 2001; **56**: 880–887.

Juhl C, Lund H, Roos EM, Zhang W, Christensen R. A hierarchy of patient-reported outcomes for meta-analysis of knee osteoarthritis trials: empirical evidence from a survey of high impact journals. *Arthritis* 2012; **2012**: 136245.

Kirkham JJ, Dwan KM, Altman DG, Gamble C, Dodd S, Smyth R, Williamson PR. The impact of outcome reporting bias in randomised controlled trials on a cohort of systematic reviews. *BMJ* 2010; **340**: c365.

Kirshner B, Guyatt G. A methodological framework for assessing health indices. *Journal of Chronic Diseases* 1985; **38**: 27–36.

Martinez-Devesa P, Waddell A, Perera R, Theodoulou M. Cognitive behavioural therapy for tinnitus. *Cochrane Database of Systematic Reviews* 2007; **9**: CD005233.

Müller-Bühl U, Engeser P, Klimm H-D, Wiesemann A. Quality of life and objective disease criteria in patients with intermittent claudication in general practice. *Family Practice* 2003; **20**: 36–40.

Patrick DL, Deyo RA. Generic and disease-specific measures in assessing health status and quality of life. *Medical Care* 1989; **27**: S217–232.

Patrick DL, Burke LB, Gwaltney CJ, Leidy NK, Martin ML, Molsen E, Ring L. Content validity-establishing and reporting the evidence in newly developed patient-reported outcomes (PRO) instruments for medical product evaluation: ISPOR PRO good research practices task force report: part 1 – eliciting concepts for a new PRO instrument. *Value in Health* 2011a; **14**: 967–977.

Patrick DL, Burke LB, Gwaltney CJ, Leidy NK, Martin ML, Molsen E, Ring L. Content validity-establishing and reporting the evidence in newly developed patient-reported outcomes (PRO) instruments for medical product evaluation: ISPOR PRO Good Research Practices Task Force report: part 2 – assessing respondent understanding. *Value in Health* 2011b; **14**: 978–988.

Powers JH, 3rd, Patrick DL, Walton MK, Marquis P, Cano S, Hobart J, Isaac M, Vamvakas S, Slagle A, Molsen E, Burke LB. Clinician-reported outcome assessments of treatment benefit: report of the ISPOR Clinical Outcome Assessment Emerging Good Practices Task Force. *Value in Health* 2017; **20**: 2–14.

Prinsen CA, Vohra S, Rose MR, Boers M, Tugwell P, Clarke M, Williamson PR, Terwee CB. How to select outcome measurement instruments for outcomes included in a "Core Outcome Set" – a practical guideline. *Trials* 2016; **17**: 449.

PROMIS. Patient Reported Outcomes Measurement Information System 2018. http://www.healthmeasures.net/explore-measurement-systems/promis.

PROQOLID. Patient Reported Outcomes and Quality of Life Instruments Database 2018. https://eprovide.mapi-trust.org/about/about-proqolid.

Puhan MA, Soesilo I, Guyatt GH, Schünemann HJ. Combining scores from different patient reported outcome measures in meta-analyses: when is it justified? *Health and Quality of Life Outcomes* 2006; **4**: 94–94.

Revicki D, Hays RD, Cella D, Sloan J. Recommended methods for determining responsiveness and minimally important differences for patient-reported outcomes. *Journal of Clinical Epidemiology* 2008; **61**: 102–109.

Rutten-van Mölken M, Roos B, Van Noord JA. An empirical comparison of the St George's Respiratory Questionnaire (SGRQ) and the Chronic Respiratory Disease Questionnaire (CRQ) in a clinical trial setting. *Thorax* 1999; **54**: 995–1003.

Schünemann HJ, Best D, Vist G, Oxman AD, Group GW. Letters, numbers, symbols and words: how to communicate grades of evidence and recommendations. *Canadian Medical Association Journal* 2003; **169**: 677–680.

Schünemann HJ, Goldstein R, Mador MJ, McKim D, Stahl E, Puhan M, Griffith LE, Grant B, Austin P, Collins R, Guyatt GH. A randomised trial to evaluate the self-administered standardised chronic respiratory questionnaire. *European Respiratory Journal* 2005; **25**: 31–40.

Schünemann HJ, Akl EA, Guyatt GH. Interpreting the results of patient reported outcome measures in clinical trials: the clinician's perspective. *Health and Quality of Life Outcomes* 2006; **4**: 62.

Singh SJ, Sodergren SC, Hyland ME, Williams J, Morgan MD. A comparison of three disease-specific and two generic health-status measures to evaluate the outcome of pulmonary rehabilitation in COPD. *Respiratory Medicine* 2001; **95**: 71–77.

Smith K, Cook D, Guyatt GH, Madhavan J, Oxman AD. Respiratory muscle training in chronic airflow limitation: a meta-analysis. *American Review of Respiratory Disease* 1992; **145**: 533–539.

Tarlov AR, Ware JE, Jr., Greenfield S, Nelson EC, Perrin E, Zubkoff M. The Medical Outcomes Study. An application of methods for monitoring the results of medical care. *JAMA* 1989; **262**: 925–930.

Tendal B, Nuesch E, Higgins JP, Jüni P, Gøtzsche PC. Multiplicity of data in trial reports and the reliability of meta-analyses: empirical study. *BMJ* 2011; **343**: d4829.

Thorlund K, Walter SD, Johnston BC, Furukawa TA, Guyatt GH. Pooling health-related quality of life outcomes in meta-analysis-a tutorial and review of methods for enhancing interpretability. *Research Synthesis Methods* 2011; **2**: 188–203.

Wainer H. Estimating coefficients in linear models: it don't make no nevermind. *Psychological Bulletin* 1976; **83**: 213–217.

Ware J, Jr., Kosinski M, Keller SD. A 12-Item Short-Form Health Survey: construction of scales and preliminary tests of reliability and validity. *Medical Care* 1996; **34**: 220–233.

Ware JE, Jr., Kosinski M, Bayliss MS, McHorney CA, Rogers WH, Raczek A. Comparison of methods for the scoring and statistical analysis of SF-36 health profile and summary measures: summary of results from the Medical Outcomes Study. *Medical Care* 1995; **33**: As264–279.

Wiebe S, Guyatt G, Weaver B, Matijevic S, Sidwell C. Comparative responsiveness of generic and specific quality-of-life instruments. *Journal of Clinical Epidemiology* 2003; **56**: 52–60.

Witter JP. Introduction: PROMIS a first look across diseases. *Journal of Clinical Epidemiology* 2016; **73**: 87–88.

Yohannes AM, Roomi J, Waters K, Connolly MJ. Quality of life in elderly patients with COPD: measurement and predictive factors. *Respiratory Medicine* 1998; **92**: 1231–1236.

19

Adverse effects

Guy Peryer, Su Golder, Daniela R Junqueira, Sunita Vohra, Yoon Kong Loke; on behalf of the Cochrane Adverse Effects Methods Group

KEY POINTS

- To achieve a balanced perspective, all reviews should try to consider adverse aspects of interventions.
- A detailed analysis of adverse effects is particularly relevant when evidence on the potential for harm has a major influence on treatment or policy decisions.
- There are major challenges in specifying relevant outcomes and study designs for systematic reviews evaluating adverse effects. This is due to high diversity in the number and type of possible adverse effects, as well as variation in their definition, methods of ascertainment, incidence and time-course.
- Review authors should pre-specify their approach to reviewing studies of adverse effects within the review protocol. The approach may be confirmatory (focused on particular adverse effects of interest), exploratory (opportunistic capture of any adverse effects that happen to be reported), or a hybrid (combination of both).
- Depending on the approach used and outcomes of interest to the review, identification of relevant adverse effects data may require a bespoke search process that includes a wider selection of sources than that required to identify data on beneficial outcomes.
- Because adverse effects data are often handled with less rigour than the primary beneficial outcomes of a study, review authors must recognize the possibility of poor case definition, inadequate monitoring and incomplete reporting when synthesizing data.

19.1 Introduction to issues in addressing adverse effects

Every healthcare intervention comes with the risk, great or small, of harmful or adverse effects. A Cochrane Review that considers only the favourable outcomes of the interventions that it examines, without also assessing the adverse effects, will lack balance

This chapter should be cited as: Peryer G, Golder S, Junqueira D, Vohra S, Loke YK. Chapter 19: Adverse effects. In: Higgins JPT, Thomas J, Chandler J, Cumpston M, Li T, Page MJ, Welch VA (editors). *Cochrane Handbook for Systematic Reviews of Interventions*. 2nd Edition. Chichester (UK): John Wiley & Sons, 2019: 493–506.

and may make the intervention look more favourable than it should. All reviews should try to consider the adverse aspects of interventions.

This chapter addresses special issues about adverse effects in Cochrane Reviews. It focuses on methodological differences when assessing adverse effects compared with other outcomes.

19.1.1 Terminology and definitions

Poor standardization and usage of adverse effects terminology in study reports can produce challenges for review authors. Common, and closely related, terms include adverse event, adverse effect, serious adverse event, serious adverse effects, adverse drug reaction, side effect, complications and harms (Zorzela et al 2016). In this chapter we use the term **adverse event** for an unfavourable or harmful outcome that occurs during, or after, the use of a drug or other intervention, but is not necessarily caused by it, and an **adverse effect** (or **harm**) as an adverse event for which the causal relation between the intervention and the event is at least a reasonable possibility.

19.1.2 Special issues for addressing adverse effects

In this section we discuss some of the particular challenges when addressing adverse effects. First, there can be wide diversity across studies in how adverse events are defined, ascertained, analysed and reported. Second, adverse effects may not be known when studies were planned, so data collection processes and analytic strategies may not be in place. Third, many adverse events are too uncommon or too long-term to be observed within randomized trials.

19.1.2.1 Diversity in defining and monitoring of adverse events

A huge range of adverse events can occur in a research study, and there are multiple ways in which adverse effects can be ascertained and categorized by study investigators (Smith et al 2015). There are two broad strategies for collecting information on adverse events. Study investigators may use **active monitoring or surveillance**, which directs enquiry towards pre-defined adverse events of interest, usually following protocol-defined procedures for data collection, case definitions and adjudication. For example, if the event of interest is myocardial infarction, the study protocol might require collection of laboratory and electrocardiogram data for suspected events. These results might then be referred to an independent panel which adjudicates or ascertains the occurrence of an event. Such active monitoring usually relates to sets of potential adverse events that are either known or suspected to be associated with an intervention.

Although prospective collection of adverse event data is desirable, many adverse effects cannot be pre-specified because they are not yet known or suspected to be associated with an intervention. Thus, **spontaneous report monitoring** may occur, which involves recording all adverse events (pre-defined or not) throughout the duration of the study. Both participants and researchers recognizing any adverse event can file a report at any time. This may uncover new or unexpected adverse effects not previously associated with the intervention. For regulated products (e.g. drugs, biologics, vaccines), spontaneously reported adverse events are usually coded, grouped and categorized following established dictionaries for analysis and presentation.

Whichever monitoring method is used to collect information about adverse events, study investigators may combine adverse events into **global or composite measures**, which are often reported as total number of serious adverse events, or number of withdrawals due to adverse events, or total number of adverse events in an anatomic or organ system (e.g. gastrointestinal, cardiovascular). However, these composite measures do not give information on what exactly the events were, and so it is usually necessary to drill down for details of distinct or individual adverse events, such as nausea or rash.

Ideally, the definition and ascertainment of adverse events should be as uniform as possible across the included studies in the review. The lack of systematic monitoring or follow-up, coupled with divergent methods of seeking, verifying and classifying adverse events, can introduce heterogeneity in effect estimates among studies. Review authors will therefore need to pay close attention to outcome definition and method of monitoring when interpreting or comparing frequencies, rates and risk estimates for adverse effects.

19.1.2.2 Inconsistent and poor reporting of adverse effects

Inconsistent outcome definition and poor ascertainment are problematic for reviews that rely exclusively on published data. Information taken from published reports may be incomplete or lack specificity. Across multiple investigations of published versus unpublished studies, Golder and colleagues found a median of 43% of published studies reported adverse events data, compared with a median of 83% of unpublished studies (Golder et al 2016). A wider range of specific adverse events was found in sources other than published journal articles. In addition, when published and unpublished reports of the same study were compared, it was shown that the unpublished version was more likely to contain adverse effects data (median 95%) compared with the published version (median 46%). Similarly, a study of an obesity drug (orlistat or Xenical) by Schroll and colleagues compared study documents (protocol, clinical study report (CSR), and published report), and identified important inconsistencies (Schroll et al 2016). For example, adverse events in published studies were coded to appear less severe, with reduced incidence, compared with events reported in the unpublished CSRs. Of the total number of adverse events reported by trial investigators in CSRs, between 3% and 33% were subsequently reported in the corresponding published journal articles.

19.1.2.3 Different study designs to measure adverse events

Some adverse effects occur rarely or may only become apparent long after the start of intervention. This contrasts with adverse effects that have a higher incidence and occur soon after the intervention is delivered. A small randomized trial with only short-term follow-up may be able to capture common, immediately apparent adverse effects (e.g. skin reaction after injection) adequately. However, rare or long-term adverse effects may only be observed in non-randomized studies such as large cohort studies or case-control studies. Therefore, depending on the type of adverse outcome of interest, review authors may need to consider evidence extending beyond the time frame of randomized trials.

19.2 Formulation of the review

A starting point for assessing adverse effects of an intervention is to consider whether a review will evaluate both beneficial and adverse effects of an intervention, or just the adverse effects. Although most Cochrane Reviews look at both beneficial and adverse effects, review authors may decide to conduct a separate review of only the adverse effects of an intervention (see Box 19.2.a). Whichever strategy is taken, review authors will need to decide whether to focus only on a pre-specified set of adverse events (a 'confirmatory' approach), or analyse data on adverse events identified during the conduct of the review (an 'exploratory' approach). In practice, some review authors will use a hybrid of these two approaches. Consideration will also be needed of whether the same sources of evidence will be used to look at beneficial and adverse effects, or whether additional types of evidence will be sought to examine the adverse effects. Finally, the specific selection and definition of adverse effects will need to be considered. In this section we tackle these key considerations for formulating a review to look at adverse effects.

19.2.1 Which adverse events to look at

19.2.1.1 Confirmatory approach

In a confirmatory approach, review authors list one or more adverse effects as outcomes of interest in their review protocol. Golder and colleagues found that

Box 19.2.a Reviews of adverse effects alone

For an intervention that is given for a variety of diseases or conditions, yet whose adverse effect profile might be expected to be similar in different populations and settings, it may be reasonable to examine adverse effects regardless of the condition for which the intervention was delivered. This can be achieved in a stand-alone Cochrane Review focusing only on adverse effects.

For example, aspirin is used for many conditions, such as in patients after a stroke, with peripheral vascular disease, and with coronary artery disease. The main effects of aspirin on outcomes relevant to these different conditions would typically be addressed in separate Cochrane Reviews. However, the mechanism of harm and susceptibility to adverse effects (such as bleeding into the brain or gut) are sufficiently similar across the different disease groups that an independent review might address them together. Indeed, if trials exist on combined populations, such a question would be difficult to address in any other way.

Similarly, there may be limited adverse effects data for an intervention in a subpopulation. Analysing all available data for this subpopulation – such as adverse effects of selective serotonin reuptake inhibitors in children – may be worthwhile, even if the trials were aimed at different disease conditions.

Reviews of adverse effects alone should provide adequate cross-referencing to related reviews of intended effects of the intervention. If new safety concerns are identified when an efficacy review is updated, then the adverse effects review should be updated as soon as possible.

approximately 80% of systematic reviews of adverse effects published between 1994 and 2011 used this approach, selecting particular events, or categories of events, as their main interest (Golder et al 2013).

When adopting the confirmatory approach, review authors should aim to pre-specify adverse effects that are anticipated or already recognized to be associated with the intervention, and assumed to be measured regularly and consistently in studies. Selection of adverse effects of interest can be based on biological, physiological or psychological plausibility. For example, in a review of a surgical intervention it is plausible to pre-specify 'wound infection' as an adverse outcome of interest. Similarly, a systematic review of drug therapy that affects platelets or clotting would be justified in pre-specifying bleeding as an adverse outcome of interest. In some cases, it may be reasonable to select adverse effects for review based on previously established observation or association, although the plausible mechanism of effect has not yet been established.

A key limitation of the confirmatory approach is the inability to handle unanticipated adverse effects that are reported in the included studies.

19.2.1.2 Exploratory approach

An exploratory approach to reviewing adverse effects does not include pre-specification of any particular adverse outcomes of interest. Rather, it typically involves extracting any, or all, of the adverse event data found within the included studies. Only about 20% of reviews of adverse effects specify this as their main approach (Golder et al 2013).

The exploratory approach can identify unanticipated and rare adverse effects of an intervention. This may inform which outcomes are investigated in future reviews of pre-specified adverse events that use the confirmatory approach. In addition, the exploratory approach may provide data on possible associations between an intervention and a list of observed adverse events, which can be used to generate new signals to add to existing safety profiles.

A limitation of the exploratory approach is that the specific adverse effects reported may have been selectively analysed and reported because of the nature of the findings (e.g. based on statistical significance rather than clinical importance). Also, post-hoc or arbitrary analytic decisions regarding data extraction and analysis are often required when review authors encounter long lists of adverse events. Processes for selection and synthesis of such data need consideration in the review protocol, even if the outcomes of interest are not fully specified.

19.2.1.3 Hybrid approach

The hybrid approach combines elements of both confirmatory and exploratory approaches to capture anticipated and previously unrecognized adverse effects of an intervention. Reviews based on this approach might list a small number of adverse outcomes of interest in the protocol, whilst allowing post-hoc exploratory analyses to capture adverse events data available from the studies identified. An example is provided in Box 19.2.b.

Regardless of the approach adopted, review authors should be mindful of the potential for problems related to definition and ascertainment of adverse events when reviews are based solely on published data.

Box 19.2.b Illustration of three approaches to reviewing the adverse effects of a particular intervention: acupuncture
Confirmatory approach Review authors aim to synthesize data on the pre-specified adverse events of skin infection and pain on needle insertion. **Exploratory approach** Review authors aim to synthesize data on all or any adverse effects that are mentioned in the included studies. **Hybrid approach** Review authors aim to synthesize data on pre-specified outcomes of skin infection and total number of withdrawals due to adverse events, along with any other adverse effects found in the included studies.

19.2.2 Strategies for assessing beneficial and adverse effects in the same review

When conducting a review of both beneficial and adverse effects of interventions, review authors may:

1) use **the same eligibility criteria** to assess intended (beneficial) and unintended (adverse) effects, in terms of types of studies, types of participant and types of interventions; or
2) use **different eligibility criteria** for selecting studies that address unintended (adverse) effects compared with studies that address intended (beneficial) effects.

Using the same eligibility criteria to gather data on both types of outcome makes the review easier to conduct, not least because a single search can usually be undertaken if outcome terms are not stipulated in the search string. It also may allow for a direct comparison between beneficial and adverse effects, because the data are derived from the same types of studies (although it will not necessarily be the case that exactly the same studies report data on both beneficial and adverse effects). Two disadvantages of using the same eligibility criteria are (i) that the types of studies that are most appropriate to address the beneficial effects – typically randomized trials – may not be large enough or long enough to capture important adverse effects; and (ii) that it may lead to omission of relevant data on adverse effects if the adverse effects are also observed when the intervention is given for other conditions (see also Box 19.2.a).

Thus, review authors may apply different eligibility criteria when attempting to identify adverse effects data. The two main aspects of eligibility that may differ are the types of study design and the types of participants. It is also possible that studies performed for a different purpose may be eligible for the adverse effects component of the review.

- **Different study designs** To address adverse effects it may be necessary to seek non-randomized studies, because the effects are unlikely to be seen in randomized trials due to their size, duration or restricted eligibility for participants: see Section 19.2.3.
- **Different types of participants** Adverse effects data might be obtained from randomized trials evaluating the same or similar intervention but conducted in different populations or diseases (see also Box 19.2.a).
- **Different purposes** There may be randomized trials with adverse effects data on participants of interest to the review, but which did not measure the beneficial outcomes

relevant to the review (e.g. a pharmacokinetic study assessing drug concentrations in patients with the disease).

When different eligibility criteria are used to address beneficial and adverse effects, it will often be necessary to conduct a separate search for the two (or more) sets of studies (see Section 19.3), and it may be necessary to plan different methods in other aspects such as assessing risk of bias (see Section 19.4).

19.2.3 Selecting types of study design

Cochrane Reviews typically include randomized trials because randomization should distribute both known and unknown confounding variables equally across intervention groups (see Chapter 3, Section 3.3.1). However, the duration of follow-up in a randomized trial may not be sufficient to capture long-term adverse effects, and criteria for selecting participants into randomized trials may exclude participants at increased risk of harm (such as people with comorbidities or older adults living with frailty). Also, randomized crossover trials (see Chapter 22, Section 23.2) may not be appropriate for investigating some adverse effects, particularly if exposure to an intervention in one period results in an adverse event occurring in a later period. Non-randomized studies of interventions such as cohort studies (assembled from disease or drug/device registries) and case-control studies may be more likely than randomized trials to provide data on some types of adverse effects. However, non-randomized studies tend to be at greater risk of bias (see Chapter 24).

Spontaneous case reports or case series may assist in signalling rare and previously unknown events. However, for most Cochrane Reviews, these data sources should be used for scoping purposes only (particularly as they do not have denominator data to allow estimation of risks or rates). These spontaneous reports may guide drafting of the protocol when there is a need to choose relevant or important adverse effects as outcomes of interest.

19.2.4 Selecting adverse effects of interest

Review authors may define outcomes of interest based on severity, timing or the type of adverse effects that could occur based on the known mode of action of the intervention. Different sources may be used to inform pre-specification of adverse effects of interest. These sources include clinicians' observations in case reports, patients' reports on internet forums, scoping reviews, regulatory approved product information leaflets (e.g. from the US Food and Drug Administration) or other sources (e.g. British National Formulary, Meyler's Side Effects of Drugs).

Composite adverse outcomes are often reported by trials. Common examples include 'total number of participants with adverse events', or 'numbers of withdrawals due to adverse events'. Review authors should recognize major difficulties in interpreting composite adverse outcomes that are potentially constructed from hundreds of diverse events, because an important signal of rare serious adverse events could be masked by common, trivial adverse events. Also, review authors should hesitate to interpret data on withdrawals as surrogate markers for safety or tolerability, for the following reasons.

- The attribution of reason(s) for discontinuation is complex and may be due to mild but irritating side effects, toxicity, lack of efficacy, non-medical reasons, or a combination of causes.
- The pressures on patients and investigators under trial conditions to reduce number of withdrawals and dropouts can result in rates that do not reflect the experience of adverse events within the wider population.
- Unblinding of intervention assignment often precedes the decision to withdraw. This can lead to an over-estimate of the intervention's effect on patient withdrawal. For example, symptoms of patients in the placebo arm are less likely to lead to discontinuation. Conversely, patients in the active intervention group who complained of symptoms suggesting adverse effects may have been more readily withdrawn.

19.3 Identification of evidence

19.3.1 Search methods for adverse effects data

When considering the search process, review authors may decide to perform a single search to retrieve studies evaluating both benefits and harms. If so, the search strategy should be designed to take account of the selected approach, either confirmatory, exploratory or hybrid, and any differences in eligibility criteria for addressing beneficial and adverse effects. A single search may be reasonable if it is sufficiently broad (e.g. if it captures all studies containing a specific drug name or intervention) without being limited to specific study designs or types of participants.

In general, we recommend consideration of a separate bespoke search for data on adverse effects, particularly if the study designs that evaluate adverse effects of interest are different from those that report efficacy. It is unlikely that a single search that is focused on efficacy or effectiveness studies will be sufficient to identify evidence on all adverse effects in a comprehensive manner.

19.3.2 Allocating resources for the search

Despite significant improvements in reporting of adverse effects in primary studies, specific terms relating to adverse effects may not feature in the title, abstract, keywords or bibliographic database indexing systems. To determine the necessary work and resources involved, careful scoping when drafting the review question is recommended. This may need to account for the inclusion of unpublished data (see Section 19.3.4 and Chapter 4) and non-randomized studies (see Chapter 24).

19.3.3 Sources to search

Due to the variable content and indexing techniques of healthcare databases, it is important not to restrict adverse effect review searches to a single source, nor to a limited combination of the primary clinical research databases. Performing a search in MEDLINE alone is not recommended.

A case study reviewing adverse effects of thiazolidinedione use in patients diagnosed with type 2 diabetes mellitus tested over 60 sources (Golder and Loke 2012).The results indicated that the minimum combination of sources required to identify all relevant references included 11 sources: the pharmaceutical company website, Science Citation Index, Embase, BIOSIS Previews, British Library Direct, Medscape DrugInfo, American Hospital Formulary Service (AHFS First), Thomson Reuters Integrity, Conference Papers Index, hand searching and reference checking. In this specific example, just searching MEDLINE failed to retrieve 66% of relevant references. A search strategy conducted in MEDLINE, Embase and the Cochrane Central Register of Controlled Trials (CENTRAL) failed to retrieve 57% of relevant references. This example illustrates the breadth of sources needed to ensure identification of relevant data. Authors will need to consider sources most relevant to their clinical question; the list above is an illustration only.

Identifying adverse effects of pharmacological interventions often requires search methods that are different from those required for reviews of non-pharmacological interventions, or medical devices. Further guidance for sourcing adverse effects data is given in the online Technical Supplement to Chapter 4.

19.3.4 Including unpublished sources

Review authors should search for unpublished sources of data on adverse effects. We consider unpublished sources to be those outside of a peer-reviewed journal. This includes: clinical study reports (CSR), trials registers and regulatory agency websites. Tang and colleagues showed the value of searching ClinicalTrials.gov for data on serious adverse events (Tang et al 2015). Among 300 trials with serious adverse events mentioned in ClinicalTrials.gov, 78 (26%) did not have a corresponding publication, and for the remaining 202 trials, 26 (13%) published articles did not mention serious adverse events. Limiting search strategies to published reports may therefore not produce a balanced review, leading to underestimates of harm.

Mandatory changes applied to trials regulated by the Food and Drug Administration (FDA) regarding the submission of adverse events data to ClinicalTrials.gov, and the legislated publication of clinical data by the European Medicines Agency (EMA), means that previous accessibility limitations are steadily improving. Although accessibility is likely to continue to improve, the logistics and feasibility of routinely using such data sources for adverse effects reviews has yet to be established. Review authors should therefore report on the number of unpublished studies identified and instances where data on adverse effects were inaccessible.

19.3.5 Search methods: specific and generic outcome terms

Searching for specific adverse effects outcomes is similar to searching for specific benefit outcomes, so that search terms for the particular adverse effects outcome(s) are included in the search string. Examples of specific adverse effects terms are: 'headache', 'blood loss' or 'dysphagia'. However, it is likely that this method will lack sensitivity due to variation in reporting and indexing.

A possible option for the larger databases is to use a broad search involving two components at the same time: **generic index terms** combined with **specific free-text** searches using the 'OR' Boolean function. Both specific and generic search techniques have strengths and limitations, but the strengths are increased and limitations reduced when they are combined. It is therefore advisable to combine index terms and free-text searching (where possible) to increase search sensitivity and reduce the possibility of missing relevant material. More details are provided in the online Technical Supplement to Chapter 4.

19.4 Appraisal of evidence

19.4.1 Challenges in assessing risk of bias for adverse effects data

Assessing risk of bias for pre-specified adverse effects that are actively monitored in included studies is generally the same as for the pre-specified beneficial effects. However, adverse effects are seldom specified as primary outcomes, and often are not pre-specified at all, so there is often lack of clarity in the methods used to obtain adverse effects data. Thus, different susceptibilities to bias can arise for adverse effects due to the way in which they are measured, recorded and reported. It is important that the outcome measure is appropriate for detection of the adverse effect, and that the outcomes are measured or ascertained using a method that is comparable across intervention groups (see Chapter 8, Section 8.7). Study participants prematurely stopping assigned intervention or withdrawing from the study (due to adverse events) can result in dissimilar observation times for ascertaining future adverse events. When assessing the risk of bias for missing outcome data, it is important to consider the possibility of differential follow-up and informative censoring. A particular challenge when assessing risk of bias for adverse effects data is that of selective reporting. Results based on spontaneously reported adverse outcomes may lead to concerns that these were selected post hoc based on the finding being noteworthy. Similarly, unusual composite outcomes may be reported to hide or emphasize particular findings.

19.4.2 Recommended tools for assessing risk of bias in adverse effects data

Review authors should use the currently recommended risk-of-bias tools, the RoB 2 tool for randomized trials (see Chapter 8), and the ROBINS-I tool for non-randomized studies (see Chapter 25). Although these tools are most easily directed at outcomes that have been pre-specified by the review team, they are suitable for any type of quantitative outcome analysed in a review. Where adverse effects are extracted post hoc from included trials in an exploratory approach, it may not be possible to list important co-interventions or confounding variables in the review protocol, as would usually be expected for using the ROBINS-I tool.

Particular issues in assessing risk of bias for adverse effects data include outcome definition and methods of monitoring adverse effects. These warrant special attention when there are significant concerns over bias towards the null stemming from poor definition, ascertainment or reporting of harms. This is particularly important for new or unexpected adverse events that have not been pre-specified as outcomes of interest in the trials, and where monitoring and reporting may be potentially inadequate. Additional resources such as the McHarm tool (Chou et al 2010) and the Agency for Healthcare Research and Quality (AHRQ) assessment tool (Chou et al 2007, Viswanathan and Berkman 2012) provide further discussion of these issues.

19.4.3 Selective outcome reporting bias of adverse effects data

Selective outcome reporting refers to authors reporting a subset of variables, based on the results, from among all the outcomes originally analysed (see Chapter 7). Selective outcome reporting distorts the body of available evidence on which to conduct data synthesis and can lead to a high risk of bias (Kicinski et al 2015). Missing or partially reported adverse effects data are common in systematic reviews evaluating adverse effects (Saini et al 2014).

There is evidence that Cochrane Reviews may suffer from reporting bias. Kicinski and colleagues explored the potential impact of reporting bias on meta-analyses in Cochrane Reviews published between 1990 and 2005 (Kicinski et al 2015). They applied hypothesized mechanisms of reporting bias to 802 meta-analyses of efficacy and 304 meta-analyses of safety that each combined at least 10 individual estimates. The results from their model indicated that statistically significant results favouring treatment were more likely to be included in meta-analyses of efficacy than non-significant results. In contrast, results showing no evidence of adverse effect had greater probability of inclusion in a meta-analysis of safety than statistically significant results of adverse effects. Reporting bias therefore, may lead to the erroneous conclusion that an intervention is safe or relatively free from adverse effects.

19.5 Synthesis and interpretation of evidence

19.5.1 Estimating intervention effects from adverse effects

Review authors can have greater confidence in their interpretation of adverse effects data when outcomes are defined, monitored and reported as pre-specified outcomes in the research studies. In contrast, where the adverse effects are unexpected or ascertained ad hoc through spontaneous reporting, review authors will have to make more cautious interpretations regarding perceived safety or lack of harm, unless there is evidence that monitoring and reporting were sufficiently robust to have accurately captured any events of concern (Loke and Mattishent 2015).

It is important to evaluate the consistency and similarity of case definitions and methods of ascertainment for harms outcomes from the various included studies before comparing or synthesizing adverse effects data across studies. An important source of potential heterogeneity in effect estimates for adverse effects is variation in outcome definition and measurement. Review authors should ask study authors to resolve any ambiguity by providing additional data, or disaggregated data, which can be reanalysed more consistently.

Important analytical challenges relating to imprecision of estimates and rare events are covered in Chapter 10 (Section 10.4.4); see also Section 19.5.2 for particular challenges of determining whether there were zero adverse events.

Grouping adverse effects together in a composite measure (e.g. total number of adverse effects) can only give a broad impression, and may lead to genuine differences between the interventions in individual adverse effects being obscured. Owing to differences in coding and categorization of adverse effects between studies, review authors should avoid trying to increase numbers of events available for analysis by constructing composite categories that have not been reported in the primary studies. Conversely, review authors should be alert to situations in which the coding of adverse effects splits data unnecessarily (e.g. pain in leg, pain in arm), which may dilute the signal of a more global effect (e.g. all patients affected by pain).

Review authors should include at least one adverse effect outcome in the 'Summary of findings' table. If the review did not focus on detailed evaluation of any adverse effects, then the review authors should make an explicit statement that harms were not assessed, rather than say (or imply) the intervention appears to be safe.

19.5.2 Synthesizing and interpreting 'zero events'

It can be difficult, or unwise, to determine that there were no adverse events of a specific type. Although trial reports may provide tables detailing withdrawals (and reasons) or serious adverse effects, they will not necessarily include all events of interest to the review authors. New or unexpected adverse events may have been missed if ascertainment relied solely on spontaneous reporting. Furthermore, trials may report statements such as "no serious harms were found" without specifying their definition of serious harms, or that "there was no evidence of significant adverse effects", without giving the numbers of events on which such a conclusion is based.

If a serious adverse event of interest, such as heart failure, was not explicitly mentioned in the text or the serious adverse effects tables, the question then arises as to whether it is reasonable to interpret this as zero heart failure events. We generally recommend against extracting data as 'zero' unless it is clearly listed as such in the study report. Even where heart failure is explicitly reported as 'zero', we suggest that review authors carefully check the methods section of the included study for details on the rigour of monitoring for the adverse outcome (e.g. specific active surveillance for heart failure, versus reliance only on spontaneous reports that are prone to underreporting). Ambiguity frequently crops up in the extraction and interpretation of absence of harms, so review authors should record how they reached a decision of 'zero events'.

19.6 Chapter information

Authors: Guy Peryer, Su Golder, Daniela Junqueira, Sunita Vohra, Yoon Kong Loke; on behalf of the Cochrane Adverse Effects Methods Group

Acknowledgements: We thank Julian Higgins, Jamie Kirkham and Barbara Jennings.

Funding: This work was supported by Cochrane Methods Innovation Fund.

19.7 References

Chou R, Fu R, Carson S, Saha S, Helfand M. Methodological shortcomings predicted lower harm estimates in one of two sets of studies of clinical interventions. *Journal of Clinical Epidemiology* 2007; **60**: 18–28.

Chou R, Aronson N, Atkins D, Ismaila AS, Santaguida P, Smith DH, Whitlock E, Wilt TJ, Moher D. AHRQ series paper 4: assessing harms when comparing medical interventions: AHRQ and the effective health-care program. *Journal of Clinical Epidemiology* 2010; **63**: 502–512.

Golder S, Loke YK. The contribution of different information sources for adverse effects data. *International Journal of Technology Assessment in Health Care* 2012; **28**: 133–137.

Golder S, Loke YK, Zorzela L. Some improvements are apparent in identifying adverse effects in systematic reviews from 1994 to 2011. *Journal of Clinical Epidemiology* 2013; **66**: 253–260.

Golder S, Loke YK, Wright K, Norman G. Reporting of adverse events in published and unpublished studies of health care interventions: a systematic review. *PLoS Medicine* 2016; **13**: e1002127.

Kicinski M, Springate DA, Kontopantelis E. Publication bias in meta-analyses from the Cochrane Database of Systematic Reviews. *Statistics in Medicine* 2015; **34**: 2781–2793.

Loke YK, Mattishent K. If nothing happens, is everything all right? Distinguishing genuine reassurance from a false sense of security. *CMAJ: Canadian Medical Association Journal* 2015; **187**: 15–16.

Saini P, Loke YK, Gamble C, Altman DG, Williamson PR, Kirkham JJ. Selective reporting bias of harm outcomes within studies: findings from a cohort of systematic reviews. *BMJ* 2014; **349**: g6501.

Schroll JB, Penninga EI, Gøtzsche PC. Assessment of adverse events in protocols, clinical study reports, and published papers of trials of orlistat: a document analysis. *PLoS Medicine* 2016; **13**: e1002101.

Smith PG, Morrow RH, Ross DA. Outcome measures and case definition. In: *Field Trials of Health Interventions: A Toolbox*. Smith PG, Morrow RH, Ross DA, editors. Oxford (UK): Oxford University Press; 2015.

Tang E, Ravaud P, Riveros C, Perrodeau E, Dechartres A. Comparison of serious adverse events posted at ClinicalTrials.gov and published in corresponding journal articles. *BMC Medicine* 2015; **13**: 189.

Viswanathan M, Berkman ND. Development of the RTI item bank on risk of bias and precision of observational studies. *Journal of Clinical Epidemiology* 2012; **65**: 163–178.

Zorzela L, Loke YK, Ioannidis JP, Golder S, Santaguida P, Altman DG, Moher D, Vohra S, PRISMA Harms Group. PRISMA harms checklist: improving harms reporting in systematic reviews. *BMJ* 2016; **352**: i157.

20

Economic evidence

Ian Shemilt, Patricia Aluko, Erin Graybill, Dawn Craig, Catherine Henderson, Michael Drummond, Edward CF Wilson, Shannon Robalino, Luke Vale; on behalf of the Campbell and Cochrane Economics Methods Group

KEY POINTS

- Economics is the study of the optimal allocation of limited resources for the production of benefit to society and is therefore relevant to any healthcare decision.
- Optimal decisions also require best evidence on cost-effectiveness.
- This chapter describes methods for incorporating an economics view on the review question and evidence into Cochrane Reviews.
- Incorporating an economics view on the review question and evidence into Cochrane Reviews can enhance their usefulness and applicability for healthcare decision-making and new economic analyses.

20.1 Introduction

Economics is the study of the optimal allocation of limited resources for the production of benefit to society. Resources include human time and skills, equipment, buildings, energy and any other inputs used to achieve a specified course of action. These courses of action might relate, for example, to a clinical decision to refer a patient for a healthcare intervention (including management of complications and follow-up care), or a policy decision to implement a public health intervention.

In the face of limited resource availability, decision makers often need to consider not only the beneficial and adverse health effects of interventions, but the impacts on the use of healthcare resources, costs associated with use of those resources, and ultimately their value – decision makers also need information on efficiency. The need for evidence on both effectiveness and efficiency are closely aligned in healthcare

This chapter should be cited as: Shemilt I, Aluko P, Graybill E, Craig D, Henderson C, Drummond M, Wilson ECF, Robalino S, Vale L; on behalf of the Campbell and Cochrane Economics Methods Group. Chapter 20: Economic evidence. In: Higgins JPT, Thomas J, Chandler J, Cumpston M, Li T, Page MJ, Welch VA (editors). *Cochrane Handbook for Systematic Reviews of Interventions*. 2nd Edition. Chichester (UK): John Wiley & Sons, 2019: 507–524.

decision making. For these reasons, incorporating economic perspectives and evidence into Cochrane Reviews – alongside (and informed by) the evidence for beneficial and adverse effects – can make the findings of the review more useful for decision making (MacLehose et al 2012, Niessen et al 2012).

The focus of this this chapter is on methods to incorporate a health economics perspective into a Cochrane Review. Decisions about whether to include an economic perspective in a Cochrane Review should be included in the planning stage. Further support with this stage is available from the Economics Methods Group and can be found in other chapters of this *Handbook*.

A number of economics terms are used in this chapter but it is not expected that the reader will be familiar with economics terminology. Where a brief definition is possible it is provided but where a fuller definition is needed please see the glossary and supplementary material, available on the Campbell and Cochrane Economics Methods Group website.

20.1.1 Economic perspectives and economic evidence

Incorporating an economic *perspective* into a Cochrane Review involves the relatively straightforward task of placing an 'economics lens' on the health condition (population), intervention(s) and effectiveness question(s) under investigation, in order to highlight economic issues of potential importance to end-users such as the importance of a particular research question or the burden of a health condition on a society or specific group. An economic perspective might provide information about whether a more costly intervention is worth any additional benefits and whether the information could change a policy decision. In comparison, incorporating economic *evidence* into a Cochrane Review requires the application of specialized methods and procedures to include estimates of the cost or other economic effects of the interventions in the review.

In this chapter we restrict the term economic evidence to information on resource use, or costs or cost-effectiveness data taken from studies that draw comparisons for patient populations that match those of the Cochrane Review. The type of studies that we are interested in are economic evaluations. These are full economic evaluations that compare the costs and effects of two or more interventions. Partial economic evaluations are also possible and these compare only costs or effects but not both. Relevant partial economic evaluations that compare only effects would already be included in the review (under this definition a trial comparing the effects and harms of an intervention is a form of a partial economic evaluation). Partial economic evaluations that consider costs only are called cost-analyses. It is not currently recommended to include these and methodological research is needed to assess the value of including them. Further information describing how full and partial economic evaluations are defined is provided in the glossary and supplementary material, which are available on the Campbell and Cochrane Economics Methods Group website.

Two optional methodological frameworks have therefore been developed for incorporating economic evidence into reviews. The methodological and practical implications of each approach should be considered carefully at an early stage of planning the protocol for a systematic review. The two methodological frameworks are:

1) integrated full systematic review of economic evidence; and
2) brief economic commentary.

The integrated full systematic review of economic evidence is covered only briefly in this chapter. A detailed definition and description can be found on the Campbell and Cochrane Economics Methods Group website. This approach is substantially more resource intensive when implemented in full than the brief economic commentary. This is because it requires additional 'economic' methods procedures to be integrated into each stage of the main systematic review of intervention effects. Conducting an integrated full systematic review of economic evidence will also require specialist input to the author team from a health economist, with experience (or support from someone with experience) of applying the framework, at all stages of the process.

The brief economic commentary framework is less intensive but also less rigorous, and most of this chapter focuses on this approach. This framework is specifically designed to support the inclusion of economic evidence in Cochrane Reviews without requiring specialist input from health economists (beyond initial guidance and training in the method and procedures), and without placing a major additional workload burden on author teams or editorial bases. This framework can be viewed as a 'minimal framework' for incorporating economic evidence, with inherent limitations that will require appropriate caveats in the commentary.

20.1.2 Core principles for the methods for the review of economic evidence

Three core principles underpin both frameworks.

1) **Economics evidence should not be presented alone**

Full reviews or brief economic commentaries developed with the aim of summarizing evidence on the costs and/or cost-effectiveness of interventions should not in general be conducted as a standalone exercise. They must place the relevant economic evidence (in this case the impacts on resource use, costs and/or cost-effectiveness) into the context of reliable evidence for intervention effects on health and related outcomes. Failure to do so can lead to a biased summary of the evidence and a distorted assembly of data from primary studies, because data on the evidence of effects used in identified economic evaluations are highly likely to be (at best) only a subset of the data used to provide the summary of evidence of effects (including assessment of the quality of that evidence). The evidence of effects produced by a Cochrane Review will be the most up-to-date synthesis and any published economic evaluation can, at best, be based on only a subset of the data that were available at some earlier time point.

Furthermore, economic evaluations may be susceptible to a specific source of publication bias (or indeed conduct bias). For example, audits of some clinical areas have shown that clinical effect sizes in randomized trials published with a concurrent economic evaluation are systematically larger than those in randomized trials without. This may reflect the difficulty in publishing planned economic evaluations conducted alongside 'inconclusive' trials. Also, decisions made whilst planning a trial may mean that an economic evaluation is excluded (e.g. because it is felt implausible that an effective intervention could be anything other than cost-saving). However, such reasoning may not be reflected in published trial protocols or final study reports. Both of these issues compound the issue of reporting biases in randomized trials (see Chapter 13).

2) **Consider contributors to economic outcomes rather than specific resources or settings**

Given the international audience of end-users of Cochrane Reviews, any assumptions in the review about the setting for decision making (such as the availability of resources or the structure of the health system), and any specific resource estimates may not be appropriate. The primary aim of economics components of reviews should be to explain how interventions affected incremental resource use, costs, health outcomes and cost-effectiveness when implemented at specific times in specific settings (i.e. a focus on 'what happens?' (Petticrew 2015)) and what drives variation in estimates of economic and health outcomes between studies and settings. This will help end-users understand key economic trade-offs between alternatives that could be used in practice in their own setting.

3) **Consider how economics evidence may inform future research**

A key secondary aim of economics components of reviews should be to present health and economic outcome data outputs from Cochrane Reviews in formats that facilitate the reuse of these data as inputs to the subsequent, or parallel, development of new model-based economic evaluations.

20.1.3 Criteria for prioritizing inclusion of economic evidence in a Cochrane Review

20.1.3.1 Rationale and principles

Whilst all reviews could have an economic component, an economic component might not always be necessary. In general, it is more likely to be important to incorporate economic evidence into a review when important differences are expected between the intervention(s) and comparator(s) being compared in terms of their impacts on resource use and associated costs. In addition, pragmatic factors, such as the availability of specialist expertise and research resources available, may also impact on the final decision.

Some commissioners of systematic reviews have found it useful to develop decision algorithms, such as the one shown in Table 20.1.a, to help prioritize systematic reviews of the effects of health interventions for inclusion of economic evidence (Frick et al 2012).

Table 20.2.a provides three criteria to help prioritize reviews for inclusion of economic evidence:

1) the expected incremental effect of an intervention (i.e. how large is the difference in effect between intervention options likely to be? The smallest meaningful effect might correspond to the minimally important difference, or the difference in effect likely to be meaningful to patients);
2) the expected incremental cost of the intervention (i.e. what are the key elements of resource use likely to be affected, and how large is the difference likely to be in cost between intervention options? How important might this difference be to decision makers?); and
3) the likelihood that economic evidence could change potential decisions about use of an intervention (this may take into consideration other contextual factors, such as prevalence of a condition or health system factors).

Table 20.1.a Decision algorithm to help prioritize reviews for inclusion of economic evidence (reproduced from Frick et al (2012))

Expected incremental effect	Expected incremental cost	Probability economic evidence could change potential adoption decisions	Priority for incorporating economic evidence
Small	Low	Low probability	Low priority
Small	Low	High probability	Medium priority
Large	Low	Low probability	Very low priority
Large	Low	High probability	Low priority
Small	High	Low probability	Medium priority
Small	High	High probability	High priority
Large	High	Low probability	Low priority
Large	High	High probability	Medium priority

20.1.3.2 Making judgements about the criteria

Each of these criteria is dichotomized for simplicity: large or small incremental effect, high or low incremental cost, and a high or low probability that economic evidence will affect potential decisions concerning the adoption of the intervention.

It can be challenging to judge the likely size of incremental effects and costs in these broad, dichotomized terms, in advance of conducting the research. However, this is an essential first step in planning any study of intervention effects or economic evaluation, just as it is in planning systematic reviews of such studies. In practice, it may be easier to apply this algorithm when planning an update of an already published Cochrane Review. This is because the results of the current, published version may indicate potential sources of important differences in resource use and costs between the intervention(s) and comparator(s). For example, a summary effect size that shows an increased/decreased risk of a revisional procedure being required following a surgical intervention implies a difference in resource use and costs associated with performing additional/fewer revisional procedures (including those associated with management of any complications and follow-up care).

Prior to conducting the review the expected probability that economic evidence could change adoption decisions is largely a subjective judgement. This judgement is again challenging to make given the intended international audience of end-users of Cochrane Reviews. Authors are therefore encouraged to consult a health economist who can provide specialist advice to about what factors would be worth considering when making a judgement.

20.1.3.3 Using the criteria for prioritizing inclusion of economic evidence in a Cochrane Review

There are two rows in Table 20.2.a for which the decision to de-prioritize or prioritize incorporation of economic evidence is relatively clear. The first scenario is characterized by a large incremental beneficial effect, a low incremental cost, and a low probability of the economic evidence changing the decision. In this scenario, a very low priority is placed on the incorporation of economic evidence into review. This is because with a large beneficial effect on health (which is likely to translate into lower subsequent use of health services and lower associated healthcare costs) and small input costs, the intervention is likely to be cost-effective (possibly cost-saving) overall. It would, however, be important to state this reasoning in the Background section of a protocol and review.

Conversely, if the expected incremental beneficial effect is small, the expected incremental costs are high, and the economic evidence has a high probability of changing the decision, then this algorithm places a high priority on the incorporation of economic evidence.

The other rows of Table 20.2.a represent six further scenarios that fall between these two extremes. For example, the second row represents a scenario in which the incremental beneficial effect is small, the incremental cost is low, and the economic evidence has a high probability of changing the decision. This scenario may occur when, for example, the expected cost impact of the intervention is small but the health condition targeted by the intervention has a very high prevalence, such that the cumulative impact of small changes in costs across a large number of treated patients adds up to a large overall change in costs at the level of a region or a country, so affordability may be very important to a decision maker.

The decision algorithm in Table 20.2.a excludes scenarios in which the intervention is expected to be associated with negative incremental cost (i.e. net savings) and a positive incremental effect relative to the comparator (and vice versa); in other words, situations in which decisions to adopt or reject are expected to be straightforward because the intervention is clearly better or clearly worse than the comparator (i.e. it dominates, or is dominated by the comparator).

It is important to understand that if the decision algorithm shown in Table 20.2.a suggests that low (or very low) priority should be placed on incorporating economic evidence, this does not necessarily imply that doing so would provide no useful information for decision makers. Rather, it implies that a low (or very low) priority might be assigned to devoting limited research time and resources to conducting the economics component of a review.

20.2 Formulation of the review

20.2.1 Planning the economic component of the review

Regardless of which of the two methodological frameworks will be applied, authors of Cochrane Reviews aiming to incorporate economic evidence will need to plan the economics component from the very first stages. Further guidance and information on the planning can be accessed through the Campbell and Cochrane Economics Methods Group website.

The concise details of methods and procedures that will be used to develop the brief economic commentary should be planned at the protocol stage, and can be described in the 'Methods' section under a separate subheading, 'Incorporating economic evidence'.

Once a decision to include economic evidence has been taken, it is advisable to consult with a health economist with experience of Cochrane Review methods as soon as possible.

20.2.2 Formulating the objective

The economic question can be formulated with close reference to the question(s) that frame the systematic review of intervention effects. The research questions to be addressed by Cochrane Reviews of intervention effects are conventionally formulated as objectives, for example:

> To assess the effects of aspirin [*intervention*] versus placebo [*comparator*] for primary prevention of heart attacks [*condition and primary health outcome*] among adults aged > 50 years [*population*].

The questions for a brief economic commentary need to be expressed in the form of an objective, usually a secondary objective for the review. However, the most important objective in this case is to summarize the availability and principal findings in terms of costs and cost-effectiveness of eligible economic evaluations.

20.2.3 Introducing the economic perspective on the decision problem in the Background section

20.2.3.1 Purpose of introducing the economic perspective in the Background section

The aim of incorporating an economic perspective into the review is to place an 'economic lens' on the health condition (population) being addressed and the interventions being investigated in the review. This should be discussed in the Background to the review, to highlight the relevance of economic issues and context to the questions that the review will address.

Three distinct economic issues to consider highlighting in the Background section of a review are:

1) the economic burden of the health condition (i.e. the 'cost of illness');
2) potential impacts of intervention(s) on resource use (costs); and
3) general issues of intervention costs and cost-effectiveness that are relevant for the readers of the review to consider.

To address the first point, the 'Description of the condition' section of the Background can be expanded to include a discussion of the economic burden, or cost of illness of the condition being addressed. A brief literature search will be required to identify source material for this section, and guidance for this is presented in Section 20.2.3.2. The second and third points should be reported in the Background section on 'How the intervention might work' and 'Why is it important to do this review'. For the second and third points supplementary searches to identify source material are not required. Instead, the review should consider of the potential impacts of the intervention on resource use and their importance to decision making (as considered in the early planning stages and framing of the question, described in Section 20.2.2).

Depending on the scope of the cost-of-illness studies found, the commentary in the 'Description of the condition' section should include:

- a brief, general statement of the scale of economic burden/cost-of-illness to health-care systems, patients and/or their families and/or society as a whole; and

- monetized estimates of the economic burden of disease to healthcare systems, patients and/or their families and/or to societies.

We further recommend that any monetized estimates presented should include details of the country, currency and price year, if reported, in which the source studies were conducted.

An example commentary of how to summarize information on the economic burden of disease is presented in Box 20.2.a using example text extracted from a published Cochrane Review of surgery for faecal incontinence in adults (Brown et al 2013). Box 20.2.b and Box 20.2.c provide example text for potential impacts of intervention(s) on resource use (costs); and cost-effectiveness, which are taken from a published Cochrane Review of bone morphogenetic protein (BMP) for fracture healing in adults (Garrison et al 2010).

Box 20.2.a Example commentary on economic burden of the health condition (cost of illness)

Faecal incontinence...can be a debilitating problem with medical, social and economic implications... In the United States the average annual cost of treating a patient with mixed urinary and faecal incontinence in an outpatient setting was estimated at USD 17,166 (Mellgren et al 1999). During 1999 the direct costs of pads, appliances and other prescription items throughout hospitals and long-term care settings in the UK for incontinence in general was estimated at GBP 82.5 million (Integrated continence service 2000). With the rise in numbers of elderly people in the world, this condition will be an increasing challenge to both healthcare services and home carers (Brown et al 2013).

Box 20.2.b Example commentary on potential impacts of intervention(s) on resource use (costs)

From an economic perspective, it is possible that a proportion or all of the direct medical costs of fracture treatment using BMP may be offset by reductions in the subsequent direct medical costs associated with complications and/or secondary interventions and also by earlier return to productive activity. Use of BMP also has the potential to improve patients' health-related quality of life and function by avoiding donor site pain and dissatisfaction with donor site appearance associated with alternative treatments that involve bone grafts (Garrison et al 2010).

Box 20.2.c Example commentary on the general issue of intervention costs and cost-effectiveness

Given the economic impact of acute and non-union fractures and their treatment, and the need for economic decisions on the added value of adopting BMP in clinical practice, it is also important to critically evaluate and summarize current evidence on the costs (resource use) and estimated cost-effectiveness associated with use of BMP as an adjunct to, or replacement for, current standard treatments (Garrison et al 2010).

20.2.3.2 Identifying cost-of-illness studies for the Background section

The target type of health economics study (source material) needed to inform this brief commentary in the 'Description of the condition' section of the Background is the cost-of-illness study. A cost-of-illness study is a form of economic analysis that aims to describe, measure and value the total resources used in the management of a specific health condition, or within a specific patient population (Abdelhamid and Shemilt 2010) (see also the training resources on the Campbell and Cochrane Economics Methods Group website).

The objective of this search is to locate the few most useful articles that report information on the economic burden of the condition being addressed (cost-of-illness). It is not to conduct a comprehensive search of the literature and identify all relevant studies. Rather, the focus might be searching two or more databases (see below) where it is most likely a cost-of-illness study may be found. As noted above, the most useful sources of this information are likely to be found in the one or two articles that report a recently conducted cost-of-illness study, or a recently conducted review of cost-of-illness studies, focused on international comparisons, and which includes estimates of the wider economic burden not just in terms of the costs of management but also in terms of the costs of ill-health itself to an individual and to a society. In common with other material used in the Background section, a formal assessment of the quality and risk of bias of the cost-of–illness study is not conducted. However, it is still useful to know the key features that affect the validity of cost-of-illness studies (Larg and Moss 2011).

This search should be conducted when preparing the protocol for the review or when conducting an update of the review. Targeted search strategies to identify relevant cost-of-illness studies should be based on keyword search terms designed to capture 'Population' concepts, adapted from those 'Population' keyword terms used in strategies designed to search for eligible studies of effects for the main review. This set of keyword terms should be coupled (using the 'AND' operator) with a filter designed to retrieve cost-of-illness studies and run in general biomedical electronic literature databases, such as MEDLINE, EMBASE, CINAHL, PsycINFO or PubMed. We recommend a search of at least MEDLINE and EMBASE, with further databases searched if deemed relevant for the specific review topic. There are no specialist tertiary health economics electronic literature databases that currently tag records of cost-of-illness studies specifically, and no search filters designed specifically for cost-of-illness studies have been evaluated and validated (Jenkins 2004). We suggest using the search filters provided here. The search filters themselves have been piloted in the development of brief economic commentaries to successfully identify relevant cost of illness studies (Box 20.2.d, Box 20.2.e and Box 20.2.f shows the filter for MEDLINE (OvidSP), EMBASE (OvidSP) and PsycINFO, respectively).

20.2.4 Formulating eligibility criteria

For a brief economic commentary it is not necessary to include separate eligibility criteria describing the population, intervention(s), comparator(s) and outcomes (PICO) for economics studies that will be sought to inform the review. The eligibility criteria for studies that will be used to develop the commentary are the same as those set for the main systematic review of intervention effects with respect to the PICO elements.

Box 20.2.d MEDLINE (OvidSP) filter for cost-of-illness studies

1) (cost? adj2 (illness or disease or sickness)).tw.
2) (burden? adj2 (illness or disease? or condition? or economic*)).tw.
3) ("quality-adjusted life years" or "quality adjusted life years" or QALY?).tw.
4) Quality-adjusted life years/
5) "cost of illness"/
6) Health expenditures/
7) (out-of-pocket adj2 (payment? or expenditure? or cost? or spending or expense?)).tw.
8) (expenditure? adj3 (health or direct or indirect)).tw.
9) ((adjusted or quality-adjusted) adj2 year?).tw.
10) or/1-9

Box 20.2.e EMBASE (OvidSP) filter for cost-of-illness studies

1) (cost? adj2 (illness or disease or sickness)).tw.
2) (burden? adj2 (illness or disease? or condition? or economic*)).tw.
3) ("quality-adjusted life years" or "quality adjusted life years" or QALY?).tw.
4) Quality-adjusted life years/
5) "cost of illness"/
6) Exp "health care cost"/
7) (out-of-pocket adj2 (payment? or expenditure? or cost? or spending or expense?)).tw.
8) (expenditure? adj3 (health or direct or indirect)).tw.
9) ((adjusted or quality-adjusted) adj2 year?).tw.
10) or/1-9

Box 20.2.f PsycINFO filter for cost-of-illness studies

1) (cost? adj2 (illness or disease or sickness)).tw.
2) (burden? adj2 (illness or disease? or condition? or economic*)).tw.
3) ("quality-adjusted life years" or "quality adjusted life years" or QALY?).tw.
4) Health Care Economics/
5) Costs and Cost Analysis/
6) Health care costs/
7) (out-of-pocket adj2 (payment? or expenditure? or cost? or spending or expense?)).tw.
8) (expenditure? adj3 (health or direct or indirect)).tw.
9) ((adjusted or quality-adjusted) adj2 year?).tw.
10) or/1-9

To reflect this it is recommended to add a section to the Methods called 'Incorporating economic evidence', to state this clearly. This section should then go on to state supplementary criteria with respect to the type of economic evaluation study designs. For example:

> We will develop a brief economic commentary based on current methods guidelines (http://methods.cochrane.org/economics/) to summarize the availability and principal findings of [trial-based and model-based] full economic evaluations (cost-effectiveness analyses, cost-utility analyses, cost-benefit analyses)* that compare the use of aspirin versus placebo for primary prevention of heart attacks among adults aged > 50 years. This commentary will focus on the extent to which principal findings of eligible economic evaluations indicate that an intervention might be judged favourably (or unfavourably) from an economic perspective, when implemented in different settings.

* a definition of these terms can be found in the Glossary and a fuller explanation is provided in the supplementary material on the Campbell and Cochrane Economics Methods Group website.

20.3 Identification of evidence

Alongside the main search for studies for inclusion in the review, a separate search strategy should be planned (at the protocol stage for a new review or when planning an update of an existing review) and conducted during the review stage for eligible health economic evaluations to inform development of a brief economic commentary. The following elements are recommended for this supplementary search:

1) checking reference lists and conduct forward citation tracking from eligible studies of effects identified for inclusion in the main review;
2) conducting a search of NHS Economic Evaluation Database (NHS EED) using keyword terms based on intervention (and possibly comparator) concepts; and
3) applying specialist search filters to sets of records retrieved by searches of one or two selected general electronic biomedical literature databases searched for the main review of intervention effects. Examples of relevant search filters can be obtained from the Economics Methods Group.

The primary rationale for incorporating using specialist search filters is the need to identify reports of eligible full economic evaluations published since NHS EED stopped being updated at the end of 2014. If a brief economic commentary is restricted to full economic evaluations only, then we recommend using specialist searches from 1 January 2014 as the NHS EED was based on rigorous and comprehensive searches for full economic evaluations before that date.

20.3.1 Selecting studies and collecting data

For a brief economic commentary, procedures for selecting eligible full economic evaluations for inclusion are less onerous than required for an integrated full review. This reflects both the intention to minimize the workload for author teams and caveats for the discussion of the findings of identified economic evaluations (see Section 20.5.1).

Identified economic evaluations will still need to be screened against eligibility criteria relating to study population, intervention and comparator already defined for the main systematic review of intervention effects. It is recommended that this task needs to be undertaken by one review author only. One author will also need to classify each economic evaluation using the general procedure described below (including establishing any links with eligible trials included in the main review of intervention effects).

Collecting data for a brief economic commentary requires the extraction of two types of data: basic details of the characteristics of each identified economic evaluation; and brief text extracts that summarize their principal findings.

Basic data collected on the characteristics of each economic evaluation should include:

- the analytic framework (trial- or model-based) and type (*cost-effectiveness analysis, cost-utility analysis, cost-benefit analysis*) of economic evaluation to be summarized as a count of each type identified as part of the commentary (see also Section 20.5.1);
- the analytic perspective (whose costs and benefits a decision maker views as important) and time horizon (the duration over which costs and effects are assessed) adopted for costs and (if applicable) effects in each analysis;
- the main cost items included in each analysis (e.g. costs that fall under the following categories of health sector costs, other sector costs, patient and family costs and productivity impacts hospital care costs, direct health care costs; indirect non-health care costs); and
- the setting (i.e. country in which the study was performed), currency and price year used in each analysis.

It is helpful to classify cost items into four categories: health sector costs, other sector costs, patient and family costs, and productivity impacts (Drummond et al 2015) (although not all economic evaluations will follow this structure). The categories included will be driven primarily by the analytic perspective of the study. Health sector costs include the cost to the system or insurers of care provided (excluding costs directly paid by patients) and can include items such as primary care physician contacts (e.g. face-to-face visits or formal contacts via phone or via the internet, etc), prescribed medications, inpatient and outpatient hospital contacts, as well as any specialist tertiary care contacts. Other sector costs include costs borne by social services, education, local authorities, or police and criminal justice services. Patient and family costs could include any direct payment or co-payments for medications or care, or out of pocket expenses such as travel or arranging child or adult care while attending appointments. Productivity losses are the loss of output to the economy, and are usually measured in terms of time off work due to accessing care as well as morbidity or premature mortality.

For principal findings, the following data should be collected:

- verbatim text on conclusions drawn by the authors of each economic evaluation (with respect to what the study authors report as their main (base case) analysis; and
- text that summarizes uncertainty surrounding authors' principal conclusions (i.e. based on the results of any sensitivity analyses conducted).

For example, the following verbatim text was extracted from a report of a model-based cost-utility analysis that compared two interventions for preventing heart attacks and death in patients with non-ST-elevation myocardial infarction. This extract was used in the development of an exemplar brief economic commentary based on a Cochrane Review of factor Xa inhibitors for acute coronary syndromes (ACS) as part of a pilot study (Shemilt et al 2011):

> Our results suggest that the use of fondaparinux together with triple antiplatelet therapy in NSTE-ACS patients submitted to early (non-urgent) invasive therapy is cost saving. The strategy of fondaparinux was found to be dominant in almost all the scenarios considered, and the highest cost-effectiveness of fondaparinux was found in younger patients, patients at high risk of a cardiac event (high TIMI score) and patients at the highest risk of bleeding.
>
> (Latour-Perez and de Miguel Balsa 2009)

20.4 Appraisal of evidence

A brief economic commentary need not include (or report) assessments of methodological quality of included economic evaluations. This guidance reflects both the intention to minimize the additional workload burden placed on author teams and the limiting caveats that will be placed on discussion of the principal findings of identified economic evaluations in the review (see text at the end of Section 20.3.1). However, it is mandatory for this limitation to be explicitly described in the text of a brief economic commentary, for example:

> It is important to highlight that we did not subject any of the [N] identified economic evaluations to critical appraisal and we do not attempt to draw any firm or general conclusions regarding the relative costs or efficiency of ['Intervention X'] compared with ['Comparator Y'].

20.5 Synthesis and interpretation of evidence

20.5.1 Analysing and presenting results

An exemplar brief economic commentary is shown in Box 20.5.a (Shemilt et al 2011) and further examples can be found in supplementary material and training materials on the Campbell and Cochrane Economics Methods Group website.

Box 20.5.a Example brief economic commentary

To supplement the main systematic review of efficacy and safety of factor Xa inhibitors in the treatment of ACS, we sought to identify economic evaluations in which factor Xa inhibitors are compared with other anticoagulant strategies. A supplementary search of the NHS Economic Evaluation Database [insert other search methods as appropriate or refer to 'Incorporating economic evidence' section of the methods] identified three economic evaluations. Two cost-utility analyses (decision models) compared subcutaneous fondaparinux (2.5 mg/day) with SC enoxaparin (1 mg/kg 12 hourly) in patients with non ST-elevation myocardial infarction, pre-treated with triple antiplatelet therapy and early revascularization in Spain and the US respectively (Latour-Perez and de Miguel Balsa 2009, Sculpher et al 2009). Both analyses used comparative effectiveness and safety data collected from the OASIS-5 trial (Yusuf et al 2006). Both adopted a healthcare provider perspective and modelled costs and quality-adjusted life years (QALYs) over the patients' lifetimes. Both analyses found that fondaparinux dominated enoxaparin (i.e. was both less costly and generated more QALYs) over the patients' lifetime, in most scenarios considered, and across all levels of baseline risk.

A cost-effectiveness analysis (decision model) compared four anticoagulation strategies (UFH with a glycoprotein inhibitor; enoxaparin with a glycoprotein inhibitor; bivalirudin alone; and fondaparinux with a glycoprotein inhibitor) in patients with non-ST-elevation acute coronary syndrome (Maxwell et al 2009) in US secondary care. This analysis used clinical evidence collected from three randomized trials, including the OASIS-5 trial (Yusuf et al 2006). It adopted a healthcare provider perspective but the time horizon was not reported. The analysis found that bivalirudin and fondaparinux were superior in most scenarios considered and the authors concluded that bivalirudin was the least costly anticoagulation therapy amongst those compared for early invasive treatment, with fondaparinux preferred for patients undergoing conservative treatment.

We did not subject the three identified economic evaluations to critical appraisal and we do not attempt to draw any firm or general conclusions regarding the relative costs or efficiency of the anticoagulation strategies compared. However, evidence collected from these economic evaluations indicates that, from an economic perspective, use of fondaparinux is (at least) a promising strategy compared with other anticoagulation strategies in patients with non-ST-elevation acute coronary syndrome. End users of this review will need to assess the extent to which methods and results of identified economic evaluations may be applicable (or transferable) to their own setting. (Shemilt et al 2011)

The findings of the brief economic commentary should be incorporated into the Discussion (and not the Results) section of a Cochrane Review. The most appropriate place for this material is where the results of the systematic review of effects are put into context of other information and other reviews.

The overall aim of this element of the commentary is to summarize the availability and principal findings of identified eligible economic evaluations, with appropriate caveats, rather than to present the detailed results of a systematic search for evidence.

This commentary should include a brief narrative summary of:

- the electronic health economics literature databases searched;
- the number of relevant economic evaluations identified for each eligible comparison (each eligible intervention/comparison combination);
- the descriptive information collected from each study;
- principal conclusions as reported by the authors of each analysis (with respect to the base case analysis); and
- principal sources of uncertainty regarding authors' principal conclusions (based on the results of any sensitivity analyses conducted).

In a Cochrane Review, all published reports of economic analyses and/or economic evaluations used to inform the brief economic commentary should be cited as 'Additional references', not as 'Included studies', unless they are also eligible and included as part of the main review of effects.

20.5.2 Interpreting results and drawing conclusions

Discussion points in a brief economic commentary can be concise and over-interpretation of the results of this relatively modest exercise must be avoided. Interpretation and discussion points should focus on the extent to which it is judged clear, based on consistency in principal findings between identified economic evaluations, that the intervention(s) could be considered promising from an economic perspective (with appropriate caveats). In the example brief economic commentary shown in Box 20.5.a, the discussion points gave a qualified statement that one intervention (fondaparinux) appeared to be cost-saving while not inferior in terms of effects compared to other interventions measured. In this specific example, the basis for this qualified inference was evidence for consistent results favouring use of fondaparinux among full economic evaluations identified for inclusion in the brief economic commentary.

Example standard forms of words for potential use in different scenarios, depending on the profile of included economic evaluations, are shown in Box 20.5.b. "End users of this review will need to assess the extent to which methods and results of identified economic evaluations may be applicable (or transferable) to their own setting" is a recommended standard caveat for all brief economic commentaries.

20.6 Chapter information

Authors: Ian Shemilt, Patricia Aluko, Erin Graybill, Dawn Craig, Catherine Henderson, Michael Drummond, Edward CF Wilson, Shannon Robalino, Luke Vale; on behalf of the Campbell and Cochrane Economics Methods Group

Acknowledgements: The authors wish to thank Economics Methods Group Administrator, Jan Legge, for support whilst preparing this chapter, attendees at health economics group workshops that have provided valuable comments on the approaches to incorporate economics into Cochrane Reviews. We would also like to thank the peer reviewers of this chapter and the editorial team of the *Handbook* for comments and advice.

Box 20.5.b Example forms of words for concise discussion points in a brief economic commentary

Lack of evidence

The apparent shortage of relevant economic evaluations indicates that economic evidence regarding ['Intervention X'] for ['Health Condition Z'] is currently lacking.

Equivocal findings between studies

It is clear that the available economic evidence for ['Intervention X'] compared ['Comparator Y'] in the treatment of patients with ['Health Condition Z'] is, at best, equivocal.

Consistent findings between studies [1]

The available economic evidence indicates that, from an economic perspective, use of ['Intervention X'] is (at least) a promising strategy compared with ['Comparator Y'] for the secondary prevention of ['Health Condition Z'].

Consistent findings between studies [2]

Taking into account these limitations, there was consistency between economic evaluations in the finding that short-term direct healthcare costs were, on average, lower amongst patients with ['Health Condition Z'] who underwent ['Intervention X'] compared with those who underwent ['Comparator Y']. When considered alongside the principal finding from our main review of intervention effects that there is no clear difference in the primary outcomes between ['Intervention X'] and ['Comparator Y'], the available economic evidence indicates that, from an economic perspective, ['Intervention X'] may be a promising intervention, as a comparably safe and lower cost alternative to ['Comparator Y'], in patients with ['Health Condition Z'].

20.7 References

Abdelhamid A, Shemilt I. Glossary of terms. In: Shemilt I MM, Vale L, Marsh K, Donaldson C, editors. *Evidence-based Decisions and Economics: Health Care, Social Welfare, Education and Criminal Justice*. Oxford: Wiley-Blackwell; 2010.

Brown SR, Wadhawan H, Nelson RL. Surgery for faecal incontinence in adults. *Cochrane Database of Systematic Reviews* 2013; **7**: CD001757.

Drummond M, Sculpher M, Claxton K, Stoddart G, Torrance G. *Methods for Economic Evaluation of Health Care Programmes*. 4th ed. USA: Oxford University Press; 2015.

Frick K, Neissen L, Bridges J, Walker D, Wilson R, Bass E. Usefulness of Economic Evaluation Data in Systematic Reviews of Evidence. Rockville (MD): Agency for Healthcare Research and Quality (US); 2012. 12(13)-EHC114-EF. https://www.ncbi.nlm.nih.gov/books/NBK114533/

Garrison KR, Shemilt I, Donell S, Ryder JJ, Mugford M, Harvey I, Song F, Alt V. Bone morphogenetic protein (BMP) for fracture healing in adults. *Cochrane Database of Systematic Reviews* 2010; **6**: CD006950.

Gilbody S, Bower P, Sutton AJ. Randomized trials with concurrent economic evaluations reported unrepresentatively large clinical effect sizes. *Journal of Clinical Epidemiology* 2007; **60**: 781–786.

Jenkins M. Evaluation of methodological search filters: a review. *Health Information and Libraries Journal* 2004; **21**: 148–163.

Larg A, Moss JR. Cost-of-illness studies: a guide to critical evaluation. *Pharmacoeconomics* 2011; **29**: 653–671.

Latour-Perez J, de Miguel Balsa E. Cost effectiveness of fondaparinux in non-ST-elevation acute coronary syndrome. *Pharmacoeconomics* 2009; **27**: 585–595.

MacLehose H, Hilton J, Tovey D. The Cochrane Library: Revolution or evolution? Shaping the future of Cochrane content (background paper). The Cochrane Collaboration's Strategic Session; 2012; Paris, France.

Maxwell CB, Holdford DA, Crouch MA, Patel DA. Cost-effectiveness analysis of anticoagulation strategies in non-ST-elevation acute coronary syndromes. *Annals of Pharmacotherapy* 2009; **43**: 586–595.

Mellgren A, Jensen LL, Zetterstrom JP, Wong WD, Hofmeister JH, Lowry AC. Long-term cost of fecal incontinence secondary to obstetric injuries. *Diseases of the Colon and Rectum* 1999; **42**: 857–865; discussion 865–857.

Niessen L, Bridges J, Lau B, Wilson R, Sharma R, Walker D, Frick K, Bass E. Assessing the Impact of Economic Evidence on Policymakers in Health Care: A Systematic Review. Agency for Healthcare Research and Quality (US); 2012 Contract No.: No. 12(13)-EHC133-EF https://effectivehealthcare.ahrq.gov/topics/economic-evidence/research

Petticrew M. Time to rethink the systematic review catechism? Moving from 'what works' to 'what happens'. *Systematic Reviews* 2015; **4**: 36.

Sculpher MJ, Lozano-Ortega G, Sambrook J, Palmer S, Ormanidhi O, Bakhai A, Flather M, Steg PG, Mehta SR, Weintraub W. Fondaparinux versus Enoxaparin in non-ST-elevation acute coronary syndromes: short-term cost and long-term cost-effectiveness using data from the Fifth Organization to Assess Strategies in Acute Ischemic Syndromes Investigators (OASIS-5) trial. *American Heart Journal* 2009; **157**: 845–852.

Shemilt I, Mugford M, Vale L, Craig D, on behalf of the Campbell and Cochrane Economics Methods Group. Searching NHS EED and HEED to inform development of economic commentary for Cochrane intervention reviews. 2011. http://methods.cochrane.org/economics/sites/methods.cochrane.org.economics/files/public/uploads/brief_economic_commentaries_study_report.pdf

Yusuf S, Mehta SR, Chrolavicius S, Afzal R, Pogue J, Granger CB, Budaj A, Peters RJ, Bassand JP, Wallentin L, Joyner C, Fox KA. Comparison of fondaparinux and enoxaparin in acute coronary syndromes. *New England Journal of Medicine* 2006; **354**: 1464–1476.

21

Qualitative evidence

Jane Noyes, Andrew Booth, Margaret Cargo, Kate Flemming, Angela Harden, Janet Harris, Ruth Garside, Karin Hannes, Tomás Pantoja, James Thomas

KEY POINTS

- A qualitative evidence synthesis (commonly referred to as QES) can add value by providing decision makers with additional evidence to improve understanding of intervention complexity, contextual variations, implementation, and stakeholder preferences and experiences.
- A qualitative evidence synthesis can be undertaken and integrated with a corresponding intervention review; or
- Undertaken using a mixed-method design that integrates a qualitative evidence synthesis with an intervention review in a single protocol.
- Methods for qualitative evidence synthesis are complex and continue to develop. Authors should always consult current methods guidance at methods.cochrane.org/qi.

21.1 Introduction

The potential contribution of qualitative evidence to decision making is well-established (Glenton et al 2016, Booth 2017, Carroll 2017). A synthesis of qualitative evidence can inform understanding of how interventions work by:

- increasing understanding of a phenomenon of interest (e.g. women's conceptualization of what good antenatal care looks like);
- identifying associations between the broader environment within which people live and the interventions that are implemented;
- increasing understanding of the values and attitudes toward, and experiences of, health conditions and interventions by those who implement or receive them; and

This chapter should be cited as: Noyes J, Booth A, Cargo M, Flemming K, Harden A, Harris J, Garside R, Hannes K, Pantoja T, Thomas J. Chapter 21: Qualitative evidence. In: Higgins JPT, Thomas J, Chandler J, Cumpston M, Li T, Page MJ, Welch VA (editors). *Cochrane Handbook for Systematic Reviews of Interventions*. 2nd Edition. Chichester (UK): John Wiley & Sons, 2019: 525–546.

- providing a detailed understanding of the complexity of interventions and implementation, and their impacts and effects on different subgroups of people and the influence of individual and contextual characteristics within different contexts.

The aim of this chapter is to provide authors (who already have experience of undertaking qualitative research and qualitative evidence synthesis) with additional guidance on undertaking a qualitative evidence synthesis that is subsequently integrated with an intervention review. This chapter draws upon guidance presented in a series of six papers published in the *Journal of Clinical Epidemiology* (Cargo et al 2018, Flemming et al 2018, Harden et al 2018, Harris et al 2018, Noyes et al 2018a, Noyes et al 2018b) and from a further World Health Organization series of papers published in *BMJ Global Health,* which extend guidance to qualitative evidence syntheses conducted within a complex intervention and health systems and decision making context (Booth et al 2019a, Booth et al 2019b, Flemming et al 2019, Noyes et al 2019, Petticrew et al 2019).The qualitative evidence synthesis and integration methods described in this chapter supplement Chapter 17 on methods for addressing intervention complexity. Authors undertaking qualitative evidence syntheses should consult these papers and chapters for more detailed guidance.

21.2 Designs for synthesizing and integrating qualitative evidence with intervention reviews

There are two main designs for synthesizing qualitative evidence with evidence of the effects of interventions:

1) **Sequential reviews:** where one or more existing intervention review(s) has been published on a similar topic, it is possible to do a sequential qualitative evidence synthesis and then integrate its findings with those of the intervention review to create a mixed-method review. For example, Lewin and colleagues (Lewin et al 2010) and Glenton and colleagues (Glenton et al 2013) undertook sequential reviews of lay health worker programmes using separate protocols and then integrated the findings.
2) **Convergent mixed-methods review:** where no pre-existing intervention review exists, it is possible to do a full convergent 'mixed-methods' review where the trials and qualitative evidence are synthesized separately, creating opportunities for them to 'speak' to each other during development, and then integrated within a third synthesis. For example, Hurley and colleagues (Hurley et al 2018) undertook an intervention review and a qualitative evidence synthesis following a single protocol.

It is increasingly common for sequential and convergent reviews to be conducted by some or all of the same authors; if not, it is critical that authors working on the qualitative evidence synthesis and intervention review work closely together to identify and create sufficient points of integration to enable a third synthesis that integrates the two reviews, or the conduct of a mixed-method review (Noyes et al 2018a) (see Figure 21.2.a). This consideration also applies where an intervention review has already been published and there is no prior relationship with the qualitative evidence synthesis authors. We recommend that at least one joint author works across both reviews to facilitate

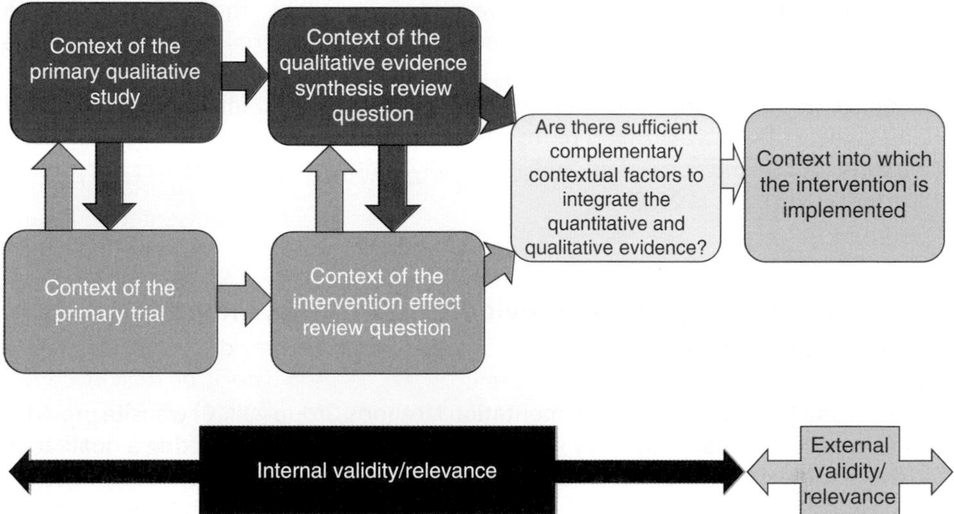

Figure 21.2.a Considering context and points of contextual integration with the intervention review or within a mixed-method review

development of the qualitative evidence synthesis protocol, conduct of the synthesis, and subsequent integration of the qualitative evidence synthesis with the intervention review within a mixed-methods review.

21.3 Defining qualitative evidence and studies

We use the term 'qualitative evidence synthesis' to acknowledge that other types of qualitative evidence (or data) can potentially enrich a synthesis, such as narrative data derived from qualitative components of mixed-method studies or free text from questionnaire surveys. We would not, however, consider a questionnaire survey to be a qualitative study and qualitative data from questionnaires should not usually be privileged over relevant evidence from qualitative studies. When thinking about qualitative evidence, specific terminology is used to describe the level of conceptual and contextual detail. Qualitative evidence that includes higher or lower levels of *conceptual* detail is described as 'rich' or 'poor'. Associated terms 'thick' or 'thin' are best used to refer to higher or lower levels of *contextual* detail. Review authors can potentially develop a stronger synthesis using rich and thick qualitative evidence but, in reality, they will identify diverse conceptually rich and poor and contextually thick and thin studies. Developing a clear picture of the type and conceptual richness of available qualitative evidence strongly influences the choice of methodology and subsequent methods. We recommend that authors undertake scoping searches to determining the type and richness of available qualitative evidence before selecting their methodology and methods.

A qualitative study is a research study that uses a qualitative method of data collection *and* analysis. Review authors should include the studies that enable them to answer their review question. When selecting qualitative studies in a review about intervention effects, two types of qualitative study are available: those that collect data from the same participants as the included trials, known as 'trial siblings'; and those that address relevant issues about the intervention, but as separate items of research – not connected to any included trials. Both can provide useful information, with trial sibling studies obviously closer in terms of their precise contexts to the included trials (Moore et al 2015), and non-sibling studies possibly contributing perspectives not present in the trials (Noyes et al 2016b).

21.4 Planning a qualitative evidence synthesis linked to an intervention review

The Cochrane Qualitative and Implementation Methods Group (QIMG) website provides links to practical guidance and key steps for authors who are considering a qualitative evidence synthesis (methods.cochrane.org/qi). The RETREAT framework outlines seven key considerations that review authors should systematically work through when planning a review (Booth et al 2016, Booth et al 2018) (Box 21.4.a). Flemming and colleagues (Flemming et al 2019) further explain how to factor in such considerations when undertaking a qualitative evidence synthesis within a complex intervention and decision making context when complexity is an important consideration.

Box 21.4.a RETREAT considerations when selecting an appropriate method for qualitative synthesis

Review question – first, consider the complexity of the review question. Which elements contribute most to complexity (e.g. the condition, the intervention or the context)? Which elements should be prioritized as the focal point for attention? (Squires et al 2013, Kelly et al 2017).

Epistemology – consider the philosophical foundations of the primary studies. Would it be appropriate to favour a method such as thematic synthesis that it is less reliant on epistemological considerations? (Barnett-Page and Thomas 2009).

Time frame – consider what type of qualitative evidence synthesis will be feasible and manageable within the time frame available (Booth et al 2016).

Resources – consider whether the ambition of the review matches the available resources. Will the extent of the scope and the sampling approach of the review need to be limited? (Benoot et al 2016, Booth et al 2016).

Expertise – consider access to expertise, both within the review team and among a wider group of advisors. Does the available expertise match the qualitative evidence synthesis approach chosen? (Booth et al 2016).

Audience and purpose – consider the intended audience and purpose of the review. Does the approach to question formulation, the scope of the review and the intended outputs meet their needs? (Booth et al 2016).

Type of data – consider the type of data present in typical studies for inclusion. To what extent are candidate studies conceptually rich and contextually thick in their detail?

21.5 Question development

The review question is critical to development of the qualitative evidence synthesis (Harris et al 2018). Question development affords a key point for integration with the intervention review. Complementary guidance supports novel thinking about question development, application of question development frameworks and the types of questions to be addressed by a synthesis of qualitative evidence (Cargo et al 2018, Harris et al 2018, Noyes et al 2018a, Booth et al 2019b, Flemming et al 2019).

Research questions for quantitative reviews are often mapped using structures such as PICO. Some qualitative reviews adopt this structure, or use an adapted variation of such a structure (e.g. SPICE (Setting, Perspective, Intervention or Phenomenon of Interest, Comparison, Evaluation) or SPIDER (Sample, Phenomenon of Interest, Design, Evaluation, Research type); Cooke et al 2012). Booth and colleagues (Booth et al 2019b) propose an extended question framework (PerSPecTIF) to describe both wider context and immediate setting that is particularly suited to qualitative evidence synthesis and complex intervention reviews (see Table 21.5.a).

Detailed attention to the question and specification of context at an early stage is critical to many aspects of qualitative synthesis (see Petticrew et al 2019 and Booth et al 2019a for a more detailed discussion). By specifying the context a review team is able to identify opportunities for integration with the intervention review, or opportunities for maximizing use and interpretation of evidence as a mixed-method review progresses (see Figure 21.2.a), and informs both the interpretation of the observed effects and assessment of the strength of the evidence available in addressing the review question (Noyes et al 2019). Subsequent application of GRADE CERQual (Lewin et al 2015, Lewin et al 2018), an approach to assess the confidence in synthesized qualitative findings, requires further specification of context in the review question.

Table 21.5.a PerSPecTIF Question formulation framework for qualitative evidence syntheses (Booth et al 2019b). Reproduced with permission of BMJ Publishing Group

Per	S	P	E	(C)	Ti	F
Perspective	Setting	Phenomenon of interest/ Problem	Environment	Comparison (optional)	Time/ Timing	Findings
From the perspective of a pregnant woman	In the setting of rural communities	How does facility-based care	Within an environment of poor transport infrastructure and distantly located facilities	Compare with traditional birth attendants at home	Up to and including delivery	In relation to the woman's perceptions and experiences?

21.6 Questions exploring intervention implementation

Additional guidance is available on formulation of questions to understand and assess intervention implementation (Cargo et al 2018). A strong understanding of how an intervention is thought to work, and how it should be implemented in practice, will enable a critical consideration of whether any observed lack of effect might be due to a poorly conceptualized intervention (i.e. theory failure) or a poor intervention implementation (i.e. implementation failure). Heterogeneity needs to be considered for both the underlying theory and the ways in which the intervention was implemented. An a priori scoping review (Levac et al 2010), concept analysis (Walker and Avant 2005), critical review (Grant and Booth 2009) or textual narrative synthesis (Barnett-Page and Thomas 2009) can be undertaken to classify interventions and/or to identify the programme theory, logic model or implementation measures and processes. The intervention Complexity Assessment Tool for Systematic Reviews iCAT_SR (Lewin et al 2017) may be helpful in classifying complexity in interventions and developing associated questions.

An existing intervention model or framework may be used within a new topic or context. The 'best-fit framework' approach to synthesis (Carroll et al 2013) can be used to establish the degree to which the source context (from where the framework was derived) resembles the new target context (see Figure 21.2.a). In the absence of an explicit programme theory and detail of how implementation relates to outcomes, an a priori realist review, meta-ethnography or meta-interpretive review can be undertaken (Booth et al 2016). For example, Downe and colleagues (Downe et al 2016) undertook an initial meta-ethnography review to develop an understanding of the outcomes of importance to women receiving antenatal care.

However, these additional activities are very resource-intensive and are only recommended when the review team has sufficient resources to supplement the planned qualitative evidence syntheses with an additional explanatory review. Where resources are less plentiful a review team could engage with key stakeholders to articulate and develop programme theory (Kelly et al 2017, De Buck et al 2018).

21.6.1 Using logic models and theories to support question development

Review authors can develop a more comprehensive representation of question features through use of logic models, programme theories, theories of change, templates and pathways (Anderson et al 2011, Kneale et al 2015, Noyes et al 2016a) (see also Chapter 17, Section 17.2.1 and Chapter 2, Section 2.5.1). These different forms of social theory can be used to visualize and map the research question, its context, components, influential factors and possible outcomes (Noyes et al 2016a, Rehfuess et al 2018).

21.6.2 Stakeholder engagement

Finally, review authors need to engage stakeholders, including consumers affected by the health issue and interventions, or likely users of the review from clinical or policy contexts. From the preparatory stage, this consultation can ensure that the review scope and question is appropriate and resulting products address implementation concerns of decision makers (Kelly et al 2017, Harris et al 2018).

21.7 Searching for qualitative evidence

In comparison with identification of quantitative studies (see also Chapter 4), procedures for retrieval of qualitative research remain relatively under-developed. Particular challenges in retrieval are associated with non-informative titles and abstracts, diffuse terminology, poor indexing and the overwhelming prevalence of quantitative studies within data sources (Booth et al 2016).

Principal considerations when planning a search for qualitative studies, and the evidence that underpins them, have been characterized using a 7S framework from Sampling and Sources through Structured questions, Search procedures, Strategies and filters and Supplementary strategies to Standards for Reporting (Booth et al 2016).

A key decision, aligned to the purpose of the qualitative evidence synthesis is whether to use the comprehensive, exhaustive approaches that characterize quantitative searches or whether to use purposive sampling that is more sensitive to the qualitative paradigm (Suri 2011). The latter, which is used when the intent is to generate an interpretative understanding, for example, when generating theory, draws upon a versatile toolkit that includes theoretical sampling, maximum variation sampling and intensity sampling. Sources of qualitative evidence are more likely to include book chapters, theses and grey literature reports than standard quantitative study reports, and so a search strategy should place extra emphasis on these sources. Local databases may be particularly valuable given the criticality of context (Stansfield et al 2012).

Another key decision is whether to use study filters or simply to conduct a topic-based search where qualitative studies are identified at the study selection stage. Search filters for qualitative studies lack the specificity of their quantitative counterparts. Nevertheless, filters may facilitate efficient retrieval by study type (e.g. qualitative (Rogers et al 2017) or mixed methods (El Sherif et al 2016) or by perspective (e.g. patient preferences (Selva et al 2017)) particularly where the quantitative literature is overwhelmingly large and thus increases the number needed to retrieve. Poor indexing of qualitative studies makes citation searching (forward and backward) and the Related Articles features of electronic databases particularly useful (Cooper et al 2017). Further guidance on searching for qualitative evidence is available (Booth et al 2016, Noyes et al 2018a). The CLUSTER method has been proposed as a specific named method for tracking down associated or sibling reports (Booth et al 2013). The BeHEMoTh approach has been developed for identifying explicit use of theory (Booth and Carroll 2015).

21.7.1 Searching for process evaluations and implementation evidence

Four potential approaches are available to identify process evaluations.

1) Identify studies at the point of study selection rather than through tailored search strategies. This involves conducting a sensitive topic search without any study design filter (Harden et al 1999), and identifying all study designs of interest during the screening process. This approach can be feasible when a review question involves multiple publication types (e.g. randomized trial, qualitative research and economic evaluations), which then do not require separate searches.

2) Restrict included process evaluations to those conducted within randomized trials, which can be identified using standard search filters (see Chapter 4, Section 4.4.7). This method relies on reports of process evaluations also describing the surrounding randomized trial in enough detail to be identified by the search filter.
3) Use unevaluated filter terms (such as 'process evaluation', 'program(me) evaluation', 'feasibility study', 'implementation' or 'proof of concept' etc) to retrieve process evaluations or implementation data. Approaches using strings of terms associated with the study type or purpose are considered experimental. There is a need to develop and test such filters. It is likely that such filters may be derived from the study type (process evaluation), the data type (process data) or the application (implementation) (Robbins et al 2011).
4) Minimize reliance on topic-based searching and rely on citations-based approaches to identify linked reports, published or unpublished, of a particular study (Booth et al 2013) which may provide implementation or process data (Bonell et al 2013).

More detailed guidance is provided by Cargo and colleagues (Cargo et al 2018).

21.8 Assessing methodological strengths and limitations of qualitative studies

Assessment of the methodological strengths and limitations of qualitative research remains contested within the primary qualitative research community (Garside 2014). However, within systematic reviews and evidence syntheses it is considered essential, even when studies are not to be excluded on the basis of quality (Carroll et al 2013). One review found almost 100 appraisal tools for assessing primary qualitative studies (Munthe-Kaas et al 2019). Limitations included a focus on reporting rather than conduct and the presence of items that are separate from, or tangential to, consideration of study quality (e.g. ethical approval).

Authors should distinguish between assessment of study quality and assessment of risk of bias by focusing on assessment of methodological strengths and limitations as a marker of study rigour (what we term a 'risk to rigour' approach (Noyes et al 2019)). In the absence of a definitive risk to rigour tool, we recommend that review authors select from published, commonly used and validated tools that focus on the assessment of the methodological strengths and limitations of qualitative studies (see Box 21.8.a). Pragmatically, we consider a 'validated' tool as one that has been subjected to evaluation. Issues such as inter-rater reliability are afforded less importance given that identification of complementary or conflicting perspectives on risk to rigour is considered more useful than achievement of consensus per se (Noyes et al 2019).

The CASP tool for qualitative research (as one example) maps onto the domains in Box 21.8.a (CASP 2013). Tools **not** meeting the criterion of focusing on assessment of methodological strengths and limitations include those that integrate assessment of the quality of reporting (such as scoring of the title and abstract, etc) into an overall assessment of methodological strengths and limitations. As with other risk of bias assessment tools, we strongly recommend against the application of scores to domains or calculation of total quality scores. We encourage review authors to discuss the studies

Box 21.8.a Example domains that provide an assessment of methodological strengths and limitations to determine study rigour

Clear aims and research question
Congruence between the research aims/question and research design/method(s)
Rigour of case and or participant identification, sampling and data collection to address the question
Appropriate application of the method
Richness/conceptual depth of findings
Exploration of deviant cases and alternative explanations
Reflexivity of the researchers*

* Reflexivity encourages qualitative researchers and reviewers to consider the actual and potential impacts of the researcher on the context, research participants and the interpretation and reporting of data and findings (Newton et al 2012). Being reflexive entails making conflicts of interest transparent, discussing the impact of the reviewers and their decisions on the review process and findings and making transparent any issues discussed and subsequent decisions.

Adapted from Noyes et al (2019) and Alvesson and Sköldberg (2009)

and their assessments of 'risk to rigour' for each paper and how the study's methodological limitations may affect review findings (Noyes et al 2019). We further advise that qualitative 'sensitivity analysis', exploring the robustness of the synthesis and its vulnerability to methodologically limited studies, be routinely applied regardless of the review authors' overall confidence in synthesized findings (Carroll et al 2013). Evidence suggests that qualitative sensitivity analysis is equally advisable for mixed methods studies from which the qualitative component is extracted (Verhage and Boels 2017).

21.8.1 Additional assessment of methodological strengths and limitations of process evaluation and intervention implementation evidence

Few assessment tools explicitly address rigour in process evaluation or implementation evidence. For qualitative primary studies, the 8-item process evaluation tool developed by the EPPI-Centre (Rees et al 2009, Shepherd et al 2010) can be used to supplement tools selected to assess methodological strengths and limitations and risks to rigour in primary qualitative studies. One of these items, a question on usefulness (framed as '*how well the intervention processes were described and whether or not the process data could illuminate why or how the interventions worked or did not work*') offers a mechanism for exploring process mechanisms (Cargo et al 2018).

21.9 Selecting studies to synthesize

Decisions about inclusion or exclusion of studies can be more complex in qualitative evidence syntheses compared to reviews of trials that aim to include all relevant studies. Decisions on whether to include all studies or to select a sample of studies depend on a range of general and review specific criteria that Noyes and colleagues (Noyes et al 2019) outline in detail. The number of qualitative studies selected needs to be consistent with a manageable synthesis, and the contexts of the included studies should enable integration with the trials in the effectiveness analysis (see Figure 21.2.a). The guiding principle is transparency in the reporting of all decisions and their rationale.

21.10 Selecting a qualitative evidence synthesis and data extraction method

Authors will typically find that they cannot select an appropriate synthesis method until the pool of available qualitative evidence has been thoroughly scoped. Flexible options concerning choice of method may need to be articulated in the protocol.

The INTEGRATE-HTA guidance on selecting methodology and methods for qualitative evidence synthesis and health technology assessment offers a useful starting point when selecting a method of synthesis (Booth et al 2016, Booth et al 2018). Some methods are designed primarily to develop findings at a descriptive level and thus directly feed into lines of action for policy and practice. Others hold the capacity to develop new theory (e.g. meta-ethnography and theory building approaches to thematic synthesis). Noyes and colleagues (Noyes et al 2019) and Flemming and colleagues (Flemming et al 2019) elaborate on key issues for consideration when selecting a method that is particularly suited to a Cochrane Review and decision making context (see Table 21.10.a). Three qualitative evidence synthesis methods (thematic synthesis, framework synthesis and meta-ethnography) are recommended to produce syntheses that can subsequently be integrated with an intervention review or analysis.

21.11 Data extraction

Qualitative findings may take the form of quotations from participants, subthemes and themes identified by the study's authors, explanations, hypotheses or new theory, or observational excerpts and author interpretations of these data (Sandelowski and Barroso 2002). Findings may be presented as a narrative, or summarized and displayed as tables, infographics or logic models and potentially located in any part of the paper (Noyes et al 2019).

Methods for qualitative data extraction vary according to the synthesis method selected. Data extraction is not sequential and linear; often, it involves moving backwards and forwards between review stages. Review teams will need regular meetings to discuss and further interrogate the evidence and thereby achieve a shared understanding. It may be helpful to draw on a key stakeholder group to help in interpreting the evidence and in formulating key findings. Additional approaches (such as subgroup analysis) can be used to explore evidence from specific contexts further.

Irrespective of the review type and choice of synthesis method, we consider it best practice to extract detailed contextual and methodological information on each study and to report this information in a table of 'Characteristics of included studies' (see

Table 21.10.a Recommended methods for undertaking a qualitative evidence synthesis for subsequent integration with an intervention review, or as part of a mixed-method review (adapted from an original source developed by convenors (Flemming et al 2019, Noyes et al 2019))

Methodology	Explanation
Likely to be most suitable	
Thematic synthesis (Thomas and Harden 2008)	*Pros:* Most accessible form of synthesis. Clear approach, can be used with 'thin' data to produce descriptive themes and with 'thicker' data to develop descriptive themes in to more in-depth analytic themes. Themes are then integrated within the quantitative synthesis.
	Cons: May be limited in interpretive 'power' and risks over-simplistic use and thus not truly informing decision making such as guidelines. Complex synthesis process that requires an experienced team. Theoretical findings may combine empirical evidence, expert opinion and conjecture to form hypotheses. More work is needed on how GRADE CERQual to assess confidence in synthesized qualitative findings (see Section 21.12) can be applied to theoretical findings. May lack clarity on how higher-level findings translate into actionable points.
Requires some caution in its use	
Framework synthesis (Oliver et al 2008, Dixon-Woods 2011) Best-fit framework synthesis (Carroll et al 2011)	*Pros:* Works well within reviews of complex interventions by accommodating complexity within the framework, including representation of theory. The framework allows a clear mechanism for integration of qualitative and quantitative evidence in an aggregative way – see Noyes et al (2018a). Works well where there is broad agreement about the nature of interventions and their desired impacts.
	Cons: Requires identification, selection and justification of framework. A framework may be revealed as inappropriate only once extraction/synthesis is underway. Risk of simplistically forcing data into a framework for expedience.
Requires more caution in its use	
Meta-ethnography (Noblit and Hare 1988)	*Pros:* Primarily interpretive synthesis method leading to creation of descriptive as well as new high order constructs. Descriptive and theoretical findings can help inform decision making such as guidelines. Explicit reporting standards have been developed.
	Cons: Complex methodology and synthesis process that requires highly experienced team. Can take more time and resources than other methodologies. Theoretical findings may combine empirical evidence, expert opinion and conjecture to form hypotheses. May not satisfy requirements for an audit trail (although new reporting guidelines will help overcome this (France et al 2019). More work is needed to determine how CERQual can be applied to theoretical findings. May be unclear how higher-level findings translate into actionable points.

Table 21.11.a). The template for intervention description and replication TIDieR checklist (Hoffmann et al 2014) and ICAT_SR tool may help with specifying key information for extraction (Lewin et al 2017). Review authors must ensure that they preserve the context of the primary study data during the extraction and synthesis process to prevent misinterpretation of primary studies (Noyes et al 2019).

Table 21.11.a Contextual and methodological information for inclusion within a table of 'Characteristics of included studies'. From Noyes et al (2019). Reproduced with permission of BMJ Publishing Group

Data extraction field	Information extracted
Context and participants	Important elements of study context, relevant to addressing the review question and locating the context of the primary study; for example, the study setting, population characteristics, participants and participant characteristics, the intervention delivered (if appropriate), etc.
Study design and methods used	Methodological design and approach taken by the study; methods for identifying the sample recruitment; the specific data collection and analysis methods utilized; and any theoretical models used to interpret or contextualize the findings.

Noyes and colleagues (Noyes et al 2019) provide additional guidance and examples of the various methods of data extraction. It is usual for review authors to select one method. In summary, extraction methods can be grouped as follows.

- ***Using a bespoke universal, standardized or adapted data extraction template*** Review authors can develop their own review-specific data extraction template, or select a generic data extraction template by study type (e.g. templates developed by the National Institute for Health and Clinical Excellence (National Institute for Health Care Excellence 2012).
- ***Using an a priori theory or predetermined framework to extract data*** Framework synthesis, and its subvariant 'Best Fit' Framework approach, involve extracting data from primary studies against an a priori framework in order to better understand a phenomenon of interest (Carroll et al 2011, Carroll et al 2013). For example, Glenton and colleagues (Glenton et al (2013) extracted data against a modified SURE Framework (2011) to synthesize factors affecting the implementation of lay health worker interventions. The SURE framework enumerates possible factors that may influence the implementation of health system interventions (The SURE (Supporting the Use of Research Evidence) Collaboration 2011, Glenton et al 2013). Use of the 'PROGRESS' (place of residence, race/ethnicity/culture/language, occupation, gender/sex, religion, education, socioeconomic status, and social capital) framework also helps to ensure that data extraction maintains an explicit equity focus (O'Neill et al 2014). A logic model can also be used as a framework for data extraction.
- ***Using a software program to code original studies inductively*** A wide range of software products have been developed by systematic review organizations (such as EPPI-Reviewer (Thomas et al 2010)). Most software for the analysis of primary qualitative data – such as NVivo (www.qsrinternational.com/nvivo/home) and others – can be used to code studies in a systematic review (Houghton et al 2017). For example, one method of data extraction and thematic synthesis involves coding the original studies using a software program to build inductive descriptive themes and a theoretical explanation of phenomena of interest (Thomas and Harden 2008). Thomas and Harden (2008) provide a worked example to demonstrate coding and developing a new understanding of children's choices and motivations to eating fruit and vegetables from included primary studies.

21.12 Assessing the confidence in qualitative synthesized findings

The GRADE system has long featured in assessing the certainty of quantitative findings and application of its qualitative counterpart, GRADE-CERQual, is recommended for Cochrane qualitative evidence syntheses (Lewin et al 2015). CERQual has four components (relevance, methodological limitations, adequacy and coherence) which are used to formulate an overall assessment of confidence in the synthesized qualitative finding. Guidance on its components and reporting requirements have been published in a series in *Implementation Science* (Lewin et al 2018).

21.13 Methods for integrating the qualitative evidence synthesis with an intervention review

A range of methods and tools is available for data integration or mixed-method synthesis (Harden et al 2018, Noyes et al 2019). As noted at the beginning of this chapter, review authors can integrate a qualitative evidence synthesis with an existing intervention review published on a similar topic (sequential approach), or conduct a new intervention review and qualitative evidence syntheses in parallel before integration (convergent approach). Irrespective of whether the qualitative synthesis is sequential or convergent to the intervention review, we recommend that qualitative and quantitative evidence be synthesized separately using appropriate methods before integration (Harden et al 2018). The scope for integration can be more limited with a pre-existing intervention review unless review authors have access to the data underlying the intervention review report.

Harden and colleagues and Noyes and colleagues outline the following methods and tools for integration with an intervention review (Harden et al 2018, Noyes et al 2019):

- ***Juxtaposing findings in a matrix*** Juxtaposition is driven by the findings from the qualitative evidence synthesis (e.g. intervention components related to the acceptability or feasibility of the interventions) and these findings form one side of the matrix. Findings on intervention effects (e.g. improves outcome, no difference in outcome, uncertain effects) form the other side of the matrix. Quantitative studies are grouped according to findings on intervention effects and the presence or absence of features specified by the hypotheses generated from the qualitative synthesis (Candy et al 2011). Observed patterns in the matrix are used to explain differences in the findings of the quantitative studies and to identify gaps in research (van Grootel et al 2017). (See, for example, Ames et al 2017, Munabi-Babigumira et al 2017, Hurley et al 2018.)
- ***Analysing programme theory*** Theories articulating how interventions are expected to work are analysed. Findings from quantitative studies, testing the effects of interventions, and from qualitative and process evaluation evidence are used together to examine how the theories work in practice (Greenhalgh et al 2007). The value of different theories is assessed or new/revised theory developed. Factors that enhance or reduce intervention effectiveness are also identified.

- ***Using logic models or other types of conceptual framework*** A logic model (Glenton et al 2013) or other type of conceptual framework, which represents the processes by which an intervention produces change provides a common scaffold for integrating findings across different types of evidence (Booth and Carroll 2015). Frameworks can be specified a priori from the literature or through stakeholder engagement or newly developed during the review. Findings from quantitative studies testing the effects of interventions and those from qualitative evidence are used to develop and/or further refine the model.
- ***Testing hypotheses derived from syntheses of qualitative evidence*** Quantitative studies are grouped according to the presence or absence of the proposition specified by the hypotheses to be tested and subgroup analysis is used to explore differential findings on the effects of interventions (Thomas et al 2004).
- ***Qualitative comparative analysis (QCA)*** Findings from a qualitative synthesis are used to identify the range of *features* that are important for successful interventions, and the *mechanisms* through which these features operate. A QCA then tests whether or not the features are associated with effective interventions (Kahwati et al 2016). The analysis unpicks multiple potential pathways to effectiveness accommodating scenarios where the same intervention feature is associated *both* with effective and less effective interventions, depending on context. QCA offers potential for use in integration; unlike the other methods and tools presented here it does not yet have sufficient methodological guidance available. However, exemplar reviews using QCA are available (Thomas et al 2014, Harris et al 2015, Kahwati et al 2016).

Review authors can use the above methods in combination (e.g. patterns observed through juxtaposing findings within a matrix can be tested using subgroup analysis or QCA). Analysing programme theory, using logic models and QCA would require members of the review team with specific skills in these methods. Using subgroup analysis and QCA are not suitable when limited evidence is available (Harden et al 2018, Noyes et al 2019). (See also Chapter 17 on intervention complexity.)

21.14 Reporting the protocol and qualitative evidence synthesis

Reporting standards and tools designed for intervention reviews (such as Cochrane's MECIR standards (http://methods.cochrane.org/mecir) or the PRISMA Statement (Liberati et al 2009), may not be appropriate for qualitative evidence syntheses or an integrated mixed-method review. Additional guidance on how to choose, adapt or create a hybrid reporting tool is provided as a 5-point 'decision flowchart' (Figure 21.14.a) (Flemming et al 2018). Review authors should consider whether: a specific set of reporting guidance is available (e.g. eMERGe for meta-ethnographies (France et al 2015)); whether generic guidance (e.g. ENTREQ (Tong et al 2012)) is suitable; or whether additional checklists or tools are appropriate for reporting a specific aspect of the review.

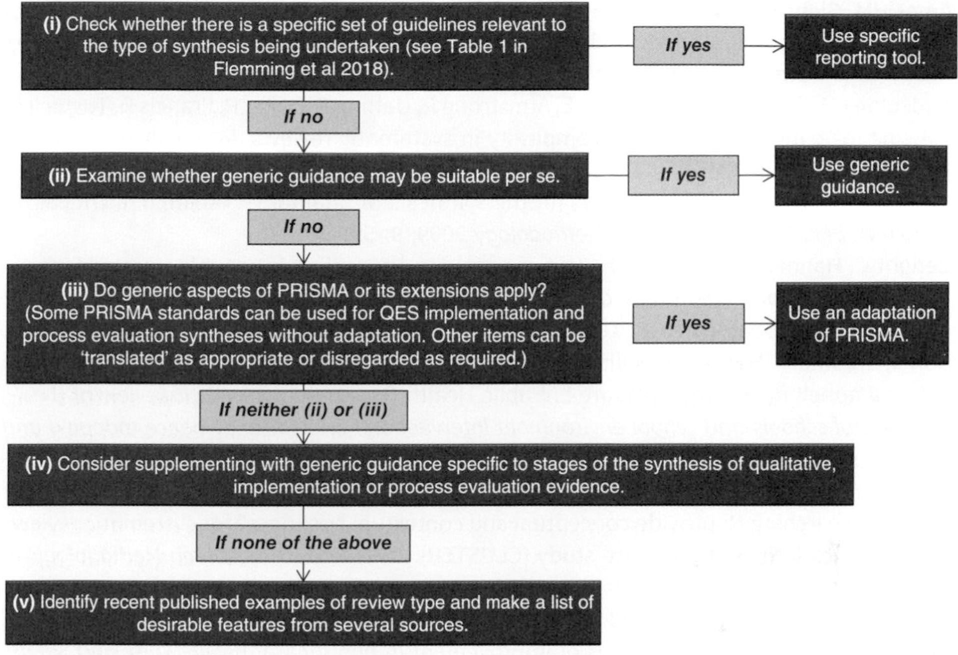

Figure 21.14.a Decision flowchart for choice of reporting approach for syntheses of qualitative, implementation or process evaluation evidence (Flemming et al 2018). Reproduced with permission of Elsevier

21.15 Chapter information

Authors: Jane Noyes, Andrew Booth, Margaret Cargo, Kate Flemming, Angela Harden, Janet Harris, Ruth Garside, Karin Hannes, Tomás Pantoja, James Thomas

Acknowledgements: This chapter replaces Chapter 20 in the first edition of this *Handbook* (2008) and subsequent Version 5.2. We would like to thank the previous Chapter 20 authors Jennie Popay and Alan Pearson. Elements of this chapter draw on previous supplemental guidance produced by the Cochrane Qualitative and Implementation Methods Group Convenors, to which Simon Lewin contributed.

Funding: JT is supported by the National Institute for Health Research (NIHR) Collaboration for Leadership in Applied Health Research and Care North Thames at Barts Health NHS Trust. The views expressed are those of the author(s) and not necessarily those of the NHS, the NIHR or the Department of Health.

21.16 References

Alvesson M, Sköldberg K. *Reflexive Methodology: New Vistas for Qualitative Research*. 2nd ed. London, UK: Sage; 2009.

Ames HM, Glenton C, Lewin S. Parents' and informal caregivers' views and experiences of communication about routine childhood vaccination: a synthesis of qualitative evidence. *Cochrane Database of Systematic Reviews* 2017; **2**: CD011787.

Anderson LM, Petticrew M, Rehfuess E, Armstrong R, Ueffing E, Baker P, Francis D, Tugwell P. Using logic models to capture complexity in systematic reviews. *Research Synthesis Methods* 2011; **2**: 33–42.

Barnett-Page E, Thomas J. Methods for the synthesis of qualitative research: a critical review. *BMC Medical Research Methodology* 2009; **9**: 59.

Benoot C, Hannes K, Bilsen J. The use of purposeful sampling in a qualitative evidence synthesis: a worked example on sexual adjustment to a cancer trajectory. *BMC Medical Research Methodology* 2016; **16**: 21.

Bonell C, Jamal F, Harden A, Wells H, Parry W, Fletcher A, Petticrew M, Thomas J, Whitehead M, Campbell R, Murphy S, Moore L. Public Health Research. *Systematic review of the effects of schools and school environment interventions on health: evidence mapping and synthesis*. Southampton (UK): NIHR Journals Library; 2013.

Booth A, Harris J, Croot E, Springett J, Campbell F, Wilkins E. Towards a methodology for cluster searching to provide conceptual and contextual "richness" for systematic reviews of complex interventions: case study (CLUSTER). *BMC Medical Research Methodology* 2013; **13**: 118.

Booth A, Carroll C. How to build up the actionable knowledge base: the role of 'best fit' framework synthesis for studies of improvement in healthcare. *BMJ Quality and Safety* 2015; **24**: 700–708.

Booth A, Noyes J, Flemming K, Gerhardus A, Wahlster P, van der Wilt GJ, Mozygemba K, Refolo P, Sacchini D, Tummers M, Rehfuess E. Guidance on choosing qualitative evidence synthesis methods for use in health technology assessment for complex interventions 2016. https://www.integrate-hta.eu/wp-content/uploads/2016/02/Guidance-on-choosing-qualitative-evidence-synthesis-methods-for-use-in-HTA-of-complex-interventions.pdf

Booth A. Qualitative evidence synthesis. In: Facey K, editor. *Patient involvement in Health Technology Assessment*. Singapore: Springer; 2017. p. 187–199.

Booth A, Noyes J, Flemming K, Gehardus A, Wahlster P, Jan van der Wilt G, Mozygemba K, Refolo P, Sacchini D, Tummers M, Rehfuess E. Structured methodology review identified seven (RETREAT) criteria for selecting qualitative evidence synthesis approaches. *Journal of Clinical Epidemiology* 2018; **99**: 41–52.

Booth A, Moore G, Flemming K, Garside R, Rollins N, Tuncalp Ö, Noyes J. Taking account of context in systematic reviews and guidelines considering a complexity perspective. *BMJ Global Health* 2019a; **4**: e000840.

Booth A, Noyes J, Flemming K, Moore G, Tuncalp O, Shakibazadeh E. Formulating questions to address the acceptability and feasibility of complex interventions in qualitative evidence synthesis. *BMJ Global Health* 2019b; **4**: e001107.

Candy B, King M, Jones L, Oliver S. Using qualitative synthesis to explore heterogeneity of complex interventions. *BMC Medical Research Methodology* 2011; **11**: 124.

Cargo M, Harris J, Pantoja T, Booth A, Harden A, Hannes K, Thomas J, Flemming K, Garside R, Noyes J. Cochrane Qualitative and Implementation Methods Group guidance series-paper 4: methods for assessing evidence on intervention implementation. *Journal of Clinical Epidemiology* 2018; **97**: 59–69.

Carroll C, Booth A, Cooper K. A worked example of “best fit” framework synthesis: a systematic review of views concerning the taking of some potential chemopreventive agents. *BMC Medical Research Methodology* 2011; **11**: 29.

Carroll C, Booth A, Leaviss J, Rick J. “Best fit” framework synthesis: refining the method. *BMC Medical Research Methodology* 2013; **13**: 37.

Carroll C. Qualitative evidence synthesis to improve implementation of clinical guidelines. *BMJ* 2017; **356**: j80.

CASP. Making sense of evidence: 10 questions to help you make sense of qualitative research: Public Health Resource Unit, England; 2013. http://media.wix.com/ugd/dded87_29c5b002d99342f788c6ac670e49f274.pdf.

Cooke A, Smith D, Booth A. Beyond PICO: the SPIDER tool for qualitative evidence synthesis. *Qualitative Health Research* 2012; **22**: 1435–1443.

Cooper C, Booth A, Britten N, Garside R. A comparison of results of empirical studies of supplementary search techniques and recommendations in review methodology handbooks: a methodological review. *Systematic Reviews* 2017; **6**: 234.

De Buck E, Hannes K, Cargo M, Van Remoortel H, Vande Veegaete A, Mosler HJ, Govender T, Vandekerckhove P, Young T. Engagement of stakeholders in the development of a Theory of Change for handwashing and sanitation behaviour change. *International Journal of Environmental Research and Public Health* 2018; **28**: 8–22.

Dixon-Woods M. Using framework-based synthesis for conducting reviews of qualitative studies. *BMC Medicine* 2011; **9**: 39.

Downe S, Finlayson K, Tuncalp, Metin Gulmezoglu A. What matters to women: a systematic scoping review to identify the processes and outcomes of antenatal care provision that are important to healthy pregnant women. *BJOG: An International Journal of Obstetrics and Gynaecology* 2016; **123**: 529–539.

El Sherif R, Pluye P, Gore G, Granikov V, Hong QN. Performance of a mixed filter to identify relevant studies for mixed studies reviews. *Journal of the Medical Library Association* 2016; **104**: 47–51.

Flemming K, Booth A, Hannes K, Cargo M, Noyes J. Cochrane Qualitative and Implementation Methods Group guidance series-paper 6: reporting guidelines for qualitative, implementation, and process evaluation evidence syntheses. *Journal of Clinical Epidemiology* 2018; **97**: 79–85.

Flemming K, Booth A, Garside R, Tuncalp O, Noyes J. Qualitative evidence synthesis for complex interventions and guideline development: clarification of the purpose, designs and relevant methods. *BMJ Global Health* 2019; **4**: e000882.

France EF, Ring N, Noyes J, Maxwell M, Jepson R, Duncan E, Turley R, Jones D, Uny I. Protocol-developing meta-ethnography reporting guidelines (eMERGe). *BMC Medical Research Methodology* 2015; **15**: 103.

France EF, Cunningham M, Ring N, Uny I, Duncan EAS, Jepson RG, Maxwell M, Roberts RJ, Turley RL, Booth A, Britten N, Flemming K, Gallagher I, Garside R, Hannes K, Lewin S, Noblit GW, Pope C, Thomas J, Vanstone M, Higginbottom GMA, Noyes J. Improving reporting of meta-ethnography: the eMERGe Reporting Guidance. *BMC Medical Research Methodology* 2019; **19**: 25.

Garside R. Should we appraise the quality of qualitative research reports for systematic reviews, and if so, how? *Innovation: European Journal of Social Science Research* 2014; **27**: 67–79.

Glenton C, Colvin CJ, Carlsen B, Swartz A, Lewin S, Noyes J, Rashidian A. Barriers and facilitators to the implementation of lay health worker programmes to improve access to maternal and child health: qualitative evidence synthesis. *Cochrane Database of Systematic Reviews* 2013; **10**: CD010414.

Glenton C, Lewin S, Norris S. Chapter 15: Using evidence from qualitative research to develop WHO guidelines. In: Norris S, editor. *World Health Organization Handbook for Guideline Development*. 2nd ed. Geneva: WHO; 2016.

Grant MJ, Booth A. A typology of reviews: an analysis of 14 review types and associated methodologies. *Health Information and Libraries Journal* 2009; **26**: 91–108.

Greenhalgh T, Kristjansson E, Robinson V. Realist review to understand the efficacy of school feeding programmes. *BMJ* 2007; **335**: 858.

Harden A, Oakley A, Weston R. *A review of the effectiveness and appropriateness of peer-delivered health promotion for young people*. London: Institute of Education, University of London; 1999.

Harden A, Thomas J, Cargo M, Harris J, Pantoja T, Flemming K, Booth A, Garside R, Hannes K, Noyes J. Cochrane Qualitative and Implementation Methods Group guidance series-paper 5: methods for integrating qualitative and implementation evidence within intervention effectiveness reviews. *Journal of Clinical Epidemiology* 2018; **97**: 70–78.

Harris JL, Booth A, Cargo M, Hannes K, Harden A, Flemming K, Garside R, Pantoja T, Thomas J, Noyes J. Cochrane Qualitative and Implementation Methods Group guidance series-paper 2: methods for question formulation, searching, and protocol development for qualitative evidence synthesis. *Journal of Clinical Epidemiology* 2018; **97**: 39–48.

Harris KM, Kneale D, Lasserson TJ, McDonald VM, Grigg J, Thomas J. School-based self management interventions for asthma in children and adolescents: a mixed methods systematic review (Protocol). *Cochrane Database of Systematic Reviews* 2015; **4**: CD011651.

Hoffmann TC, Glasziou PP, Boutron I, Milne R, Perera R, Moher D, Altman DG, Barbour V, Macdonald H, Johnston M, Lamb SE, Dixon-Woods M, McCulloch P, Wyatt JC, Chan AW, Michie S. Better reporting of interventions: template for intervention description and replication (TIDieR) checklist and guide. *BMJ* 2014; **348**: g1687.

Houghton C, Murphy K, Meehan B, Thomas J, Brooker D, Casey D. From screening to synthesis: using nvivo to enhance transparency in qualitative evidence synthesis. *Journal of Clinical Nursing* 2017; **26**: 873–881.

Hurley M, Dickson K, Hallett R, Grant R, Hauari H, Walsh N, Stansfield C, Oliver S. Exercise interventions and patient beliefs for people with hip, knee or hip and knee osteoarthritis: a mixed methods review. *Cochrane Database of Systematic Reviews* 2018; **4**: CD010842.

Kahwati L, Jacobs S, Kane H, Lewis M, Viswanathan M, Golin CE. Using qualitative comparative analysis in a systematic review of a complex intervention. *Systematic Reviews* 2016; **5**: 82.

Kelly MP, Noyes J, Kane RL, Chang C, Uhl S, Robinson KA, Springs S, Butler ME, Guise JM. AHRQ series on complex intervention systematic reviews-paper 2: defining complexity, formulating scope, and questions. *Journal of Clinical Epidemiology* 2017; **90**: 11–18.

Kneale D, Thomas J, Harris K. Developing and optimising the use of logic models in systematic reviews: exploring practice and good practice in the use of programme theory in reviews. *PloS One* 2015; **10**: e0142187.

Levac D, Colquhoun H, O'Brien KK. Scoping studies: advancing the methodology. *Implementation Science* 2010; **5**: 69.

Lewin S, Munabi-Babigumira S, Glenton C, Daniels K, Bosch-Capblanch X, van Wyk BE, Odgaard-Jensen J, Johansen M, Aja GN, Zwarenstein M, Scheel IB. Lay health workers in primary and community health care for maternal and child health and the management of infectious diseases. *Cochrane Database of Systematic Reviews* 2010; **3**: CD004015.

Lewin S, Glenton C, Munthe-Kaas H, Carlsen B, Colvin CJ, Gulmezoglu M, Noyes J, Booth A, Garside R, Rashidian A. Using qualitative evidence in decision making for health and social interventions: an approach to assess confidence in findings from qualitative evidence syntheses (GRADE-CERQual). *PLoS Medicine* 2015; **12**: e1001895.

Lewin S, Hendry M, Chandler J, Oxman AD, Michie S, Shepperd S, Reeves BC, Tugwell P, Hannes K, Rehfuess EA, Welch V, McKenzie JE, Burford B, Petkovic J, Anderson LM, Harris J, Noyes J. Assessing the complexity of interventions within systematic reviews: development, content and use of a new tool (iCAT_SR). *BMC Medical Research Methodology* 2017; **17**: 76.

Lewin S, Booth A, Glenton C, Munthe-Kaas H, Rashidian A, Wainwright M, Bohren MA, Tuncalp O, Colvin CJ, Garside R, Carlsen B, Langlois EV, Noyes J. Applying GRADE-CERQual to qualitative evidence synthesis findings: introduction to the series. *Implementation Science* 2018; **13**: 2.

Liberati A, Altman DG, Tetzlaff J, Mulrow C, Gøtzsche PC, Ioannidis JPA, Clarke M, Devereaux PJ, Kleijnen J, Moher D. The PRISMA statement for reporting systematic reviews and meta-analyses of studies that evaluate healthcare interventions: explanation and elaboration. *BMJ* 2009; **339**: b2700.

Moore G, Audrey S, Barker M, Bond L, Bonell C, Harderman W, et al. Process evaluation of complex interventions: Medical Research Council guidance. *BMJ* 2015; **350**: h1258.

Munabi-Babigumira S, Glenton C, Lewin S, Fretheim A, Nabudere H. Factors that influence the provision of intrapartum and postnatal care by skilled birth attendants in low- and middle-income countries: a qualitative evidence synthesis. *Cochrane Database of Systematic Reviews* 2017; **11**: CD011558.

Munthe-Kaas H, Glenton C, Lewin S, Noyes J, Booth A. Systematic mapping of existing tools to appraise methodological strengths and limitations of qualitative research: Preliminary development of the CAMELOT tool. *BMC Medical Research Methodology* 2019; **19**: 113.

National Institute for Health Care Excellence. NICE Process and Methods Guides. *Methods for the Development of NICE Public Health Guidance*. London: National Institute for Health and Care Excellence (NICE); 2012.

Newton BJ, Rothlingova Z, Gutteridge R, LeMarchand K, Raphael JH. No room for reflexivity? Critical reflections following a systematic review of qualitative research. *Journal of Health Psychology* 2012; **17**: 866–885.

Noblit GW, Hare RD. *Meta-Ethnography: Synthesizing Qualitative Studies*. Newbury Park: Sage Publications, Inc; 1988.

Noyes J, Hendry M, Booth A, Chandler J, Lewin S, Glenton C, Garside R. Current use was established and Cochrane guidance on selection of social theories for systematic reviews of complex interventions was developed. *Journal of Clinical Epidemiology* 2016a; **75**: 78–92.

Noyes J, Hendry M, Lewin S, Glenton C, Chandler J, Rashidian A. Qualitative “trial-sibling” studies and “unrelated” qualitative studies contributed to complex intervention reviews. *Journal of Clinical Epidemiology* 2016b; **74**: 133–143.

Noyes J, Booth A, Flemming K, Garside R, Harden A, Lewin S, Pantoja T, Hannes K, Cargo M, Thomas J. Cochrane Qualitative and Implementation Methods Group guidance series-paper 3: methods for assessing methodological limitations, data extraction and synthesis, and confidence in synthesized qualitative findings. *Journal of Clinical Epidemiology* 2018a; **97**: 49–58.

Noyes J, Booth A, Cargo M, Flemming K, Garside R, Hannes K, Harden A, Harris J, Lewin S, Pantoja T, Thomas J. Cochrane Qualitative and Implementation Methods Group guidance series-paper 1: introduction. *Journal of Clinical Epidemiology* 2018b; **97**: 35–38.

Noyes J, Booth A, Moore G, Flemming K, Tuncalp O, Shakibazadeh E. Synthesising quantitative and qualitative evidence to inform guidelines on complex interventions: clarifying the purposes, designs and outlining some methods. *BMJ Global Health* 2019; **4 (**Suppl 1**)**: e000893.

O'Neill J, Tabish H, Welch V, Petticrew M, Pottie K, Clarke M, Evans T, Pardo Pardo J, Waters E, White H, Tugwell P. Applying an equity lens to interventions: using PROGRESS ensures consideration of socially stratifying factors to illuminate inequities in health. *Journal of Clinical Epidemiology* 2014; **67**: 56–64.

Oliver S, Rees R, Clarke-Jones L, Milne R, Oakley A, Gabbay J, Stein K, Buchanan P, Gyte G. A multidimensional conceptual framework for analysing public involvement in health services research. *Health Expectations* 2008; **11**: 72–84.

Petticrew M, Knai C, Thomas J, Rehfuess E, Noyes J, Gerhardus A, Grimshaw J, Rutter H. Implications of a complexity perspective for systematic reviews and guideline development in health decision making. *BMJ Global Health* 2019; **4 (**Suppl 1**)**: e000899.

Rees R, Oliver K, Woodman J, Thomas J. *Children's views about obesity, body size, shape and weight: a systematic review*. London: EPPI-Centre, Social Science Research Unit, Institute of Education, University of London; 2009.

Rehfuess EA, Booth A, Brereton L, Burns J, Gerhardus A, Mozygemba K, Oortwijn W, Pfadenhauer LM, Tummers M, van der Wilt GJ, Rohwer A. Towards a taxonomy of logic models in systematic reviews and health technology assessments: a priori, staged, and iterative approaches. *Research Synthesis Methods* 2018; **9**: 13–24.

Robbins SCC, Ward K, Skinner SR. School-based vaccination: a systematic review of process evaluations. *Vaccine* 2011; **29**: 9588–9599.

Rogers M, Bethel A, Abbott R. Locating qualitative studies in dementia on MEDLINE, EMBASE, CINAHL, and PsycINFO: a comparison of search strategies. *Research Synthesis Methods* 2018; **9**: 579–586.

Sandelowski M, Barroso J. Finding the findings in qualitative studies. *Journal of Nursing Scholarship* 2002; **34**: 213–219.

Selva A, Sola I, Zhang Y, Pardo-Hernandez H, Haynes RB, Martinez Garcia L, Navarro T, Schünemann H, Alonso-Coello P. Development and use of a content search strategy for retrieving studies on patients' views and preferences. *Health and Quality of Life Outcomes* 2017; **15**: 126.

Shepherd J, Kavanagh J, Picot J, Cooper K, Harden A, Barnett-Page E, Jones J, Clegg A, Hartwell D, Frampton GK, Price A. The effectiveness and cost-effectiveness of behavioural interventions for the prevention of sexually transmitted infections in young people aged 13-19: a systematic review and economic evaluation. *Health Technology Assessment* 2010; **14**: 1–206, iii–iv.

Squires JE, Valentine JC, Grimshaw JM. Systematic reviews of complex interventions: framing the review question. *Journal of Clinical Epidemiology* 2013; **66**: 1215–1222.

Stansfield C, Kavanagh J, Rees R, Gomersall A, Thomas J. The selection of search sources influences the findings of a systematic review of people's views: a case study in public health. *BMC Medical Research Methodology* 2012; **12**: 55.

SURE (Supporting the Use of Research Evidence) Collaboration. SURE Guides for Preparing and Using Evidence-based Policy Briefs: 5 Identifying and Addressing Barriers to Implementing the Policy Options. Version 2.1, updated November 2011. http://global.evipnet.org/SURE-Guides/.

Suri H. Purposeful sampling in qualitative research synthesis. *Qualitative Research Journal* 2011; **11**: 63–75.

Thomas J, Harden A, Oakley A, Oliver S, Sutcliffe K, Rees R, Brunton G, Kavanagh J. Integrating qualitative research with trials in systematic reviews. *BMJ* 2004; **328**: 1010–1012.

Thomas J, Harden A. Methods for the thematic synthesis of qualitative research in systematic reviews. *BMC Medical Research Methodology* 2008; **8**: 45.

Thomas J, Brunton J, Graziosi S. EPPI-Reviewer 4.0: software for research synthesis [Software]. EPPI-Centre Software. Social Science Research Unit, Institute of Education, University of London UK; 2010. https://eppi.ioe.ac.uk/CMS/Default.aspx?alias=eppi.ioe.ac.uk/cms/er4&.

Thomas J, O'Mara-Eves A, Brunton G. Using qualitative comparative analysis (QCA) in systematic reviews of complex interventions: a worked example. *Systematic Reviews* 2014; **3**: 67.

Tong A, Flemming K, McInnes E, Oliver S, Craig J. Enhancing transparency in reporting the synthesis of qualitative research: ENTREQ. *BMC Medical Research Methodology* 2012; **12**: 181.

van Grootel L, van Wesel F, O'Mara-Eves A, Thomas J, Hox J, Boeije H. Using the realist perspective to link theory from qualitative evidence synthesis to quantitative studies: broadening the matrix approach. *Research Synthesis Methods* 2017; **8**: 303–311.

Verhage A, Boels D. Critical appraisal of mixed methods research studies in a systematic scoping review on plural policing: assessing the impact of excluding inadequately reported studies by means of a sensitivity analysis. *Quality and Quantity* 2017; **51**: 1449–1468.

Walker LO, Avant KC. *Strategies for Theory Construction in Nursing*. Upper Saddle River (NJ): Pearson Prentice Hall; 2005.

SURE (Supporting the Use of Research Evidence) Collaboration. SURE Guides for Preparing and Using Evidence-based Policy Briefs: 5 Identifying and Addressing Barriers to Implementing the Policy Options. Version 2.1 [updated November 2011]. [illegible]evipnet.org/SURE-Guides/.

Suri H. Purposeful sampling in qualitative research synthesis. Qualitative Research Journal 2011; 11: 63–75.

Thomas J, Harden A, Oakley A, Oliver S, Sutcliffe K, Rees R, Brunton G, Kavanagh J. Integrating qualitative research with trials in systematic reviews. BMJ 2004; 328: 1010–1012.

Thomas J, Harden A. Methods for the thematic synthesis of qualitative research [illegible]

[illegible]

Part Three

Further topics

22

Prospective approaches to accumulating evidence

James Thomas, Lisa M Askie, Jesse A Berlin, Julian H Elliott, Davina Ghersi, Mark Simmonds, Yemisi Takwoingi, Jayne F Tierney, Julian PT Higgins

KEY POINTS

- Cochrane Reviews should reflect the state of current knowledge, but maintaining their currency is a challenge due to resource limitations. It is difficult to know when a given review might become out of date, but tools are available to assist in identifying when a review might need updating.
- Living systematic reviews are systematic reviews that are continually updated, with new evidence being incorporated as soon as it becomes available. They are useful in rapidly evolving fields where research is published frequently. New technologies and better processes for data storage and reuse are being developed to facilitate the rapid identification and synthesis of new evidence.
- A prospective meta-analysis is a meta-analysis of studies (usually randomized trials) that were identified or even collectively planned to be eligible for the meta-analysis before the results of the studies became known. They are usually undertaken by a collaborative group including authors of the studies to be included, and they usually collect and analyse individual participant data.
- Formal sequential statistical methods are discouraged for standard updated meta-analyses in most circumstances for Cochrane Reviews. They should not be used for the main analyses, or to draw main conclusions. Sequential methods may, however, be used in the context of a prospectively planned series of randomized trials.

22.1 Introduction

Iain Chalmers' vision of "a library of trial overviews which will be updated when new data become available" (Chalmers 1986), became the mission and founding purpose of Cochrane. Thousands of systematic reviews are now published in the *Cochrane Database of Systematic Reviews*, presenting critical summaries of the evidence. However,

This chapter should be cited as: Thomas J, Askie LM, Berlin JA, Elliott JH, Ghersi D, Simmonds M, Takwoingi Y, Tierney JF, Higgins HPT. Chapter 22: Prospective approaches to accumulating evidence. In: Higgins JPT, Thomas J, Chandler J, Cumpston M, Li T, Page MJ, Welch VA (editors). *Cochrane Handbook for Systematic Reviews of Interventions*. 2nd Edition. Chichester (UK): John Wiley & Sons, 2019: 549–568.

maintaining the currency of these reviews through periodic updates, consistent with Chalmers' vision, has been a challenge. Moreover, as the global community of researchers has begun to see research in a cumulative way, rather than in terms of individual studies, the idea of 'prospective' meta-analyses has emerged. A prospective meta-analysis (PMA) begins with the idea that future studies will be integrated within a systematic review and works backwards to plan a programme of trials with the explicit purpose of their future integration.

The first part of this chapter covers methods for keeping abreast of the accumulating evidence to help a review team understand when a systematic review might need updating (see Section 22.2). This includes the processes that can be put into place to monitor relevant publications, and algorithms that have been proposed to determine whether or when it is appropriate to revisit the review to incorporate new findings. We outline a vision for regularly updated reviews, known as 'living' systematic reviews, which are continually updated, with new evidence being identified and incorporated as soon as it becomes available.

While evidence surveillance and living systematic reviews may require some modifications to review processes, and can dramatically improve the delivery time and currency of updates, they are still essentially following a retrospective model of reviewing the existing evidence base. The retrospective nature of most systematic reviews poses an inevitable challenge, in that the selection of what types of evidence to include may be influenced by authors' knowledge of the context and findings of the available studies. This might introduce bias into any aspect of the review's eligibility criteria including the selection of a target population, the nature of the intervention(s), choice of comparator and the outcomes to be assessed. The best way to overcome this problem is to identify evidence entirely prospectively, that is before the results of the studies are known. Section 22.3 describes such prospectively planned meta-analyses.

Finally, Section 22.4 addresses concerns about the regular repeating of statistical tests in meta-analyses as they are updated over time. Cochrane actively discourages use of the notion of statistical significance in favour of reporting estimates and confidence intervals, so such concerns should not arise. Nevertheless, sequential approaches are an established method in randomized trials, and may play a role in a prospectively planned series of trials in a prospective meta-analysis.

22.2 Evidence surveillance: active monitoring of the accumulating evidence

22.2.1 Maintaining the currency of systematic reviews

Cochrane Reviews were conceived with the vision that they be kept up to date. For many years, a policy was in place of updating each Cochrane Review at least every two years. This policy was not closely followed due to a range of issues including: a lack of resources; the need to balance starting new reviews with maintaining older ones; the rapidly growing volume of research in some areas of health care and the paucity of new evidence in others; and challenges in knowing at any given point in time whether a systematic review was out of date and therefore possibly giving misleading, and potentially harmful, advice.

Maintaining the currency of systematic reviews by incorporating new evidence is important in many cases. For example, one study suggested that while the conclusions of most reviews might be valid for five or more years, the findings of 23% might be out of date within two years, and 7% were outdated at the time of their publication (Shojania et al 2007). Systematic reviews in rapidly evolving fields are particularly at risk of becoming out of date, leading to the development of a range of methods for identifying when a systematic review might need to be updated.

22.2.2 Signals for updating

Strategies for prioritizing updates, and for updating only reviews that warrant it, have been developed (Martinez Garcia et al 2017) (see Chapter 2, Section 2.4.1). A multi-component tool was proposed by Takwoingi and colleagues in 2013 (Takwoingi et al 2013). Garner and colleagues have refined this tool and described a staged process that starts by assessing the extent to which the review is up to date (including relevance of the question, impact of the review and implementation of appropriate and up-to-date methods), then examines whether relevant new evidence or new systematic review methodology are available, and then assesses the potential impact of updating the review in terms of whether the findings are likely to change (Garner et al 2016). For a detailed discussion of updating Cochrane Reviews, see online Chapter IV.

Information about the availability of new (or newly identified) evidence may come from a variety of sources and use a diverse range of approaches (Garner et al 2016), including:

- re-running the full search strategies in the original review;
- using an abbreviated search strategy;
- using literature notification services;
- developing machine-learning algorithms based on study reports identified for the original review;
- tracking studies in clinical trials (and other) registries;
- checking studies included in related systematic reviews; and
- other formal surveillance methods.

Searches of bibliographic databases may be streamlined by using literature notification services ('alerts'), whereby searches are run automatically at regular intervals, with potentially relevant new research being provided ('pushed') to the review authors (see Chapter 4, Section 4.4.9). Alternatively, it may be possible to run automated searches via an application programming interface (API). Unfortunately, only some databases offer notification services and, of those that do not, only some offer an open API that allows review authors to set up their own automated searches. Thus, this approach is most useful when the studies likely to be relevant to the review are those indexed in systems that will work within a 'push' model (typically, large mainstream biomedical databases such as MEDLINE). A further key challenge, which is lessening over time, is that trials and other registries, websites and other unpublished sources typically require manual searches, so it is inappropriate to rely entirely on 'push' services to identify all new evidence. See Section 22.2.4 for further information on technological approaches to ameliorate this.

Statistical methods have been proposed to assess the extent to which new evidence might affect the findings of a systematic review. Sample size calculations can incorporate the result of a current meta-analysis, thus providing information about how additional studies of a particular sample size could have an impact on the results of an updated meta-analysis (Sutton et al 2007, Roloff et al 2013). These methods demonstrate in many cases that new evidence may have very little impact on a random-effects meta-analysis if there is heterogeneity across studies, and they require assumptions that the future studies will be similar to the existing studies. Their practical use in deciding whether to update a systematic review may therefore be limited.

As part of their development of the aforementioned tool, Takwoingi and colleagues created a prediction equation based on findings from a sample of 65 updated Cochrane Reviews (Takwoingi et al 2013). They collated a list of numerical 'signals' as candidate predictors of changing conclusions on updating (including, for example, heterogeneity statistics in the original meta-analysis, presence of a large new study, and various measures of the amount of information in the new studies versus the original meta-analysis). Their prediction equation involved two of these signals: the ratio of statistical information (inverse variance) in the new versus the original studies, and the number of new studies. Further work is required to develop ways to operationalize this approach efficiently, as it requires detailed knowledge of the new evidence; once this is in place, much of the effort to perform the update has already been expended.

22.2.3 'Living' systematic reviews

A 'living' systematic review (LSR) is a systematic review that is continually updated, with new (or newly identified) evidence incorporated as soon as it becomes available (Elliott et al 2014, Elliott et al 2017). Such regular and frequent updating has been suggested for reviews of high priority to decision makers, when certainty in the existing evidence is low or very low, and when there is likely to be new research evidence (Elliott et al 2017).

Continual surveillance for new research evidence is undertaken by frequent searches (e.g. monthly), and new information is incorporated into the review in a timely manner (e.g. within a month of its identification). Ongoing developments in technology, which we overview in Section 22.2.4, can facilitate this (Thomas et al 2017). An important issue when setting up an LSR is that the search methods and anticipated frequency of review updates are made explicit in the review protocol. This transparency is helpful for end-users, giving them the opportunity to plan downstream decisions around the expected dates of new versions, and reducing the need for others to plan or undertake review updates. The maintenance of LSRs offers the possibility for decision makers to update their processes in line with evidence updates from the LSR; for example, facilitating 'living' guidelines (Akl et al 2017), although ongoing challenges include the clear communication to authors, editors and users on what has changed when evidence is updated, and how to implement frequently updated guidelines. Practical guidance on initiating and maintaining LSRs has been developed by the Living Evidence Network.

22.2.4 Technologies to support evidence surveillance

Moving towards more regular updates of reviews may yield benefits in terms of their currency (Elliott et al 2014), but streamlining the necessary increase in searching is required if they are not to consume more resources than traditional approaches. Fortunately, new developments in information and computer science offer some potential for reductions in manual effort through automation. (For an overview of a range of these technologies see Chapter 4, Section 4.6.6.2.)

New systems (such as the Epistemonikos database, which contains the results of regular searches of multiple datasets), offer potential reductions in the number of databases that individuals need to search, as well as reducing duplication of effort across review teams. In addition, the growth in interest of open access publications has led to the creation of large datasets of open access bibliographic records, such as OpenCitation, CrossRef and Microsoft Academic. As these datasets continue to grow to contain all relevant records in their respective areas, they may also reduce the need for author teams to search as many different sources as they currently need to.

Undertaking regular searches also requires the regular screening of records retrieved for eligibility. Once the review has been set up and initial searches screened, subsequent updates can reduce manual screening effort using automation tools that 'learn' the review's eligibility criteria based on previous screening decisions by the review authors. Automation tools that are built on large numbers of records for more generic use are also available, such as Cochrane's RCT Classifier, which can be used to filter studies that are unlikely to be randomized trials from a set of records (Thomas et al 2017). Cochrane has also developed Cochrane Crowd, which crowdsources decisions classifying studies as randomized trials, (see Chapter 4, Section 4.6.6.2).

Later stages of the review process can also be assisted using new technologies. These include risk-of-bias assessment, the extraction of structured data from tables in PDF files, information extraction from reports (such as identifying the number of participants in a study and characteristics of the intervention) and even the writing of review results. These technologies are less well-advanced than those used for study identification.

These various tools aim to reduce manual effort at specific points in the standard systematic review process. However, Cochrane is also setting up systems that aim to change the study selection process quite substantially, as depicted in Figure 22.2.a. These developments begin with the prospective identification of relevant evidence, outside of the context of any given review, including bibliographic and trial registry records, through centralized routine searches of appropriate sources. These records flow through a 'pipeline' which classifies the records in detail using a combination of machine learning and human effort (including Cochrane Crowd). First, the type of study is determined and, if it is likely to be a randomized trial, then the record proceeds to be classified in terms of its review topic and its PICO elements using terms from the Cochrane Linked Data ontology. Finally, relevant data are extracted from the full text report. The viability of such a system depends upon its accuracy, which is contingent on human decisions being consistent and correct. For this reason, the early focus on randomized trials is appropriate, as a clear and widely understood definition exists for this type of study. Overall, the accuracy of Cochrane Crowd for identification of randomized trials exceeds 99%; and the machine learning system is similarly calibrated to achieve over 99% recall (Wallace et al 2017, Marshall et al 2018).

Setting up such a system for centralized study discovery is yielding benefits through economies of scale. For example, in the past the same decisions about the same studies have been made multiple times across different reviews because previously there was no way of sharing these decisions between reviews. Duplication in manual effort is

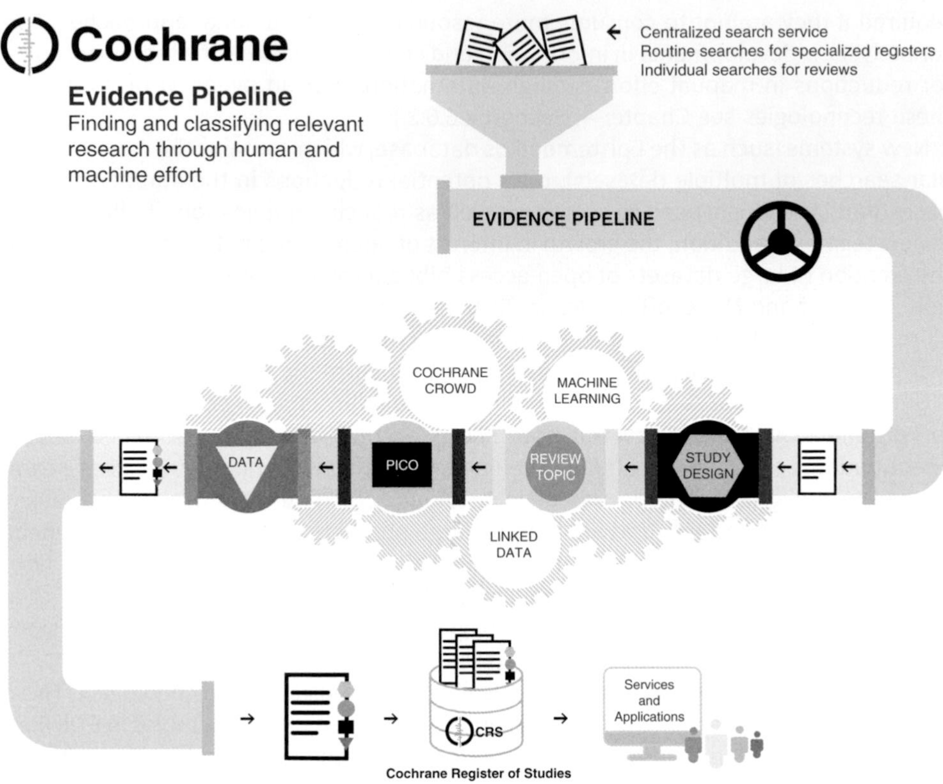

Figure 22.2.a Evidence Pipeline

being reduced substantially by ensuring that decisions made about a given record (e.g. whether or not it describes a randomized trial) are only made once. These decisions are then reflected in the inclusion of studies in the Cochrane Register of Studies, which can then be searched more efficiently for future reviews. The system benefits further from its scale by learning that if a record is relevant for one review, it is unlikely to be relevant for reviews with quite different eligibility criteria. Ultimately, the aim is for randomized trials to be identified for reviews through a single search of their PICO classifications in the central database, with new studies for existing reviews being identified automatically.

22.3 Prospectively planned meta-analysis

22.3.1 What is a prospective meta-analysis?

A properly conducted systematic review defines the question to be addressed in advance of the identification of potentially eligible trials. Systematic reviews are by nature, however, retrospective because the trials included are usually identified after the trials have been completed and the results reported. A prospective meta-analysis

(PMA) is a systematic review and meta-analysis of studies that are identified, evaluated and determined to be eligible for the meta-analysis before the relevant results of any of those studies become known. Most experience of PMA comes from their application to randomized trials. In this section we focus on PMAs of trials, although most of the same considerations will also apply to systematic reviews of other types of studies.

PMA can help to overcome some of the problems of retrospective meta-analyses of individual participant data or of aggregate data by enabling:

1) hypotheses to be specified without prior knowledge of the results of individual trials (including hypotheses underlying subgroup analyses);
2) selection criteria to be applied to trials prospectively; and
3) analysis methods to be chosen before the results of individual trials are known, avoiding potential difficulties in interpretation arising from data-dependent decisions.

PMAs are usually initiated when trials have already started recruiting, and are carried out by collaborative groups including representatives from each of the participating trials. They have tended to involve collecting individual participant data (IPD), such that they have many features in common with retrospective IPD meta-analyses (see also Chapter 26).

If initiated early enough, PMA provides an opportunity for trial design, data collection and other trial processes to be standardized across the eligible ongoing trials. For example, the investigators may agree to use the same instrument to measure a particular outcome, and to measure the outcome at the same time-points in each trial. In a Cochrane Review of interventions for preventing obesity in children, for example, the diversity and unreliability of some of the outcome measures made it difficult to combine data across trials (Summerbell et al 2005). A PMA of this question proposed a set of shared standards so that some of the issues raised by lack of standardization could be addressed (Steinbeck et al 2006).

PMAs based on IPD have been conducted by trialists in cardiovascular disease (Simes 1995, WHO-ISI Blood Pressure Lowering Treatment Trialists' Collaboration 1998), childhood leukaemia (Shuster and Gieser 1996, Valsecchi and Masera 1996), childhood and adolescent obesity (Askie et al 2010, Steinbeck et al 2006) and neonatology (Askie et al 2018). There are areas such as infectious diseases, however, where the opportunity to use PMA has largely been missed (Ioannidis and Lau 1999).

Where resources are limited, it may still be possible to undertake a prospective systematic review and meta-analysis based on aggregate data, rather than IPD, as we discuss in Section 22.3.6. In practice, these are often initiated at a later stage during the course of the trials, so there is less opportunity to standardize conduct of the trials. However, it is possible to harmonize data for inclusion in meta-analysis.

22.3.1.1 What is the difference between a prospective meta-analysis and a large multicentre trial?

PMAs based on IPD are similar to multicentre clinical trials and have similar advantages, including increased sample size, increased diversity of treatment settings and populations, and the ability to examine heterogeneity of intervention effects across multiple settings. However, whereas traditional multicentre trials implement a single protocol across all sites to reduce variability in trial conduct among centres, PMAs allow investigators greater flexibility in how their trial is conducted. Sites can follow a local protocol appropriate to local circumstances, with the local protocol being aligned with elements of a PMA protocol that are common to all included trials.

PMAs may be an attractive alternative when a single, adequately sized trial is infeasible for practical or political reasons (Simes 1987, Probstfield and Applegate 1998). They may also be useful when two or more trials addressing the same question are started with the investigators ignorant of the existence of the other trial(s): once these similar trials are identified, investigators can plan prospectively to combine their results in a meta-analysis.

Variety in the design of the included trials is a potentially desirable feature of PMA as it may improve generalizability. For example, FICSIT (Frailty and Injuries: Cooperative Studies of Intervention Techniques) was a pre-planned meta-analysis of eight trials of exercise-based interventions in a frail elderly population (Schechtman and Ory 2001). The eight FICSIT sites defined their own interventions using site-specific endpoints and evaluations and differing entry criteria (except that all participants were elderly).

22.3.1.2 Negotiating collaboration

As with retrospective IPD meta-analyses, negotiating and establishing a strong collaboration with the participating trialists is essential to the success of a PMA (see Chapter 26, Sections 26.1.3 and 26.2.1). The collaboration usually has a steering group or secretariat that manages the project on a day-to-day basis. Because the collaboration must be formed before the results of any trial are known, an important focus of a PMA's collaborative efforts is often on reaching agreement on trial population, design and data collection methods for each of the participating trials. Ideally, the collaborative group will agree on a core common protocol and data items (including operational definitions) that will be collected across all trials. While individual trials can include local protocol amendments or additional data items, the investigators should ensure that these will not compromise the core common protocol elements.

It is advisable for the collaborative group to obtain an explicit (and signed) collaboration agreement from each of the trial groups. This should also encourage substantive contributions by the individual investigators, ensure 'buy-in' to the concept of the PMA, and facilitate input into the protocol.

22.3.1.3 Confidentiality of individual participant data and results

Confidentiality issues regarding data anonymity and security are similar to those for IPD meta-analyses (see Chapter 26, Section 26.2.4). Specific issues for PMA include planning how to deal with trials as they reach completion and publish their results, and how to manage issues relating to data and safety monitoring, including the impact of interim analyses of individual trials in the PMA, or possibly a pooled interim analysis of the PMA (see also Section 22.3.5).

22.3.2 Writing a protocol for a prospective meta-analysis

All PMAs should be registered on PROSPERO or a similar registry, and have a publicly available protocol. For an example protocol, see the NeOProM Collaboration protocol (Askie et al 2011). Developing a protocol for a PMA is conceptually similar to the process for a systematic review with a traditional meta-analysis component (Moher et al 2015). However, some considerations are unique to a PMA, as follows.

Objectives, eligibility and outcomes As for any systematic review or meta-analysis, the protocol for a PMA should specify its objectives and eligibility criteria for inclusion of the trials (including trial design, participants, interventions and comparators). In addition, it should specify which outcomes will be measured by *all* trials in the PMA, and when and how these should be measured. Additionally, details of subgroup analysis variables should be specified.

Search methods Just as for a retrospective systematic review, a systematic search should be performed to identify *all* eligible ongoing trials, in order to maximize precision. The protocol should describe in detail the efforts made to identify ongoing, or planned trials, or to identify trialists with a common interest in developing a PMA, including how potential collaborators have been (or will be) located and approached to participate.

Trial details Details of trials already identified for inclusion should be listed in the protocol, including their trial registration identifiers, the anticipated number of participants and timelines for each participating trial. The protocol should state whether a signed agreement to collaborate has been obtained from the appropriate representative of each trial (e.g. the sponsor or principal investigator). The protocol should include a statement that, at the time of inclusion in the PMA, no trial results related to the PMA research question were known to anyone outside each trial's own data monitoring committee. If eligible trials are identified but not included in the PMA because their results related to the PMA research question are already known, the PMA protocol should outline how these data will be dealt with. For example, sensitivity analyses including data from these trials might be planned. The protocol should describe actions to be taken if subsequent trials are located while the PMA is in progress.

Data collection and analysis The protocol should outline the plans for the collection and analyses of data in a similar manner to that of a standard, aggregate data meta-analysis or an IPD meta-analysis. Details of overall sample size and power calculations, interim analyses (if applicable) and subgroup analyses should be provided. For a prospectively planned series of trials, a sequential approach to the meta-analysis may be reasonable (see Section 22.4).

In an IPD-PMA, the protocol should describe what will happen if the investigators of some trials within the PMA are unable (or unwilling) to provide participant-level data. Would the PMA secretariat, for example, accept appropriate summary data? The protocol should specify whether there is an intention to update the PMA data at regular intervals via ongoing cycles of data collection (e.g. five yearly). A detailed statistical analysis plan should be agreed and made public before the receipt or analysis of any data to be included in the PMA.

Management and co-ordination The PMA protocol should outline details of project management structure (including any committees, see Section 22.3.1.2), the procedures for data management (how data are to be collected, the format required, when data will be required to be submitted, quality assurance procedures, etc; see Chapter 26, Section 26.2), and who will be responsible for the statistical analyses.

Publication policy It is important to have an authorship policy in place for the PMA (e.g. specifying that publications will be in the group name, but also including a list of individual authors), and a policy on manuscript preparation (e.g. formation of a writing committee, opportunities to comment on draft papers).

A unique issue that arises within the context of the PMA (which would generally not arise for a multicentre trial or a retrospective IPD meta-analysis) is whether or not individual trials should publish their own results separately and, if so, the timing of those publications. In addition to contributing to the PMA, it is likely that investigators will prefer trial-specific publications to appear before the combined PMA results are published. It is recommended that PMA publication(s) clearly indicate the sources of the included data and refer to prior publications of the individual included trials.

22.3.3 Data collection in a prospective meta-analysis

Participating trials in a PMA usually agree to supply individual participant data once their individual trials are completed and published. As trialists prospectively decide which data they will collect and in what format, the need to re-define and re-code supplied data should be less problematic than is often the case with a retrospective IPD meta-analysis.

Once data are received by the PMA secretariat, they should be rigorously checked using the same procedures as for IPD meta-analyses, including checking for missing or duplicated data, conducting data plausibility checks, assessing patterns of randomization, and ensuring the information supplied is up to date (see Chapter 26, Section 26.3). Data queries will be resolved by direct consultation with the individual trialists before being included in the final combined dataset for analysis.

22.3.4 Data analysis in prospective meta-analysis

Most PMAs will use similar analysis methods to those employed in retrospective IPD meta-analyses (see Chapter 26, Section 26.4). The use of participant-level data also permits more statistically powerful investigations of whether intervention effects vary according to participant characteristics, and in some cases allow prognostic modelling.

22.3.5 Interim analysis and data monitoring in prospective meta-analysis

Individual clinical trials frequently include a plan for interim analyses of data, particularly to monitor safety of the interventions. PMA offers a unique opportunity to perform these interim analyses using data contributed by *all* trials. Under the auspices of an over-arching data safety monitoring committee (DSMC) for the PMA, available data may be combined from all trials for an interim analysis, or assessed separately by each trial and the results then shared amongst the DSMCs of all the participating trials.

The ability to perform combined interim analyses raises some ethical issues. Is it, for example, appropriate to continue randomization within individual trials if an overall net benefit of an intervention has been demonstrated in the combined analysis? When results are not known in the subgroups of clinical interest, or for less common endpoints, should the investigators continue to proceed with the PMA to obtain further information regarding overall net clinical benefit? If each trial has its own DSMC, then communication amongst committees would be beneficial in this situation, as recommended by Hillman and Louis (Hillman and Louis 2003). This would be helpful, for example, in deciding whether or not to close an individual trial early because of evidence of efficacy from the combined interim data. It could be argued that knowledge of emerging, concerning, combined safety data from *all* participating trials might actually *reduce* the chances of spurious early stopping of an individual trial. It would be helpful, therefore, for the individual trial DSMCs within the PMA to adopt a common agreement that individual trials should not be stopped until the aims of the PMA, with respect to subgroups and uncommon endpoints (or 'net clinical benefit'), are achieved.

Another possible option might be to consider limiting enrolment in the continuing trials to participants in a particular subgroup of interest if such a decision makes clinical and statistical sense. In any case, it might be appropriate to apply the concepts of sequential meta-analysis methodology, as discussed in Section 22.4, to derive stringent stopping rules for the PMA as individual trial results become available.

22.3.6 Prospective approaches based on aggregate data: the Framework for Adaptive Meta-analysis (FAME)

The Framework for Adaptive Meta-analysis (FAME) is a combination of 'traditional' and prospective elements that is suitable for aggregate data (rather than IPD) meta-analysis and is responsive to emerging trial results. In the FAME approach, all methods are defined in a publicly available systematic review protocol ideally before all trial results are known. The approach aims to take all eligible trials into account, including those that have been completed (and analysed) and those that are yet to complete or report (Tierney et al 2017). FAME can be used to anticipate the earliest opportunity for a reliable aggregate data meta-analysis, which may be well in advance of all relevant results becoming available. The key steps of FAME are as follows.

1) **Start the systematic review process whilst most trials are ongoing or yet to report**

This makes it possible to plan the objectives, eligibility criteria, outcomes and analyses with little or no knowledge of eligible trial results, and also to anticipate the emergence of trial results so that completion of the review and meta-analysis can be aligned accordingly.

2) **Search comprehensively for published, unpublished and ongoing eligible trials**

This ensures that the meta-analysis planning is based on all potential trial data and that results can be placed in the context of all the current and likely future evidence. Conference proceedings, study registers and investigator networks are therefore important sources of information. Although unpublished and ongoing studies should be examined for any systematic review, evidence suggests that it is not standard practice (Page et al 2016).

3) **Liaise with trialists to develop and maintain a detailed understanding of these trials**

Liaising with trialists provides information on how trials are progressing and when results are likely to be available, but it also provides information on trial design, conduct and analysis, bringing greater clarity to eligibility screening and accuracy to risk-of-bias assessments (Vale et al 2013).

4) **Predict if and when sufficient results will be available for reliable and robust meta-analysis (typically using aggregate data)**

The information from steps 2 and 3 about how results will emerge over time allows a prospective assessment of the feasibility and timing of a reliable meta-analysis. A first indicator of reliability is that the projected amount of participants or events that would be available for the meta-analysis would constitute an 'optimal information size' (Pogue and Yusuf 1997). In other words they would provide sufficient power to detect realistic effects of the intervention under investigation, on the basis of standard methods of sample size calculation. A second indicator of reliability is that the anticipated participants or events would comprise a substantial proportion of the total eligible ('relative information size'). This serves to minimize the likelihood of reporting or other data availability biases. Such predictions and decisions for FAME should be outlined in the systematic review protocol.

5) **Conduct meta-analysis and interpret results, taking account of available and unavailable data**

Interpretation should consider how representative the actual data obtained are, and the potential impact of the results of unpublished or ongoing trials that were not included. This is in addition to the direction and precision of the meta-analysis result and consistency of effects across trials, as is standard.

6) **Assess the value of updating the systematic review and meta-analysis in the future**

If the results of a meta-analysis are not deemed definitive, it is important to ascertain whether there is likely to be value in updating with trial results that will emerge in the future and, if so, whether aggregate data will suffice or IPD might be needed.

FAME has been used to evaluate reliably the effects of prostate cancer interventions well in advance of all trial results being available (Vale et al 2016, Rydzewska et al 2017). In these reviews, collaboration with trial investigators provided access to pre-publication results, expediting the review process further and allowing publication in the same time frame as key trial results, increasing the visibility and potential impact of both. It also enabled access to additional outcome, subgroup and toxicity analyses, which allowed a more consistent and thorough analysis than is often possible with aggregate data. Such an approach requires a suitable non-disclosure agreement between the review authors and the trial authors.

Additionally, FAME could be used in the living systematic review context (Crequit et al 2016, Elliott et al 2017, Nikolakopoulou et al 2018), either to provide a suitable baseline meta-analysis, or to predict when a living update might be definitive. Combining multiple FAME reviews in a network meta-analysis (Vale et al 2018) offers an alternative to living network meta-analysis for the timely synthesis of competing treatments (Crequit et al 2016, Nikolakopoulou et al 2018).

22.4 Statistical analysis of accumulating evidence

22.4.1 Statistical issues arising from repeating meta-analyses

In any prospective or updated systematic review the body of evidence may grow over time, and meta-analyses may be repeated with the addition of new studies. If each meta-analysis is interpreted through the use of a statistical test of significance (e.g. categorizing a finding as 'statistically significant' if the P value is less than 0.05 or 'not statistically significant' otherwise), then on each occasion the conclusion has a 5% chance of being incorrect if the null hypothesis (that there is no difference between experimental and comparator interventions on average) is true. Such an incorrect conclusion is often called a type I error. If significance tests are repeated each time a meta-analysis is updated with new studies, then the probability that at least one of the repeated meta-analyses will produce a P value lower than 0.05 under the null hypothesis (i.e. the probability of a type I error) is somewhat higher than 5% (Berkey et al 1996). This has led some researchers to be concerned about the statistical methods they were using when meta-analyses are repeated over time, for fear they were leading to spurious findings.

A related concern is that we may wish to determine when there is enough evidence in the meta-analysis to be able to say that the question is sufficiently well-answered. Traditionally, 'enough evidence' has been interpreted as information with enough statistical power (e.g. 80% or 90% power) to detect a specific magnitude of effect using a significance test. This requires that attention be paid to type II error, which is the chance that a true (non-null) effect will fail to be picked up by the test. When meta-analyses are repeated over time, statistical power may be expected to increase as new studies are added. However, just as type I error is not controlled across repeated analyses, neither is type II error.

Statistical methods for meta-analysis have been proposed to address these concerns. They are known as **sequential approaches**, and are derived from methods commonly used in clinical trials. The appropriateness of applying sequential methods in the context of a systematic review has been hotly debated. We describe the main methods in brief in Section 22.4.2, and in Section 22.4.3 we explain that the use of sequential methods is explicitly discouraged in the context of a Cochrane Review, but may be reasonable in the context of a PMA.

22.4.2 Sequential statistical methods for meta-analysis

Interim analyses are often performed in randomized trials, so the trial can be stopped early if there is convincing evidence that the intervention is beneficial or harmful. Sequential methods have been developed that aim to control type I and II errors in the context of a clinical trial. These methods have been adapted for prospectively adding studies to a meta-analysis, rather than prospectively adding participants to a trial.

The main methods involve pre-specification of a **stopping rule**. The stopping rule is informed by considerations of (i) type I error; (ii) type II error; (c) a clinically important magnitude of effect; and (iv) the desired properties of the stopping rule (e.g. whether it is particularly important to avoid stopping too soon). To control type II error, it is necessary to quantify the amount of information that has accumulated to date. This can be measured using sample size (number of participants) or using statistical information (i.e. the sum of the inverse-variance weights in the meta-analysis).

Implementation of the stopping rule can be done in several ways. One possibility is to perform a statistical test in the usual way but to lower the threshold for interpreting the result as statistically significant. This penalization of the type I error rate at each analysis may be viewed as 'spending' (or distributing) proportions of the error over the repeated analyses. The amount of penalization is specified to create the stopping rule, and is referred to as an 'alpha spending function' (because alpha is often used as shorthand for the acceptable type I error rate).

An alternative way of implementing a stopping rule is to plot the path of the accumulating evidence. Specifically, the plot is a scatter plot of a cumulative measure of effect magnitude (one convenient option is the sum of the study effect estimates times their meta-analytic weights) against a cumulative measure of statistical information (a convenient option is the sum of the meta-analytic weights) at each update. The plotted points are compared with a plot 'boundary', which is determined uniquely by the four pre-specified considerations of a stopping rule noted above. A conclusive result is deemed to be achieved if a point in the plot falls outside the boundary. For meta-analysis, a rectangular boundary has been recommended, as this reduces the chance of crossing a boundary very early; this also produces a scheme that is equivalent to the most popular alpha-spending approach proposed by O'Brien and Fleming (O'Brien and Fleming 1979). Additional stopping boundaries can be added to test for futility, so the updating process can be stopped if it is unlikely that a meaningful effect will be found.

Methods translate directly from sequential clinical trials to a sequential fixed-effect meta-analysis. Random-effects meta-analyses are more problematic. For sequential methods based on statistical weights, the between-study variation (heterogeneity) is naturally incorporated. For methods based on sample size, adjustments can be made to the target sample size to reflect the impact of between-study variation. Either way, there are important technical problems with the methods because between-study variation impacts on the results of a random-effects meta-analysis and it is impossible to anticipate how much between-study variation there will be in the accumulating evidence. Whereas it would be natural to expect that adding studies to a meta-analysis increases precision, this is not necessarily the case under a random-effects model. Specifically, if a new set of studies is added to a meta-analysis among which there is substantially more heterogeneity than in the previous studies, then the estimated between-study variance will go up, and the confidence interval for the new totality of studies may get wider rather than narrower. Possibilities to reduce the impact of this include: (i) using a fixed value (a prior guess) for the amount of between-study heterogeneity throughout the sequential scheme; and (ii) using a high estimate of the amount of heterogeneity during the early stages of the sequential scheme.

Sequential approaches can be inverted to produce a series of confidence intervals, one for each update, which reflects the sequential scheme. This allows representation of the results in a conventional forest plot. The interpretation of these confidence intervals is that we can be 95% confident that all confidence intervals in the entire series of adjusted confidence intervals (across all updates) contain the true intervention effect. The adjusted confidence interval excludes the null value only if a stopping boundary is crossed. This is a somewhat technical interpretation that is unlikely to be helpful in the interpretation of results within any particular update of a review.

There are several choices to make when deciding on a sequential approach to meta-analysis. Two particular sets of choices have been articulated in papers by Wetterslev, Thorlund, Brok and colleagues, and by Whitehead, Higgins and colleagues.

The first group refer to their methods as 'trials sequential analysis' (TSA). They use the principle of alpha spending and articulate the desirable total amount of information in terms of sample size (Wetterslev et al 2008, Brok et al 2009, Thorlund et al 2009). This sample size is calculated in the same way as if the meta-analysis was a single clinical trial, by setting a desired type I error, an assumed effect size, and the desired statistical power to detect that effect. They recommended that the sample size be adjusted for heterogeneity, using either some pre-specified estimate of heterogeneity or the best current estimate of heterogeneity in the meta-analysis. The adjustment is generally made using a statistic called D^2, which produces a larger required sample size, although the more widely used I^2 statistic may be used instead (Wetterslev et al 2009).

Whitehead and Higgins implemented a boundaries approach and represent information using statistical information (specifically, the sum of the meta-analytic weights) (Whitehead 1997, Higgins et al 2011). As noted, this implicitly adjusts for heterogeneity because as heterogeneity increases, the information contained in the meta-analysis decreases. In this approach, the cumulative information can decrease between updates as well as increase (i.e. the path can go backwards in relation to the boundary). These authors propose a parallel Bayesian approach to updating the estimate of between-study heterogeneity, starting with an informative prior distribution, to reduce the risk that the path will go backwards (Higgins et al 2011). If the prior estimate of heterogeneity is suitably large, the method can account for underestimation of heterogeneity early in the updating process.

22.4.3 Using sequential approaches to meta-analysis in Cochrane Reviews

Formal sequential meta-analysis approaches are discouraged for updated meta-analyses in most circumstances within the Cochrane context. They should not be used for the main analyses, or to draw main conclusions. This is for the following reasons.

1) The results of each meta-analysis, conducted at any point in time, indicate the current best evidence of the estimated intervention effect and its accompanying uncertainty. These results need to stand on their own merit. Decision makers should use the currently available evidence, and their decisions should not be influenced by previous meta-analyses or plans for future updates.
2) Cochrane Review authors should interpret evidence on the basis of the estimated magnitude of the effect of intervention and its uncertainty (usually quantified using a confidence interval) and not on the basis of statistical significance (see Chapter 15, Section 15.3.1). In particular, Cochrane Review authors should not draw binary interpretations of intervention effects as present or absent, based on defining results as 'significant' or 'non-significant' (see Chapter 15, Section 15.3.2).
3) There are important differences between the context of an individual trial and the context of a meta-analysis. Whereas a trialist is in control of recruitment of further participants, the meta-analyst (except in the context of a prospective meta-analysis) has no control over designing or affecting trials that are eligible for the meta-

analysis, so it would be impossible to construct a set of workable stopping rules which require a pre-planned set of interim analyses. Conversely, planned adjustments for future updates may be unnecessary if new evidence does not appear.

4) A meta-analysis will not usually relate to a single decision or single decision maker, so that a sequential adjustment will not capture the complexity of the decision making process. Furthermore, Cochrane summarizes evidence for the benefit of multiple end users including patients, health professionals, policy decision makers and guideline developers. Different decision makers may choose to use the evidence differently and reach different decisions based on different priorities and contexts. They might not agree with sequential adjustments or stopping rules set up by review authors.
5) Heterogeneity is prevalent in meta-analyses and random-effects models are commonly used when heterogeneity is present. Sequential methods have important methodological limitations when heterogeneity is present.

It remains important for review authors to avoid over-optimistic conclusions being drawn from a small number of studies. Review authors need to be particularly careful not to over-interpret promising findings when there is very little evidence. Such findings could be due to chance, to bias, or to use of meta-analytic methods that have poor properties when there are few studies (see Chapter 10, Section 10.10.4), and might be overturned at later updates of the review. Evaluating the confidence in the body of evidence, for example using the GRADE framework, should highlight when there is insufficient information (i.e. too much imprecision) for firm conclusions to be drawn.

Sequential approaches to meta-analysis may be used in Cochrane Reviews in two situations.

1) Sequential methods may be used in the context of a prospectively planned series of clinical trials, when the primary analysis is a meta-analysis of the findings across trials, as discussed in Section 22.3. In this case, the meta-analysts are in control of the production of new data and crossing a boundary in a sequential scheme would indicate that no further data need to be collected.
2) Sequential methods may be performed as secondary analyses in Cochrane Reviews, to provide an additional interpretation of the data from a specific perspective. If sequential approaches are to be applied, then (i) they must be planned prospectively (and not retrospectively), with a full analysis plan provided in the protocol; and (ii) the assumptions underlying the sequential design must be clearly conveyed and justified, including the parameters determining the design such as the clinically important effect size, assumptions about heterogeneity, and *both* the type I and type II error rates.

22.5 Chapter information

Authors: James Thomas, Lisa M Askie, Jesse A Berlin, Julian H Elliott, Davina Ghersi, Mark Simmonds, Yemisi Takwoingi, Jayne F Tierney, Julian PT Higgins

Acknowledgements: The following contributed to the policy on use of sequential approaches to meta-analysis: Christopher Schmid, Stephen Senn, Jonathan Sterne, Elena Kulinskaya, Martin Posch, Kit Roes and Joanne McKenzie.

Funding: JFT's work is funded by the UK Medical Research Council (MC_UU_12023/24). JT is supported by the National Institute for Health Research (NIHR) Collaboration for Leadership in Applied Health Research and Care North Thames at Barts Health NHS Trust. JHE is supported by a Career Development Fellowship from the Australian National Health and Medical Research Council (APP1126434). Development of Cochrane's Evidence Pipeline and RCT Classifier was supported by Cochrane's Game Changer Initiative and the Australian National Health and Medical Research Council through a Partnership Project Grant (APP1114605). JPTH is a member of the NIHR Biomedical Research Centre at University Hospitals Bristol NHS Foundation Trust and the University of Bristol. JPTH received funding from National Institute for Health Research Senior Investigator award NF-SI-0617-10145. The views expressed are those of the author(s) and not necessarily those of the NHS, the NIHR or the Department of Health and Social Care.

22.6 References

Akl EA, Meerpohl JJ, Elliott J, Kahale LA, Schunemann HJ, Living Systematic Review N. Living systematic reviews: 4. Living guideline recommendations. *Journal of Clinical Epidemiology* 2017; **91**: 47–53.

Askie LM, Baur LA, Campbell K, Daniels L, Hesketh K, Magarey A, Mihrshahi S, Rissel C, Simes RJ, Taylor B, Taylor R, Voysey M, Wen LM, on behalf of the EPOCH Collaboration. The Early Prevention of Obesity in CHildren (EPOCH) Collaboration –an Individual Patient Data Prospective Meta-Analysis [study protocol]. *BMC Public Health* 2010; **10**: 728.

Askie LM, Brocklehurst P, Darlow BA, Finer N, Schmidt B, Tarnow-Mordi W. NeOProM: Neonatal Oxygenation Prospective Meta-analysis Collaboration study protocol. *BMC Pediatrics* 2011; **11**: 6.

Askie LM, Darlow BA, Finer N, et al. Association between oxygen saturation targeting and death or disability in extremely preterm infants in the neonatal oxygenation prospective meta-analysis collaboration. *JAMA* 2018; **319**: 2190–2201.

Berkey CS, Mosteller F, Lau J, Antman EM. Uncertainty of the time of first significance in random effects cumulative meta-analysis. *Controlled Clinical Trials* 1996; **17**: 357–371.

Brok J, Thorlund K, Wetterslev J, Gluud C. Apparently conclusive meta-analyses may be inconclusive: trial sequential analysis adjustment of random error risk due to repetitive testing of accumulating data in apparently conclusive neonatal meta-analyses. *International Journal of Epidemiology* 2009; **38**: 287–298.

Chalmers I. Electronic publications for updating controlled trial reviews. *Lancet* 1986; **328**: 287.

Crequit P, Trinquart L, Yavchitz A, Ravaud P. Wasted research when systematic reviews fail to provide a complete and up-to-date evidence synthesis: the example of lung cancer. *BMC Medicine* 2016; **14**: 8.

Elliott JH, Turner T, Clavisi O, Thomas J, Higgins JPT, Mavergames C, Gruen RL. Living systematic reviews: an emerging opportunity to narrow the evidence-practice gap. *PLoS Medicine* 2014; **11**: e1001603.

Elliott JH, Synnot A, Turner T, Simmonds M, Akl EA, McDonald S, Salanti G, Meerpohl J, MacLehose H, Hilton J, Tovey D, Shemilt I, Thomas J, Living Systematic Review N. Living systematic review: 1. Introduction-the why, what, when, and how. *Journal of Clinical Epidemiology* 2017; **91**: 23–30.

Garner P, Hopewell S, Chandler J, MacLehose H, Schünemann HJ, Akl EA, Beyene J, Chang S, Churchill R, Dearness K, Guyatt G, Lefebvre C, Liles B, Marshall R, Martinez Garcia L, Mavergames C, Nasser M, Qaseem A, Sampson M, Soares-Weiser K, Takwoingi Y, Thabane L, Trivella M, Tugwell P, Welsh E, Wilson EC, Schünemann HJ, Panel for Updating Guidance for Systematic Reviews (PUGs). When and how to update systematic reviews: consensus and checklist. *BMJ* 2016; **354**: i3507.

Higgins JPT, Whitehead A, Simmonds M. Sequential methods for random-effects meta-analysis. *Statistics in Medicine* 2011; **30**: 903–921.

Hillman DW, Louis TA. DSMB case study: decision making when a similar clinical trial is stopped early. *Controlled Clinical Trials* 2003; **24**: 85–91.

Ioannidis JPA, Lau J. State of the evidence: current status and prospects of meta-analysis in infectious diseases. *Clinical Infectious Diseases* 1999; **29**: 1178–1185.

Marshall IJ, Noel-Storr A, Kuiper J, Thomas J, Wallace BC. Machine learning for identifying Randomized Controlled Trials: An evaluation and practitioner's guide. *Research Synthesis Methods* 2018; **9**: 602–614.

Martínez García L, Pardo-Hernandez H, Superchi C, Niño de Guzman E, Ballesteros M, Ibargoyen Roteta N, McFarlane E, Posso M, Roqué IFM, Rotaeche Del Campo R, Sanabria AJ, Selva A, Solà I, Vernooij RWM, Alonso-Coello P. Methodological systematic review identifies major limitations in prioritization processes for updating. *Journal of Clinical Epidemiology* 2017; **86**: 11–24.

Moher D, Shamseer L, Clarke M, Ghersi D, Liberati A, Petticrew M, Shekelle P, Stewart LA. Preferred reporting items for systematic review and meta-analysis protocols (PRISMA-P) 2015 statement. *Systematic Reviews* 2015; **4**: 1.

Nikolakopoulou A, Mavridis D, Furukawa TA, Cipriani A, Tricco AC, Straus SE, Siontis GCM, Egger M, Salanti G. Living network meta-analysis compared with pairwise meta-analysis in comparative effectiveness research: empirical study. *BMJ* 2018; **360**: k585.

O'Brien PC, Fleming TR. A multiple testing procedure for clinical trials. *Biometrics* 1979; **35**: 549–556.

Page MJ, Shamseer L, Altman DG, Tetzlaff J, Sampson M, Tricco AC, Catalá-López F, Li L, Reid EK, Sarkis-Onofre R, Moher D. Epidemiology and reporting characteristics of systematic reviews of biomedical research: a cross-sectional study. *PLoS Medicine* 2016; **13**: e1002028.

Pogue JM, Yusuf S. Cumulating evidence from randomized trials: utilizing sequential monitoring boundaries for cumulative meta-analysis. *Controlled Clinical Trials* 1997; **18**: 580–593; discussion 661–586.

Probstfield J, Applegate WB. Prospective meta-analysis: Ahoy! A clinical trial? *Journal of the American Geriatrics Society* 1998; **43**: 452–453.

Roloff V, Higgins JPT, Sutton AJ. Planning future studies based on the conditional power of a meta-analysis. *Statistics in Medicine* 2013; **32**: 11–24.

Rydzewska LHM, Burdett S, Vale CL, Clarke NW, Fizazi K, Kheoh T, Mason MD, Miladinovic B, James ND, Parmar MKB, Spears MR, Sweeney CJ, Sydes MR, Tran N, Tierney JF, STOPCaP Abiraterone Collaborators. Adding abiraterone to androgen deprivation therapy in men with metastatic hormone-sensitive prostate cancer: a systematic review and meta-analysis. *European Journal of Cancer* 2017; **84**: 88–101.

Schechtman K, Ory M. The effects of exercise on the quality of life of frail older adults: a preplanned meta-analysis of the FICSIT trials. *Annals of Behavioural Medicine* 2001; **23**: 186–197.

Shojania KG, Sampson M, Ansari MT, Ji J, Doucette S, Moher D. How quickly do systematic reviews go out of date? A survival analysis. *Annals of Internal Medicine* 2007; **147**: 224–233.

Shuster JJ, Gieser PW. Meta-analysis and prospective meta-analysis in childhood leukemia clinical research. *Annals of Oncology* 1996; **7**: 1009–1014.

Simes RJ. Confronting publication bias: a cohort design for meta-analysis. *Statistics in Medicine* 1987; **6**: 11–29.

Simes RJ. Prospective meta-analysis of cholesterol-lowering studies: the Prospective Pravastatin Pooling (PPP) Project and the Cholesterol Treatment Trialists' (CTT) Collaboration. *American Journal of Cardiology* 1995; **76**: 122c–126c.

Steinbeck KS, Baur LA, Morris AM, Ghersi D. A proposed protocol for the development of a register of trials of weight management of childhood overweight and obesity. *International Journal of Obesity* 2006; **30**: 2–5.

Summerbell CD, Waters E, Edmunds LD, Kelly S, Brown T, Campbell KJ. *Interventions For Preventing Obesity in Children*. 3rd ed. 2005.

Sutton AJ, Cooper NJ, Jones DR, Lambert PC, Thompson JR, Abrams KR. Evidence-based sample size calculations based upon updated meta-analysis. *Statistics in Medicine* 2007; **26**: 2479–2500.

Takwoingi Y, Hopewell S, Tovey D, Sutton AJ. A multicomponent decision tool for prioritising the updating of systematic reviews. *BMJ* 2013; **347**: f7191.

Thomas J, Noel-Storr A, Marshall I, Wallace B, McDonald S, Mavergames C, Glasziou P, Shemilt I, Synnot A, Turner T, Elliott J, Living Systematic Review N. Living systematic reviews: 2. Combining human and machine effort. *Journal of Clinical Epidemiology* 2017; **91**: 31–37.

Thorlund K, Devereaux PJ, Wetterslev J, Guyatt G, Ioannidis JPA, Thabane L, Gluud LL, Als-Nielsen B, Gluud C. Can trial sequential monitoring boundaries reduce spurious inferences from meta-analyses? *International Journal of Epidemiology* 2009; **38**: 276–286.

Tierney J, Vale CL, Burdett S, Fisher D, Rydzewska L, Parmar MKB. Timely and reliable evaluation of the effects of interventions: a framework for adaptive meta-analysis (FAME). *Trials* 2017; **18 (**Suppl 1**)**: 200.

Vale CL, Tierney JF, Burdett S. Can trial quality be reliably assessed from published reports of cancer trials: evaluation of risk of bias assessments in systematic reviews. *BMJ* 2013; **346**: f1798.

Vale CL, Burdett S, Rydzewska LHM, Albiges L, Clarke NW, Fisher D, Fizazi K, Gravis G, James ND, Mason MD, Parmar MKB, Sweeney CJ, Sydes MR, Tombal B, Tierney JF, STOpCaP Steering Group. Addition of docetaxel or bisphosphonates to standard of care in men with localised or metastatic, hormone-sensitive prostate cancer: a systematic review and meta-analyses of aggregate data. *Lancet Oncology* 2016; **17**: 243–256.

Vale CL, Fisher DJ, White IR, Carpenter JR, Burdett S, Clarke NW, Fizazi K, Gravis G, James ND, Mason MD, Parmar MKB, Rydzewska LH, Sweeney CJ, Spears MR, Sydes MR, Tierney JF. What is the optimal systemic treatment of men with metastatic, hormone-naive prostate cancer? A STOPCAP systematic review and network meta-analysis. *Annals of Oncology* 2018; **29**: 1249–1257.

Valsecchi MG, Masera G. A new challenge in clinical research in childhood ALL: the prospective meta-analysis strategy for intergroup collaboration. *Annals of Oncology* 1996; **7**: 1005–1008.

Wallace BC, Noel-Storr A, Marshall IJ, Cohen AM, Smalheiser NR, Thomas J. Identifying reports of randomized controlled trials (RCTs) via a hybrid machine learning and crowdsourcing approach. *Journal of the American Medical Informatics Association* 2017; **24**: 1165–1168.

Wetterslev J, Thorlund K, Brok J, Gluud C. Trial sequential analysis may establish when firm evidence is reached in cumulative meta-analysis. *Journal of Clinical Epidemiology* 2008; **61**: 64–75.

Wetterslev J, Thorlund K, Brok J, Gluud C. Estimating required information size by quantifying diversity in random-effects model meta-analyses. *BMC Medical Research Methodology* 2009; **9**: 86.

Whitehead A. A prospectively planned cumulative meta-analysis applied to a series of concurrent clinical trials. *Statistics in Medicine* 1997; **16**: 2901–2913.

WHO-ISI Blood Pressure Lowering Treatment Trialists' Collaboration. Protocol for prospective collaborative overviews of major randomised trials of blood-pressure-lowering treatments. *Journal of Hypertension* 1998; **16**: 127–137.

23

Including variants on randomized trials

Julian PT Higgins, Sandra Eldridge, Tianjing Li

KEY POINTS

- Non-standard designs, such as cluster-randomized trials and crossover trials, should be analysed using methods appropriate to the design.
- If the authors of studies included in the review fail to account for correlations among outcome data that arise because of the design, approximate methods can often be applied by review authors.
- A variant of the risk-of-bias assessment tool is available for cluster-randomized trials. Special attention should be paid to the potential for bias arising from how individual participants were identified and recruited within clusters.
- A variant of the risk-of-bias assessment tool is available for crossover trials. Special attention should be paid to the potential for bias arising from carry-over of effects from one period to the subsequent period of the trial, and to the possibility of 'period effects'.
- To include a study with more than two intervention groups in a meta-analysis, a recommended approach is (i) to omit groups that are not relevant to the comparison being made, and (ii) to combine multiple groups that are eligible as the experimental or comparator intervention to create a single pair-wise comparison. Alternatively, multi-arm studies are dealt with appropriately by network meta-analysis.

23.1 Cluster-randomized trials

23.1.1 Introduction

In **cluster-randomized trials**, groups of individuals rather than individuals are randomized to different interventions. We say the 'unit of allocation' is the cluster, or the group. The groups may be, for example, schools, villages, medical practices or families. Cluster-randomized trials may be done for one of several reasons. It may be to evaluate

This chapter should be cited as: Higgins JPT, Eldridge S, Li T (editors). Chapter 23: Including variants on randomized trials. In: Higgins JPT, Thomas J, Chandler J, Cumpston M, Li T, Page MJ, Welch VA (editors). *Cochrane Handbook for Systematic Reviews of Interventions*. 2nd Edition. Chichester (UK): John Wiley & Sons, 2019: 569–594.

the group effect of an intervention, for example herd-immunity of a vaccine. It may be to avoid 'contamination' across interventions when trial participants are managed within the same setting, for example in a trial evaluating training of clinicians in a clinic. A cluster-randomized design may be used simply for convenience.

One of the main consequences of a cluster design is that participants within any one cluster often tend to respond in a similar manner, and thus their data can no longer be assumed to be independent. It is important that the analysis of a cluster-randomized trial takes this issue into account. Unfortunately, many studies have in the past been incorrectly analysed as though the unit of allocation had been the individual participants (Eldridge et al 2008). This is often referred to as a 'unit-of-analysis error' (Whiting-O'Keefe et al 1984) because the unit of analysis is different from the unit of allocation. If the clustering is ignored and cluster-randomized trials are analysed as if individuals had been randomized, resulting confidence intervals will be artificially narrow and P values will be artificially small. This can result in false-positive conclusions that the intervention had an effect. In the context of a meta-analysis, studies in which clustering has been ignored will receive more weight than is appropriate.

In some trials, individual people are allocated to interventions that are then applied to multiple parts of those individuals (e.g. to both eyes or to several teeth), or repeated observations are made on a participant. These body parts or observations are then clustered within individuals in the same way that individuals can be clustered within, for example, medical practices. If the analysis is by the individual units (e.g. each tooth or each observation) without taking into account that the data are clustered within participants, then a unit-of-analysis error can occur.

There are several useful sources of information on cluster-randomized trials (Murray and Short 1995, Donner and Klar 2000, Eldridge and Kerry 2012, Campbell and Walters 2014, Hayes and Moulton 2017). A detailed discussion of incorporating cluster-randomized trials in a meta-analysis is available (Donner and Klar 2002), as is a more technical treatment of the problem (Donner et al 2001). Evidence suggests that many cluster-randomized trials have not been analysed appropriately when included in Cochrane Reviews (Richardson et al 2016).

23.1.2 Assessing risk of bias in cluster-randomized trials

A detailed discussion of risk-of-bias issues is provided in Chapter 7, and for the most part the Cochrane risk-of-bias tool for randomized trials, as outlined in Chapter 8, applies to cluster-randomized trials.

A key difference between cluster-randomized trials and individually randomized trials is that the individuals of interest (those within the clusters) may not be directly allocated to one intervention or another. In particular, sometimes the individuals are recruited into the study (or otherwise selected for inclusion in the analysis) after the interventions have been allocated to clusters, creating the potential for knowledge of the allocation to influence whether individuals are recruited or selected into the analysis (Puffer et al 2003, Eldridge et al 2008). The bias that arises when this occurs is referred to in various ways, but we use the term **identification/recruitment bias**, which distinguishes it from other types of bias. Careful trial design can protect against this bias (Hahn et al 2005, Eldridge et al 2009a).

A second key difference between cluster-randomized trials and individually randomized trials is that identifying who the 'participants' are is not always straightforward in cluster-randomized trials. The reasons for this are that in some trials:

1) there may be no formal recruitment of participants;
2) there may be two or more different groups of participants on whom different outcomes are measured (e.g. outcomes measured on clinicians and on patients); or
3) data are collected at two or more time points on different individuals (e.g. measuring physical activity in a community using a survey, which reaches different individuals at baseline and after the intervention).

For the purposes of an assessment of risk of bias using the RoB 2 tool (see Chapter 8) we define participants in cluster-randomized trials as those on whom investigators seek to measure the outcome of interest.

The RoB 2 tool has a variant specifically for cluster-randomized trials. To avoid very general language, it focuses mainly on cluster-randomized trials in which groups of individuals form the clusters (rather than body parts or time points). Because most cluster-randomized trials are pragmatic in nature and aim to support high-level decisions about health care, the tool currently considers only the effect of assignment to intervention (and not the effect of adhering to the interventions as they were intended). Special issues in assessing risk of bias in cluster-randomized trials using RoB 2 are provided in Table 23.1.a.

Table 23.1.a Issues addressed in the Cochrane risk-of-bias tool for cluster-randomized trials

Bias domain	Additional or different issues compared with individually randomized trials
Bias arising from the randomization process	• Processes for randomizing clusters vary: clusters may be randomized sequentially, in batches or all at once. Minimization is quite common and should be treated as equivalent to randomization. Cluster randomization is often performed at a single point in time by a methodologist, who may have less motivation or knowledge to subvert randomization. • The number of clusters can be relatively small, so chance imbalances are more common than in individually randomized trials. Such chance imbalances should not be interpreted as evidence of risk of bias.
Bias arising from the timing of identification and recruitment of participants	• This bias domain is specific to cluster-randomized trials. • It is important to consider when individual participants were identified and recruited in relation to the timing of randomization. • If identification or recruitment of any participants in the trial happened after randomization of the cluster, then their recruitment could have been affected by knowledge of the intervention, introducing bias.

(*Continued*)

Table 23.1.a (Continued)

Bias domain	Additional or different issues compared with individually randomized trials
	• Baseline imbalances in characteristics of participants (rather than of clusters) can suggest a problem with identification/recruitment bias.
Bias due to deviations from intended interventions	*When the review authors' interest is in the effect of assignment to intervention* (see Chapter 8, Section 8.4): • If participants are not aware that they are in a trial, then there will not be deviations from the intended intervention that arise because of the trial context. It is these deviations that we are concerned about in this domain. • If participants, carers or people delivering interventions are aware of the assigned intervention, then the issues are the same as for individually randomized trials.
Bias due to missing outcome data	• Data may be missing for clusters or for individuals within clusters. • Considerations when addressing either type of missing data are the same as for individually randomized trials, but review authors should ensure that they cover both.
Bias in measurement of the outcome	• If outcome assessors are not aware that a trial is taking place, then their assessments should not be affected by intervention assignment. • If outcome assessors are aware of the assigned intervention, then the issues are the same as for individually randomized trials.
Bias in selection of the reported result	• The issues are the same as for individually randomized trials.

* For the precise wording of signalling questions and guidance for answering each one, see the full risk-of-bias tool at www.riskofbias.info.

23.1.3 Methods of analysis for cluster-randomized trials

One way to avoid a unit-of-analysis error in a cluster-randomized trial is to conduct the analysis at the same level as the allocation. That is, the data could be analysed as if each cluster was a single individual, using a summary measurement from each cluster. Then the sample size for the analysis is the number of clusters. However, this strategy might unnecessarily reduce the precision of the effect estimate if the clusters vary in their size.

Alternatively, statistical analysis at the level of the individual can lead to an inappropriately high level of precision in the analysis, unless methods are used to account for the clustering in the data. The ideal information to extract from a cluster-randomized trial is a direct estimate of the required effect measure (e.g. an odds ratio with its confidence interval) from an analysis that properly accounts for the cluster design. Such an analysis might be based on a multilevel model or may use generalized estimating equations, among other techniques. Statistical advice is recommended to determine whether the method used is appropriate. When the study authors have not conducted such an analysis, there are two approximate approaches that can be used by review authors to adjust the results (see Sections 23.1.4 and 23.1.5).

Effect estimates and their standard errors from correct analyses of cluster-randomized trials may be meta-analysed using the generic inverse-variance approach (e.g. in RevMan).

23.1.4 Approximate analyses of cluster-randomized trials for a meta-analysis: effective sample sizes

Unfortunately, many cluster-randomized trials have in the past failed to report appropriate analyses. They are commonly analysed as if the randomization was performed on the individuals rather than the clusters. If this is the situation, approximately correct analyses may be performed if the following information can be extracted:

- the number of clusters (or groups) randomized to each intervention group and the total number of participants in the study; or the average (mean) size of each cluster;
- the outcome data ignoring the cluster design for the total number of individuals (e.g. the number or proportion of individuals with events, or means and standard deviations for continuous data); and
- an estimate of the intracluster (or intraclass) correlation coefficient (ICC).

The ICC is an estimate of the relative variability within and between clusters (Eldridge and Kerry 2012). Alternatively it describes the 'similarity' of individuals within the same cluster (Eldridge et al 2009b). In spite of recommendations to report the ICC in all trial reports (Campbell et al 2012), ICC estimates are often not available in published reports.

A common approach for review authors is to use external estimates obtained from similar studies, and several resources are available that provide examples of ICCs (Ukoumunne et al 1999, Campbell et al 2000, Health Services Research Unit 2004), or use an estimate based on known patterns in ICCs for particular types of cluster or outcome. ICCs may appear small compared with other types of correlations: values lower than 0.05 are typical. However, even small values can have a substantial impact on confidence interval widths (and hence weights in a meta-analysis), particularly if cluster sizes are large. Empirical research has observed that clusters that tend to be naturally larger have smaller ICCs (Ukoumunne et al 1999). For example, for the same outcome, regions are likely to have smaller ICCs than towns, which are likely to have smaller ICCs than families.

An approximately correct analysis proceeds as follows. The idea is to reduce the size of each trial to its 'effective sample size' (Rao and Scott 1992). The effective sample size of a single intervention group in a cluster-randomized trial is its original sample size divided by a quantity called the 'design effect'. The design effect is approximately

$$1 + (M - 1) \times \text{ICC},$$

where M is the average cluster size and ICC is the intracluster correlation coefficient. When cluster sizes vary, M can be estimated more appropriately in other ways (Eldridge et al 2006). A common design effect is usually assumed across intervention groups. For dichotomous data, both the number of participants and the number experiencing the event should be divided by the same design effect. Since the resulting data must be rounded to whole numbers for entry into meta-analysis software such as RevMan, this approach may be unsuitable for small trials. For continuous data, only the sample size need be reduced; means and standard deviations should remain unchanged. Special considerations for analysis of standardized mean differences from cluster-randomized trials are discussed by White and Thomas (White and Thomas 2005).

23.1.4.1 Example of incorporating a cluster-randomized trial

As an example, consider a cluster-randomized trial that randomized 10 school classrooms with 295 children into a treatment group and 11 classrooms with 330 children into a control group. Suppose the numbers of successes among the children, ignoring the clustering, are:

$$\text{Treatment}: 63/295$$

$$\text{Control}: 84/330.$$

Imagine an intracluster correlation coefficient of 0.02 has been obtained from a reliable external source or is expected to be a good estimate, based on experience in the area. The average cluster size in the trial is

$$(295 + 330) \div (10 + 11) = 29.8.$$

The design effect for the trial as a whole is then

$$1 + (\text{M} - 1)\,\text{ICC} = 1 + (29.8 - 1) \times 0.02 = 1.576.$$

The effective sample size in the treatment group is

$$295 \div 1.576 = 187.2$$

and for the control group is

$$330 \div 1.576 = 209.4.$$

Applying the design effects also to the numbers of events (in this case, successes) produces the following modified results:

$$\text{Treatment}: 40.0/187.2$$

$$\text{Control}: 53.3/209.4.$$

Once trials have been reduced to their effective sample size, the data may be entered into statistical software such as RevMan as, for example, dichotomous outcomes or continuous outcomes. Rounding the results to whole numbers, the results from the example trial may be entered as:

$$\text{Treatment}: 40/187$$

$$\text{Control}: 53/209.$$

23.1.5 Approximate analyses of cluster-randomized trials for a meta-analysis: inflating standard errors

A clear disadvantage of the method described in Section 23.1.4 is the need to round the effective sample sizes to whole numbers. A slightly more flexible approach, which is equivalent to calculating effective sample sizes, is to multiply the standard error of the effect estimate (from an analysis ignoring clustering) by the square root of the design effect. The standard error may be calculated from the confidence interval of any effect estimate derived from an analysis ignoring clustering (see Chapter 6, Section 6.3.1). Standard analyses of dichotomous or continuous outcomes may be used to obtain these confidence intervals using standard meta-analysis software (e.g. RevMan). The meta-analysis using the inflated variances may be performed using the generic inverse-variance method.

As an example, the odds ratio (OR) from a study with the results

$$\text{Treatment}: 63/295$$

$$\text{Control}: 84/330$$

is OR = 0.795 (95% CI 0.548 to 1.154). Using methods described in Chapter 6 (Section 6.1.3.2), we can determine from these results that the log odds ratio is lnOR = –0.23 with standard error 0.19. Using the same design effect of 1.576 as in Section 23.1.4.1, an inflated standard error that accounts for clustering is given by $0.19 \times \sqrt{1.576} = 0.24$. The log odds ratio (–0.23) and this inflated standard error (0.24) may be used as the basis for a meta-analysis using a generic inverse-variance approach.

23.1.6 Issues in the incorporation of cluster-randomized trials

Cluster-randomized trials may, in principle, be combined with individually randomized trials in the same meta-analysis. Consideration should be given to the possibility of important differences in the effects being evaluated between the different types of trial. There are often good reasons for performing cluster-randomized trials and these should be examined. For example, in the treatment of infectious diseases an intervention applied to all individuals in a community may be more effective than treatment applied to select (randomized) individuals within the community, since it may reduce the possibility of re-infection (Eldridge and Kerry 2012).

Authors should always identify any cluster-randomized trials in a review and explicitly state how they have dealt with the data. They should conduct sensitivity analyses to investigate the robustness of their conclusions, especially when ICCs have been borrowed from external sources (see Chapter 10, Section 10.14). Statistical support is recommended.

23.1.7 Stepped-wedge trials

In a stepped-wedge trial, randomization is by cluster. However, rather than assign a predefined proportion of the clusters to the experimental intervention and the rest to a comparator intervention, a stepped-wedge design starts with all clusters allocated to the comparator intervention and sequentially randomizes individual clusters (or groups of clusters) to switch to the experimental intervention. By the end of the trial, all clusters are implementing the experimental intervention (Hemming et al 2015). Stepped-wedge trials are increasingly used to evaluate health service and policy interventions, and are often attractive to policy makers because all clusters can expect to receive (or implement) the experimental intervention.

The analysis of a stepped-wedge trial must take into account the possibility of time trends. A naïve comparison of experimental intervention periods with comparator intervention periods will be confounded by any variables that change over time, since more clusters are receiving the experimental intervention during the later stages of the trial.

The RoB 2 tool for cluster-randomized trials can be used to assess risk of bias in a stepped-wedge trial. However, the tool does not address the need to adjust for time trends in the analysis, which is an important additional source of potential bias in a stepped-wedge trial.

23.1.8 Individually randomized trials with clustering

Issues related to clustering can also occur in individually randomized trials. This can happen when the same health professional (e.g. doctor, surgeon, nurse or therapist) delivers the intervention to a number of participants in the intervention group. This type of clustering raises issues similar to those in cluster-randomized trials in relation to the analysis (Lee and Thompson 2005, Walwyn and Roberts 2015, Walwyn and Roberts 2017), and review authors should consider inflating the variance of the intervention effect estimate using a design effect, as for cluster-randomized trials.

23.2 Crossover trials

23.2.1 Introduction

Parallel-group trials allocate each participant to a single intervention for comparison with one or more alternative interventions. In contrast, **crossover trials** allocate each participant to a sequence of interventions. A simple randomized crossover design is an 'AB/BA' design in which participants are randomized initially to intervention A or intervention B, and then 'cross over' to intervention B or intervention A, respectively. It can be seen that data from the first period of a crossover trial represent a parallel-group trial, a feature referred to in Section 23.2.6. In keeping with the rest of the *Handbook*, we will use E and C to refer to interventions, rather than A and B.

Crossover designs offer a number of possible advantages over parallel-group trials. Among these are that:

1) each participant acts as his or her own control, significantly reducing between-participant variation;
2) consequently, fewer participants are usually required to obtain the same precision in estimation of intervention effects; and
3) every participant receives every intervention, which allows the determination of the best intervention or preference for an individual participant.

In some trials, randomization of interventions takes place within individuals, with different interventions being applied to different body parts (e.g. to the two eyes or to teeth in the two sides of the mouth). If body parts are randomized and the analysis is by the multiple parts within an individual (e.g. each eye or each side of the mouth) then the analysis should account for the pairing (or matching) of parts within individuals in the same way that pairing of intervention periods is recognized in the analysis of a crossover trial.

A readable introduction to crossover trials is given by Senn (Senn 2002). More detailed discussion of meta-analyses involving crossover trials is provided by Elbourne and colleagues (Elbourne et al 2002), and some empirical evidence on their inclusion in systematic reviews by Lathyris and colleagues (Lathyris et al 2007). Evidence suggests that many crossover trials have not been analysed appropriately when included in Cochrane Reviews (Nolan et al 2016).

23.2.2 Assessing suitability of crossover trials

Crossover trials are suitable for evaluating interventions with a temporary effect in the treatment of stable, chronic conditions (at least over the time period under study). They are employed, for example, in the study of interventions to relieve asthma, rheumatoid arthritis and epilepsy. There are many situations in which a crossover trial is not appropriate. These include:

1) if the medical condition evolves over time, such as a degenerative disorder, a temporary condition that will resolve within the time frame of the trial, or a cyclic disorder;
2) when an intervention (or its cessation) can lead to permanent or long-term modification (e.g. a vaccine). In this situation, either a participant will be unable (or ineligible) to enter a subsequent period of the trial; or a 'carry-over' effect is likely (see Section 23.2.3);
3) if the elimination half-life of a drug is very long so that a 'carry-over' effect is likely (see Section 23.2.3); and
4) if wash-out itself induces a withdrawal or rebound effect in the second period.

In considering the inclusion of crossover trials in meta-analysis, authors should first address the question of whether a crossover trial is a suitable method for the condition and intervention in question. For example, one group of authors decided that crossover trials were inappropriate for studies in Alzheimer's disease (although they are frequently employed in the field) due to the degenerative nature of the condition, and included only data from the first period of crossover trials in their systematic review (Qizilbash et al 1998). The second question to be addressed is whether there is a likelihood of serious carry-over, which relies largely on judgement since the statistical techniques to demonstrate carry-over are far from satisfactory. The nature of the interventions and the length of any wash-out period are important considerations.

It is only justifiable to exclude crossover trials from a systematic review if the design is inappropriate to the clinical context. Very often, however, even where the design has been appropriate, it is difficult or impossible to extract suitable data from a crossover trial. In Section 23.2.6 we outline some considerations and suggestions for including crossover trials in a meta-analysis.

23.2.3 Assessing risk of bias in crossover trials

The principal problem associated with crossover trials is that of **carry-over** (a type of period-by-intervention interaction). Carry-over is the situation in which the effects of an intervention given in one period persist into a subsequent period, thus interfering with the effects of the second intervention. These effects may be because the first intervention itself persists (such as a drug with a long elimination half-life), or because the effects of the intervention persist. An extreme example of carry-over is when a key outcome of interest is irreversible or of long duration, such as mortality, or pregnancy in a subfertility study. In this case, a crossover study is generally considered to be inappropriate. A carry-over effect means that the observed difference between the treatments depends upon the order in which they were received; hence the estimated overall treatment effect will be affected (usually under-estimated, leading to a bias towards the null). Many crossover trials include a period between interventions known as a **wash-out period** as a means of reducing carry-over.

A second problem that may occur in crossover trials is **period effects**. Period effects are systematic differences between responses in the second period compared with responses in the first period that are not due to different interventions. They may occur, for example, when the condition changes systematically over time, or if there are changes in background factors such as underlying healthcare strategies. For an AB/BA design, period effects can be overcome by ensuring the same number of participants is randomized to the two sequences of interventions or by including period effects in the statistical model.

A third problem for crossover trials is that the trial might report only analyses based on the first period. Although the first period of a crossover trial is in effect a parallel group comparison, use of data from only the first period will be biased if, as is likely, the decision to use first period data is based on a test for carry-over. Such a 'two-stage analysis' has been discredited but is still used (Freeman 1989). This is because the test for carry-over is affected by baseline differences in the randomized groups at the start of the crossover trial, so a statistically significant result might reflect such baseline differences. Reporting only the first period data in this situation is particularly problematic. Crossover trials for which only first period data are available should be considered to be at risk of bias, especially when the investigators explicitly report using a two-stage analysis strategy.

Another potential problem with crossover trials is the risk of dropout due to their longer duration compared with comparable parallel-group trials. The analysis techniques for crossover trials with missing observations are limited.

The Cochrane risk-of-bias tool for randomized trials (RoB 2, see Chapter 8) has a variant specifically for crossover trials. It focuses on crossover trials with two intervention periods rather than with two body parts. Carry-over effects are addressed specifically. Period effects are addressed through examination of the allocation ratio and the approach to analysis. The tool also addresses the possibility of selective reporting of first period results in the domain 'Bias in selection of the reported result'. Special issues in assessing risk of bias in a crossover trials using RoB 2 are provided in Table 23.2.a.

Table 23.2.a Issues addressed in version 2 of the Cochrane risk-of-bias tool for randomized crossover trials

Bias domain	Additional or different issues addressed compared with parallel-group trials
Bias arising from the randomization process	• The issues surrounding methods of randomization are the same as for parallel-group trials. • If an equal proportion of participants is randomized to each intervention sequence, then any period effects will cancel out in the analysis (providing there is not differential missing data). • If unequal proportions of participants are randomized to the different intervention sequences, then period effects should be included in the analysis to avoid bias. • When using baseline differences to infer a problem with the randomization process, this should be based on differences at the start of the first period only.
Bias due to deviations from intended interventions	• Carry-over is the key concern when assessing risk of bias in a crossover trial. Carry-over effects should not affect outcomes measured in the second period. A long period of wash-out between periods can avoid this but is not essential. The important consideration is whether sufficient time passes before outcome measurement in the second period, such that any carry-over effects have disappeared. • All other issues are the same as for parallel-group trials.
Bias due to missing outcome data	• The issues are the same as for parallel-group trials. Use of last observation carried forward imputation may be particularly problematic if the observations being carried forward were made before carry-over effects had disappeared. Some analyses of crossover trials will automatically exclude (for an AB/BA design) all patients with missing data in either period.
Bias in measurement of the outcome	• The issues are the same as for parallel-group trials.
Bias in selection of the reported result	• An additional concern is the selective reporting of first period data on the basis of a test for carry-over.

* For the precise wording of signalling questions and guidance for answering each one, see the full risk-of-bias tool at www.riskofbias.info.

23.2.4 Using only the first period of a crossover trial

One option when crossover trials are anticipated in a review is to plan from the outset that only data from the first periods will be used. Including only the first intervention period of a crossover trial discards more than half of the information in the study, and often substantially more than half. A sound rationale is therefore needed for this approach, based on the inappropriateness of a crossover design (see Section 23.2.2), and not based on lack of methodological expertise.

If the review intends (from the outset) to look only at the first period of any crossover trial, then review authors should use the standard version of the RoB 2 tool for parallel group randomized trials. Review authors must, however, be alert to the potential impact of selective reporting if first-period data are reported only when carry-over is detected by the trialists. Omission of trials reporting only paired analyses (i.e. not reporting data for the first period separately) may lead to bias at the meta-analysis level. The bias will not be picked up using study-level assessments of risk of bias.

23.2.5 Methods of analysis for crossover trials

If neither carry-over nor period effects are thought to be a problem, then an appropriate analysis of continuous data from a two-period, two-intervention crossover trial is a paired t-test. This evaluates the value of 'measurement on experimental intervention (E)' minus 'measurement on control intervention (C)' separately for each participant. The mean and standard error of these difference measures are the building blocks of an effect estimate and a statistical test. The effect estimate may be included in a meta-analysis using a generic inverse-variance approach (e.g. in RevMan).

A paired analysis is possible if the data in any one of the following bullet points is available:

- individual participant data from the paper or by correspondence with the trialist;
- the mean and standard deviation (or standard error) of the participant-level differences between experimental intervention (E) and comparator intervention (C) measurements;
- the mean difference and one of the following: (i) a t-statistic from a paired t-test; (ii) a P value from a paired t-test; (iii) a confidence interval from a paired analysis;
- a graph of measurements on experimental intervention (E) and comparator intervention (C) from which individual data values can be extracted, as long as matched measurements for each individual can be identified as such.

For details see Elbourne and colleagues (Elbourne et al 2002).

Crossover trials with dichotomous outcomes require more complicated methods and consultation with a statistician is recommended (Elbourne et al 2002).

If results are available broken into subgroups by the particular sequence each participant received, then analyses that adjust for period effects are straightforward (e.g. as outlined in Chapter 3 of Senn (Senn 2002)).

23.2.6 Methods for incorporating crossover trials into a meta-analysis

Unfortunately, the reporting of crossover trials has been very variable, and the data required to include a paired analysis in a meta-analysis are often not published (Li et al 2015). A common situation is that means and standard deviations (or standard errors) are available only for measurements on E and C separately. A simple approach to incorporating crossover trials in a meta-analysis is thus to take all measurements from intervention E periods and all measurements from intervention C periods and analyse these as if the trial were a parallel-group trial of E versus C. This approach gives rise to a unit-of-analysis error (see Chapter 6, Section 6.2) and should be avoided. The reason for this is that confidence intervals are likely to be too wide, and the trial will receive too little weight, with the possible consequence of disguising clinically important heterogeneity. Nevertheless, this incorrect analysis is conservative, in that studies are under-weighted rather than over-weighted. While some argue against the inclusion of crossover trials in this way, the unit-of-analysis error might be regarded as less serious than some other types of unit-of-analysis error.

A second approach to incorporating crossover trials is to include only data from the first period. This might be appropriate if carry-over is thought to be a problem, or if a crossover design is considered inappropriate for other reasons. However, it is possible that available data from first periods constitute a biased subset of all first period data. This is because reporting of first period data may be dependent on the trialists having found statistically significant carry-over.

A third approach to incorporating inappropriately reported crossover trials is to attempt to approximate a paired analysis, by imputing missing standard deviations. We address this approach in detail in Section 23.2.7.

23.2.7 Approximate analyses of crossover trials for a meta-analysis

Table 23.2.b presents some results that might be available from a report of a crossover trial, and presents the notation we will use in the subsequent sections. We review straightforward methods for approximating appropriate analyses of crossover trials to obtain mean differences or standardized mean differences for use in meta-analysis. Review authors should consider whether imputing missing data is preferable to excluding crossover trials completely from a meta-analysis. The trade-off will depend on the confidence that can be placed on the imputed numbers, and on the robustness of the meta-analysis result to a range of plausible imputed results.

23.2.7.1 Mean differences

The point estimate of mean difference for a paired analysis is usually available, since it is the same as for a parallel-group analysis (the mean of the differences is equal to the difference in means):

$$\mathrm{MD} = M_E - M_C.$$

The standard error of the mean difference is obtained as

$$\mathrm{SE}(\mathrm{MD}) = \frac{\mathrm{SD_{diff}}}{\sqrt{N}},$$

where N is the number of participants in the trial, and $\mathrm{SD_{diff}}$ is the standard deviation of *within-participant differences between E and C measurements*. As indicated in

Table 23.2.b Some possible data available from the report of a crossover trial

Data relate to	Core statistics	Related, commonly reported statistics
Intervention E	N, M_E, SD_E	Standard error of M_E.
Intervention C	N, M_C, SD_C	Standard error of M_C.
Difference between E and C	N, MD, SD_{diff}	Standard error of MD; Confidence interval for MD; Paired t-statistic; P value from paired t-test.

Section 23.2.5, the standard error can also be obtained directly from a confidence interval for MD, from a paired t-statistic, or from the P value from a paired t-test. The quantities MD and SE(MD) may be entered into a meta-analysis under the generic inverse-variance outcome type (e.g. in RevMan).

When the standard error is not available directly and the standard deviation of the differences is not presented, a simple approach is to impute the standard deviation, as is commonly done for other missing standard deviations (see Chapter 6, Section 6.5.2.7). Other studies in the meta-analysis may present standard deviations of differences, and as long as the studies use the same measurement scale, it may be reasonable to borrow these from one study to another. As with all imputations, sensitivity analyses should be undertaken to assess the impact of the imputed data on the findings of the meta-analysis (see Chapter 10, Section 10.14).

If no information is available from any study on the standard deviations of the within-participant differences, imputation of standard deviations can be achieved by assuming a particular correlation coefficient. The correlation coefficient describes how similar the measurements on interventions E and C are within a participant, and is a number between −1 and 1. It may be expected to lie between 0 and 1 in the context of a crossover trial, since a higher than average outcome for a participant while on E will tend to be associated with a higher than average outcome while on C. If the correlation coefficient is zero or negative, then there is no statistical benefit of using a crossover design over using a parallel-group design.

A common way of presenting results of a crossover trial is as if the trial had been a parallel-group trial, with standard deviations for each intervention separately (SD_E and SD_C; see Table 23.2.b). The desired standard deviation of the differences can be estimated using these intervention-specific standard deviations and an imputed correlation coefficient (Corr):

$$\mathrm{SD_{diff}} = \sqrt{\mathrm{SD}_E^2 + \mathrm{SD}_C^2 - (2 \times \mathrm{Corr} \times \mathrm{SD}_E \times \mathrm{SD}_C)}.$$

23.2.7.2 Standardized mean difference

The most appropriate standardized mean difference (SMD) from a crossover trial divides the mean difference by the standard deviation of measurements (and not by the standard deviation of the differences). A SMD can be calculated by pooled intervention-specific standard deviations as follows:

$$\mathrm{SMD} = \frac{\mathrm{MD}}{\mathrm{SD_{pooled}}},$$

where

$$\mathrm{SD_{pooled}} = \sqrt{\frac{\mathrm{SD}_E^2 + \mathrm{SD}_C^2}{2}}.$$

A correlation coefficient is required for the standard error of the SMD:

$$\mathrm{SE(SMD)} = \sqrt{\frac{1}{N} + \frac{\mathrm{SMD}^2}{2N}} \times \sqrt{2(1-\mathrm{Corr})}.$$

Alternatively, the SMD can be calculated from the MD and its standard error, using an imputed correlation:

$$\text{SMD} = \frac{\text{MD}}{\text{SE(MD)} \times \sqrt{\frac{N}{2(1-\text{Corr})}}}.$$

In this case, the imputed correlation impacts on the magnitude of the SMD effect estimate itself (rather than just on the standard error, as is the case for MD analyses in Section 23.2.7.1). Imputed correlations should therefore be used with great caution for estimation of SMDs.

23.2.7.3 Imputing correlation coefficients

The value for a correlation coefficient might be imputed from another study in the meta-analysis (see below), it might be imputed from a source outside of the meta-analysis, or it might be hypothesized based on reasoned argument. In all of these situations, a sensitivity analysis should be undertaken, trying different plausible values of Corr, to determine whether the overall result of the analysis is robust to the use of imputed correlation coefficients.

Estimation of a correlation coefficient is possible from another study in the meta-analysis if that study presents all three standard deviations in Table 23.2.b. The calculation assumes that the mean and standard deviation of measurements for intervention E is the same when it is given in the first period as when it is given in the second period (and similarly for intervention C).

$$\text{Corr} = \frac{\text{SD}_E^2 + \text{SD}_C^2 - \text{SD}_{\text{diff}}^2}{2 \times \text{SD}_E \times \text{SD}_C}.$$

Before imputation is undertaken it is recommended that correlation coefficients are computed for as many studies as possible and compared. If these correlations vary substantially then sensitivity analyses are particularly important.

23.2.7.4 Example

As an example, suppose a crossover trial reports the following data:

Intervention E (sample size 10)	$M_E = 7.0$, $SD_E = 2.38$
Intervention C (sample size 10)	$M_C = 6.5$, $SD_C = 2.21$

Mean difference, imputing SD of differences (SD_{diff})

The estimate of the mean difference is MD = 7.0 – 6.5 = 0.5. Suppose that a typical standard deviation of differences had been observed from other trials to be 2. Then we can estimate the standard error of MD as

$$\text{SE(MD)} = \frac{\text{SD}_{\text{diff}}}{\sqrt{N}} = \frac{2}{\sqrt{10}} = 0.632.$$

The numbers 0.5 and 0.632 may be entered into RevMan as the estimate and standard error of a mean difference, under a generic inverse-variance outcome.

Mean difference, imputing correlation coefficient (Corr)

The estimate of the mean difference is again MD = 0.5. Suppose that a correlation coefficient of 0.68 has been imputed. Then we can impute the standard deviation of the differences as:

$$\begin{aligned}\text{SD}_{\text{diff}} &= \sqrt{\text{SD}_E^2 + \text{SD}_C^2 - (2 \times \text{Corr} \times \text{SD}_E \times \text{SD}_C)} \\ &= \sqrt{2.38^2 + 2.21^2 - (2 \times 0.68 \times 2.38 \times 2.21)} = 1.846.\end{aligned}$$

The standard error of MD is then

$$\text{SE(MD)} = \frac{\text{SD}_{\text{diff}}}{\sqrt{N}} = \frac{1.8426}{\sqrt{10}} = 0.583.$$

The numbers 0.5 and 0.583 may be entered into a meta-analysis as the estimate and standard error of a mean difference, under a generic inverse-variance outcome. Correlation coefficients other than 0.68 should be used as part of a sensitivity analysis.

Standardized mean difference, imputing correlation coefficient (Corr)

The standardized mean difference can be estimated directly from the data:

$$\text{SMD} = \frac{\text{MD}}{\text{SD}_{\text{pooled}}} = \frac{\text{MD}}{\sqrt{\frac{\text{SD}_E^2 + \text{SD}_C^2}{2}}} = \frac{0.5}{\sqrt{\frac{2.38^2 + 2.21^2}{2}}} = 0.218.$$

The standard error is obtained thus:

$$\text{SE(SMD)} = \sqrt{\frac{1}{N} + \frac{\text{SMD}^2}{2N}} \times \sqrt{2(1-\text{Corr})} = \sqrt{\frac{1}{10} + \frac{0.218^2}{20}} \times \sqrt{2(1-0.68)} = 0.256.$$

The numbers 0.218 and 0.256 may be entered into a meta-analysis as the estimate and standard error of a standardized mean difference, under a generic inverse-variance outcome.

We could also have obtained the SMD from the MD and its standard error:

$$\text{SMD} = \frac{\text{MD}}{\text{SE(MD)} \times \sqrt{\frac{N}{2(1-\text{Corr})}}} = \frac{0.5}{0.583 \times \sqrt{\frac{10}{2(1-0.68)}}} = 0.217.$$

The minor discrepancy arises due to the slightly different ways in which the two formulae calculate a pooled standard deviation for the standardizing.

23.2.8 Issues in the incorporation of crossover trials

Crossover trials may, in principle, be combined with parallel-group trials in the same meta-analysis. Consideration should be given to the possibility of important differences in other characteristics between the different types of trial. For example, crossover trials may have shorter intervention periods or may include participants with less severe illness. It is generally advisable to meta-analyse parallel-group and crossover trials in separate subgroups, irrespective of whether they are also combined.

Review authors should explicitly state how they have dealt with data from crossover trials and should conduct sensitivity analyses to investigate the robustness of their conclusions, especially when correlation coefficients have been borrowed from external sources (see Chapter 10, Section 10.14). Statistical support is recommended.

23.2.9 Cluster crossover trials

A cluster crossover trial combines aspects of a cluster-randomized trial (Section 23.1.1) and a crossover trial (Section 23.2.1). In a two-period, two-intervention cluster crossover trial, clusters are randomized to either the experimental intervention or the comparator intervention. At the end of the first period, clusters on the experimental intervention cross over to the comparator intervention for the second period, and clusters on the comparator intervention cross over to the experimental intervention for the second period (Rietbergen and Moerbeek 2011, Arnup et al 2017). The clusters may involve the same individuals in both periods, or different individuals in the two periods. The design introduces the advantages of a crossover design into situations in which interventions are most appropriately implemented or evaluated at the cluster level.

The analysis of a cluster crossover trial should consider both the pairing of intervention periods within clusters and the similarity of individuals within clusters. Unfortunately, many trials have not performed appropriate analyses (Arnup et al 2016), so review authors are encouraged to seek statistical advice.

The RoB 2 tool does not currently have a variant for cluster crossover trials.

23.3 Studies with more than two intervention groups

23.3.1 Introduction

It is not uncommon for clinical trials to randomize participants to one of several intervention groups. A review of randomized trials published in December 2000 found that a quarter had more than two intervention groups (Chan and Altman 2005). For example, there may be two or more experimental intervention groups with a common comparator group, or two comparator intervention groups such as a placebo group and a standard treatment group. We refer to these studies as 'multi-arm' studies. A special case is a factorial trial, which addresses two or more simultaneous intervention comparisons using four or more intervention groups (see Section 23.3.6).

Although a systematic review may include several intervention comparisons (and hence several meta-analyses), almost all meta-analyses address pair-wise comparisons.

There are three separate issues to consider when faced with a study with more than two intervention groups.

1) Determine which intervention groups are relevant to the systematic review.
2) Determine which intervention groups are relevant to a particular meta-analysis.
3) Determine how the study will be included in the meta-analysis if more than two groups are relevant.

23.3.2 Determining which intervention groups are relevant

For a particular multi-arm study, the intervention groups of relevance to a *systematic review* are all those that could be included in a pair-wise comparison of intervention groups that would meet the criteria for including studies in the review. For example, a review addressing only a comparison of nicotine replacement therapy versus placebo for smoking cessation might identify a study comparing nicotine gum versus behavioural therapy versus placebo gum. Of the three possible pair-wise comparisons of interventions in this study, only one (nicotine gum versus placebo gum) addresses the review objective, and no comparison involving behavioural therapy does. Thus, the behavioural therapy group is not relevant to the review, and can be safely left out of any syntheses. However, if the study had compared nicotine gum plus behavioural therapy versus behavioural therapy plus placebo gum versus placebo gum alone, then a comparison of the first two interventions might be considered relevant (with behavioural therapy provided as a consistent co-intervention to both groups of interest), and the placebo gum alone group might not.

As an example of multiple comparator groups, a review addressing the comparison 'acupuncture versus no acupuncture' might identify a study comparing 'acupuncture versus sham acupuncture versus no intervention'. The review authors would ask whether, on the one hand, a study of 'acupuncture versus sham acupuncture' would be included in the review and, on the other hand, a study of 'acupuncture versus no intervention' would be included. If both of them would, then all three intervention groups of the study are relevant to the review.

As a general rule, and to avoid any confusion for the reader over the identity and nature of each study, it is recommended that all intervention groups of a multi-intervention study be mentioned in the table of 'Characteristics of included studies'. However, it is necessary to provide detailed descriptions of only the intervention groups relevant to the review, and only these groups should be used in analyses.

The same considerations of relevance apply when determining which intervention groups of a study should be included in a particular *meta-analysis*. Each meta-analysis addresses only a single pair-wise comparison, so review authors should consider whether a study of each possible pair-wise comparison of interventions in the study would be eligible for the meta-analysis. To draw the distinction between the review-level decision and the meta-analysis-level decision, consider a review of 'nicotine therapy versus placebo or other comparators'. All intervention groups of a study of 'nicotine gum versus behavioural therapy versus placebo gum' might be relevant to the review. However, the presence of multiple interventions may not pose any problem for meta-analyses, since it is likely that 'nicotine gum versus placebo gum', and 'nicotine gum versus behavioural therapy' would be addressed in different meta-analyses.

Conversely, all groups of the study of 'acupuncture versus sham acupuncture versus no intervention' might be considered eligible for the same meta-analysis. This would be the case if the meta-analysis would otherwise include both studies of 'acupuncture versus sham acupuncture' and studies of 'acupuncture versus no intervention', treating sham acupuncture and no intervention both as relevant comparators. We describe methods for dealing with the latter situation in Section 23.3.4.

23.3.3 Risk of bias in studies with more than two groups

Bias may be introduced in a multiple-intervention study if the decisions regarding data analysis are made after seeing the data. For example, groups receiving different doses of the same intervention may be combined only after looking at the results. Also, decisions about the selection of outcomes to report may be made after comparing different pairs of intervention groups and examining the findings. These issues would be addressed in the domain 'Bias due to selection of the reported result' in the Cochrane risk-of-bias tool for randomized trials (RoB 2, see Chapter 8).

Juszczak and colleagues reviewed 60 multiple-intervention randomized trials, of which over a third had at least four intervention arms (Juszczak et al 2003). They found that only 64% reported the same comparisons of groups for all outcomes, suggesting selective reporting analogous to selective outcome reporting in a two-arm trial. Also, 20% reported combining groups in an analysis. However, if the summary data are provided for each intervention group, it does not matter how the groups had been combined in reported analyses; review authors do not need to analyse the data in the same way as the study authors.

23.3.4 How to include multiple groups from one study

There are several possible approaches to including a study with multiple intervention groups in a particular meta-analysis. One approach that must be avoided is simply to enter several comparisons into the meta-analysis so that the same comparator intervention group is included more than once. This 'double-counts' the participants in the intervention group(s) shared across more than one comparison, and creates a unit-of-analysis error due to the unaddressed correlation between the estimated intervention effects from multiple comparisons (see Chapter 6, Section 6.2). An important distinction is between situations in which a study can contribute several *independent* comparisons (i.e. with no intervention group in common) and when several comparisons are *correlated* because they have intervention groups, and hence participants, in common. For example, consider a study that randomized participants to four groups: 'nicotine gum' versus 'placebo gum' versus 'nicotine patch' versus 'placebo patch'. A meta-analysis that addresses the broad question of whether nicotine replacement therapy is effective might include the comparison 'nicotine gum versus placebo gum' as well as the independent comparison 'nicotine patch versus placebo patch', with no unit of analysis error or double-counting. It is usually reasonable to include independent comparisons in a meta-analysis as if they were from different studies, although there are subtle complications with regard to random-effects analyses (see Section 23.3.5).

Approaches to overcoming a unit-of-analysis error for a study that could contribute multiple, correlated, comparisons include the following.

- Combine groups to create a single pair-wise comparison (recommended).
- Select one pair of interventions and exclude the others.
- Split the 'shared' group into two or more groups with smaller sample size, and include two or more (reasonably independent) comparisons.
- Include two or more correlated comparisons and account for the correlation.
- Undertake a *network meta-analysis* (see Chapter 11).

The recommended method in most situations is to combine all relevant experimental intervention groups of the study into a single group, and to combine all relevant comparator intervention groups into a single comparator group. As an example, suppose that a meta-analysis of 'acupuncture versus no acupuncture' would consider studies of either 'acupuncture versus sham acupuncture' or studies of 'acupuncture versus no intervention' to be eligible for inclusion. Then a study with three intervention groups (acupuncture, sham acupuncture and no intervention) would be included in the meta-analysis by combining the participants in the 'sham acupuncture' group with participants in the 'no intervention' group. This combined comparator group would be compared with the 'acupuncture' group in the usual way. For dichotomous outcomes, both the sample sizes and the numbers of people with events can be summed across groups. For continuous outcomes, means and standard deviations can be combined using methods described in Chapter 6 (Section 6.5.2.10).

The alternative strategy of selecting a single pair of interventions (e.g. choosing either 'sham acupuncture' or 'no intervention' as the comparator) results in a loss of information and is open to results-related choices, so is not generally recommended.

A further possibility is to include each pair-wise comparison separately, but with shared intervention groups divided out approximately evenly among the comparisons. For example, if a trial compares 121 patients receiving acupuncture with 124 patients receiving sham acupuncture and 117 patients receiving no acupuncture, then two comparisons (of, say, 61 'acupuncture' against 124 'sham acupuncture', and of 60 'acupuncture' against 117 'no intervention') might be entered into the meta-analysis. For dichotomous outcomes, both the number of events and the total number of patients would be divided up. For continuous outcomes, only the total number of participants would be divided up and the means and standard deviations left unchanged. This method only partially overcomes the unit-of-analysis error (because the resulting comparisons remain correlated) so is not generally recommended. A potential advantage of this approach, however, would be that approximate investigations of heterogeneity across intervention arms are possible (e.g. in the case of the example here, the difference between using sham acupuncture and no intervention as a comparator group).

Two final options are to account for the correlation between correlated comparisons from the same study in the analysis, and to perform a network meta-analysis. The former involves calculating an average (or weighted average) of the relevant pair-wise comparisons from the study, and calculating a variance (and hence a weight) for the study, taking into account the correlation between the comparisons (Borenstein et al 2008). It will typically yield a similar result to the recommended method of combining across experimental and comparator intervention groups. Network meta-analysis allows for the simultaneous analysis of multiple interventions, and so naturally allows for multi-arm studies. Network meta-analysis is discussed in more detail in Chapter 11.

23.3.5 Heterogeneity considerations with multiple-intervention studies

Two possibilities for addressing heterogeneity between studies are to allow for it in a random-effects meta-analysis, and to investigate it through subgroup analyses or meta-regression (Chapter 10, Section 10.11). Some complications arise when including multiple-intervention studies in such analyses. First, it will not be possible to investigate certain intervention-related sources of heterogeneity if intervention groups are combined as in the recommended approach in Section 23.3.4. For example, subgrouping according to 'sham acupuncture' or 'no intervention' as a comparator group is not possible if these two groups are combined prior to the meta-analysis. The simplest method for allowing an investigation of this difference, across studies, is to create two or more comparisons from the study (e.g. 'acupuncture versus sham acupuncture' and 'acupuncture versus no intervention'). However, if these contain a common intervention group (here, acupuncture), then they are not independent and a unit-of-analysis error will occur, even if the sample size is reduced for the shared intervention group(s). Nevertheless, splitting up the sample size for the shared intervention group remains a practical means of performing approximate investigations of heterogeneity.

A more subtle problem occurs in random-effects meta-analyses if multiple comparisons are included from the same study. A random-effects meta-analysis allows for variation by assuming that the effects underlying the studies in the meta-analysis follow a distribution across studies. The intention is to allow for study-to-study variation. However, if two or more estimates come from the same study then the same variation is assumed across comparisons within the study and across studies. This is true whether the comparisons are independent or correlated (see Section 23.3.4). One way to overcome this is to perform a fixed-effect meta-analysis across comparisons within a study, and a random-effects meta-analysis across studies. Statistical support is recommended; in practice the difference between different analyses is likely to be trivial.

23.3.6 Factorial trials

In a factorial trial, two (or more) intervention comparisons are carried out simultaneously. Thus, for example, participants may be randomized to receive aspirin or placebo, and also randomized to receive a behavioural intervention or standard care. Most factorial trials have two 'factors' in this way, each of which has two levels; these are called 2 × 2 factorial trials. Occasionally 3 × 2 trials may be encountered, or trials that investigate three, four, or more interventions simultaneously. Often only one of the comparisons will be of relevance to any particular review. The following remarks focus on the 2 × 2 case but the principles extend to more complex designs.

In most factorial trials the intention is to achieve 'two trials for the price of one', and the assumption is made that the effects of the different active interventions are independent, that is, there is no interaction (synergy). Occasionally a trial may be carried out specifically to investigate whether there is an interaction between two treatments. That aspect may more often be explored in a trial comparing each of two active treatments on its own with both combined, without a placebo group. Such three intervention group trials are not factorial trials.

The 2 × 2 factorial design can be displayed as a 2 × 2 table, with the rows indicating one comparison (e.g. aspirin versus placebo) and the columns the other (e.g. behavioural intervention versus standard care):

Randomization of A		Randomization of B	
		Behavioural intervention (B)	**Standard care (not B)**
	Aspirin (A)	A and B	A, not B
	Placebo (not A)	B, not A	Not A, not B

A 2 × 2 factorial trial can be seen as two trials addressing different questions. It is important that both parts of the trial are reported as if they were just a two-arm parallel-group trial. Thus, we expect to see the results for aspirin versus placebo, including all participants regardless of whether they had behavioural intervention or standard care, and likewise for the behavioural intervention. These results may be seen as relating to the margins of the 2 × 2 table. We would also wish to evaluate whether there may have been some interaction between the treatments (i.e. effect of A depends on whether B or 'not B' was received), for which we need to see the four cells within the table (McAlister et al 2003). It follows that the practice of publishing two separate reports, possibly in different journals, does not allow the full results to be seen.

McAlister and colleagues reviewed 44 published reports of factorial trials (McAlister et al 2003). They found that only 34% reported results for each cell of the factorial structure. However, it will usually be possible to derive the marginal results from the results for the four cells in the 2 × 2 structure. In the same review, 59% of the trial reports included the results of a test of interaction. On re-analysis, 2/44 trials (6%) had $P < 0.05$, which is close to expectation by chance (McAlister et al 2003). Thus, despite concerns about unrecognized interactions, it seems that investigators are appropriately restricting the use of the factorial design to those situations in which two (or more) treatments do not have the potential for substantive interaction. Unfortunately, many review authors do not take advantage of this fact and include only half of the available data in their meta-analysis (e.g. including only aspirin versus placebo among those that *were not* receiving behavioural intervention, and excluding the valid investigation of aspirin among those that *were* receiving behavioural intervention).

When faced with factorial trials, review authors should consider whether both intervention comparisons are relevant to a meta-analysis. If only one of the comparisons is relevant, then the full comparison of all participants for that comparison should be used. If both comparisons are relevant, then both full comparisons can be included in a meta-analysis without a need to account for the double counting of participants. Additional considerations may apply if important interaction has been found between the interventions.

23.4 Chapter information

Editors: Julian PT Higgins, Sandra Eldridge, Tianjing Li

Acknowledgements: We are grateful to Doug Altman, Marion Campbell, Michael Campbell, François Curtin, Amy Drahota, Bruno Giraudeau, Barnaby Reeves, Stephen Senn and Nandi Siegfried for contributions to the material in this chapter.

23.5 References

Arnup SJ, Forbes AB, Kahan BC, Morgan KE, McKenzie JE. Appropriate statistical methods were infrequently used in cluster-randomized crossover trials. *Journal of Clinical Epidemiology* 2016; **74**: 40–50.

Arnup SJ, McKenzie JE, Hemming K, Pilcher D, Forbes AB. Understanding the cluster randomised crossover design: a graphical illustraton of the components of variation and a sample size tutorial. *Trials* 2017; **18**: 381.

Borenstein M, Hedges LV, Higgins JPT, Rothstein HR. *Introduction to Meta-analysis*. Chichester (UK): John Wiley & Sons; 2008.

Campbell M, Grimshaw J, Steen N. Sample size calculations for cluster randomised trials. Changing Professional Practice in Europe Group (EU BIOMED II Concerted Action). *Journal of Health Services Research and Policy* 2000; **5**: 12–16.

Campbell MJ, Walters SJ. *How to design, Analyse and Report Cluster Randomised Trials in Medicine and Health Related Research*. Chichester (UK): John Wiley & Sons; 2014.

Campbell MK, Piaggio G, Elbourne DR, Altman DG, Group C. Consort 2010 statement: extension to cluster randomised trials. *BMJ* 2012; **345**: e5661.

Chan AW, Altman DG. Epidemiology and reporting of randomised trials published in PubMed journals. *Lancet* 2005; **365**: 1159–1162.

Donner A, Klar N. *Design and Analysis of Cluster Randomization Trials in Health Research*. London (UK): Arnold; 2000.

Donner A, Piaggio G, Villar J. Statistical methods for the meta-analysis of cluster randomized trials. *Statistical Methods in Medical Research* 2001; **10**: 325–338.

Donner A, Klar N. Issues in the meta-analysis of cluster randomized trials. *Statistics in Medicine* 2002; **21**: 2971–2980.

Elbourne DR, Altman DG, Higgins JPT, Curtin F, Worthington HV, Vaillancourt JM. Meta-analyses involving cross-over trials: methodological issues. *International Journal of Epidemiology* 2002; **31**: 140–149.

Eldridge S, Ashby D, Bennett C, Wakelin M, Feder G. Internal and external validity of cluster randomised trials: systematic review of recent trials. *BMJ* 2008; **336**: 876–880.

Eldridge S, Kerry S, Torgerson DJ. Bias in identifying and recruiting participants in cluster randomised trials: what can be done? *BMJ* 2009a; **339**: b4006.

Eldridge S, Kerry S. *A Practical Guide to Cluster Randomised Trials in Health Services Research*. Chichester (UK): John Wiley & Sons; 2012.

Eldridge SM, Ashby D, Kerry S. Sample size for cluster randomized trials: effect of coefficient of variation of cluster size and analysis method. *International Journal of Epidemiology* 2006; **35**: 1292–1300.

Eldridge SM, Ukoumunne OC, Carlin JB. The intra-cluster correlation coefficient in cluster randomized trials: a review of definitions. *International Statistical Review* 2009b; **77**: 378–394.

Freeman PR. The performance of the two-stage analysis of two-treatment, two-period cross-over trials. *Statistics in Medicine* 1989; **8**: 1421–1432.

Hahn S, Puffer S, Torgerson DJ, Watson J. Methodological bias in cluster randomised trials. *BMC Medical Research Methodology* 2005; **5**: 10.

Hayes RJ, Moulton LH. *Cluster Randomised Trials*. Boca Raton (FL): CRC Press; 2017.

Health Services Research Unit. Database of ICCs: Spreadsheet (Empirical estimates of ICCs from changing professional practice studies) [page last modified 11 Aug 2004] 2004. http://www.abdn.ac.uk/hsru/epp/cluster.shtml.

Hemming K, Haines TP, Chilton PJ, Girling AJ, Lilford RJ. The stepped wedge cluster randomised trial: rationale, design, analysis, and reporting. *BMJ* 2015; **350**: h391.

Juszczak E, Altman D, Chan AW. A review of the methodology and reporting of multi-arm, parallel group, randomised clinical trials (RCTs). 3rd Joint Meeting of the International Society for Clinical Biostatistics and Society for Clinical Trials; London (UK) 2003.

Lathyris DN, Trikalinos TA, Ioannidis JP. Evidence from crossover trials: empirical evaluation and comparison against parallel arm trials. *International Journal of Epidemiology* 2007; **36**: 422–430.

Lee LJ, Thompson SG. Clustering by health professional in individually randomised trials. *BMJ* 2005; **330**: 142–144.

Li T, Yu T, Hawkins BS, Dickersin K. Design, analysis, and reporting of crossover trials for inclusion in a meta-analysis. *PloS One* 2015; **10**: e0133023.

McAlister FA, Straus SE, Sackett DL, Altman DG. Analysis and reporting of factorial trials: a systematic review. *JAMA* 2003; **289**: 2545–2553.

Murray DM, Short B. Intraclass correlation among measures related to alcohol-use by young-adults – estimates, correlates and applications in intervention studies. *Journal of Studies on Alcohol* 1995; **56**: 681–694.

Nolan SJ, Hambleton I, Dwan K. The use and reporting of the cross-over study design in clinical trials and systematic reviews: a systematic assessment. *PloS One* 2016; **11**: e0159014.

Puffer S, Torgerson D, Watson J. Evidence for risk of bias in cluster randomised trials: review of recent trials published in three general medical journals. *BMJ* 2003; **327**: 785–789.

Qizilbash N, Whitehead A, Higgins J, Wilcock G, Schneider L, Farlow M. Cholinesterase inhibition for Alzheimer disease: a meta-analysis of the tacrine trials. *JAMA* 1998; **280**: 1777–1782.

Rao JNK, Scott AJ. A simple method for the analysis of clustered binary data. *Biometrics* 1992; **48**: 577–585.

Richardson M, Garner P, Donegan S. Cluster tandomised trials in Cochrane Reviews: evaluation of methodological and reporting practice. *PloS One* 2016; **11**: e0151818.

Rietbergen C, Moerbeek M. The design of cluster randomized crossover trials. *Journal of Educational and Behavioral Statistics* 2011; **36**: 472–490.

Senn S. *Cross-over Trials in Clinical Research*. 2nd ed. Chichester (UK): John Wiley & Sons; 2002.

Ukoumunne OC, Gulliford MC, Chinn S, Sterne JA, Burney PG. Methods for evaluating area-wide and organisation-based interventions in health and health care: a systematic review. *Health Technology Assessment* 1999; **3**: 5.

Walwyn R, Roberts C. Meta-analysis of absolute mean differences from randomised trials with treatment-related clustering associated with care providers. *Statistics in Medicine* 2015; **34**: 966–983.

Walwyn R, Roberts C. Meta-analysis of standardised mean differences from randomised trials with treatment-related clustering associated with care providers. *Statistics in Medicine* 2017; **36**: 1043–1067.

White IR, Thomas J. Standardized mean differences in individually-randomized and cluster-randomized trials, with applications to meta-analysis. *Clinical Trials* 2005; **2**: 141–151.

Whiting-O'Keefe QE, Henke C, Simborg DW. Choosing the correct unit of analysis in medical care experiments. *Medical Care* 1984; **22**: 1101–1114.

Walwyn R, Roberts C. Meta-analysis of standardised mean differences from randomised trials with treatment-related clustering associated with care providers. *Statistics in Medicine* 2017; 36: 1043–1067.

White IR, Thomas J. Standardized mean differences in individually-randomized and cluster-randomized trials, with applications to meta-analysis. *Clinical Trials* 2005; 2: 141–151.

Whiting-O'Keefe QE, Henke C, Simborg DW. Choosing the correct unit of analysis in medical care experiments. *Medical Care* 1984; 22: 1101–1114.

24

Including non-randomized studies on intervention effects

Barnaby C Reeves, Jonathan J Deeks, Julian PT Higgins, Beverley Shea, Peter Tugwell, George A Wells; on behalf of the Cochrane Non-Randomized Studies of Interventions Methods Group

KEY POINTS

- For some Cochrane Reviews, the question of interest cannot be answered by randomized trials, and review authors may be justified in including non-randomized studies.
- Potential biases are likely to be greater for non-randomized studies compared with randomized trials when evaluating the effects of interventions, so results should always be interpreted with caution when they are included in reviews and meta-analyses.
- Non-randomized studies of interventions vary in their ability to estimate a causal effect; key design features of studies can distinguish 'strong' from 'weak' studies.
- Biases affecting non-randomized studies of interventions vary depending on the features of the studies.
- We recommend that eligibility criteria, data collection and assessment of included studies place an emphasis on specific features of study design (e.g. which parts of the study were prospectively designed) rather than 'labels' for study designs (such as case-control versus cohort).
- Review authors should consider how potential confounders, and how the likelihood of increased heterogeneity resulting from residual confounding and from other biases that vary across studies, are addressed in meta-analyses of non-randomized studies.

24.1 Introduction

This chapter aims to support review authors who are considering including non-randomized studies of interventions (NRSI) in a Cochrane Review. NRSI are defined here as any quantitative study estimating the effectiveness of an intervention (harm or benefit) that does not use randomization to allocate units (individuals or clusters of

This chapter should be cited as: Reeves BC, Deeks JJ, Higgins JPT, Shea B, Tugwell P, Wells GA. Chapter 24: Including non-randomized studies on intervention effects. In: Higgins JPT, Thomas J, Chandler J, Cumpston M, Li T, Page MJ, Welch VA (editors). *Cochrane Handbook for Systematic Reviews of Interventions*. 2nd Edition. Chichester (UK): John Wiley & Sons, 2019: 595–620.

individuals) to intervention groups. Such studies include those in which allocation occurs in the course of usual treatment decisions or according to peoples' choices (i.e. studies often called *observational*). (The term observational is used in various ways and, therefore, we discourage its use with respect to NRSI studies; see Box 24.2.a and Section 24.2.1.3.) Review authors have a duty to patients, practitioners and policy makers to do their best to provide these groups with a summary of available evidence balancing harms against benefits, albeit qualified with a certainty assessment. Some of this evidence, especially about harms of interventions, will often need to come from NRSI.

NRSI are used by researchers to evaluate numerous types of interventions, ranging from drugs and hospital procedures, through diverse community health interventions, to health systems implemented at a national level. There are many types of NRSI. Common labels attached to them include cohort studies, case-control studies, controlled before-and-after studies and interrupted-time-series studies (see Section 24.5.1 for a discussion of why these labels are not always clear and can be problematic). We also consider controlled trials that use inappropriate strategies of allocating interventions (sometimes called quasi-randomized studies), and specific types of analysis of non-randomized data, such as instrumental variable analysis and regression discontinuity analysis, to be NRSI. We prefer to characterize NRSI with respect to specific study design features (see Section 24.2.2 and Box 24.2.a) rather than study design labels. A mapping of features to some commonly used study design labels can be found in Reeves and colleagues (Reeves et al 2017).

Including NRSI in a Cochrane Review allows, in principle, the inclusion of non-randomized studies in which the use of an intervention occurs in the course of usual health care or daily life. These include interventions that a study participant chooses to take (e.g. an over-the-counter preparation or a health education session). Such studies also allow exposures to be studied that are not obviously 'interventions', such as nutritional choices, and other behaviours that may affect health. This introduces a grey area between evidence about effectiveness and aetiology.

An intervention review needs to distinguish carefully between aetiological and effectiveness research questions related to a particular exposure. For example, nutritionists may be interested in the health-related effects of a diet that includes a minimum of five portions of fruit or vegetables per day ('five-a-day'), an aetiological question. On the other hand, public health professionals may be interested in the health-related effects of interventions to promote a change in diet to include 'five-a-day', an effectiveness question. NRSI addressing the former type of question are often perceived as being more direct than randomized trials because of other differences between studies addressing these two kinds of question (e.g. compared with the randomized trials, NRSI of health behaviours may be able to investigate longer durations of follow-up and outcomes than become apparent in the short term). However, it is important to appreciate that they are addressing fundamentally different research questions. Cochrane Reviews target effects of interventions, and interventions have a defined start time.

This chapter has been prepared by the Cochrane Non-Randomized Studies of Interventions Methods Group (NRSMG). It aims to describe the particular challenges that arise if NRSI are included in a Cochrane Review. Where evidence or established theory indicates a suitable strategy, we propose this strategy; where it does not, we sometimes offer our recommendations about what to do. Where we do not make any recommendations, we aim to set out the pros and cons of alternative actions and to identify questions for further methodological research.

Review authors who are considering including NRSI in a Cochrane Review should not start with this chapter unless they are already familiar with the process of preparing a systematic review of randomized trials. The format and basic steps of a Cochrane Review should be the same irrespective of the types of study included. The reader is referred to Chapters 1 to 15 of the *Handbook* for a detailed description of these steps. Every step in carrying out a systematic review is more difficult when NRSI are included and the review team should include one or more people with expert knowledge of the subject and of NRSI methods.

24.1.1 Why consider non-randomized studies of interventions?

Cochrane Reviews of interventions have traditionally focused mainly on systematic reviews of randomized trials because they are more likely to provide unbiased information about the differential effects of alternative health interventions than NRSI. Reviews of NRSI are generally undertaken when the question of interest cannot be answered by a review of randomized trials. Broadly, we consider that there are two main justifications for including NRSI in a systematic review, covered by the flow diagram shown in Figure 24.1.a:

1) To provide evidence of the effects (benefit or harm) of interventions that can feasibly be studied in randomized trials, but for which available randomized trials address the review question indirectly or incompletely (an element of the GRADE approach to assessing the certainty of the evidence, see Chapter 14, Section 14.2) (Schünemann et al 2013). Such non-randomized evidence might address, for example, long-term or rare outcomes, different populations or settings, or ways of delivering interventions that better match the review question.
2) To provide evidence of the effects (benefit or harm) of interventions that *cannot* be randomized, or that are extremely unlikely to be studied in randomized trials. Such non-randomized evidence might address, for example, population-level interventions (e.g. the effects of legislation; Macpherson and Spinks 2008) or interventions about which prospective study participants are likely to have strong preferences, preventing randomization (Li et al 2016).

A third justification for including NRSI in a systematic review is reasonable, but is unlikely to be a strong reason in the context of a Cochrane Review:

3) To examine the case for undertaking a randomized trial by providing an explicit evaluation of the weaknesses of available NRSI. The findings of a review of NRSI may also be useful to inform the design of a subsequent randomized trial (e.g. through the identification of relevant subgroups).

Two other reasons sometimes described for including NRSI in systematic reviews are:

4) When an intervention effect is very large.
5) To provide evidence of the effects (benefit or harm) of interventions that can feasibly be studied in randomized trials, but for which only a small number of randomized trials is available (or likely to be available).

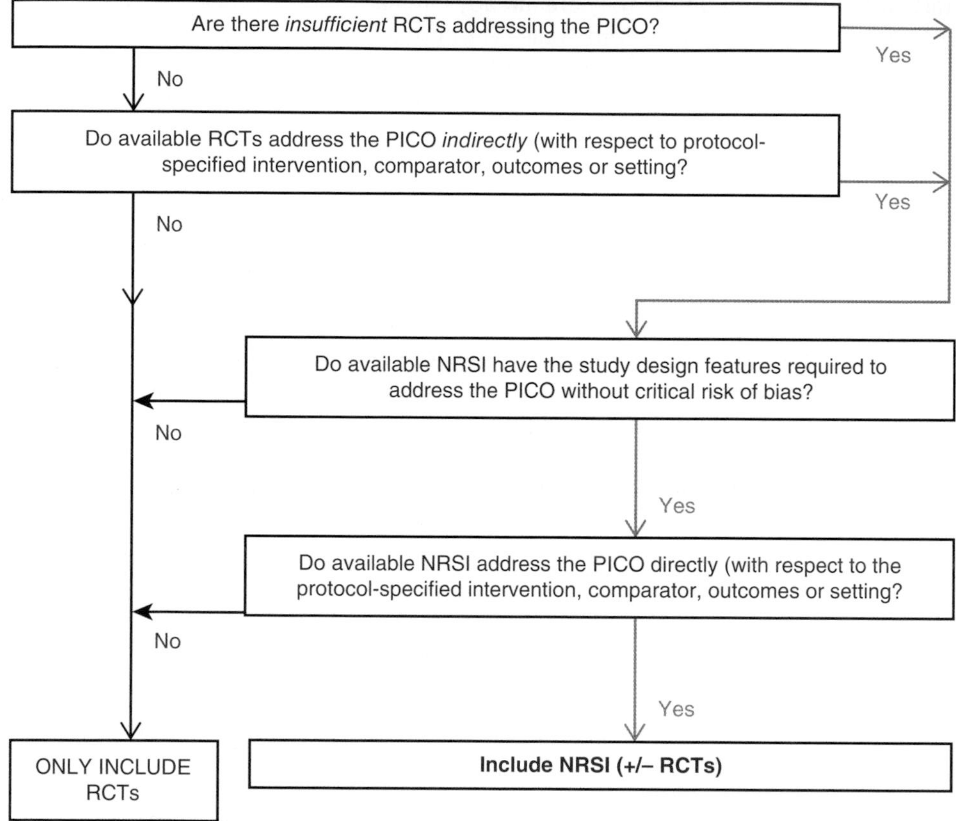

Figure 24.1.a Algorithm to decide whether a review should include non-randomized studies of an intervention or not

We urge caution in invoking either of these justifications. Reason 4, that an effect is large, is implicitly a result-driven or post-hoc argument, since some evidence or opinion would need to be available to inform the judgement about the likely size of the effect. Whilst it can be argued that large effects are less likely to be completely explained by bias than small effects (Glasziou et al 2007), clinical and economic decisions still need to be informed by unbiased estimates of the magnitude of these large effects (Reeves 2006). Randomized trials are the appropriate design to quantify large effects (and the trials need not be large if the effects are truly large). Of course, there may be ethical opposition to randomized trials of interventions already suspected to be associated with a large benefit, making it difficult to randomize participants, and interventions postulated to have large effects may also be difficult to randomize for other reasons (e.g. surgery versus no surgery). However, the justification for a systematic review including NRSI in these circumstances can be classified as reason 2 above (i.e. interventions that are unlikely to be randomized).

The appropriateness of reason 5 depends to a large extent on expectations of how the review will be used in practice. Most Cochrane Reviews seek to identify highly trustworthy evidence (typically only randomized trials) and if none is found then the review can be published as an 'empty review'. However, as Cochrane Reviews also seek to inform clinical and policy decisions, it can be necessary to draw on the 'best available' evidence rather than the 'highest tier' of evidence for questions that have a high priority. While acknowledging the priority to inform decisions, it remains important that the challenges associated with appraising, synthesizing and interpreting evidence from NRSI, as discussed in the remainder of this chapter, are well-appreciated and addressed in this situation. See also Section 24.2.1.3 for further discussion of these issues. Reason 5 is a less appropriate justification in a review that is not a priority topic where there is a paucity of evidence from randomized trials alone; in such instances, the potential of NRSI to inform the review question directly and without a critical risk of bias are paramount.

Review authors may need to apply different eligibility criteria in order to answer different review questions about harms as well as benefits (Chapter 19, Section 19.2.2). In some reviews the situation may be still more complex, since NRSI specified to answer questions about benefits may have different design features from NRSI specified to answer questions about harms (see Section 24.2). A further complexity arises in relation to the specification of eligible NRSI in the protocol and the desire to avoid an empty review (depending on the justification for including NRSI).

Whenever review authors decide that NRSI are required to answer one or more review questions, the review protocol must specify appropriate methods for reviewing NRSI. If a review aims to include both randomized trials and NRSI, the protocol must specify methods appropriate for both. Since methods for reviewing NRSI can be complex, **we recommend that review authors scope the available NRSI evidence**, after registering a title but in advance of writing a protocol, allowing review authors to check that relevant NRSI exist and to specify NRSI with the most appropriate study design features in the protocol (Reeves et al 2013). If the registered title is broadly conceived, this may require detailed review questions to be formulated in advance of scoping: these are the **PICOs for each synthesis** as discussed in Chapter 3 (Section 3.2). Scoping also allows the directness of the available evidence to be assessed against specific review questions (see Figure 24.1.a). Basing protocol decisions on scoping creates a small risk that different kinds of studies are found to be necessary at a later stage to answer the review questions. In such instances, we recommend completing the review as specified and including other studies in a planned update, to allow timelines for the completion of a review to be set.

An alternative approach is to write a protocol that describes the review methods to be used for both randomized trials and NRSI (and all types of NRSI) and to specify the study design features of eligible NRSI after carrying out searches for both types of study. We recommend against this approach in a Cochrane Review, largely to minimize the work required to write the protocol, carry out searches and examine study reports, and to allow timelines for the completion of a review to be set.

24.1.2 Key issues about the inclusion of non-randomized studies of interventions in a Cochrane Review

Randomized trials are the preferred design for studying the effects of healthcare interventions because, in most circumstances, a high-quality randomized trial is the study design that is least likely to be biased. All Cochrane Reviews must consider the risk of bias in individual primary studies, whether randomized trials or NRSI (see Chapters 7, 8 and 25). Some biases apply to both randomized trials and NRSI. However, some biases are specific (or particularly important) to NRSI, such as biases due to confounding or selection of participants into the study (see Chapter 25). The key advantage of a high-quality randomized trial is its ability to estimate the causal relationship between an experimental intervention (relative to a comparator) and outcome. Review authors will need to consider (i) the strengths of the design features of the NRSI that have been used (such as noting their potential to estimate causality, in particular by inspecting the assumptions that underpin such estimation); and (ii) the execution of the studies through a careful assessment of their risk of bias. The review team should be constituted so that it can judge suitability of the design features of included studies and implement a careful assessment of risk of bias.

Potential biases are likely to be greater for NRSI compared with randomized trials because some of the protections against bias that are available for randomized trials are not established for NRSI. Randomization is an obvious example. Randomization aims to balance prognostic factors across intervention groups, thus preventing confounding (which occurs when there are common causes of intervention group assignment and outcome). Other protections include a detailed protocol and a pre-specified statistical analysis plan which, for example, should define the primary and secondary outcomes to be studied, their derivation from measured variables, methods for managing protocol deviations and missing data, planned subgroup and sensitivity analyses and their interpretation.

24.1.3 The importance of a protocol for a Cochrane Review that includes non-randomized studies of interventions

Chapter 1 (Section 1.5) establishes the importance of writing a protocol before carrying out the review. Because the methodological choices made during a review including NRSI are complex and may affect the review findings, a protocol is even more important for such a review. The rationale for including NRSI (see Section 24.1.1) should be documented in the protocol. The protocol should include much more detail than for a review of randomized trials, pre-specifying key methodological decisions about the methods to be used and the analyses that are planned. The protocol needs to specify details that are not as relevant for randomized trials (e.g. potential confounding domains, important co-interventions, details of the risk-of-bias assessment and analysis of the NRSI), as well as providing more detail about standard steps in the review process that are more difficult when including NRSI (e.g. specification of eligibility criteria and the search strategy for identifying eligible studies).

We recognize that it may not be possible to pre-specify all decisions about the methods used in a review. Nevertheless, review authors should aim to make all decisions about the methods for the review without reference to the *findings* of primary studies, and report methodological decisions that had to be made or modified after collecting data about the study findings.

24.2 Developing criteria for including non-randomized studies of interventions

24.2.1 What is different when including non-randomized studies of interventions?

24.2.1.1 Evaluating benefits and harms

Cochrane Reviews aim to quantify the effects of healthcare interventions, both beneficial and harmful, and both expected and unexpected. The expected benefits of an intervention can often be assessed in randomized trials. Randomized trials may also report some of the harms of an intervention, either those that were expected and which a trial was designed to assess, or those that were not expected but which were collected in a trial as part of standard monitoring of safety. However, many serious harms of an intervention are rare or do not arise during the follow-up period of randomized trials, preventing randomized trials from providing high-quality evidence about these effects, even when combined in a meta-analysis (see Chapter 19 for further discussion of adverse events). Therefore, one of the most important reasons to include NRSI in a review is to assess potential unexpected or rare harms of interventions (reason 1 in Section 24.1.1).

Although widely accepted criteria for selecting appropriate studies for evaluating rare or long-term adverse and unexpected effects have not been established, some design features are preferred to reduce the risk of bias. In cohort studies, a preferred design feature is the ascertainment of outcomes of interest (e.g. an adverse event) from the onset of an exposure (i.e. the start of intervention); these are sometimes referred to as inception cohorts. The relative strengths and weaknesses of different study design features do not differ in principle between beneficial and harmful outcomes, but the choice of study designs to include may depend on both the frequency of an outcome and its importance. For example, for some rare or delayed adverse outcomes only case series or case-control studies may be available. NRSI with some study design features that are more susceptible to bias may be acceptable for evaluation of serious adverse events in the absence of better evidence, but the risk of bias must still be assessed and reported.

Confounding (see Chapter 25, Section 25.2.1) may be less of a threat to the validity of a review when researching rare harms or unexpected effects of interventions than when researching expected effects, since it may be argued that 'confounding by indication' mainly influences treatment decisions with respect to outcomes about which the clinicians are primarily concerned. However, confounding can never be ruled out because the same factors that are confounders for the expected effects may also be direct confounders for the unexpected effects, or be correlated with factors that are confounders.

A related issue is the need to distinguish between *quantifying* and *detecting* an effect of an intervention. Quantifying the intended benefits of an intervention – maximizing the precision of the estimate and minimizing susceptibility to bias – is critical when weighing up the relative merits of alternative interventions for the same condition. A review should also try to quantify the harms of an intervention, minimizing susceptibility to bias as far as possible. However, if a review can establish beyond reasonable doubt that an intervention causes a particular harm, the precision and susceptibility to bias of the estimated effect may not be essential. In other words, the seriousness of the harm may outweigh any benefit from the intervention. This situation is more likely to occur when there are competing interventions for a condition.

24.2.1.2 Including both randomized trials and non-randomized studies of interventions

When both randomized trials and NRSI are identified that appear to address the same underlying research question, it is important to check carefully that this is indeed the case. There are often systematic differences between randomized trials and NRSI in the PICO elements (MacLehose et al 2000), which may become apparent when considering the directness (e.g. applicability or generalizability) of the primary studies (see Chapter 14, Section 14.2.2).

A NRSI can be viewed as an attempt to emulate a hypothetical randomized trial answering the same question. Hernán and Robins have referred to this as a 'target' trial; the target trial is usually a hypothetical pragmatic randomized trial comparing the health effects of the same interventions, conducted on the same participant group and without features putting it at risk of bias (Hernán and Robins 2016). Importantly, a target randomized trial need not be feasible or ethical. This concept is the foundation of the risk-of-bias assessment for NRSI, and helps a review author to distinguish between the risk of bias in a NRSI (see Chapter 25) and a lack of directness of a NRSI with respect to the review question (see Chapter 14, Section 14.2.2). A lack of directness among randomized trials may be a motivation for including NRSI that address the review question more directly. In this situation, review authors need to recognize that discrepancies in intervention effects between randomized trials and NRSI (and, potentially, between NRSI with different study design features) may arise either from differential risk of bias or from differences in the specific PICO questions evaluated by the primary studies.

A single review may include different types of study to address different outcomes, for example, randomized trials for evaluating benefits and NRSI to evaluate harms; see Section 24.2.1.1 and Chapter 19 (Section 19.2). Scoping in advance of writing a protocol should allow review authors to identify whether NRSI are required to address directly one or more of the PICO questions for a review comparison. In time, as a review is updated, the NRSI may be dropped if randomized trials addressing these questions become available.

24.2.1.3 Determining which non-randomized studies of interventions to include

A randomized trial is a prospective, experimental study design specifically involving random allocation of participants to interventions. Although there are variations in randomized trial design (see Chapter 23), they constitute a distinctive study category. By contrast, NRSI embrace a number of fundamentally different design principles, several of which were originally conceived in the context of aetiological epidemiology; some studies combine different principles. As we discuss in Section 24.2.2, study design labels such as 'cohort' or 'prospective study' are not consistently applied. The diversity of NRSI designs raises two related questions. First, should all NRSI relevant to a PICO question for a planned synthesis be included in a review, irrespective of their study design features? Second, if review authors do not include all NRSI, what study design features should be used as criteria to decide which NRSI to include and which to exclude?

NRSI vary with respect to their intrinsic ability to estimate the causal effect of an intervention (Reeves et al 2017, Tugwell et al 2017). Therefore, to reach reliable conclusions, review authors should include only 'strong' NRSI that can estimate causality with minimal risk of bias. It is not helpful to include primary studies in a review when the results of the studies are highly likely to be biased even if there is no better evidence (except for justification 3, i.e. to examine the case for performing a randomized trial by describing the weakness of the NRSI evidence; see Section 24.1.1). This is because a misleading effect estimate from a systematic review may be more harmful to future patients than no estimate at all, particularly if the people using the evidence to make decisions are unaware of its limitations (Doll 1993, Peto et al 1995). Systematic reviews have a privileged status in the evidence base (Reeves et al 2013), typically sitting between primary research studies and guidelines (which frequently cite them). There may be long-term undesirable consequences of reviewing evidence when it is inadequate: an evidence synthesis may make it less likely that less biased research will be carried out in the future, increasing the risk that more poorly informed decisions will be made than would otherwise have been the case (Stampfer and Colditz 1991, Siegfried et al 2005).

There is not currently a general framework for deciding which kinds of NRSI will be used to answer a specific PICO question. One possible strategy is to limit included NRSI to those that have used a strong design (NRSI with specified design features; Reeves et al 2017, Tugwell et al 2017). This should give reasonably valid effect estimates, subject to assessment of risk of bias. An alternative strategy is to include the best available NRSI (i.e. those with the strongest design features among those that have been carried out) to answer the PICO question. In this situation, we recommend scoping available NRSI in advance of finalizing study eligibility for a specific review question and defining eligibility with respect to study design features (Reeves et al 2017). Widespread adoption of the first strategy might result in reviews that consistently include NRSI with the same design features, but some reviews would include no studies at all. The second strategy would lead to different reviews including NRSI with different study design features according to what is available. Whichever strategy is adopted, it is important to explain the choice of included studies in the protocol. For example, review authors might be justified in using different eligibility criteria when reviewing the harms, compared with the benefits, of an intervention (see Chapter 19, Section 19.2).

We advise caution in assessing NRSI according to existing 'evidence hierarchies' for studies of effectiveness (Eccles et al 1996, National Health and Medical Research Council 1999, Oxford Centre for Evidence-based Medicine 2001). These appear to have arisen largely by applying hierarchies for aetiological research questions to effectiveness questions and refer to study design labels. NRSI used for studying the effects of interventions are very diverse and complex (Shadish et al 2002) and may not be easily assimilated into existing evidence hierarchies. NRSI with different study design features are susceptible to different biases, and it is often unclear which biases have the greatest impact and how they vary between healthcare contexts. We recommend including at least one expert with knowledge of the subject and NRSI methods (with previous experience of estimating an intervention effect from NRSI similar to the ones of interest) on a review team to help to address these complexities.

24.2.2 Guidance and resources available to support review authors

Review authors should scope the available NRSI evidence between deciding on the specific synthesis PICOs that the review will address and finalizing the review protocol (see Section 24.1.1). Review authors may need to consult with stakeholders about the specific PICO questions of interest to ensure that scoping is informative. With this information, review authors can then use the algorithm (Figure 24.1.a) to decide whether the review needs to include NRSI and for which questions, enabling review authors to justify their decision(s) to include or exclude NRSI in their protocol. It will be important to ensure that the review team includes informed methodologists. Review authors intending to review the adverse effects (harms) of an intervention should consult Chapter 19.

We recommend that review authors use explicit study design features (NB: not study design labels) when deciding which types of NRSI to include in a review. A checklist of study design features was first drawn up for the designs most frequently used to evaluate healthcare interventions (Higgins et al 2013). This checklist has since been revised to include designs often used to evaluate health systems (Reeves et al 2017) and combines the previous two checklists (for studies with individual and cluster-level allocation, respectively). Thirty-two items are grouped under seven headings, characterizing key features of strong and weak study designs (Box 24.2.a). The paper also sets out which features are associated with NRSI study design labels (acknowledging that these labels can be used inconsistently). We propose that the checklist be used in the processes of data collection and as part of the assessment of the studies (Sections 24.4.2 and 24.6.2).

Box 24.2.a Checklist of study features. Responses to each item should be recorded as: yes, no, or can't tell (Reeves et al 2017). Reproduced with permission of Elsevier

1) Was the intervention/comparator (answer 'yes' to more than one item, if applicable):
   - allocated to (provided for/administered to/chosen by) individuals?
   - allocated to (provided for/administered to/chosen by) clusters of individuals?[a]
   - clustered in the way it was provided (by practitioner or organizational unit)?[b]
2) Were outcome data available (answer 'yes' to only one item):
   - after intervention/comparator only (same individuals)?
   - after intervention/comparator only (not all same individuals)?
   - before (once) AND after intervention/comparator (same individuals)?
   - before (once) AND after intervention/comparator (not all same individuals)?
   - multiple times before AND multiple times after intervention/comparator (same individuals)?
   - multiple times before AND multiple times after intervention/comparator (not all same individuals)?
3) Was the intervention effect estimated by (answer 'yes' to only one item):
   - change over time (same individuals at different time-points)?
   - change over time (not all same individuals at different time-points)?
   - difference between groups (of individuals or clusters receiving either intervention or comparator)[c]?

4) Did the researchers aim to control for confounding (design or analysis) (answer 'yes' to only one item):
   - using methods that control in principle for any confounding?
   - using methods that control in principle for time invariant unobserved confounding?
   - using methods that control only for confounding by observed covariates?
5) Were groups of individuals or clusters formed by (answer 'yes' to more than one item, if applicable)[d]:
   - randomization?
   - quasi-randomization?
   - explicit rule for allocation based on a threshold for a variable measured on a continuous or ordinal scale or boundary (in conjunction with identifying the variable dimension, below)?
   - some other action of researchers?
   - time differences?
   - location differences?
   - healthcare decision makers/practitioners?
   - participants' preferences?
   - policy maker?
   - on the basis of outcome?[e]
   - some other process? (specify)
6) Were the following features of the study carried out after the study was designed (answer 'yes' to more than one item, if applicable):
   - characterization of individuals/clusters before intervention?
   - actions/choices leading to an individual/cluster becoming a member of a group?[e]
   - assessment of outcomes?
7) Were the following variables measured before intervention (answer 'yes' to more than one item, if applicable):
   - potential confounders?
   - outcome variable(s)?

[a] This item describes 'explicit' clustering. In randomized controlled trials, participants can be allocated individually or by virtue of 'belonging to a cluster such as a primary care practice or a village.
[b] This item describes 'implicit' clustering. In randomized controlled trials, participants can be allocated individually but with the intervention being delivered in clusters (e.g. group cognitive therapy); similarly, in a cluster-randomized trial (by general practice), the provision of an intervention could also be clustered by therapist, with several therapists providing 'group' therapy.
[c] A study should be classified as 'yes' for this feature, even if it involves comparing the extent of change over time between groups.
[d] The distinction between these options is to do with the exogeneity of the allocation.
[e] For (nested) case-control studies, group refers to the case/control status of an individual. This option is not applicable when interventions are allocated to (provided for/administered to/chosen by) clusters.

Some Cochrane Reviews have limited inclusion of NRSI by study design labels, sometimes in combination with considerations of methodological quality. For example, Cochrane Effective Practice and Organisation of Care accepts protocols that include interrupted time series (ITS) and controlled before-and-after (CBA) studies, and specifies some minimum criteria for these types of studies. The risks of using design labels are highlighted by a recent review that showed that Cochrane Reviews inconsistently labelled CBA and ITS studies, and included studies that used these labels in highly inconsistent ways (Polus et al 2017). We believe that these issues will be addressed by applying the study feature checklist.

Our proposal is that:

1) the review team decides which study design features are desirable in a NRSI to address a specific PICO question;
2) scoping will indicate the study design features of the NRSI that are available; and
3) the review team sets eligibility criteria based on study design features that represent an appropriate balance between the priority of the question and the likely strength of the available evidence.

When both randomized trials and NRSI of an intervention exist in relation to a specific PICO question and, for one or more of the reasons given in Section 24.1.1, both are defined as eligible, the results for randomized trials and for NRSI should be presented and analysed separately. Alternatively, if there is an adequate number of randomized trials to inform the main analysis for a review question, comments about relevant NRSI can be included in the Discussion section of a review although the reader needs to be reassured that NRSI studies are not selectively cited.

24.3 Searching for non-randomized studies of interventions

24.3.1 What is different when including non-randomized studies of interventions?

24.3.1.1 Identifying non-randomized studies in searches

Searching for NRSI is less straightforward than searching for randomized trials. A broad search strategy – with search strings for the population and disease characteristics, the intervention and possibly the comparator – can potentially identify all evidence about an intervention. When a review aims to include randomized trials only, various approaches are available to focus the search strategy towards randomized trials (see Chapter 4, Section 4.4):

1) implement the search within resources, such as the Cochrane Central Register of Controlled Trials (CENTRAL), that are 'rich' in randomized trials;
2) use methodological filters and indexing fields, such as publication type in MEDLINE, to limit searches to studies that are likely to be randomized trials; and
3) search trials registers.

Restricting the search to NRSI with specific study design features is more difficult. Of the above approaches, only 1 is likely to be helpful. Some Cochrane Review Groups maintain specialized trials registers that also include NRSI, only some of which will also be found in CENTRAL, and authors of Cochrane Reviews can search these registers where they are likely to be relevant (e.g. the register of Cochrane Effective Practice and Organisation of Care). There are no databases of NRSI similar to CENTRAL.

Some review authors have tried to develop and validate methodological filters for NRSI (strategy 2) but with limited success because NRSI design labels are not reliably indexed by bibliographic databases and are used inconsistently by authors of primary studies (Wieland and Dickersin 2005, Fraser et al 2006, Furlan et al 2006). Furthermore, study design features, which are the preferred approach to determining eligibility of NRSI for a review, suffer from the same problems. Review authors have also sought to optimize search strategies for adverse effects (see Chapter 19, Section 19.3) (Golder et al 2006c, Golder et al 2006b). Because of the time-consuming nature of systematic reviews that include NRSI, attempts to develop search strategies for NRSI have not investigated large numbers of review questions. Therefore, review authors should be cautious about assuming that previous strategies can be applied to new topics.

Finally, although trials registers such as ClinicalTrials.gov do include some NRSI, their coverage is very low so strategy 3 is unlikely to be very fruitful.

Searching using 'snowballing' methods may be helpful, if one or more publications of relevance or importance are known (Wohlin 2014), although it is likely to identify other evidence about the research question in general rather than studies with similar design features.

24.3.1.2 Non-reporting biases for non-randomized studies

We are not aware of evidence that risk of bias due to missing evidence affects randomized trials and NRSI differentially. However, it is difficult to believe that publication bias could affect NRSI *less* than randomized trials, given the increasing number of safeguards associated with carrying out and reporting randomized trials that act to prevent reporting biases (e.g. pre-specified protocols, ethical approval including progress and final reports, the CONSORT statement (Moher et al 2001), trials registers and indexing of publication type in bibliographic databases). These safeguards are much less applicable to NRSI, which may not have been executed according to a pre-specified protocol, may not require explicit ethical approval, are unlikely to be registered, and do not always have a research sponsor or funder. The likely magnitude and determinants of publication bias for NRSI are not known.

24.3.1.3 Practical issues in selecting non-randomized studies for inclusion

Section 24.2.1.3 points out that NRSI include diverse study design features, and that there is difficulty in categorizing them. Assuming that review authors set specific criteria against which potential NRSI should be assessed for eligibility (e.g. study features), many of the potentially eligible NRSI will report insufficient information to allow them to be classified.

There is a further problem in defining exactly when a NRSI comes into existence. For example, is a cohort study that has collected data on the interventions and outcome of interest, but that has not examined their association, an eligible NRSI? Is computer output in a filing cabinet that includes a calculated odds ratio for the relevant association an eligible NRSI? Consequently, it is difficult to define a 'finite population of NRSI' for a particular review question. Many NRSI that have been done may not be traceable at all, that is, they are not to be found even in the proverbial 'bottom drawer'.

Given these limitations of NRSI evidence, it is tempting to question the benefits of comprehensive searching for NRSI. It is possible that the studies that are the hardest to find are the most biased – if being hard to find is associated with design features that are susceptible to bias – to a greater extent than has been shown for randomized trials for some topics. It is likely that search strategies can be developed that identify eligible studies with reasonable precision (see Chapter 4, Section 4.4.3) and are replicable, but which are not comprehensive (i.e. lack sensitivity). Unfortunately, the risk of bias to review findings with such strategies has not been researched and their acceptability would depend on pre-specifying the strategy without knowledge of influential results, which would be difficult to achieve.

24.3.2 Guidance and resources available to support review authors

We do not recommend limiting search strategies by index terms relating to study design labels. However, review authors may wish to contact information specialists with expertise in searching for NRSI, researchers who have reported some success in developing efficient search strategies for NRSI (see Section 24.3.1) and other review authors who have carried out Cochrane Reviews (or other systematic reviews) of NRSI for review questions similar to their own.

When searching for NRSI, review authors are advised to search for studies investigating all effects of an intervention and not to limit search strategies to specific outcomes (Chapter 4, Section 4.4.2). When searching for NRSI of specific rare or long-term (usually adverse or unintended) outcomes of an intervention, including free text and MeSH terms for specific outcomes in the search strategy may be justified (see Chapter 19, Section 19.3).

Review authors should check with their Cochrane Review Group editors whether the Group-specific register includes NRSI with particular study design features and should seek the advice of information retrieval experts within the Group and in the Information Retrieval Methods Group (see also Chapter 4).

24.4 Selecting studies and collecting data

24.4.1 What is different when including non-randomized studies?

Search results obtained using search strategies without study design filters are often much more numerous, and contain large numbers of irrelevant records. Also, abstracts of NRSI reports often do not provide adequate detail about NRSI study design features (which are likely to be required to judge eligibility), or some secondary outcomes measured (such as adverse effects). Therefore, more so than when reviewing randomized trials, very many full reports of studies may need to be obtained and read in order to identify eligible studies.

Review authors need to collect the same types of data required for a systematic review of randomized trials (see Chapter 5, Section 5.3) and will also need to collect data specific to the NRSI. For a NRSI, review authors should extract the estimate of intervention effect together with a measure of precision (e.g. a confidence interval) and information about how the estimate was derived (e.g. the confounders controlled for). Relevant results can then be meta-analysed using standard software.

If both unadjusted and adjusted intervention effects are reported, then adjusted effects should be preferred. It is straightforward to extract an adjusted effect estimate and its standard error for a meta-analysis if a single adjusted estimate is reported for a particular outcome in a primary NRSI. However, some NRSI report multiple adjusted estimates from analyses including different sets of covariates. **If multiple adjusted estimates of intervention effect are reported, the one that is judged to minimize the risk of bias due to confounding should be chosen** (see Chapter 25, Section 25.2.1). (Simple numerators and denominators, or means and standard errors, for intervention and control groups cannot control for confounding unless the groups have been matched on all important confounding domains at the design stage.)

Anecdotally, the experience of review authors is that NRSI are poorly reported so that the required information is difficult to find, and different review authors may extract different information from the same paper. Data collection forms may need to be customized to the research question being investigated. Restricting included studies to those that share specific features can help to reduce their diversity and facilitate the design of customized data collection forms.

As with randomized trials, results of NRSI may be presented using different measures of effect and uncertainty or statistical significance. **Before concluding that information required to describe an intervention effect has not been reported, review authors should seek statistical advice about whether reported information can be transformed or used in other ways to provide a consistent effect measure across studies** so that this can be analysed using standard software (see Chapter 6). Data collection sheets need to be able to handle the different kinds of information about study findings that review authors may encounter.

24.4.2 Guidance and resources available to support review authors

Data collection for each study needs to cover the following.

1) Data about study design features to demonstrate the eligibility of included studies against criteria specified in the review protocol. The study design feature checklist can help to do this (see Section 24.2.2). When using this checklist, whether to decide on eligibility or for data extraction, the intention should be to document what researchers did in the primary studies, rather than what researchers called their studies or think they did. Further guidance on using the checklist is included with the description of the tool (Reeves et al 2017).
2) Variables measured in a study that characterize confounding domains of interest; the ROBINS-I tool provides a template for collecting this information (see Chapter 25, Section 25.3) (Sterne et al 2016).
3) The availability of data for experimental and comparator intervention groups, and about the co-interventions; the ROBINS-I tool provides a template for collecting information about co-interventions (see Chapter 25).
4) Data to characterize the directness with which the study addresses the review question (i.e. the PICO elements of the study). We recommend that review authors record this information, then apply a simple template that has been published for doing this (Schünemann et al 2013, Wells et al 2013), judging the directness of each

element as 'sufficient' on a 4-point categorical scale. (This tool could be used for scoping and can be applied to randomized trials as well as NRSI.)

5) Data describing the study results (see Section 24.6.1). Capturing these data is likely to be challenging and data collection will almost certainly need to be customized to the research question being investigated. Review authors are strongly advised to pilot the methods they plan to use with studies that cover the expected diversity; developing the data collection form may require several iterations. It is almost impossible to finalize these forms in advance. Methods developed at the outset (e.g. forms or database) may need to be amended to record additional important information identified when appraising NRSI but overlooked at the outset. Review authors should record when required data are not available due to poor reporting, as well as data that are available. Data should be captured describing both unadjusted and adjusted intervention effects.

24.5 Assessing risk of bias in non-randomized studies

24.5.1 What is different when including non-randomized studies?

Biases in non-randomized studies are a major threat to the validity of findings from a review that includes NRSI. Key challenges affecting NRSI include the appropriate consideration of confounding in the absence of randomization, less consistent development of a comprehensive study protocol in advance of the study, and issues in the analysis of routinely collected data.

Assessing the risk of bias in a NRSI has long been a challenge and has not always been performed or performed well. Indeed, two studies of systematic reviews that included NRSI have commented that only a minority of reviews assessed the methodological quality of included studies (Audigé et al 2004, Golder et al 2006a).

The process of assessing risk of bias in NRSI is hampered in practice by the quality of reporting of many NRSI, and – in most cases – by the lack of availability of a protocol. A protocol is a tool to protect against bias; when registered in advance of a study starting, it proves that aspects of study design and analysis were considered in advance of starting to recruit (or acquiring historical data), and that data definitions and methods for standardizing data collection were defined. Primary NRSI rarely report whether the methods are based on a protocol and, therefore, these protections often do not apply to NRSI. An important consequence of not having a protocol is the lack of constraint on researchers with respect to 'cherry-picking' outcomes, subgroups and analyses to report; this can be a source of bias even in randomized trials where protocols exist (Chan et al 2004).

24.5.2 Guidance and resources available to support review authors

The recommended tool for assessing risk of bias in NRSI included in Cochrane Reviews is the ROBINS-I tool, described in detail in Chapter 25 (Sterne et al 2016). If review authors choose not to use ROBINS-I, they should demonstrate that their chosen method of assessment covers the range of biases assessed by ROBINS-I.

The ROBINS-I tool involves some preliminary work when writing the protocol. Notably, review authors will need to specify important confounding domains and co-interventions. There is no established method for identifying a pre-specified set of important confounding domains. The list of potential confounding domains should not be generated solely on the basis of factors considered in primary studies included in the review (at least, not without some form of independent validation), since the number of suspected confounders is likely to increase over time (hence, older studies may be out of date) and researchers themselves may simply choose to measure confounders considered in previous studies. Rather, the list should be based on evidence (although undertaking a systematic review to identify all potential prognostic factors is extreme) and expert opinion from members of the review team and advisors with content expertise.

The ROBINS-I assessment involves consideration of several bias domains. Each domain is judged as low, moderate, serious or critical risk of bias. A judgement of low risk of bias for a NRSI using ROBINS-I equates to a low risk-of-bias judgement for a high-quality randomized trial. Few circumstances around a NRSI are likely to give a similar level of protection against confounding as randomization, and few NRSI have detailed statistical analysis plans in advance of carrying out analyses. We therefore consider it very unlikely that any NRSI will be judged to be at low risk of bias overall.

Although the bias domains are common to all types of NRSI, specific issues can arise for certain types of study, such as analyses of routinely collected data, pharmacoepidemiological studies. Review authors are advised to consider carefully whether a methodologist with knowledge of the kinds of study to be included should be recruited to the review team to help to identify key areas of weakness.

24.6 Synthesis of results from non-randomized studies

24.6.1 What is different when including non-randomized studies?

Review authors should expect greater heterogeneity in a systematic review of NRSI than a systematic review of randomized trials. This is partly due to the diverse ways in which non-randomized studies may be designed to investigate the effects of interventions, and partly due to the increased potential for methodological variation between primary studies and the resulting variation in their risk of bias. It is very difficult to interpret the implications of this diversity in the analysis of primary studies. Some methodological diversity may give rise to bias, for example different methods for measuring exposure and outcome, or adjustment for more versus fewer important confounding domains. There is no established method for assessing how, or the extent to which, these biases affect primary studies (but see Chapters 7 and 25).

Unlike for randomized trials, it will usually be appropriate to analyse adjusted, rather than unadjusted, effect estimates (i.e. analyses should be selected that attempt to control for confounding). Review authors may have to choose between alternative adjusted estimates reported for one study and should choose the one that minimizes the risk of bias due to confounding (see Chapter 25, Section 25.2.1). In principle, any effect measure used in meta-analysis of randomized trials can also be used in meta-analysis of non-randomized studies (see Chapter 6). The odds ratio will commonly be used as it is the only effect measure for dichotomous outcomes that can be estimated from case-control studies, and is estimated when logistic regression is used to adjust for confounders.

One danger is that a very large NRSI of poor methodological quality (e.g. based on routinely collected data) may dominate the findings of other smaller studies at less risk of bias (perhaps carried out using customized data collection). Review authors need to remember that the confidence intervals for effect estimates from larger NRSI are less likely to represent the true uncertainty of the observed effect than are the confidence intervals for smaller NRSI (Deeks et al 2003), although there is no way of estimating or correcting for this. Review authors should exclude from analysis any NRSI judged to be at critical risk of bias and may choose to include only studies that are at moderate or low risk of bias, specifying this choice a priori in the review protocol.

24.6.2 Guidance and resources available to support review authors

24.6.2.1 Combining studies

If review authors judge that included NRSI are at low to moderate overall risk of biases and relatively homogeneous in other respects, then they may combine results across studies using meta-analysis (Taggart et al 2001). Decisions about combining results at serious risk of bias are more difficult to make, and any such syntheses will need to be presented with very clear warnings about the likelihood of bias in the findings. As stated earlier, results considered to be at critical risk of bias using the ROBINS-I tool should be excluded from analyses.

Estimated intervention effects for NRSI with different study design features can be expected to be influenced to varying degrees by different sources of bias (see Section 24.6). Results from NRSI with different combinations of study design features should be expected to differ systematically, resulting in increased heterogeneity. Therefore, we recommend that NRSI that have very different design features should be analysed separately. **This recommendation implies that, for example, randomized trials and NRSI should not be combined in a meta-analysis**, and that cohort studies and case-control studies should not be combined in a meta-analysis if they address different research questions.

An illustration of many of these points is provided by a review of the effects of some childhood vaccines on overall mortality. The authors analysed randomized trials separately from NRSI. However, they decided that the cohort studies and case-control studies were asking sufficiently similar questions to be combined in meta-analyses, while results from any NRSI that were judged to be at a very high risk of bias were excluded from the syntheses (Higgins et al 2016). In many other situations, it may not be reasonable to combine results from cohort studies and case-control studies.

Meta-analysis methods based on estimates and standard errors, and in particular the generic inverse-variance method, will be suitable for NRSI (see Chapter 10, Section 10.3). Given that heterogeneity between NRSI is expected to be high because of their diversity, the random-effects meta-analysis approach should be the default choice; a clear rationale should be provided for any decision to use the fixed-effect method.

24.6.2.2 Analysis of heterogeneity

The exploration of possible sources of heterogeneity between studies should be part of any Cochrane Review, and is discussed in detail in Chapter 10 (Section 10.11). Non-randomized studies may be expected to be more heterogeneous than randomized trials, given the extra sources of methodological diversity and bias. Researchers do not always make the same decisions concerning confounding factors, so the extent of residual confounding is an important source of heterogeneity between studies. There may be differences in the confounding factors considered, the method used to control for confounding and the precise way in which confounding factors were measured and included in analyses.

The simplest way to display the variation in results of studies is by drawing a forest plot (see Chapter 10, Section 10.2.1). Providing that sufficient intervention effect estimates are available, it may be valuable to undertake meta-regression analyses to identify important determinants of heterogeneity, even in reviews when studies are considered too heterogeneous to combine. Such analyses could include study design *features* believed to be influential, to help to identify methodological features that systematically relate to observed intervention effects, and help to identify the subgroups of studies most likely to yield valid estimates of intervention effects. Investigation of key study design features should preferably be pre-specified in the protocol, based on scoping.

24.6.2.3 When combining results is judged not to be appropriate

Before undertaking a meta-analysis, review authors should ask themselves the standard question about whether primary studies are 'similar enough' to justify combining results (see Chapter 9, Section 9.3.2). Forest plots allow the presentation of estimates and standard errors for each study, and in most software (including RevMan) it is possible to omit summary estimates from the plots, or include them only for subgroups of studies. Providing that effect estimates from the included studies can be expressed using consistent effect measures, we recommend that review authors display individual study results for NRSI with similar study design features using forest plots, as a standard feature. If consistent effect measures are not available or calculable, then additional tables should be used to present results in a systematic format (see also Chapter 12, Section 12.3).

If the features of studies are not sufficiently similar to combine in a meta-analysis (which is expected to be the norm for reviews that include NRSI), we recommend displaying the results of included studies in a forest plot but suppressing the summary estimate (see Chapter 12, Section 12.3.2). For example, in a review of the effects of circumcision on risk of HIV infection, a forest plot illustrated the result from each study without synthesizing them (Siegfried et al 2005). Studies may be sorted in the forest plot (or shown in separate forest plots) by study design feature, or their risk of bias. For example, the circumcision studies were separated into cohort studies, cross-sectional studies and case-control studies. Heterogeneity diagnostics and investigations (e.g. testing and quantifying heterogeneity, the I^2 statistic and meta-regression analyses) are worthwhile even when a judgement has been made that calculating a pooled estimate of effect is not (Higgins et al 2003, Siegfried et al 2003).

Non-statistical syntheses of quantitative intervention effects (see Chapter 12) are challenging, however, because it is difficult to set out or describe results without being selective or emphasizing some findings over others. Ideally, authors should set out in the review protocol how they plan to use narrative synthesis to report the findings of primary studies.

24.7 Interpretation and discussion

24.7.1 What is different when including non-randomized studies?

As highlighted at the outset, review authors have a duty to summarize available evidence about interventions, balancing harms against benefits and qualified with a certainty assessment. Some of this evidence, especially about harms of interventions, will often need to come from NRSI. Nevertheless, obtaining definitive results about the likely effects of an intervention based on NRSI alone can be difficult (Deeks et al 2003). Many reviews of NRSI conclude that an 'average' effect is not an appropriate summary (Siegfried et al 2003), that evidence from NRSI does not provide enough certainty to demonstrate effectiveness or harm (Kwan and Sandercock 2004) and that randomized trials should be undertaken (Taggart et al 2001). Inspection of the risk-of-bias judgements for the individual domains addressed by the ROBINS-I tool should help interpretation, and may highlight the main ways in which NRSI are limited (Sterne et al 2016).

Challenges arise at all stages of conducting a review of NRSI: deciding which study design features should be specified as eligibility criteria, searching for studies, assessing studies for potential bias, and deciding how to synthesize results. A review author needs to satisfy the reader of the review that these challenges have been adequately addressed, or should discuss how and why they cannot be met. In this section, the challenges are illustrated with reference to issues raised in the different sections of this chapter. The Discussion section of the review should address the extent to which the challenges have been met.

24.7.1.1 Have important and relevant studies been included?

Even if the choice of eligible study design features can be justified, it may be difficult to show that all relevant studies have been identified because of poor indexing and inconsistent use of study design labels or poor reporting of design features by researchers. Comprehensive search strategies that focus only on the health condition and intervention of interest are likely to result in a very long list of bibliographic records including relatively few eligible studies; conversely, restrictive strategies will inevitably miss some eligible studies. In practice, available resources may make it impossible to process the results from a comprehensive search, especially since review authors will often have to read full papers rather than abstracts to determine eligibility. The implications of using a more or less comprehensive search strategy are not known.

24.7.1.2 Has the risk of bias to included studies been adequately assessed?

Interpretation of the results of a review of NRSI should include consideration of the likely direction and magnitude of bias, although this can be challenging to do. Some of the biases that affect randomized trials also affect NRSI but typically to a greater extent. For example, attrition in NRSI is often worse (and poorly reported), intervention and outcome assessment are rarely conducted according to standardized protocols, outcomes are rarely assessed blind to the allocation to intervention and comparator, and there is typically little protection against selection of the reported result. Too often these limitations of NRSI are seen as part of doing a NRSI, and their implications for risk of bias are not properly considered. For example, some users of evidence may consider NRSI that investigate long-term outcomes to have 'better quality' than randomized trials of short-term outcomes, simply on the basis of their directness without appraising their risk of bias; long-term outcomes may address the review question(s) more directly, but may do so with a considerable risk of bias.

We recommend using the ROBINS-I tool to assess the risk of bias because of the consensus among a large team of developers that it covers all important bias domains. This is not true of any other tool to assess the risk of bias in NRSI. The importance of individual bias domains may vary according to the review question; for example, confounding may be less likely to arise in NRSI studies of long-term or adverse effects, or some public health primary prevention interventions.

As with randomized trials, one clue to the presence of bias is notable between-study heterogeneity. Although heterogeneity can arise through differences in participants, interventions and outcome assessments, the possibility that bias is the cause of heterogeneity in reviews of NRSI must be seriously considered. However, lack of heterogeneity does not indicate lack of bias, since it is possible that a consistent bias applies in all studies.

Predicting the direction of bias (within each bias domain) is an optional element of the ROBINS-I tool. This is a subject of ongoing research which is attempting to gather empirical evidence on factors (such as study design features and intervention type) that determine the size and direction of the biases. The ability to predict both the likely magnitude of bias and the likely direction of bias would greatly improve the usefulness of evidence from systematic reviews of NRSI. There is currently some evidence that in limited circumstances the direction, at least, can be predicted (Henry et al 2001).

24.7.2 Evaluating the strength of evidence provided by reviews that include non-randomized studies

Assembling the evidence from NRSI on a particular health question enables informed debate about its meaning and importance, and the certainty that can be attributed to it. Critically, there needs to be a debate about whether the findings could be misleading. Formal hierarchies of evidence all place NRSI lower than randomized trials, but above those of clinical opinion (Eccles et al 1996, National Health and Medical Research Council 1999, Oxford Centre for Evidence-based Medicine 2001). This emphasizes the general concern about biases in NRSI, and the difficulties of attributing causality to the observed associations between intervention and outcome.

In preference to these traditional hierarchies, the GRADE approach is recommended for assessing the certainty of a body of evidence in Cochrane Reviews, and is summarized in Chapter 14 (Section 14.2). There are four levels of certainty: 'high', 'moderate', 'low' and 'very low'. A collection of studies begins with an assumption of 'high' certainty (with the introduction of ROBINS-I, this includes collections of NRSI) (Schünemann et al 2018). The certainty is then rated down in the presence of serious concerns about study limitations (risk of bias), indirectness of evidence, heterogeneity, imprecision or publication bias. In practice, the final rating for a body of evidence based on NRSI is typically rated as 'low' or 'very low'.

Application of the GRADE approach to systematic reviews of NRSI requires expertise about the design of NRSI due to the nature of the biases that may arise. For example, the strength of evidence for an association may be enhanced by a subset of primary studies that have tested considerations about causality not usually applied to randomized trial evidence (Bradford Hill 1965), or use of negative controls (Jackson et al 2006). In some contexts, little prognostic information may be known, limiting identification of possible confounding (Jefferson et al 2005).

Whether the debate concludes that the evidence from NRSI is adequate for informed decision making or that there is a need for randomized trials will depend on the value placed on the uncertainty arising through use of potentially biased NRSI, and the collective value of the observed effects. The GRADE approach interprets certainty as the certainty that the effect of the intervention is large enough to reach a threshold for action. This value may depend on the wider healthcare context. It may not be possible to include assessments of the value within the review itself, and it may become evident only as part of the wider debate following publication.

For example, is evidence from NRSI of a rare serious adverse effect adequate to decide that an intervention should not be used? The evidence has low certainty (due to a lack of randomized trials) but the value of knowing that there is the possibility of a potentially serious harm is considerable, and may be judged sufficient to withdraw the intervention. (It is worth noting that the judgement about withdrawing an intervention may depend on whether equivalent benefits can be obtained from elsewhere without such a risk; if not, the intervention may still be offered but with full disclosure of the potential harm.) Where evidence of benefit is also uncertain, the value attached to a systematic review of NRSI of harm may be even greater.

In contrast, evidence of a small benefit of a novel intervention from a systematic review of NRSI may not be sufficient for decision makers to recommend widespread implementation in the face of the uncertainty of the evidence and the costs arising from provision of the intervention. In these circumstances, decision makers may conclude that randomized trials should be undertaken to improve the certainty of the evidence if practicable and if the investment in the trial is likely to be repaid in the future.

24.7.3 Guidance for potential review authors

Carrying out a systematic review of NRSI is likely to require complex decisions, often necessitating members of the review team with content knowledge and methodological expertise about NRSI at each stage of the review. Potential review authors should therefore seek to collaborate with methodologists, irrespective of whether a review aims to investigate harms or benefits, short-term or long-term outcomes, frequent or rare events.

Review teams may be keen to include NRSI in systematic reviews in areas where there are few or no randomized trials because they have the ambition to improve the evidence-base in their specialty areas (a key motivation for many Cochrane Reviews). However, for reviews of NRSI to estimate the effects of an intervention on short-term and expected outcomes, review authors should also recognize that the resources required to do a systematic review of NRSI are likely to be much greater than for a systematic review of randomized trials. Inclusion of NRSI to address some review questions will be invaluable in addressing the broad aims of a review; however, the conclusions in relation to some review questions are likely to be much weaker and may make a relatively small contribution to the topic. Therefore, review authors and Cochrane Review Group editors need to decide at an early stage whether the investment of resources is likely to be justified by the priority of the research question.

Bringing together the required team of healthcare professionals and methodologists may be easier for systematic reviews of NRSI to estimate the effects of an intervention on long-term and rare adverse outcomes, for example when considering the side effects of drugs. A review of this kind is likely to provide important missing evidence about the effects of an intervention in a priority area (i.e. adverse effects). However, these reviews may require the input of additional specialist authors, for example with relevant content pharmacological expertise. There is a pressing need in many health conditions to supplement traditional systematic reviews of randomized trials of effectiveness with systematic reviews of adverse (unintended) effects. It is likely that these systematic reviews will usually need to include NRSI.

24.8 Chapter information

Authors: Barnaby C Reeves, Jonathan J Deeks, Julian PT Higgins, Beverley Shea, Peter Tugwell, George A Wells; on behalf of the Cochrane Non-Randomized Studies of Interventions Methods Group

Acknowledgements: We gratefully acknowledge Ole Olsen, Peter Gøtzsche, Angela Harden, Mustafa Soomro and Guido Schwarzer for their early drafts of different sections. We also thank Laurent Audigé, Duncan Saunders, Alex Sutton, Helen Thomas and Gro Jamtved for comments on previous drafts.

Funding: BCR is supported by the UK National Institute for Health Research Biomedical Research Centre at University Hospitals Bristol NHS Foundation Trust and the University of Bristol. JJD receives support from the National Institute for Health Research (NIHR) Birmingham Biomedical Research Centre at the University Hospitals Birmingham NHS Foundation Trust and the University of Birmingham. JPTH is a member of the NIHR Biomedical Research Centre at University Hospitals Bristol NHS Foundation Trust and the University of Bristol. The views expressed are those of the author(s) and not necessarily those of the NHS, the NIHR or the Department of Health.

24.9 References

Audigé L, Bhandari M, Griffin D, Middleton P, Reeves BC. Systematic reviews of nonrandomized clinical studies in the orthopaedic literature. *Clinical Orthopaedics and Related Research* 2004: 249–257.

Bradford Hill A. The environment and disease: association or causation? *Proceedings of the Royal Society of Medicine* 1965; **58**: 295–300.

Chan AW, Hróbjartsson A, Haahr MT, Gøtzsche PC, Altman DG. Empirical evidence for selective reporting of outcomes in randomized trials: comparison of protocols to published articles. *JAMA* 2004; **291**: 2457–2465.

Deeks JJ, Dinnes J, D'Amico R, Sowden AJ, Sakarovitch C, Song F, Petticrew M, Altman DG. Evaluating non-randomised intervention studies. *Health Technology Assessment* 2003; **7**: 27.

Doll R. Doing more good than harm: the evaluation of health care interventions. Summation of the conference. *Annals of the New York Academy of Sciences* 1993; **703**: 310–313.

Eccles M, Clapp Z, Grimshaw J, Adams PC, Higgins B, Purves I, Russel I. North of England evidence based guidelines development project: methods of guideline development. *BMJ* 1996; **312**: 760–762.

Fraser C, Murray A, Burr J. Identifying observational studies of surgical interventions in MEDLINE and EMBASE. *BMC Medical Research Methodology* 2006; **6**: 41.

Furlan AD, Irvin E, Bombardier C. Limited search strategies were effective in finding relevant nonrandomized studies. *Journal of Clinical Epidemiology* 2006; **59**: 1303–1311.

Glasziou P, Chalmers I, Rawlins M, McCulloch P. When are randomised trials unnecessary? Picking signal from noise. *BMJ* 2007; **334**: 349–351.

Golder S, Loke Y, McIntosh HM. Room for improvement? A survey of the methods used in systematic reviews of adverse effects. *BMC Medical Research Methodology* 2006a; **6**: 3.

Golder S, McIntosh HM, Duffy S, Glanville J, Centre for Reviews and Dissemination and UK Cochrane Centre Search Filters Design Group. Developing efficient search strategies to identify reports of adverse effects in MEDLINE and EMBASE. *Health Information and Libraries Journal* 2006b; **23**: 3–12.

Golder S, McIntosh HM, Loke Y. Identifying systematic reviews of the adverse effects of health care interventions. *BMC Medical Research Methodology* 2006c; **6**: 22.

Henry D, Moxey A, O'Connell D. Agreement between randomized and non-randomized studies: the effects of bias and confounding. 9th Cochrane Colloquium; 2001; Lyon (France).

Hernán MA, Robins JM. Using big data to emulate a target trial when a randomized trial is not available. *American Journal of Epidemiology* 2016; **183**: 758–764.

Higgins JPT, Thompson SG, Deeks JJ, Altman DG. Measuring inconsistency in meta-analyses. *BMJ* 2003; **327**: 557–560.

Higgins JPT, Ramsay C, Reeves BC, Deeks JJ, Shea B, Valentine JC, Tugwell P, Wells G. Issues relating to study design and risk of bias when including non-randomized studies in systematic reviews on the effects of interventions. *Research Synthesis Methods* 2013; **4**: 12–25.

Higgins JPT, Soares-Weiser K, López-López JA, Kakourou A, Chaplin K, Christensen H, Martin NK, Sterne JA, Reingold AL. Association of BCG, DTP, and measles containing vaccines with childhood mortality: systematic review. *BMJ* 2016; **355**: i5170.

Jackson LA, Jackson ML, Nelson JC, Neuzil KM, Weiss NS. Evidence of bias in estimates of influenza vaccine effectiveness in seniors. *International Journal of Epidemiology* 2006; **35**: 337–344.

Jefferson T, Smith S, Demicheli V, Harnden A, Rivetti A, Di Pietrantonj C. Assessment of the efficacy and effectiveness of influenza vaccines in healthy children: systematic review. *Lancet* 2005; **365**: 773–780.

Kwan J, Sandercock P. In-hospital care pathways for stroke. *Cochrane Database of Systematic Reviews* 2004; **4**: CD002924.

Li X, You R, Wang X, Liu C, Xu Z, Zhou J, Yu B, Xu T, Cai H, Zou Q. Effectiveness of prophylactic surgeries in BRCA1 or BRCA2 mutation carriers: a meta-analysis and systematic review. *Clinical Cancer Research* 2016; **22**: 3971–3981.

MacLehose RR, Reeves BC, Harvey IM, Sheldon TA, Russell IT, Black AM. A systematic review of comparisons of effect sizes derived from randomised and non-randomised studies. *Health Technology Assessment* 2000; **4**: 1–154.

Macpherson A, Spinks A. Bicycle helmet legislation for the uptake of helmet use and prevention of head injuries. *Cochrane Database of Systematic Reviews* 2008; **3**: CD005401.

Moher D, Schulz KF, Altman DG. The CONSORT Statement: revised recommendations for improving the quality of reports of parallel-group randomised trials. *Lancet* 2001; **357**: 1191–1194.

National Health and Medical Research Council. *A guide to the development, implementation and evaluation of clinical practice guidelines [Endorsed 16 November 1998]*. Canberra (Australia): Commonwealth of Australia; 1999.

Oxford Centre for Evidence-based Medicine. Levels of Evidence. 2001. http://www.cebm.net/index.aspx?o=1047.

Peto R, Collins R, Gray R. Large-scale randomized evidence: large, simple trials and overviews of trials. *Journal of Clinical Epidemiology* 1995; **48**: 23–40.

Polus S, Pieper D, Burns J, Fretheim A, Ramsay C, Higgins JPT, Mathes T, Pfadenhauer LM, Rehfuess EA. Heterogeneity in application, design, and analysis characteristics was found for controlled before-after and interrupted time series studies included in Cochrane reviews. *Journal of Clinical Epidemiology* 2017; **91**: 56–69.

Reeves BC. Parachute approach to evidence based medicine: as obvious as ABC. *BMJ* 2006; **333**: 807–808.

Reeves BC, Higgins JPT, Ramsay C, Shea B, Tugwell P, Wells GA. An introduction to methodological issues when including non-randomised studies in systematic reviews on the effects of interventions. *Research Synthesis Methods* 2013; **4**: 1–11.

Reeves BC, Wells GA, Waddington H. Quasi-experimental study designs series-paper 5: a checklist for classifying studies evaluating the effects on health interventions – a taxonomy without labels. *Journal of Clinical Epidemiology* 2017; **89**: 30–42.

Schünemann HJ, Tugwell P, Reeves BC, Akl EA, Santesso N, Spencer FA, Shea B, Wells G, Helfand M. Non-randomized studies as a source of complementary, sequential or replacement evidence for randomized controlled trials in systematic reviews on the effects of interventions. *Research Synthesis Methods* 2013; **4**: 49–62.

Schünemann HJ, Cuello C, Akl EA, Mustafa RA, Meerpohl JJ, Thayer K, Morgan RL, Gartlehner G, Kunz R, Katikireddi SV, Sterne J, Higgins JPT, Guyatt G, Grade Working Group. GRADE guidelines: 18. How ROBINS-I and other tools to assess risk of bias in nonrandomized studies should be used to rate the certainty of a body of evidence. *Journal of Clinical Epidemiology* 2018. doi: 10.1016/j.jclinepi.2018.01.012.

Shadish WR, Cook TD, Campbell DT. *Experimental and Quasi-Experimental Designs for Generalized Causal Inference*. Boston (MA): Houghton Mifflin; 2002.

Siegfried N, Muller M, Volmink J, Deeks J, Egger M, Low N, Weiss H, Walker S, Williamson P. Male circumcision for prevention of heterosexual acquisition of HIV in men. *Cochrane Database of Systematic Reviews* 2003; **3**: CD003362.

Siegfried N, Muller M, Deeks J, Volmink J, Egger M, Low N, Walker S, Williamson P. HIV and male circumcision: a systematic review with assessment of the quality of studies. *Lancet Infectious Diseases* 2005; **5**: 165–173.

Stampfer MJ, Colditz GA. Estrogen replacement therapy and coronary heart disease: a quantitative assessment of the epidemiologic evidence. *Preventive Medicine* 1991; **20**: 47–63.

Sterne JAC, Hernán MA, Reeves BC, Savović J, Berkman ND, Viswanathan M, Henry D, Altman DG, Ansari MT, Boutron I, Carpenter JR, Chan AW, Churchill R, Deeks JJ, Hróbjartsson A, Kirkham J, Jüni P, Loke YK, Pigott TD, Ramsay CR, Regidor D, Rothstein HR, Sandhu L, Santaguida PL, Schünemann HJ, Shea B, Shrier I, Tugwell P, Turner L, Valentine JC, Waddington H, Waters E, Wells GA, Whiting PF, Higgins JPT. ROBINS-I: a tool for assessing risk of bias in non-randomized studies of interventions. *BMJ* 2016; **355**: i4919.

Taggart DP, D'Amico R, Altman DG. Effect of arterial revascularisation on survival: a systematic review of studies comparing bilateral and single internal mammary arteries. *Lancet* 2001; **358**: 870–875.

Tugwell P, Knottnerus JA, McGowan J, Tricco A. Big-5 Quasi-Experimental designs. *Journal of Clinical Epidemiology* 2017; **89**: 1–3.

Wells GA, Shea B, Higgins JPT, Sterne J, Tugwell P, Reeves BC. Checklists of methodological issues for review authors to consider when including non-randomized studies in systematic reviews. *Research Synthesis Methods* 2013; **4**: 63–77.

Wieland S, Dickersin K. Selective exposure reporting and Medline indexing limited the search sensitivity for observational studies of the adverse effects of oral contraceptives. *Journal of Clinical Epidemiology* 2005; **58**: 560–567.

Wohlin C. Guidelines for snowballing in systematic literature studies and a replication in software engineering. EASE '14 Proceedings of the 18th International Conference on Evaluation and Assessment in Software Engineering; London, UK 2014.

25

Assessing risk of bias in a non-randomized study

Jonathan AC Sterne, Miguel A Hernán, Alexandra McAleenan, Barnaby C Reeves, Julian PT Higgins

KEY POINTS

- The Risk Of Bias In Non-randomized Studies of Interventions (ROBINS-I) tool is recommended for assessing the risk of bias in non-randomized studies of interventions included in Cochrane Reviews.
- Review authors should specify important confounding domains and co-interventions of concern in their protocol.
- At the start of a ROBINS-I assessment of a study, review authors should describe a 'target trial', which is a hypothetical pragmatic randomized trial of the interventions compared in the study, conducted on the same participant group and without features putting it at risk of bias.
- Assessment of risk of bias in a non-randomized study should address pre-intervention, at-intervention, and post-intervention features of the study. The issues related to post-intervention features are similar to those in randomized trials.
- Many features of ROBINS-I are shared with the RoB 2 tool for assessing risk of bias in randomized trials. It focuses on a specific result, is structured into a fixed set of domains of bias, includes signalling questions that inform risk of bias judgements and leads to an overall risk-of-bias judgement.
- Based on answers to the signalling questions, judgements for each bias domain, and for overall risk of bias, can be 'Low', 'Moderate', 'Serious' or 'Critical' risk of bias.
- The full guidance documentation for the ROBINS-I tool, including the latest variants for different study designs, is available at www.riskofbias.info.

This chapter should be cited as: Sterne JAC, Hernán MA, McAleenan A, Reeves BC, Higgins JPT. Chapter 25: Assessing risk of bias in a non-randomized study. In: Higgins JPT, Thomas J, Chandler J, Cumpston M, Li T, Page MJ, Welch VA (editors). *Cochrane Handbook for Systematic Reviews of Interventions*. 2nd Edition. Chichester (UK): John Wiley & Sons, 2019: 621–642.

25.1 Introduction

Cochrane Reviews often include non-randomized studies of interventions (NRSI), as discussed in detail in Chapter 24. Risk of bias should be assessed for each included study (see Chapter 7). The Risk Of Bias In Non-randomized Studies of Interventions (ROBINS-I) tool (Sterne et al 2016) is recommended for assessing risk of bias in a NRSI: it provides a framework for assessing the risk of bias in a single result (an estimate of the effect of an experimental intervention compared with a comparator intervention on a particular outcome). Many features of ROBINS-I are shared with the RoB 2 tool for assessing risk of bias in randomized trials (see Chapter 8).

Evaluating risk of bias in results of NRSI requires both methodological and content expertise. The process is more involved than for randomized trials, and the participation of both methodologists with experience in the relevant study designs or design features, and health professionals with knowledge of prognostic factors that influence intervention decisions for the target patient or population group, is recommended (see Chapter 24). At the planning stage, the review question must be clearly articulated, and important potential problems in NRSI relevant to the review should be identified. This includes a preliminary specification of important confounders and co-interventions (see Section 25.3.1). Each study should then be carefully examined, considering all the ways in which its results might be put at risk of bias.

In this chapter we summarize the biases that can affect NRSI and describe the main features of the ROBINS-I tool. Since the initial version of the tool was published in 2016 (Sterne et al 2016), developments to it have continued. At the time of writing, a new version is under preparation, with variants for several types of NRSI design. **The full guidance documentation for the ROBINS-I tool, including the latest variants for different study designs, is available at** www.riskofbias.info.

25.1.1 Defining bias in a non-randomized study

We define bias as the systematic difference between the study results obtained from an NRSI and a pragmatic randomized trial (both with a very large sample size), addressing the same question and conducted on the same participant group, that had no flaws in its conduct. Defined in this way, bias is distinct from issues of indirectness (applicability, generalizability or transportability to types of individuals who were not included in the study; see Chapter 14) and distinct from chance. For example, restricting the study sample to individuals free of comorbidities may limit the utility of its findings because they cannot be generalized to clinical practice, where comorbidities are common. However, such restriction does not bias the results of the study in relation to individuals free of comorbidities.

Evaluations of risk of bias in the results of NRSI are thus facilitated by considering each NRSI as an attempt to emulate (mimic) a hypothetical **'target' randomized trial** (see also Section 25.3.2). This is the hypothetical pragmatic randomized trial that compares the health effects of the same interventions, conducted on the same participant group and without features putting it at risk of bias (Institute of Medicine 2012, Hernán and Robins 2016). Importantly, a target randomized trial need not be feasible or ethical. For example, there would be no problem specifying a target trial that randomized individuals to receive tobacco cigarettes or no cigarettes to examine the effects of smoking, even though such a trial would not be ethical in practice. Similarly, there would be no problem specifying a target trial that randomized multiple countries to implement a ban on smoking in public places, even though this would not be feasible in practice.

25.2 Biases in non-randomized studies

When a systematic review includes randomized trials, its results correspond to the causal effects of the interventions studied provided that the trials have no bias. Randomization is used to avoid an influence of either known or unknown prognostic factors (factors that predict the outcome, such as severity of illness or presence of comorbidities) on intervention group assignment. There is greater potential for bias in NRSI than in randomized trials. A key concern is the possibility of **confounding** (see Section 25.2.1). NRSI may also be affected by biases that are referred to in the epidemiological literature as **selection bias** (see Section 25.2.2) and **information bias** (see Section 25.2.3). Furthermore, we are at least as concerned about **reporting biases** as we are when including randomized trials (see Section 25.2.4).

25.2.1 Confounding

Confounding occurs when there are common causes of the choice of intervention and the outcome of interest. In the presence of confounding, the association between intervention and outcome differs from its causal effect. This difference is known as **confounding bias**. A **confounding domain** (or, more loosely, a 'confounder') is a pre-intervention prognostic factor (i.e. a variable that predicts the outcome of interest) that also predicts whether an individual receives one or the other interventions of interest. Some common examples are severity of pre-existing disease, presence of comorbidities, healthcare use, physician prescribing practices, adiposity, and socio-economic status.

Investigators measure specific variables (often also referred to as confounders) in an attempt to control fully or partly for these confounding domains. For example, baseline immune function and recent weight loss may be used to adjust for disease severity; hospitalizations and number of medical encounters in the six months preceding baseline may be used to adjust for healthcare use; geographic measures to adjust for physician prescribing practices; body mass index and waist-to-hip ratio to adjust for adiposity; and income and education to adjust for socio-economic status.

The confounding domains that are important in the context of particular interventions may vary across study settings. For example, socio-economic status might be an important confounder in settings where cost or having insurance cover affects access to health care, but might not introduce confounding in studies conducted in countries in which access to the interventions of interest is universal and therefore socio-economic status does not influence intervention received.

Confounding may be overcome, in principle, either by design (e.g. by restricting eligibility to individuals who all have the same value of the baseline confounders) or – more commonly – through statistical analyses that adjust ('control') for the confounder(s). Adjusting for factors that are *not* confounders, and in particular adjusting for variables that could be affected by intervention ('post-intervention' variables), may introduce bias.

In practice, confounding is not fully overcome. First, **residual confounding** occurs when a confounding domain is measured with error, or when the relationship between the confounding domain and the outcome or exposure (depending on the analytic approach being used) is imperfectly modelled. For example, in a NRSI comparing two antihypertensive drugs, we would expect residual confounding if pre-intervention blood pressure was measured three months before the start of intervention, but the blood pressures used by clinicians to decide between the drugs at the point of intervention were not available in our dataset. Second, **unmeasured confounding** occurs when a confounding domain has not been measured at all, or is not controlled for in the analysis. This would be the case if no pre-intervention blood pressure measurements were available, or if the analysis failed to control for pre-intervention blood pressure despite it being measured. Unmeasured confounding can usually not be excluded, because we are seldom certain that we know all the confounding domains.

When NRSI are to be included in a review, review authors should attempt to pre-specify important confounding domains in their protocol. The identification of potential confounding domains requires subject-matter knowledge. For example, experts on surgery are best-placed to identify prognostic factors that are likely to be related to the choice of a surgical strategy. We recommend that subject-matter experts be included in the team writing the review protocol, and we encourage the listing of confounding domains in the review protocol, based on initial discussions among the review authors and existing knowledge of the literature.

25.2.2 Selection bias

Selection bias occurs when some eligible participants, or some follow-up time of some participants, or some outcome events, are excluded in a way that leads to the association between intervention and outcome in the NRSI differing from the association that would have been observed in the target trial. This phenomenon is distinct from that of confounding, although the term selection bias is sometimes used to mean confounding. Selection biases occur in NRSI either due to selection of participants or follow-up time *into the study* (addressed in the 'Bias in selection of participants into the study' domain), or selection of participants or follow-up time *out of the study* (addressed in the 'Bias due to missing data' domain).

Our use of the term 'selection bias' is intended to refer only to bias that would arise even if the effect of interest were null, that is, biases that are internal to the study, and not to issues of indirectness (generalizability, applicability or transferability to people who were excluded from the study) (Schünemann et al 2013).

Selection bias occurs when selection of participants or follow-up time is **related to both intervention and outcome**. For example, studies of folate supplementation during pregnancy to prevent neural tube defects in children were biased because they only included mothers and children if children were born alive (Hernán et al 2002). The bias arose because having a live birth (rather than a stillbirth or therapeutic abortion, for which outcome data were not available) is related to both the intervention (because folate supplementation increases the chance of a live birth) and the outcome (because the presence of neural tube defects makes a live birth less likely) (Velie and Shaw 1996, Hernán et al 2002).

Selection bias can also occur when some follow-up time is excluded from the analysis. For example, there is potential for bias when prevalent users of an intervention (those already receiving the intervention), rather than incident (new) users are included in analyses comparing them with non-users. This is a type of selection bias that has also been termed **inception bias** or **lead time bias**. If participants are not followed from assignment of the intervention (inception), as they would be in a randomized trial, then a period of follow-up has been excluded, and individuals who experienced the outcome soon after starting the intervention will be missing from analyses.

Selection bias may also arise because of **missing data** due to, among other reasons, attrition (loss to follow-up), missed appointments, incomplete data collection and by participants being excluded from analysis by primary investigators. In NRSI, data may be missing for baseline characteristics (including interventions received or baseline confounders), for pre-specified co-interventions, for outcome measurements, for other variables involved in the analysis or a combination of these. Specific considerations for missing data broadly follow those established for randomized trials and described in the RoB 2 tool for randomized trials (see Chapter 8).

25.2.3 Information bias

Bias may be introduced if intervention status is misclassified, or if outcomes are misclassified or measured with error. Such bias is often referred to as **information bias** or measurement bias. Errors in classification (or measurement) may be **non-differential** or **differential**, and in general we are more concerned about such errors when they are differential. **Differential misclassification of intervention status** occurs when misclassifications are related to subsequent outcome or to risk of the outcome. **Differential misclassification (or measurement error) in outcomes** occurs when it is related to intervention status.

Misclassification of intervention status is seldom a problem in randomized trials and other experimental studies, because interventions are actively assigned by the researcher and their accurate recording is a key feature of the study. However, in observational studies information about interventions allocated or received must be ascertained. To prevent differential misclassification of intervention status it is important that, wherever possible, interventions are defined and categorized without knowledge of subsequent outcomes. A well-known example of differential misclassification, when knowledge of subsequent outcomes might affect classification of interventions, is **recall bias** in a case-control study: cases may be more likely than controls to recall potentially important events or report exposure to risk factors they believe to be responsible for their disease. Differential misclassification of intervention status can occur in cohort studies if it is obtained retrospectively. This can happen if information (or availability of information) on intervention status is influenced by outcomes: for example a cohort study in elderly people in which the outcome is dementia, and participants' recall of past intervention status at study inception was affected by pre-existing mild cognitive impairment. Such problems can be avoided if information about intervention status is collected at the time of the intervention and the information is complete and accessible to those undertaking the NRSI.

Bias in measurement of the outcome is often referred to as **detection bias**. Examples of situations in which such bias can arise are if (i) outcome assessors are aware of intervention status (particularly when assessment of the outcome is subjective); (ii) different methods (or intensities of observation) are used to assess outcomes in the different intervention groups; and (iii) measurement errors are related to intervention status (or to a confounder of the intervention-outcome relationship). Blinding of outcome assessors aims to prevent systematic differences in measurements between intervention groups but is frequently not possible or not performed in NRSI.

25.2.4 Reporting bias

Concerns over **selection of the reported results** from NRSI reflect the same concerns as for randomized trials (see Chapter 7 and Chapter 8, Section 8.7). Selective reporting typically arises from a desire for findings to be newsworthy, or sufficiently noteworthy to merit publication: this could be the case if previous evidence (or a prior hypothesis) is either supported or contradicted. Although there is a lack of empirical evidence of selective reporting in NRSI compared with randomized trials, it is difficult to imagine that the problem is any less serious for NRSI. Many NRSI do not have written protocols, and many are exploratory so – by design – involve inspecting many associations between intervention and outcome.

Selection of the reported result will lead to bias if it is based on the P value, magnitude or direction of the intervention effect estimate. Bias due to **selection of the outcome measure** occurs when an effect estimate for a particular outcome is selected from among multiple measurements, for example when a measurement is made at a number of time points or using multiple scales. Bias due to **selection of the analysis** occurs when the reported results are selected from intervention effects estimated in multiple ways, such as analyses of both change scores and post-intervention scores adjusted for baseline, or multiple analyses with adjustment for different sets of potential confounders. Finally, there may be **selective reporting of a subgroup of participants**, selected from a larger NRSI, for which results are reported on the basis of a more interesting finding.

The separate issue of bias due to missing results, where non-reporting of study outcomes or whole studies is related to the P value, magnitude or direction of the intervention effect estimate, is addressed outside the framework of the ROBINS-I tool, and is described in detail in Chapter 13.

25.3 The ROBINS-I tool

25.3.1 At protocol stage: listing the confounding domains and the possible co-interventions

Review authors planning a ROBINS-I assessment should list important confounding domains in their protocol. Relevant confounding domains are the prognostic factors (predictors of the outcome) that also predict whether an individual receives one or the other intervention of interest.

Review authors are also encouraged to list important co-interventions in their protocol. Relevant co-interventions are the interventions or exposures that individuals might receive after or with initiation of the intervention of interest, which are related to the intervention received and which are prognostic for the outcome of interest. Therefore, co-interventions are a type of confounder, which we consider separately to highlight its importance.

Important confounders and co-interventions are likely to be identified both through the knowledge of subject-matter experts who are members of the review team, and through initial (scoping) reviews of the literature. Discussions with health professionals who make intervention decisions for the target patient or population groups may also be helpful. Assessment of risk of bias may, for some domains, rely heavily on expert opinion rather than empirical data: this means that consensus may not be reached among experts with different opinions. Nonetheless use of ROBINS-I should help structure discussions about risk of bias and make disagreements explicit.

25.3.2 Specifying a target trial specific to the study

ROBINS-I requires that review authors explicitly identify the interventions that would be compared in the hypothetical target trial that the NRSI is trying to emulate (see Section 25.1.1). Often the description of these interventions will require subject-matter knowledge, because information provided by the investigators of the observational study is insufficient to define the target trial. For example, NRSI authors may refer to 'use of therapy [A],' which does not directly correspond to the intervention 'prescribe therapy [A]' that would be tested in an intention-to-treat analysis of the target trial. Meaningful assessment of risk of bias is problematic in the absence of well-defined interventions.

25.3.3 Specifying the nature of the effect of interest

In the target trial, the effect of interest will be either the effect of **assignment** to the interventions at baseline, regardless of the extent to which the interventions were received as intended, or the effect of **adhering to** the interventions as specified in the study protocol (see Chapter 8, Section 8.2.2). Risk of bias will be assessed in relation to one of these effects. The choice of effect of interest is a decision of the review authors. However, it may be influenced by the analyses that produced the NRSI result being assessed, because the result may correspond more closely to one of the effects of interest and would, therefore, be at greater risk of bias with respect to the alternative effect of interest.

In a randomized trial, these two effects may be interpreted as the **intention-to-treat (ITT) effect** and the **per protocol effect** (see also Chapter 8, Section 8.2.2). Analogues of these effects can be defined for NRSI. For example, the ITT effect can be approximated by the effect of *prescribing* experimental intervention versus *prescribing* comparator intervention. When prescription information is not available, the ITT effect can be approximated by the effect of *starting* the experimental intervention versus *starting* comparator intervention, which corresponds to the ITT effect in a trial in which participants assigned to an intervention always start the intervention. An analogue of the effect of adhering to the intervention as described in the trial protocol is (starting and) *adhering to* experimental intervention versus (starting and) *adhering to* comparator intervention unless medical reasons (e.g. toxicity) indicate discontinuation.

For both NRSI and randomized trials, unbiased estimation of the effect of adhering to sustained interventions (interventions that continue over time, such as daily ingestion of a drug intervention) requires appropriate adjustment for prognostic factors ('time-varying confounders') that predict deviations from the intervention after the start of follow-up (baseline). Review authors should seek specialist advice when assessing intervention effects estimated using methods that adjust for time-varying confounding.

When the effect of interest is that of assignment to the intervention (or starting intervention at baseline), risk-of-bias assessments need not be concerned with post-baseline deviations from intended interventions that reflect the natural course of events. For example, a departure from an allocated intervention that was clinically necessary because of a sudden worsening of the patient's condition does not lead to bias. The only post-baseline deviation that may lead to bias are the potentially biased actions of researchers arising from the experimental context. Observational studies estimating the effect of assignment to intervention from routine data should therefore have no concerns about post-baseline deviations from intended interventions.

By contrast, when the effect of interest is adhering to the intended intervention, risk-of-bias assessments of both NRSI and randomized trials should consider post-baseline deviations from the intended interventions, including lack of adherence and differences in additional interventions (co-interventions) between intervention groups.

25.3.4 Domains of bias

The domains included in ROBINS-I cover all types of bias that are currently understood to affect the results of NRSI. Each domain is mandatory, and no additional domains should be added. Table 25.3.a lists the bias domains covered by the tool for most types of NRSI. Versions of the tool are available, or in development, for several types of NRSI, and the variant selected should be appropriate to the key features of the study being assessed (see latest details at www.riskofbias.info).

In common with RoB 2 (Chapter 8, Section 8.2.3), the tool comprises, for each domain:

1) a series of 'signalling questions';
2) a judgement about risk of bias for the domain, which is facilitated by an algorithm that maps responses to the signalling questions to a proposed judgement;
3) free text boxes to justify responses to the signalling questions and risk-of-bias judgements; and
4) an option to predict (and explain) the likely direction of bias.

The **signalling questions** aim to elicit information relevant to the risk-of-bias judgement for the domain, and work in the same way as for RoB 2 (see Chapter 8, Section 8.2.3). The response options are:

- yes;
- probably yes;
- probably no;
- no;
- no information.

Table 25.3.a Bias domains included in the ROBINS-I tool

Bias domain	Category of bias	Explanation
Pre-intervention domains		
Bias due to confounding	Confounding	Baseline confounding occurs when one or more prognostic variables (factors that predict the outcome of interest) also predicts the intervention received at baseline. ROBINS-I can also address time-varying confounding, which occurs when post-baseline prognostic factors affect the intervention received after baseline.
Bias in selection of participants into the study	Selection bias	When exclusion of some eligible participants, or the initial follow-up time of some participants, or some outcome events, is related to both intervention and outcome, there will be an association between interventions and outcome even if the effect of interest is truly null. This type of bias is distinct from confounding. A specific example is bias due to the inclusion of prevalent users, rather than new users, of an intervention.
At-intervention domain		
Bias in classification of interventions	Information bias	Bias introduced by either differential or non-differential misclassification of intervention status. Non-differential misclassification is unrelated to the outcome and will usually bias the estimated effect of intervention towards the null. Differential misclassification occurs when misclassification of intervention status is related to the outcome or the risk of the outcome.
Post-intervention domains		
Bias due to deviations from intended interventions	Confounding	Bias that arises when there are systematic differences between experimental intervention and comparator groups in the care provided, which represent a deviation from the intended intervention(s). Assessment of bias in this domain will depend on the effect of interest (either the effect of assignment to intervention or the effect of adhering to intervention).
Bias due to missing data	Selection bias	Bias that arises when later follow-up is missing for individuals initially included and followed (e.g. differential loss to follow-up that is affected by prognostic factors); bias due to exclusion of individuals with missing information about intervention status or other variables such as confounders.

(*Continued*)

Table 25.3.a (Continued)

Bias domain	Category of bias	Explanation
Bias in measurement of the outcome	Information bias	Bias introduced by either differential or non-differential errors in measurement of outcome data. Such bias can arise when outcome assessors are aware of intervention status, if different methods are used to assess outcomes in different intervention groups, or if measurement errors are related to intervention status or effects.
Bias in selection of the reported result	Reporting bias	Selective reporting of results from among multiple measurements of the outcome, analyses or subgroups in a way that depends on the findings.

Table 25.3.b Reaching a risk-of-bias judgement for an individual bias domain

Risk-of-bias judgement	Interpretation
Low risk of bias	The study is comparable to a well-performed randomized trial with regard to this domain.
Moderate risk of bias	The study is sound for a non-randomized study with regard to this domain but cannot be considered comparable to a well-performed randomized trial.
Serious risk of bias	The study has some important problems in this domain.
Critical risk of bias	The study is too problematic in this domain to provide any useful evidence on the effects of intervention.
No information	No information on which to base a judgement about risk of bias for this domain.

Based on these responses to the signalling questions, the options for a domain-level **risk-of-bias judgement** are 'Low', 'Moderate', 'Serious' or 'Critical' risk of bias, with an additional option of 'No information' (see Table 25.3.b). These differ from the risk-of-bias judgements for the RoB 2 tool (Chapter 8, Section 8.2.3).

Note that a judgement of 'Low risk of bias' corresponds to the absence of bias in a well-performed randomized trial, with regard to the domain being considered. This category thus provides a reference for risk-of-bias assessment in NRSI in particular for the 'pre-intervention' and 'at-intervention' domains. Because of confounding, we anticipate that only rarely will design or analysis features of a non-randomized study lead to a classification of low risk of bias when studying the intended effects of interventions (on the other hand, confounding may be a less serious concern when studying unintended effects of intervention (Institute of Medicine 2012)). By contrast, since randomization does not protect against post-intervention biases, we expect more overlap between assessments of randomized trials and assessments of NRSI for the post-intervention domains. Nonetheless other features of randomized trials that are usually not feasible in NRSI, such as blinding of participants, health professionals or outcome assessors, may make NRSI more at risk of post-intervention biases.

As for RoB 2, a **free text box** alongside the signalling questions and judgements provides space for review authors to present supporting information for each response. Brief, direct quotations from the text of the study report should be used whenever possible.

The tool includes an optional component to judge the **direction of the bias** for each domain and overall. For some domains, the bias is most easily thought of as being towards or away from the null. For example, suspicion of selective non-reporting of statistically non-significant results would suggest bias away from the null. However, for other domains (in particular confounding, selection bias and forms of measurement bias such as differential misclassification), the bias needs to be thought of as an increase or decrease in the effect estimate to favour either the experimental intervention or comparator compared with the target trial, rather than towards or away from the null. For example, confounding bias that decreases the effect estimate would be towards the null if the true risk ratio were greater than 1, and away from the null if the risk ratio were less than 1. If review authors do not have a clear rationale for judging the likely direction of the bias, they should not attempt to guess it and should leave this response blank.

25.3.5 Reaching an overall risk-of-bias judgement for a result

The response options for an **overall risk-of-bias judgement** for a result, across all domains, are the same as for individual domains. Table 25.3.c shows the approach to mapping risk-of-bias judgements within domains to an overall judgement for the outcome.

Judging a result to be at a particular level of risk of bias for an individual domain implies that the result has an overall risk of bias at least this severe. For example, a

Table 25.3.c Reaching an overall risk-of-bias judgement for a specific outcome

Overall risk-of-bias judgement	Interpretation	Criterion
Low risk of bias	The study is comparable to a well-performed randomized trial.	The study is judged to be at **low risk of bias for all domains** for this result.
Moderate risk of bias	The study appears to provide sound evidence for a non-randomized study but cannot be considered comparable to a well-performed randomized trial.	The study is judged to be at **low or moderate risk of bias for all domains.**
Serious risk of bias	The study has one or more important problems.	The study is judged to be at **serious risk of bias** in at least one domain, but not at critical risk of bias in any domain.
Critical risk of bias	The study is too problematic to provide any useful evidence and should not be included in any synthesis.	The study is judged to be at **critical risk of bias in at least one domain.**

judgement of 'Serious' risk of bias within any domain implies that the concerns identified have serious implications for the result overall, irrespective of which domain is being assessed. In practice this means that if the answers to the signalling questions yield a proposed judgement of 'Serious' or 'Critical' risk of bias, review authors should consider whether any identified problems are of sufficient concern to warrant this judgement for that result overall. If this is not the case, the appropriate action would be to retain the answers to the signalling questions but override the proposed default judgement and provide justification.

'Moderate' risk of bias in multiple domains may lead review authors to decide on an overall judgement of 'Serious' risk of bias for that outcome or group of outcomes, and 'Serious' risk of bias in multiple domains may lead review authors to decide on an overall judgement of 'Critical' risk of bias.

Once an overall judgement has been reached for an individual study result, this information should be presented in the review and reflected in the analysis and conclusions. For discussion of the presentation of risk-of-bias assessments and how they can be incorporated into analyses, see Chapter 7. Risk-of-bias assessments also feed into one domain of the GRADE approach for assessing certainty of a body of evidence, as discussed in Chapter 14.

25.4 Risk of bias in follow-up (cohort) studies

As discussed in Chapter 24 (Section 24.2), labels such as 'cohort study' can be inconsistently applied and encompass many specific study designs. For this reason, these terms are generally discouraged in Cochrane Reviews in favour of using specific features to describe how the study was designed and analysed. For the purposes of ROBINS-I, we define a category of studies, which we refer to as **follow-up studies**, that refers to studies in which participants are followed up from the start of intervention up to a later time for ascertainment of outcomes of interest. This includes inception cohort studies (in which participants are identified at the start of intervention), non-randomized controlled trials, many analyses of routine healthcare databases, and retrospective cohort studies.

The issues covered by ROBINS-I for follow-up studies are summarized in Table 25.4.a. A distinctive feature of a ROBINS-I assessment of follow-up studies is that it addresses both baseline confounding (the most familiar type) and time-varying confounding. **Baseline confounding** occurs when one or more pre-intervention prognostic factors predict the intervention received at start of follow-up. A pre-intervention variable is one that is measured before the start of interventions of interest. For example, a cohort study comparing two antiretroviral drug regimens for HIV should control for CD4 cell count measured before the start of antiretroviral therapy, because this is strongly prognostic for the outcomes AIDS and death, and is also likely to influence choice of regimen. Baseline confounding is likely to be an issue in most NRSI.

In some NRSI, particularly those based on routinely collected data, participants switch between the interventions being compared over time, and the follow-up time from these individuals is divided between the intervention groups according to the intervention received at any point in time. If post-baseline prognostic factors affect

Table 25.4.a Bias domains included in the ROBINS-I tool for follow-up studies, with a summary of the issues addressed

Bias domain	Issues addressed*
Bias due to confounding	Whether: • the review author should consider baseline confounding only, or both baseline confounding and time-varying confounding (arising in studies in which follow-up time is split according to the intervention being received); • all important confounding domains were controlled for; • the confounding domains were measured validly and reliably by the variables available; and • appropriate analysis methods were used to control for the confounding.
Bias in selection of participants into the study	Whether: • selection of participants into the study (or into the analysis) was based on participant characteristics observed after the start of intervention; • (if applicable) these characteristics were associated with intervention and influenced by outcome (or a cause of the outcome); • start of follow-up and start of intervention were the same; and • (if applicable) adjustment techniques were used to correct for the presence of selection biases.
Bias in classification of interventions	Whether: • intervention status was classified correctly for all (or nearly all) participants; • information used to classify intervention groups was recorded at the start of the intervention; and • classification of intervention status could have been influenced by knowledge of the outcome or risk of the outcome.
Bias due to deviations from intended interventions	*When the review authors' interest is in the effect of assignment to intervention* (see Section 25.3.3): Whether: • there were deviations from the intended intervention because of the experimental context (i.e. deviations that do not reflect usual practice); and, if so, whether they were balanced between groups and likely to have affected the outcome. *When the review authors' interest is in the effect of adhering to intervention* (see Section 25.3.3): Whether: • important co-interventions were balanced across intervention groups; • failures in implementing the intervention could have affected the outcome and were unbalanced across intervention groups;

(*Continued*)

Table 25.4.a (Continued)

Bias domain	Issues addressed*
	• study participants adhered to the assigned intervention regimen and if not whether non-adherence was unbalanced across intervention groups; and • (if applicable) an appropriate analysis was used to estimate the effect of adhering to the intervention.
Bias due to missing data	Whether: • the number of participants omitted from the analysis due to missing outcome data was small; • the number of participants omitted from the analysis due to missing data on intervention status was small; • the number of participants omitted from the analysis due to missing data on other variables needed for the analysis was small; • (if applicable) there was evidence that the result was not biased by missing outcome data; and • (if applicable) missingness in the outcome was likely to depend on the true value of the outcome (e.g. because of different proportions of missing outcome data, or different reasons for missing outcome data, between intervention groups).
Bias in measurement of the outcome	Whether: • the method of measuring the outcome was inappropriate; • measurement or ascertainment of the outcome could have differed between intervention groups; • outcome assessors were aware of the intervention received by study participants; and • (if applicable) assessment of the outcome could have been influenced by knowledge of intervention received; and whether this was likely.
Bias in selection of the reported result	Whether: • the numerical result being assessed is likely to have been selected, on the basis of the results, from multiple outcome measurements within the outcome domain; • the numerical result being assessed is likely to have been selected, on the basis of the results, from multiple analyses of the data; and • the numerical result being assessed is likely to have been selected, on the basis of the results, from multiple subgroups of a larger cohort.

* For the precise wording of signalling questions and guidance for answering each one, see the full ROBINS-I tool at www.riskofbias.info.

the interventions to which the participants switch, then this can lead to **time-varying confounding**. For example, suppose a study of patients treated for HIV partitions follow-up time into periods during which patients were receiving different antiretroviral regimens and compares outcomes during these periods in the analysis. Post-baseline

CD4 cell counts might influence switches between the regimens of interest. When such post-baseline prognostic variables are affected by the interventions themselves (e.g. antiretroviral regimen may influence post-baseline CD4 count), we say that there is **treatment-confounder feedback.** This implies that conventional adjustment (e.g. Poisson or Cox regression models) is not appropriate as a means of controlling for time-varying confounding. Other post-baseline prognostic factors, such as adverse effects of an intervention, may also predict switches between interventions.

Note that a change from the baseline intervention may result in switching to an intervention other than the alternative of interest in the study (i.e. from experimental intervention to something other than the comparator intervention, or from comparator intervention to something other than the experimental intervention). If follow-up time is re-allocated to the alternative intervention in the analysis that produced the result being assessed for risk of bias, then there is a potential for bias arising from time-varying confounding. If follow-up time was not allocated to the alternative intervention, then the potential for bias is considered either (i) under the domain 'Bias due to deviations from intended interventions' *if interest is in the effect of adhering to intervention and the follow-up time on the subsequent intervention is included in the analysis*, or (ii) under 'Bias due to missing data' *if the follow-up time on the subsequent intervention is excluded from the analysis.*

25.5 Risk of bias in uncontrolled before-after studies (including interrupted time series)

In some studies measurements of the outcome variable are made both before and after an intervention takes place. The measurements may be made on individuals, clusters of individuals, or administrative entities according to the unit of analysis of the study. There may be only one unit, several units or many units. Here, we consider only *uncontrolled* studies in which all units contributing to the analysis received the (same) intervention. *Controlled* versions of these studies are covered in Section 25.6.

This category of studies includes **interrupted time series** (ITS) studies (Kontopantelis et al 2015, Polus et al 2017). ITS studies collect longitudinal data measured at an aggregate level (across participants within one or more units), with several measurement times before implementation of the intervention, and several measurement times after implementation of the intervention. These studies might be characterized as uncontrolled, repeated cross-sectional designs, where the population of interest may be defined geographically or through interaction with a health service, and measures of activity or outcomes may include different individuals at each time point. A specific time point known as the 'interruption' defines the distinction between 'before' (or 'pre-intervention') and 'after' (or 'post-intervention') time points. Specifying the exact time of this interruption can be challenging, especially when an intervention has many phases or when periods of preparation of the intervention may result in progressive changes in outcomes (e.g. when there are debates and processes leading to a new law or policy). The data from an ITS are typically a single time series, and may be analysed using time series methods (e.g. ARIMA models). In an ITS analysis, the 'comparator group' is constructed by making assumptions about the trajectory of outcomes had there been no intervention (or interruption), based on patterns observed before the intervention. The intervention effect is estimated by comparing the observed outcome trajectory after intervention with the assumed trajectory had there been no intervention.

The category also includes studies in which multiple individuals are each measured before and after receiving an intervention: there may be several pre- and post-intervention measurements. These studies might be characterized as uncontrolled, longitudinal designs (alternatively they may be referred to as repeated measures studies, before-after studies, pre-post studies or reflexive control studies). One special case is a study with a single pre-intervention outcome measurement and a single post-intervention outcome measurement for each of multiple participants. Such a study will usually be judged to be at serious or critical risk of bias because it is impossible to determine whether pre-post changes are due to the intervention rather than other factors.

The main issues addressed in a ROBINS-I evaluation of an uncontrolled before-after study are summarized below and in Table 25.5.a. We address issues only for the effect of assignment to intervention, since we do not expect uncontrolled before-after studies to examine the effect of starting and adhering to the intended intervention.

- There is a possibility that **extraneous events** or changes in context occur around the time at which the intervention is introduced. Bias will be introduced if these external forces influence the outcome. This issue is addressed under the first domain of ROBINS-I ('Bias due to confounding').
- There should be sufficient data to extrapolate from outcomes before the intervention into the future. 'Sufficient' means enough time points, over a sufficient period of time, to characterize trends and patterns. This issue is also addressed under 'Bias due to confounding'.
- ITS analyses require specification of a specific time point (the '*interruption*') before which there was no intervention (pre-intervention period) and after which there has been an intervention (the post-intervention period). However, interventions do not happen instantaneously, so this time point may be before, or after, some important features of the intervention were implemented. The time point could be selected to maximize the apparent effect: this issue is covered primarily in the domain 'Bias in classification of the intervention' but is also relevant to 'Bias in selection of the reported result' since researchers could conduct analyses with different interruption points and report that which maximizes the support for their hypothesis).
- The interruption time point might be *before* important features of the intervention have been implemented, so that there is a delay before the intervention is fully effective. Such lagging of effects should not be regarded as bias, but is rather an issue of applicability of some of the measurement times. Lagging effects can be accommodated in analyses if sufficient post-intervention measurements are available, for example by excluding data from a phase-in period of the intervention.
- The interruption time point might be *after* important features of the intervention have been implemented: for example, if anticipation of a policy change alters people's behaviour so that there is early impact of the intervention before its main implementation. Such effects will attenuate differences between pre- and post-intervention outcomes. We address this issue as a type of *contamination* of the pre-intervention period by aspects of the intervention and consider it under 'Bias due to deviations from the intended intervention'.

Table 25.5.a Bias domains included in the ROBINS-I tool for (uncontrolled) before-after studies, with a summary of the issues addressed

Bias domain	Additional or different issues addressed compared with follow-up studies*
Bias due to confounding	Whether: • measurements of outcomes were made at sufficient pre-intervention time points to permit characterization of pre-intervention trends and patterns; • there are extraneous events or changes in context around the time of the intervention that could have influenced the outcome; and • the study authors used an appropriate analysis method that accounts for time trends and patterns, and controls for all the important confounding domains.
Bias in selection of participants into the study	• The issues are similar to those for follow-up studies. For studies that prospectively follow a specific group of units from pre-intervention to post-intervention, selection bias is unlikely. For repeated cross-sectional surveys of a population, there is the potential for selection bias even if the study is prospective.
Bias in classification of interventions	• Whether specification of the distinction between pre-intervention time points and post-intervention time points could have been influenced by the outcome data.
Bias due to deviations from intended interventions	*Assuming the review authors' interest is in the effect of assignment to intervention* (see Section 25.3.3): • Whether the effects of any preparatory (pre-interruption) phases of the intervention were appropriately accounted for.
Bias due to missing data	• Whether outcome data were missing for whole clusters (units of multiple individuals) as well as for individual participants.
Bias in measurement of the outcome	Whether: • methods of outcome assessment were comparable before and after the intervention; and • there were changes in systematic errors in measurement of the outcome coincident with implementation of the intervention.
Bias in selection of the reported result	• The issues are the same as for follow-up studies.

* For the precise wording of signalling questions and guidance for answering each one, see the full ROBINS-I tool at www.riskofbias.info.

- Changes in administrative procedures related to collection of outcome data (e.g. bookkeeping, changes to success criteria) may coincide with the intervention. This is addressed under 'Bias in measurement of the outcome'. Further outcome measurement issues include 'evaluation apprehension', for example, when awareness of past responses to questionnaires influences subsequent responses.

- The intervention might cause attrition from the framework or system used to measure outcomes. This is a bias due to selection out of the study, and is addressed in the domain 'Bias due to missing data'.

25.6 Risk of bias in controlled before-after studies

Studies in which: (i) units are non-randomly allocated to a group that receives an intervention or to an alternative group that receives nothing or a comparator intervention; and (ii) at least one measurement of the outcome variable is made in both groups *before and after implementation of the intervention* are often known as **controlled before-after studies** (CBAs) (Eccles et al 2003, Polus et al 2017). The comparator group(s) may be contemporaneous or not. This category also includes **controlled interrupted time series** (CITSs) (Lopez Bernal et al 2018). The units included in the study may be individuals, clusters of individuals, or administrative units. The intervention may be at the level of the individual unit or at some aggregate (cluster) level. Studies may follow the same units over time (sometimes referred to as within-person or within-unit longitudinal designs) or look at (possibly) different units at the different time points (sometimes referred to as repeated cross-sectional designs, where the population of interest may be defined geographically or through interaction with a health service, and may include different individuals over time).

A common analysis of CBA studies is a 'difference in differences' analysis, in which before-after differences in the outcome (possibly averaged over multiple units) are contrasted between the intervention and comparator groups. The outcome measurements before and after intervention may be single observations, means, or measures of trend or pattern. The assumption underlying such an analysis is that the before-after change in the intervention group is equivalent to the before-after change in the comparator group, except for any causal effects of the intervention; that is, that the pre-post intervention difference in the comparator group reflects what would have happened in the intervention group had the intervention not taken place.

The main issues addressed in a ROBINS-I evaluation of a controlled before-after study are summarized below and in Table 25.6.a.

- The occurrence of extraneous events around the time of intervention may differ between the intervention and comparator groups. This is addressed under 'Bias due to confounding'.
- Trends and patterns of the outcome over time may differ between the intervention and comparator groups. The plausibility of this threat to validity can be assessed if more than one pre-intervention measurement of the outcome is available: the more measurements, the better the pre-intervention trends can be modelled and compared between groups. This issue is also addressed under 'Bias due to confounding'.
- If the definition of the intervention and comparator groups depends on pre-intervention outcome measurements (e.g. if individuals with high values are selected for intervention and those with low values for the comparator), regression to the mean may be confused with a treatment effect. The plausibility of this threat can be assessed by having more than one pre-intervention measurement. This is addressed under 'Bias due to confounding'.

Table 25.6.a Bias domains included in the ROBINS-I tool for controlled before-after studies, with a summary of the issues addressed

Bias domain	Additional or different issues addressed compared with follow-up studies*
Bias due to confounding	Whether: • measurements of outcomes were made at sufficiently many time points, in both the intervention and comparator groups, to permit characterization of pre-intervention trends and patterns; • any extraneous events or changes in context around the time of the intervention that could have influenced the outcome were experienced equally by both intervention groups; and • pre-intervention trends and patterns in outcomes were analysed appropriately and found to be similar across the intervention and comparator groups.
Bias in selection of participants into the study	• The issues are similar to those for follow-up studies. For repeated cross-sectional surveys of a population, there is the potential for selection bias if changes in the types of participants/units included in repeated surveys differ between intervention and comparator groups.
Bias in classification of interventions	• Whether classification of time points as before versus after intervention could have been influenced by post-intervention outcome data.
Bias due to deviations from intended interventions	*Assuming the review authors' interest is in the effect of assignment to intervention* (see Section 25.3.3): • The issues are the same as for follow-up studies.
Bias due to missing data	• Whether outcome data were missing for whole clusters as well as for individual participants.
Bias in measurement of the outcome	Whether: • methods of outcome assessment were comparable across intervention groups *and* before and after the intervention; and • there were changes in systematic errors in measurement of the outcome coincident with implementation of the intervention.
Bias in selection of the reported result	• The issues are the same as for follow-up studies.

* For the precise wording of signalling questions and guidance for answering each one, see the full ROBINS-I tool at www.riskofbias.info.

- There is a risk of selection bias in repeated cross-sectional surveys if the types of participants/units included in repeated surveys changes over time, and such changes differ between intervention and comparator groups. Changes might occur contemporaneously with the intervention if it causes (or requires) attrition from the measurement framework. These issues are addressed under 'Bias due to selection of participants into the study' and 'Bias due to missing data'.
- Outcome measurement methods might change between pre- and post-intervention periods. This issue may complicate analyses if it occurs in the intervention and

comparator groups at the same time but is a threat to validity if it differs between them. This is addressed under 'Bias due to measurement of the outcome'.

- Poor specification of the time point before which there was no intervention and after which there has been an intervention may introduce bias. This is addressed under 'Bias in classification of interventions'.

25.7 Chapter information

Authors: Jonathan AC Sterne, Miguel A Hernán, Alexandra McAleenan, Barnaby C Reeves, Julian PT Higgins

Acknowledgements: ROBINS-I was developed by a large collaborative group, and we acknowledge the contributions of Jelena Savović, Nancy Berkman, Meera Viswanathan, David Henry, Douglas Altman, Mohammed Ansari, Rebecca Armstrong, Isabelle Boutron, Iain Buchan, James Carpenter, An-Wen Chan, Rachel Churchill, Jonathan Deeks, Roy Elbers, Atle Fretheim, Jeremy Grimshaw, Asbjørn Hróbjartsson, Jemma Hudson, Jamie Kirkham, Evan Kontopantelis, Peter Jüni, Yoon Loke, Luke McGuinness, Jo McKenzie, Laurence Moore, Matt Page, Theresa Pigott, Stephanie Polus, Craig Ramsay, Deborah Regidor, Eva Rehfuess, Hannah Rothstein, Lakhbir Sandhu, Pasqualina Santaguida, Holger Schünemann, Beverley Shea, Sasha Shepperd, Ian Shrier, Hilary Thomson, Peter Tugwell, Lucy Turner, Jeffrey Valentine, Hugh Waddington, Elizabeth Waters, George Wells, Penny Whiting and David Wilson.

Funding: Development of ROBINS-I was funded by a Methods Innovation Fund grant from Cochrane and by Medical Research Council (MRC) grant MR/M025209/1. JACS, BCR and JPTH are members of the National Institute for Health Research (NIHR) Biomedical Research Centre at University Hospitals Bristol NHS Foundation Trust and the University of Bristol, the NIHR Collaboration for Leadership in Applied Health Research and Care West (CLAHRC West) at University Hospitals Bristol NHS Foundation Trust, and the MRC Integrative Epidemiology Unit at the University of Bristol. JACS and JPTH received funding from NIHR Senior Investigator awards NF-SI-0611-10168 and NF-SI-0617-10145, respectively. JPTH and AM are funded in part by Cancer Research UK (grant C18281/A19169). The views expressed are those of the authors and not necessarily those of the NHS, the NIHR, the Department of Health, the MRC or Cancer Research UK.

25.8 References

Eccles M, Grimshaw J, Campbell M, Ramsay C. Research designs for studies evaluating the effectiveness of change and improvement strategies. *Quality and Safety in Health Care* 2003; **12**: 47–52.

Hernán MA, Hernandez-Diaz S, Werler MM, Mitchell AA. Causal knowledge as a prerequisite for confounding evaluation: an application to birth defects epidemiology. *American Journal of Epidemiology* 2002; **155**: 176–184.

Hernán MA, Robins JM. Using big data to emulate a target trial when a randomized trial is not available. *American Journal of Epidemiology* 2016; **183**: 758–764.

Institute of Medicine. *Ethical and Scientific Issues in Studying the Safety of Approved Drugs*. Washington (DC): The National Academies Press; 2012.

Kontopantelis E, Doran T, Springate DA, Buchan I, Reeves D. Regression based quasi-experimental approach when randomisation is not an option: interrupted time series analysis. *BMJ* 2015; **350**: h2750.

Lopez Bernal J, Cummins S, Gasparrini A. The use of controls in interrupted time series studies of public health interventions. *International Journal of Epidemiology* 2018; **47**: 2082–2093.

Polus S, Pieper D, Burns J, Fretheim A, Ramsay C, Higgins JPT, Mathes T, Pfadenhauer LM, Rehfuess EA. Heterogeneity in application, design, and analysis characteristics was found for controlled before-after and interrupted time series studies included in Cochrane reviews. *Journal of Clinical Epidemiology* 2017; **91**: 56–69.

Schünemann HJ, Tugwell P, Reeves BC, Akl EA, Santesso N, Spencer FA, Shea B, Wells G, Helfand M. Non-randomized studies as a source of complementary, sequential or replacement evidence for randomized controlled trials in systematic reviews on the effects of interventions. *Research Synthesis Methods* 2013; **4**: 49–62.

Sterne JAC, Hernán MA, Reeves BC, Savović J, Berkman ND, Viswanathan M, Henry D, Altman DG, Ansari MT, Boutron I, Carpenter JR, Chan AW, Churchill R, Deeks JJ, Hróbjartsson A, Kirkham J, Jüni P, Loke YK, Pigott TD, Ramsay CR, Regidor D, Rothstein HR, Sandhu L, Santaguida PL, Schünemann HJ, Shea B, Shrier I, Tugwell P, Turner L, Valentine JC, Waddington H, Waters E, Wells GA, Whiting PF, Higgins JPT. ROBINS-I: a tool for assessing risk of bias in non-randomized studies of interventions. *BMJ* 2016; **355**: i4919.

Velie EM, Shaw GM. Impact of prenatal diagnosis and elective termination on prevalence and risk estimates of neural tube defects in California, 1989–1991. *American Journal of Epidemiology* 1996; **144**: 473–479.

26

Individual participant data

Jayne F Tierney, Lesley A Stewart, Mike Clarke; on behalf of the Cochrane Individual Participant Data Meta-analysis Methods Group

KEY POINTS

- Individual participant data (IPD) reviews are a specific type of systematic review that involve the collection, checking and re-analysis of the original data for each participant in each study. Data may be obtained either from study investigators or via data-sharing repositories or platforms.
- IPD reviews should be considered when the available published or other aggregate data do not permit a good quality review, or are insufficient for a thorough analysis. In certain situations, aggregate data synthesis might be an appropriate first step.
- The IPD approach can bring substantial improvements to the quality of data available and offset inadequate reporting of individual studies. Risk of bias can be assessed more thoroughly and IPD enables more detailed and flexible analysis than is possible in systematic reviews of aggregate data.
- Access to IPD offers scope to analyse data and report results in many different ways, so analytical methods should be pre-specified in detail and reporting should follow the PRISMA-IPD guideline.
- Most commonly, IPD reviews are carried out by a collaborative group, comprising a project management team, the researchers who contribute their study data, and an advisory group.
- An IPD review usually takes longer and costs more than a conventional systematic review of the same question, and requires a range of skills to obtain, manage and analyse data. Thus, they are difficult to do without dedicated time and funding.

26.1 Introduction

26.1.1 What is an IPD review?

Systematic reviews incorporating individual participant data (IPD) include the original data from each eligible study. The IPD will usually contain de-identified demographic

This chapter should be cited as: Tierney JF, Stewart LA, Clarke M. Chapter 26: Individual participant data. In: Higgins JPT, Thomas J, Chandler J, Cumpston M, Li T, Page MJ, Welch VA (editors). *Cochrane Handbook for Systematic Reviews of Interventions*. 2nd Edition. Chichester (UK): John Wiley & Sons, 2019: 643–658.

information for each participant such as age, sex, nature of their health condition, as well as information about treatments or tests received and outcomes observed (Stewart et al 1995, Stewart and Tierney 2002). These data can then be checked and analysed centrally and, if appropriate, combined in meta-analyses (Stewart et al 1995, Stewart and Tierney 2002). Most commonly, IPD are sought directly from the study investigators, but access through data-sharing platforms and data repositories may increase in the coming years.

Advantages of an IPD approach are summarized in Table 26.1.a. Compared with aggregate data, the collection of IPD can bring about substantial improvements to

Table 26.1.a Advantages of the IPD approach to systematic review and meta-analysis. Adapted from Tierney et al (2015a). (https://journals.plos.org/plosmedicine/article?id=10.1371/journal.pmed.1001855 licensed under CC BY 4.0).

Aspect of systematic review/meta-analysis	Advantages of the IPD approach
Study inclusion	Asking the IPD collaborative group (of study investigators and other experts in the clinical field) to supplement list of identified studies.* Clarify study eligibility with trial investigators.*
Data quality	Include studies that are unpublished or not reported in full. Include unreported data (e.g. more outcomes per study, and more complete information on those outcomes, data on participants excluded from study analyses). Check the integrity of study IPD and resolve any queries with investigators. Derive standardized outcome definitions across studies or translate different definitions to a common scale. Derive standardized classifications of participant characteristics or their disease/condition or translate different definitions to a common scale. Update follow-up of time-to-event or other outcomes beyond that reported.
Risk of bias	Clarify study design, conduct and analysis methods with trial investigators.* Check risk of bias of study IPD and obtain extra data where necessary.
Analysis	Analyse all important outcomes. Determine validity of analysis assumptions with IPD (e.g. proportionality of hazards for a Cox model). Derive measures of effect directly from the IPD. Use a consistent unit of analysis for each study. Apply a consistent method of analysis for each study. Conduct more detailed analysis of time-to-event outcomes (e.g. generating Kaplan-Meier curves). Achieve greater power for assessing interactions between effects of interventions and participant or disease/condition characteristics. Conduct more complex analyses not (usually) possible with aggregate data (e.g. simultaneous assessment of the relationship between multiple study and/or participant characteristics and effects of interventions). Use non-standard models or measures of effect. Account for missing data at the patient level (e.g. using multiple imputation). Use IPD to address secondary clinical questions (e.g. to explore the natural history of disease, prognostic factors or surrogate outcomes).
Interpretation	Discuss implications for clinical practice and research with a multidisciplinary group of collaborators including study investigators who supplied data.

* These may also be done for non-IPD reviews.

the quantity and quality of data, for example, through the inclusion of more trials, participants and outcomes (Debray et al 2015a, Tierney et al 2015a). A Cochrane Methodology Review of empirical research shows some of these advantages (Tudur Smith et al 2016). IPD also affords greater scope and flexibility in the analyses, including the ability to investigate how participant-level covariates such as age or severity of disease might alter the impact of the treatment, exposure or test under investigation (Debray et al 2015a, Debray et al 2015b, Tierney et al 2015a). With such better-quality data and analysis, IPD reviews can help to provide in-depth explorations and robust meta-analysis results, which may differ from those based on aggregate data (Tudur Smith et al 2016). Not surprisingly then, IPD reviews have had a substantial impact on clinical practice and research, but could be better used to inform treatment guidelines (Vale et al 2015), and new studies (Tierney et al 2015b). However, IPD reviews can take longer than other reviews; those evaluating the effects of therapeutic interventions typically taking at least two years to complete. Also, they usually require a skilled team with dedicated time and specific funding.

This chapter provides an overview of the IPD approach to systematic reviews, to help authors decide whether collecting IPD might be useful and feasible for their review. As most IPD reviews have assessed the efficacy of interventions, and have been based on randomized trials, this is the focus of the chapter. However, the approach also offers particular advantages for the synthesis of diagnostic and prognostic studies (Debray et al 2015a) and many of the principles described will apply to these sorts of synthesis. The chapter does not provide detailed guidance on practical or statistical methods, which are summarized elsewhere (Stewart et al 1995, Stewart and Tierney 2002, Debray et al 2015b, Tierney et al 2015a). Therefore, anyone contemplating carrying out their first IPD meta-analysis as part of a Cochrane Review should seek appropriate advice and guidance from experienced researchers through the IPD Meta-analysis Methods Group.

26.1.2 How do IPD and standard Cochrane Review methods differ?

The general approach to an IPD review is the same as for an aggregate data systematic review, and the only substantial differences relate to data collection, checking and analysis (Stewart and Tierney 2002). Thus, a detailed protocol should be prepared and include: the objectives for the review; the specific questions to be addressed; the reasons why IPD are being sought; study and any participant eligibility criteria; which descriptive, baseline and outcome data will be collected and how this will be managed, and the planned analyses, as well as other standard review methods. Because IPD reviews offer the potential for a greater number of analyses, they pose a greater risk of data being interrogated repeatedly until the desired results are obtained. Therefore, it is particularly important that analyses methods are pre-specified in the protocol, or a separate analysis plan.

Involving the investigators responsible for the primary studies can highlight additional eligible studies done by or known to them, and help to clarify the design and conduct of included studies, thereby improving the reliability of risk of bias assessments (Vale et al 2013). Moreover, the ability to directly check IPD and seek additional data may alleviate some of the biases associated with aggregate data reviews (Stewart et al 2005).

The project should culminate in the preparation and dissemination of a structured report, following PRISMA-IPD (Stewart et al 2015) where possible. This is a stand-alone extension to PRISMA that is geared to the IPD approach and, while it focuses on reviews of efficacy, many elements are applicable to other types of IPD review.

Systematic reviews based on IPD require expertise in data management and statistical analysis, as well as skills in managing research collaborations, and they often take longer and require more resource than a conventional aggregate data systematic review of the same question. Therefore, IPD reviews are difficult to conduct in review authors' 'spare time', and are likely to require dedicated resources and staff.

26.1.3 How are IPD reviews organized?

IPD reviews are usually carried out as collaborative projects whereby all study investigators contributing data from their studies, together with the research team managing and carrying out the project, become part of an active collaboration (Stewart et al 1995, Stewart and Tierney 2002). Ideally, this collaboration should be structured so as to keep the research team at 'arm's length' from the trialists' group. Such a group might comprise a project team who lead and are responsible for all aspects of design and conduct; an advisory group who provide clinical and methodological guidance and aid strategic decisions; and the trialists, who provide trial information and IPD and comment on the draft manuscript. Projects led solely by study investigators, or by a single group or company with a vested interest, are at greater risk of (real or perceived) bias, and findings of such projects may be viewed as less credible.

Often, the research team convenes a meeting of all collaborators to present and discuss preliminary results, and can draw on these discussions when drafting manuscripts. Results are usually published in the name of the collaborative group, with all collaborators being listed as co-authors of the review publication, and all contributions and conflicts should be clearly described therein.

26.1.4 Which healthcare areas have used IPD reviews?

IPD meta-analyses have an established history in cardiovascular disease and cancer (Clarke et al 1998), where the methodology has been developing steadily since the late 1980s, and most are still conducted in these fields (Simmonds et al 2015). However, IPD have also been collected for systematic reviews in many other fields (Simmonds et al 2005, Simmonds et al 2015), including diabetes, infections, mental health, dementia, epilepsy, hernia and respiratory disease. The Cochrane IPD Meta-analysis Methods Group website (https://methods.cochrane.org/ipdma/) includes publications of ongoing and completed IPD reviews conducted by members of the Group.

26.1.5 When is an IPD review appropriate?

Generally, IPD reviews should be considered in circumstances where the available published or other aggregate data do not permit a good quality review. Specifically, it is worth considering carefully what value the collection of IPD will bring over the traditional aggregate data approach, in terms of the aims, data quantity and quality, and analyses required (Tudur Smith et al 2015) (Table 26.1.a). This means it will often be necessary to conduct or consult an aggregate data systematic review as a first step (Tudur Smith et al 2015). Alternatively, if it is known that a key objective is to explore subpopulations and potential effect modification, then proceeding directly to an IPD review and meta-analysis may be warranted.

Another important consideration is whether sufficient IPD are likely to be available to permit credible analysis. For example, some study data may have been destroyed or lost, some outcomes, such as adverse effects or quality of life may not have been collected systematically for all studies, or study investigators may not wish to collaborate (although this may not be known at the outset). Also, it may not be possible to complete an IPD review in a suitable time frame for the question of interest and, in some situations, the additional resource required may be prohibitive. Weighing up these various factors will help determine when the IPD approach is likely to bring most benefit.

Before embarking on an IPD review, review authors need to think carefully about which skills and resources will be required for the project to succeed, and seek advice and training. The Cochrane IPD Meta-analysis Methods Group is a good first point of contact.

26.2 Collecting IPD

26.2.1 Obtaining data from the original researchers

Typically, systematic reviews based on IPD are international collaborative projects anchored on addressing one or more pre-specified questions (Stewart et al 1995, Stewart and Tierney 2002). They might be initiated by systematic review authors in collaboration with clinicians, but increasingly they may arise from trialists' consortia or via specific calls from funders.

Negotiating and maintaining collaboration with study investigators from different countries, settings and disciplines can take considerable time and effort. For example, it can be difficult to trace the people responsible for eligible studies, and they may be initially reluctant to participate in the meta-analysis. Often the first approach will be by email or letter to the principal investigator, inviting collaboration, explaining the project, describing what participation will entail and how the meta-analysis will be managed and published. A protocol is generally supplied at this stage to provide more detailed information, but data are not usually sought in the first correspondence. It may also be necessary to establish additional contact with the data centre or research organization responsible for management of the study data, and to whom data queries will be sent; the principal investigator can advise who would be most appropriate.

In encouraging study investigators to take part in the IPD review, it is important to be as supportive and flexible as possible, to take the time required to build relationships and to keep all collaborators involved and informed of progress. Regular newsletters, e-mail updates or a website can be useful, especially as the project may take place over a prolonged period. A randomized trial has examined different ways establishing these connections and obtaining the IPD (Veroniki et al 2016, Veroniki et al 2019).

26.2.2 Obtaining data from sources other than the original researchers

A number of initiatives are helping to increase the availability of IPD from both academic and industry-led studies, either through generic data sharing platforms such as Yale Open Data, Clinical Study Data Request, DataSphere or Vivli. These have been in response to calls from federal agencies (e.g. NIH), funders (e.g. MRC), journal editors, the AllTrials campaign and Cochrane to make results and IPD from clinical studies more readily available.

As the focus of these efforts is to make the data from individual studies available, formatting and coding are not necessarily standard or consistent across the different study datasets. Some platforms offer fully unrestricted access to IPD and others moderated access, with release subject to approval of a project proposal. Also, while some sources allow transfer of IPD directly to the research team conducting the review, others limit the use of IPD to within a secure area within a platform. Therefore, for any given review, the availability of study IPD from these platforms may be patchy, the modes of access variable, and the usual process of re-formatting and re-coding data in a consistent way will likely be required. Thus, although promising, as yet they do not provide a viable alternative to the traditional collaborative IPD approach. As the culture of data sharing gathers pace, the increased availability and accessibility of IPD should benefit the production of IPD reviews.

26.2.3 Establishing ‘topic-based’ repositories with the original researchers

An alternative to an IPD review with a narrow focus, or broad-based data sharing repositories, is to establish a retrospective or prospective repository of IPD from all studies of relevance to a particular healthcare area or topic. Previously, such repositories have been built from existing collaborative IPD reviews and generate a unique resource for looking investigating clinical questions in depth and potentially tackling additional questions.

For instance, since 1985, the Early Breast Cancer Trialists’ Collaborative Group has amassed the majority of trials in early breast cancer and collected extended follow-up, in order to evaluate the effects of all the key interventions in the long term (http://gas.ndph.ox.ac.uk/ebctcg). For example, they have shown that women with oestrogen-receptor positive breast cancer still face a substantial risk of cancer recurrence more than 20 years after their endocrine treatment (Pan et al 2017). The ACCENT repository built on existing colorectal cancer IPD reviews has been used to identify disease-free survival as a surrogate for overall survival (Sargent et al 2007), and show the prognostic impact of baseline body mass index on survival (Sinicrope et al 2013), and a network meta-analysis of multiple IPD reviews of drug monotherapy for epilepsy, shows the most suitable first-line treatments for partial onset and generalized tonic-clonic seizures (Nevitt et al 2017).

A considerable advantage of such repositories is that data items can be coded to a common format from the outset, facilitating subsequent re-use of data, and the IPD can be checked by those with topic expertise. The benefits of working with study investigators are also retained. Of course, the retention and re-use of IPD should comply with the same data security and confidentiality measures as for the original review, and new ethics approval and data use agreements should be sought if required. It is vitally important that any new analyses follow a new pre-specified protocol and/or analysis plan.

26.2.4 Data security and confidentiality

Study investigators naturally expect there to be safeguards that ensure their study data will be transferred, stored and used appropriately. For this reason, a data sharing or data use agreement between the original investigators and the IPD review team is usually required. The details of such agreements vary, but most will state that data will be held securely, accessed only by authorized members of the project team and will not be copied or distributed elsewhere. It is also important to request that individual participants are adequately de-identified in the supplied data, by removing or recoding identifiers, and data use agreements should prohibit researchers from attempting to re-identify individuals. The degree of de-identification required may be dictated by the data protection legislation of the country from which the study originates. For example, it may be necessary to also remove or redact free-text verbatim terms, and remove explicit information on the dates of events. Note that full anonymization, whereby all links between the de-identified datasets and the original datasets are destroyed, limits the utility of IPD for systematic reviews and therefore is not recommended. All participant data should be transferred via a secure data transfer site or by encrypted email.

Historically, ethical review was not sought for IPD reviews, on the premise that they were addressing the same research question as the original studies for which participants already gave their informed consent. However, evolving data protection regulations (e.g. the EU General Data Protection Regulation) and changing attitudes to data sharing mean that, in some circumstances, formal ethical approval will be required by the Institutes holding IPD and be expected by those supplying data. This should be explored with the ethics committee/board under whose jurisdiction the research team operate, and even if formal review is not required, it may be useful to send written confirmation of this to those providing data. It is perhaps more likely that ethical review will be required if review authors are using IPD to address a different question from the original studies, or when seeking data from a research study that was not subject to prior ethical review and did not obtain formal patient consent, such as clinical audit data. This does not imply, however, that new consent will need to be obtained from the participants in the original study; de-identification of data usually means this is not necessary. Moreover, in many circumstances it would be difficult or impossible to obtain consent retrospectively, for example in older studies (because participants would be difficult to trace) or, in studies of life-limiting conditions (because many participants will have died).

26.2.5 Deciding which data items to collect

When deciding on the data items (or variables) to collect for an IPD review, it is sensible to consider the planned analyses carefully. This minimizes the possibility that information essential to the analyses will not be sought or that data will be collected unnecessarily. Understandably, the original researchers may be aggrieved if they go to the trouble of providing data that are not subsequently analysed and reported.

In addition, the aim should be to maximize the quality of the data and so enhance the analyses. For example, data on all participants and outcomes included in studies should be sought irrespective of whether they were part of the reported analyses. Thus, before embarking on data collection, it is worthwhile checking the study protocols and/or with the original researchers to determine which data are actually available. In many cases it will only be necessary to collect outcomes and participant characteristics as defined in the individual studies. However, additional variables might be required to provide greater granularity (e.g. subscales in quality of life instruments), or to allow outcomes or other variables to be defined in a consistent way for each study. For example, to redefine pre-eclampsia according to a common definition, data on systolic and diastolic blood pressure and proteinurea are needed (Askie et al 2007).

IPD provides the most practical way to synthesize data for time-to-event outcomes, such as time to recovery, time free of seizures, or time to death. Therefore, it is important to collect data on whether an event (e.g. death) has happened, the date of the event (e.g. date of death) and the date of last follow-up for those not experiencing an event. As a bare minimum, whether an event happened and the time that each individual spent 'event-free' may suffice. IPD also allows follow-up to be updated sometimes substantially beyond the point of publication (Stewart et al 1995, Stewart and Tierney 2002), which has been particularly important in evaluating the long-term effects of therapies in the cancer field (Pan et al 2017).

26.2.6 Obtaining sufficient data

It is not always possible to obtain all the desired data for an IPD review. For example, it might be difficult to obtain IPD for all relevant trials because trial investigators cannot be traced or no longer have access to the data. If investigators do not respond or refuse to participate, it might be to suppress unfavourable results, and therefore not including such trials could bias the meta-analysis. On the other hand, if it is to avoid providing trials of poor quality, then not including these trials might make a meta-analysis more robust. Aiming to obtain a large proportion of the eligible trials and participants will both counter bias (Tierney et al 2015a) and enable exploration of any quality issues (Ahmed et al 2012), and so will help to provide a reliable and precise assessment of the effects of an intervention. Another factor is whether the IPD will likely provide sufficient power to detect an effect reliably, but to date this has received little attention (Ensor et al 2018).

26.3 Managing and checking IPD

26.3.1 Re-coding and re-defining data

Inevitably, the different studies included in an IPD review will have collected and defined data in different ways. However, it is relatively straightforward to re-code data items into a common format and it should be possible to harmonize, for example, definitions of staging, grading, ranking or other scoring systems in a consistent way, to facilitate pooling of data across studies. Thus, as well as giving investigators clear instructions on which data are needed and the process for secure data transfer, the preferred data format and coding for each variable should be supplied (Stewart et al 1995). Of course, if study investigators are unwilling or unable to prepare data according to this pre-specified format, the review team should accept data in whichever format is most convenient, and recode it as necessary. A copy of the data, as supplied, should be archived before carrying out conversions or modifications to the data, and it is vital that any alterations made are properly logged.

26.3.2 Checking the completeness and integrity of incoming data

The aims of checking and 'cleaning' data are to ensure that included data are accurate, valid and internally consistent (Stewart et al 1995, Stewart and Tierney 2002, Tierney et al 2015a). Independent scrutiny of data by the review team may also increase project credibility. When data files are first received, it is important to confirm that they can be read and loaded into the central storage/analysis system. For example, if data arrive electronically, they should be checked to ensure that the files can be opened and that data are for the correct study. Furthermore, it is useful to confirm that all participants recruited or randomized are included, and that there are no obvious omissions or duplicates in the sequence of patient identifiers. More in-depth checks for missing, invalid, out of range or inconsistent items might highlight, for example, records of unusually old or young patients or those with abnormally high or low levels of important biomarkers.

Also, the data supplied should be checked against any relevant study publications or results repositories to highlight any inconsistencies in, for example, the distribution of baseline characteristics, the number of participants and the outcome results. However, it should be borne in mind that differences might arise because of continued enrolment or further follow-up subsequent to publication.

26.3.3 Checking the risk of bias of included studies

Just as for other types of systematic review, assessing risk of bias of included studies (Higgins et al 2011, Sterne et al 2016) is recommended for IPD reviews. With the collaborative IPD approach, additional information obtained from protocols, codebooks and forms supplied by study investigators can increase the clarity of risk of bias assessments compared to those based on study reports (Mhaskar et al 2012, Vale et al 2013). Also, checking the IPD directly can provide further insight into potential biases, some of which might be reduced or not transpire when updated or additional data are obtained. These checks are best established for reviews of randomized trials (Stewart et al 1995, Stewart and Tierney 2002, Tierney et al 2015a) and are outlined next.

26.3.3.1 Checking randomization and allocation sequence concealment

For randomized trials it is important to check the IPD to ensure that the methods of randomization and allocation sequence concealment appear appropriate, so as to guard against the inclusion of non-randomized studies or participants. The pattern of treatment allocation can be checked directly, and in various ways, for any unusual patterns (Stewart et al 1995, Stewart and Tierney 2002, Tierney et al 2015a).

26.3.3.2 Checking for attrition

IPD should be checked to ensure that data on all or as many randomized participants as possible are included for each outcome, and that they are assigned to their allocated intervention. This helps to minimize bias associated with the dropout of participants or their exclusion from study analyses (Tierney and Stewart 2005), and allows an intention-to-treat analysis of all randomized participants, avoiding the potential bias of a per-protocol analysis.

26.3.3.3 Checking outcomes included

An IPD review should collect all the outcomes of relevance to the review question whether reported or not. This will help to overcome the biases that can be associated with differential reporting of outcomes (Kirkham et al 2010), and provide a more balanced view of benefits and harms. Precisely because some measured outcomes may not be reported, it is worth checking the study protocol, trial registry entry and with investigators to firmly establish which outcomes might be available (Dwan et al 2011).

For time-to-event outcomes, where events are observed over a prolonged period, for example survival in cancer trials, it is important to also check that follow-up is sufficient and balanced by randomized group. By requesting follow-up that is as up to date as possible, and which may be substantially beyond the results reported in trial publications, transitory effects can be avoided and any benefits or harms of interventions that take a long time to accrue, such as late side effects of treatment or late recurrence of disease, can be picked up. For example, in an IPD meta-analysis of chemotherapy for soft tissue sarcoma (Sarcoma Meta-analysis Collaboration 1997), the median follow-up for trials reporting it ranged from 16 to 64 months, but increased to between 74 and 204 months when updated IPD were obtained (Stewart et al 2005).

26.3.4 Assessing the overall quality of a study

For any individual study, the results of the data and risk of bias checks should be considered together in order to build up an overall picture of the quality of the data supplied and study design and conduct. Any concerns should be brought diplomatically to the attention of the responsible study team, and any subsequent changes or updates to study data should be properly recorded. Many data issues turn out to be simple errors or misunderstandings that have minimal impact on the study or meta-analysis results (Burdett and Stewart 2002), and major problems are rare. However, these checks serve to improve understanding of the peculiarities of each study, and safeguard against occurrences of major problems in study data (Burdett and Stewart 2002). If such problems exist, or it is anticipated that the design or conduct of a study might introduce significant bias into the meta-analysis, it may need to be excluded.

26.4 Analysis of IPD

26.4.1 Analysis advantages

Having access to IPD for each study enables checking of analytical assumptions, thorough exploration of the data and consistent analysis across trials (Table 26.1.a). Also, outcomes and measures of risk and effect are derived directly from analysis of the IPD, so there is no need to rely on interpreting information and analyses presented in published reports, or to combine summary statistics from studies that have been analysed in different ways. Re-analysis of IPD also avoids any problems or limitations with the original analyses. For example, it should be possible to carry out analyses according to intention-to-treat principles, even if the original/published trial analyses did not, use more appropriate effect measures, and perform sophisticated analyses to account for missing data.

As IPD offers the potential to analyse data in many different ways, it is particularly important that all methods relating to analysis are pre-specified in detail in the review protocol or analysis plan (Tierney et al 2015a) and are clearly reported in publications (Stewart et al 2015). This should include: outcomes and their definitions; methods for checking IPD and assessing risk of bias of included studies; methods for evaluating treatments effects, risks or test accuracy (including those for exploring variations by trial or patient characteristics) and methods for quantifying and accounting for heterogeneity. Unplanned analyses can still play an important role in explaining or adding to the results, but such exploratory analyses should be justified and clearly reported as such.

Statistical methods for the analysis of IPD can be complex and are described in more detail elsewhere (Debray et al 2015b). These methods are less well developed for prognostic or diagnostic test accuracy reviews than for interventions reviews based on randomized trials, so we outline some key principles for the re-analysis of IPD from randomized trials.

26.4.2 Assessing overall effects of interventions

It is important to stratify or account for clustering of participants in an IPD meta-analysis (Abo-Zaid et al 2013), because participants will have been recruited according to different study protocols. Combining IPD across studies, as though part of single 'mega' trial, could lead to biased comparisons of interventions and over-precise estimates of effect (Tierney et al 2015a). To date, most IPD meta-analyses have used a two-stage approach to analysis (Simmonds et al 2005, Bowden et al 2011, Simmonds et al 2015), whereby each individual study is analysed independently in the first stage, reducing the IPD to summary statistics (i.e. aggregate data). In the second stage, these are combined to provide a pooled estimate of effect, in much the same way as for a conventional systematic review (Simmonds et al 2005). Thus, standard statistics and forest plots can be produced.

A one-stage model is typically a regression that estimates intervention effects, while stratifying by study (e.g. including an indicator variable for each study), but does require a higher degree of statistical expertise to implement, and interpretation is not as straightforward as the more familiar two-stage approach. Although one- and two-stage meta-analyses often produce similar results, variations do occur, but may arise because of different modelling assumptions rather than the choice of one- versus two-stage (Burke et al 2017, Morris et al 2018). Yet, for some, a one-stage model seems preferable, and their use has increased dramatically in recent years (Simmonds et al 2015, Fisher et al 2017). As it is difficult to derive standard meta-analysis statistics directly from a one-stage model, a compromise is to do one-stage analysis to obtain estimates of effect, and a two-stage analysis to obtain further statistics and forest plots. Whichever approach is taken, it is important that the choice is specified in advance or that results for both approaches are reported (Stewart et al 2012).

26.4.3 Assessing if effects vary by trial characteristics

Exploring whether intervention effects vary by study characteristics is an important aspect of any meta-analysis, and can be readily investigated with IPD, using the same analytical approaches that are used for aggregate data (Deeks et al 2011). Thus, subgroup analysis might be used, whereby studies are grouped according to a particular characteristic such as drug type, and the effects compared indirectly between these groups. Alternatively, meta-regression might be used to explore whether the overall effect of an intervention varies in relation to a study treatment characteristic such as drug dose.

26.4.4 Assessing if effects vary by participant characteristics

Collecting IPD is the most reliable and often the only way to investigate whether intervention effects vary by participant characteristics, for example, whether an intervention is more or less effective in women compared to men (Stewart et al 1995, Stewart and Tierney 2002). Again, this can be done in two stages. In the first stage, interactions between gender and the intervention effect at the individual participant-level are estimated within each study, and in the second stage these interactions are pooled across studies using standard meta-analysis techniques; so-called 'within-trial' interactions (Fisher et al 2011, Fisher et al 2017). In the widely used 'subgroup analysis' approach, each study is first split into subgroups, say men and women, and a meta-analysis of effects in men is compared with a meta-analysis of effects in women. Unfortunately, this approach conflates within and across-trial interactions, so is susceptible to bias and might best be avoided (Fisher et al 2011, Fisher et al 2017). Alternatively, a one-stage approach can be used, but to avoid bias, again care must be taken to distinguish within-study interactions from any between-study interactions (Riley et al 2008, Fisher et al 2011).

Importantly, and irrespective of the analytical method, where multiple subgroups have been investigated and/or subgroups effects lack biological plausibility, results should be viewed with caution (Clarke and Halsey 2011). Where there is no particular evidence that trial or participant characteristics impact on the results, emphasis should be placed on the overall effects.

26.4.5 Software for IPD meta-analysis

Owing to the complexity and range of analyses possible with IPD, it is difficult for any software to accommodate fully all the analyses and plots required. One-stage meta-analysis typically requires mixed-effects or multilevel regression modelling, which can be achieved in a range of statistical software (Debray et al 2015b). For the first stage of a two-stage approach, these packages can also be used, and the summary statistics then combined in the second stage using either a standard meta-analysis command (e.g. **metan** command in Stata), or input into a separate meta-analysis package such as RevMan. The user-written Stata package ipdmetan (Fisher 2015) has been developed to facilitate two-stage IPD meta-analysis, by allowing the user to specify both the regression model to apply to each study in the first stage, and the meta-analytical method to apply in the second stage.

26.5 Reporting IPD reviews

Where possible, IPD reviews should be reported in accordance with the PRISMA-IPD guideline (Stewart et al 2015). This was developed as a standalone extension to PRISMA (Preferred Reporting Items for Systematic Reviews and Meta-Analyses) (Moher et al 2009), to ensure that specific features of the IPD approach are addressed, such as the reporting of the methods used to obtain, check and synthesize IPD, and to deal with studies for which IPD were not available. PRISMA-IPD is, however, geared to IPD reviews of efficacy, but much of it is also relevant to IPD reviews of, for example, diagnostic, prognostic and observational studies (Stewart et al 2015).

26.6 Appraising the quality of IPD reviews

Although clearly they offer considerable advantages, and their use has increased across a range of healthcare areas (Simmonds et al 2015), not all IPD reviews are done or reported to the same standard (Riley et al 2010, Ahmed et al 2012). Moreover, the process of collecting, checking and analysing IPD is more complex than for aggregate data, and there are usually many more analyses to be reported, so it can be difficult to judge the quality of IPD reviews. This may, in turn, hinder their conduct, dissemination and influence guidelines (Vale et al 2015) and new trials (Tierney et al 2015b). For example, an ad hoc IPD meta-analysis of randomized trials (e.g. from a single institution or company) may not include all studies of relevance, and therefore might give a biased or otherwise unrepresentative view of the effects of a particular intervention. By contrast, the quality of the included studies might be a more important determinant of reliability in an IPD meta-analysis of prognosis or diagnosis (Debray et al 2015a). Therefore, guidance has been prepared to help researchers, clinicians, patients, policy makers, funders and publishers understand, appraise and make best use of IPD reviews of randomized trials (Tierney et al 2015a), and diagnostic and prognostic modelling studies (Debray et al 2015a).

26.7 Chapter information

Authors: Jayne F Tierney, Lesley A Stewart, Mike Clarke; on behalf of the Cochrane Individual Participant Data Meta-analysis Methods Group

Funding: JFT and coordination of the IPD Meta-analysis Methods Group are funded by the UK Medical Research Council (MC_UU_12023/24); Lesley A Stewart is funded by the University of York and Mike Clarke is funded by Queen's University Belfast.

26.8 References

Abo-Zaid G, Guo B, Deeks JJ, Debray TP, Steyerberg EW, Moons KG, Riley RD. Individual participant data meta-analyses should not ignore clustering. *Journal of Clinical Epidemiology* 2013; **66**: 865–873 e864.

Ahmed I, Sutton AJ, Riley RD. Assessment of publication bias, selection bias, and unavailable data in meta-analyses using individual participant data: a database survey. *BMJ* 2012; **344**: d7762.

Askie LM, Duley L, Henderson-Smart D, Stewart LA, on behalf of the PARIS Collaborative Group. Antiplatelet agents for prevention of pre-eclampsia: a meta-analysis of individual patient data. *Lancet* 2007; **369**: 1791–1798.

Bowden J, Tierney JF, Simmonds M, Copas AJ. Individual patient data meta-analysis of time-to-event outcomes: one-stage versus two-stage approaches for estimating the hazard ratio under a random effects model. *Research Synthesis Methods* 2011; **2**: 150–162.

Burdett S, Stewart LA. A comparison of the results of checked versus unchecked individual patient data meta-analyses. *International Journal of Technology Assessment in Health Care* 2002; **18**: 619–624.

Burke DL, Ensor J, Riley RD. Meta-analysis using individual participant data: one-stage and two-stage approaches, and why they may differ. *Statistics in Medicine* 2017; **36**: 855–875.

Clarke M, Halsey J. DICE 2: a further investigation of the effects of chance in life, death and subgroup analyses. *International Journal of Clinical Practice* 2001; **55**: 240–242.

Clarke M, Stewart L, Pignon JP, Bijnens L. Individual patient data meta-analyses in cancer. *British Journal of Cancer* 1998; **77**: 2036–2044.

Debray TP, Riley RD, Rovers MM, Reitsma JB, Moons KG, Cochrane IPD Meta-analysis Methods group. Individual participant data (IPD) meta-analyses of diagnostic and prognostic modeling studies: guidance on their use. *PLoS Medicine* 2015a; **12**: e1001886.

Debray TP, Moons KG, van Valkenhoef G, Efthimiou O, Hummel N, Groenwold RH, Reitsma JB, GetReal Methods Review Group. Get real in individual participant data (IPD) meta-analysis: a review of the methodology. *Research Synthesis Methods* 2015b; **6**: 293–309.

Deeks JJ, Higgins JPT, Altman DG. Chapter 9: Analysing data and undertaking meta-analyses. In: Higgins JPT, Green S, editors. *Cochrane Handbook for Systematic Reviews of Interventions* Version 5.1.0: The Cochrane Collaboration; 2011.

Dwan K, Altman DG, Cresswell L, Blundell M, Gamble CL, Williamson PR. Comparison of protocols and registry entries to published reports for randomised controlled trials. *Cochrane Database of Systematic Reviews* 2011; **1**: MR000031.

Ensor J, Burke DL, Snell KIE, Hemming K, Riley RD. Simulation-based power calculations for planning a two-stage individual participant data meta-analysis. *BMC Medical Research Methodology* 2018; **18**.

Fisher DJ, Copas AJ, Tierney JF, Parmar MKB. A critical review of methods for the assessment of patient-level interactions in individual patient data (IPD) meta-analysis of randomised trials, and guidance for practitioners. *Journal of Clinical Epidemiology* 2011; **64**: 949–967.

Fisher DJ. Two-stage individual participant data meta-analysis and generalized forest plots. *Stata Journal* 2015; **15**: 369–396.

Fisher DJ, Carpenter JR, Morris TP, Freeman SC, Tierney JF. Meta-analytical methods to identify who benefits most from treatments: daft, deluded, or deft approach? *BMJ* 2017; **356**: j573.

Higgins JPT, Altman DG, Gøtzsche PC, Jüni P, Moher D, Oxman AD, Savović J, Schulz KF, Weeks L, Sterne J, Cochrane Bias Methods Group, Cochrane Statistical Methods Group. The Cochrane Collaboration's tool for assessing risk of bias in randomised trials. *BMJ* 2011; **343**: d5928.

Kirkham JJ, Dwan KM, Altman DG, Gamble C, Dodd S, Smyth R, Williamson PR. The impact of outcome reporting bias in randomised controlled trials on a cohort of systematic reviews. *BMJ* 2010; **340**: c365.

Mhaskar R, Djulbegovic B, Magazin A, Soares HP, Kumar A. Published methodological quality of randomized controlled trials does not reflect the actual quality assessed in protocols. *Journal of Clinical Epidemiology* 2012; **65**: 602–609.

Moher D, Liberati A, Tetzlaff J, Altman D, PRISMA Group. Preferred reporting items for systematic reviews and meta-analyses: the PRISMA Statement. *PLoS Medicine* 2009; **6**: e1000097. doi:1000010.1001371/journal.pmed.1000097.

Morris TP, Fisher DJ, Kenward MG, Carpenter JR. Meta-analysis of Gaussian individual patient data: two-stage or not two-stage? *Statistics in Medicine* 2018; **37**: 1419–1438.

Nevitt SJ, Sudell M, Weston J, Tudur Smith C, Marson AG. Antiepileptic drug monotherapy for epilepsy: a network meta-analysis of individual participant data. *Cochrane Database of Systematic Reviews* 2017; **12**: CD011412.

Pan H, Gray R, Braybrooke J, Davies C, Taylor C, McGale P, Peto R, Pritchard KI, Bergh J, Dowsett M, Hayes DF, EBCTCG. 20-Year risks of breast-cancer recurrence after stopping endocrine therapy at 5 years. *New England Journal of Medicine* 2017; **377**: 1836–1846.

Riley RD, Lambert PC, Staessen JA, Wang J, Gueyffier F, Thijs L, Boutitie F. Meta-analysis of continuous outcomes combining individual patient data and aggregate data. *Statistics in Medicine* 2008; **27**: 1870–1893.

Riley RD, Lambert PC, Abo-Zaid G. Meta-analysis of individual participant data: rationale, conduct, and reporting. *BMJ* 2010; **340**: c221.

Sarcoma Meta-analysis Collaboration. Adjuvant chemotherapy for localised resectable soft tissue sarcoma in adults: meta-analysis of individual patient data. *Lancet* 1997; **350**: 1647–1654.

Sargent DJ, Patiyil S, Yothers G, Haller DG, Gray R, Benedetti J, Buyse M, Labianca R, Seitz JF, O'Callaghan CJ, Francini G, Grothey A, O'Connell M, Catalano PJ, Kerr D, Green E, Wieand HS, Goldberg RM, de Gramont A, ACCENT Group. End points for colon cancer adjuvant trials: observations and recommendations based on individual patient data from 20,898 patients enrolled onto 18 randomized trials from the ACCENT Group. *Journal of Clinical Oncology* 2007; **25**: 4569–4574.

Simmonds M, Stewart G, Stewart L. A decade of individual participant data meta-analyses: a review of current practice. *Contemporary Clinical Trials* 2015; **45**: 76–83.

Simmonds MC, Higgins JPT, Stewart LA, Tierney JF, Clarke MJ, Thompson SG. Meta-analysis of individual patient data from randomised trials: a review of methods used in practice. *Clinical Trials* 2005; **2**: 209–217.

Sinicrope FA, Foster NR, Yothers G, Benson A, Seitz JF, Labianca R, Goldberg RM, Degramont A, O'Connell MJ, Sargent DJ, Adjuvant Colon Cancer Endpoints Group. Body mass index at diagnosis and survival among colon cancer patients enrolled in clinical trials of adjuvant chemotherapy. *Cancer* 2013; **119**: 1528–1536.

Sterne JA, Hernan MA, Reeves BC, Savović J, Berkman ND, Viswanathan M, Henry D, Altman DG, Ansari MT, Boutron I, Carpenter JR, Chan AW, Churchill R, Deeks JJ, Hróbjartsson A, Kirkham J, Jüni P, Loke YK, Pigott TD, Ramsay CR, Regidor D, Rothstein HR, Sandhu L, Santaguida PL, Schünemann HJ, Shea B, Shrier I, Tugwell P, Turner L, Valentine JC, Waddington H, Waters E, Wells GA, Whiting PF, Higgins JPT. ROBINS-I: a tool for assessing risk of bias in non-randomised studies of interventions. *BMJ* 2016; **355**: i4919.

Stewart GB, Altman DG, Askie LM, Duley L, Simmonds MC, Stewart LA. Statistical analysis of individual participant data meta-analyses: a comparison of methods and recommendations for practice. *PloS One* 2012; **7**: e46042.

Stewart L, Tierney J, Burdett S. Do systematic reviews based on individual patient data offer a means of circumventing biases associated with trial publications? In: Rothstein H, Sutton A, Borenstein M, editors. *Publication Bias in Meta-Analysis: Prevention, Assessment and Adjustments*. Chichester: John Wiley & Sons; 2005. p. 261–286.

Stewart LA, Clarke MJ, on behalf of the Cochrane Working Party Group on Meta-analysis using Individual Patient Data. Practical methodology of meta-analyses (overviews) using updated individual patient data. *Statistics in Medicine* 1995; **14**: 2057–2079.

Stewart LA, Tierney JF. To IPD or Not to IPD? Advantages and disadvantages of systematic reviews using individual patient data. *Evaluation and the Health Professions* 2002; **25**: 76–97.

Stewart LA, Clarke M, Rovers M, Riley RD, Simmonds M, Stewart G, Tierney JF, PRISMA-IPD Development Group. Preferred reporting items for a systematic review and meta-analysis of individual participant data: the PRISMA-IPD statement. *JAMA* 2015;**313**: 1657–1665.

Tierney JF, Stewart LA. Investigating patient exclusion bias in meta-analysis. *International Journal of Epidemiology* 2005; **34**: 79–87.

Tierney JF, Vale CL, Riley R, Tudur Smith C, Stewart LA, Clarke M, Rovers M. Individual participant data (IPD) meta-analyses of randomised controlled trials: guidance on their use. *PLoS Medicine* 2015a; **12**: e1001855.

Tierney JF, Pignon J-P, Gueffyier F, Clarke M, Askie L, Vale CL, Burdett S. How individual participant data meta-analyses can influence trial design and conduct *Journal of Clinical Epidemiology* 2015b; **68**: 1325–1335.

Tudur Smith C, Clarke M, Marson T, Riley R, Stewart L, Tierney J, Vail A, Williamson P. A framework for deciding if individual participant data are likely to be worthwhile (oral session). 23rd Cochrane Colloquium; 2015; Vienna, Austria. http://2015.colloquium.cochrane.org/abstracts/framework-deciding-if-individual-participant-data-are-likely-be-worthwhile.

Tudur Smith C, Marcucci M, Nolan SJ, Iorio A, Sudell M, Riley R, Rovers MM, Williamson PR. Individual participant data meta-analyses compared with meta-analyses based on aggregate data. *Cochrane Database of Systematic Reviews* 2016; **9**: MR000007.

Vale CL, Tierney JF, Burdett S. Can trial quality be reliably assessed from published reports of cancer trials: evaluation of risk of bias assessments in systematic reviews. *BMJ* 2013; **346**: f1798.

Vale CL, Rydzewska LHM, Rovers MM, Emberson JR, Gueyffier F, Stewart LA. Uptake of systematic reviews and meta-analyses based on individual participant data in clinical practice guidelines: descriptive study. *BMJ* 2015; **350**: h1088.

Veroniki AA, Straus SE, Ashoor H, Stewart LA, Clarke M, Tricco AC. Contacting authors to retrieve individual patient data: study protocol for a randomized controlled trial. *Trials* 2016; **17**: 138.

Veroniki AA, Rios P, Le S, Mavridis D, Stewart L, Clarke M, Ashoor H, Straus S, Tricco A. Obtaining individual patient data depends on study characteristics and can take longer than a year after a positive response. *Journal of Clinical Epidemiology* 2019; in press.

Index

Note: page numbers in *italics* refer to figures; those in bold to tables

Cochrane Handbook for Systematic Reviews of Interventions. 2nd Edition. Chichester (UK): John Wiley & Sons, 2019.